Current Progress in Neurorehabilitation

Current Progress in Neurorehabilitation

Edited by Laree Rangel

hayle medical

New York

Hayle Medical,
750 Third Avenue, 9th Floor,
New York, NY 10017, USA

Visit us on the World Wide Web at:
www.haylemedical.com

ISBN: 978-1-64647-548-3

Cataloging-in-Publication Data

Current progress in neurorehabilitation / edited by Laree Rangel.
p. cm.
Includes bibliographical references and index.
ISBN 978-1-64647-548-3
1. Brain damage--Patients--Rehabilitation. 2. Brain damage--Patients--Rehabilitation.
3. Nervous system--Diseases. I. Rangel, Laree.
RC387.5 .C87 2023
617.481 044--dc23

Table of Contents

Preface

Neurorehabilitation refers to a type of medical procedure that helps in the recovery from injuries to the nervous system and neurological conditions. It can be used to treat progressive neurological conditions such as tumors, Parkinson's disease and dementia. Neurorehabilitation assists patients in rapid recovery and maximizing their functional and cognitive capacities after the acute stage of brain injury treatment is over. Therapeutic treatments, remediation treatments, psycho-education, cognitive treatments and compensatory treatments are some of the treatment options used in the neurorehabilitation process. New technological advancements in this field have resulted in the development of improved imaging techniques which enables better assessment. Video games and virtual reality are also seen as potential options for promoting cerebral development and rehabilitation. This book elucidates the concepts and innovative models around prospective developments with respect to neurorehabilitation. It presents researches and studies performed by experts across the globe. This book will serve as a reference to a broad spectrum of readers.

The information shared in this book is based on empirical researches made by veterans in this field of study. The elaborative information provided in this book will help the readers further their scope of knowledge leading to advancements in this field.

Finally, I would like to thank my fellow researchers who gave constructive feedback and my family members who supported me at every step of my research.

Editor

1

Robotic Arm Rehabilitation in Chronic Stroke Patients with Aphasia may Promote Speech and Language Recovery (but Effect is not Enhanced by Supplementary tDCS)

Adam Buchwald[1†], Carolyn Falconer[1†], Avrielle Rykman-Peltz[2,3], Mar Cortes[2,3,4], Alvaro Pascual-Leone[5,6], Gary W. Thickbroom[2,3], Hermano Igo Krebs[7], Felipe Fregni[8], Linda M. Gerber[3], Clara Oromendia[3], Johanna Chang[9], Bruce T. Volpe[9] and Dylan J. Edwards[2,3,10,11]*

[1] Department of Communicative Sciences and Disorders, New York University, New York, NY, United States, [2] Restorative Neurology Clinic, Burke Neurological Institute, White Plains, NY, United States, [3] Weill Cornell Medicine, New York City, NY, United States, [4] Icahn School of Medicine at Mount Sinai, New York City, NY, United States, [5] Berenson-Allen Center for Noninvasive Brain Stimulation, Beth Israel Deaconess Medical Center, Harvard Medical School, Boston, MA, United States, [6] Fundación Institut Guttmann, Institut Universitari de Neurorehabilitació Adscrit a la UAB, Barcelona, Spain, [7] Department of Mechanical Engineering, Massachusetts Institute of Technology, Cambridge, MA, United States, [8] Spaulding Rehabilitation Hospital, Harvard Medical School, Cambridge, MA, United States, [9] Center for Biomedical Science, Feinstein Institute for Medical Research, Manhasset, NY, United States, [10] Moss Rehabilitation Research Institute, Elkins Park, PA, United States, [11] School of Medical and Health Sciences, Edith Cowan University, Joondalup, WA, Australia

***Correspondence:**
Adam Buchwald
buchwald@nyu.edu*

† These authors have contributed equally to this work

Objective: This study aimed to determine the extent to which robotic arm rehabilitation for chronic stroke may promote recovery of speech and language function in individuals with aphasia.

Methods: We prospectively enrolled 17 individuals from a hemiparesis rehabilitation study pairing intensive robot assisted therapy with sham or active tDCS and evaluated their speech ($N = 17$) and language ($N = 9$) performance before and after a 12-week (36 session) treatment regimen. Performance changes were evaluated with paired t-tests comparing pre- and post-test measures. There was no speech therapy included in the treatment protocol.

Results: Overall, the individuals significantly improved on measures of motor speech production from pre-test to post-test. Of the subset who performed language testing ($N = 9$), overall aphasia severity on a standardized aphasia battery improved from pre-test baseline to post-test. Active tDCS was not associated with greater gains than sham tDCS.

Conclusions: This work indicates the importance of considering approaches to stroke rehabilitation across different domains of impairment, and warrants additional exploration of the possibility that robotic arm motor treatment may enhance rehabilitation for speech and language outcomes. Further investigation into the role of tDCS in the relationship of limb and speech/language rehabilitation is required, as active tDCS did not increase improvements over sham tDCS.

Keywords: aphasia, stroke rehabilitation, apraxia of speech, motor control, Neurorehabilitation, tDCS

INTRODUCTION

Following stroke, participation in professional, social, and family environments is often limited by acquired deficits affecting motor control, sensation, cognition, and communication. Treatment in each domain can promote some limited recovery, but residual disability remains a problem. Thus, there is a need for efficient interventions to expedite and enhance recovery. We explored the possibility that treatment in one domain—motor function—may benefit performance in another, untreated domain—communication—in individuals with acquired aphasia and/or apraxia of speech. Synergistic effects of treatment across domains could provide a transformational approach to stroke rehabilitation.

The possibility that robotic motor treatment preceded by tDCS may benefit speech-language recovery was raised by Hesse et al. (1). They reported that 4 of the 10 individuals with subacute stroke undergoing repetitive right upper-extremity robotic arm therapy in conjunction with transcranial direct current stimulation (tDCS) exhibited unexpected improvement on a standardized speech-language measure. The present investigation extended this examination to the chronic stage of recovery, using tDCS in conjunction with a 12-week course of right upper-extremity robotic arm therapy. To determine whether changes in the untreated speech-language domain would occur in this population, eligible individuals with chronic stroke (>6 months post onset) were prospectively enrolled. These participants were a subset of a larger randomized control trial of hemiparesis recovery using intensive robotic arm treatment preceded by tDCS.

METHODS

Participants

A subset of seventeen participants (10 M, 7 F) from a large multi-site RCT were enrolled in the speech and language study reported here (dates: 4/2013-9/2014). All treatment and assessments were conducted at Burke Medical Research Institute and Feinstein Institute for Medical Research with participants consented under IRB approval of both institutions. Eligibility criteria for the larger RCT were: a single, left-hemisphere ischemic lesion; cognitive function sufficient to understand the instructions and task in the study; and a Motor Power score ranging from 1 to 4/5, indicating that participants were neither hemiplegic nor had fully recovered motor function in the muscles of the shoulder, elbow, and/or wrist. Participants in the speech and language subset also presented with chronic aphasia and/or apraxia of speech subsequent to the same lesion. Speech-language testing occurred prior to the beginning of motor therapy (pre-test baseline) and again after the conclusion of the therapy sessions (post-test). All 17 speech-language participants were administered a speech motor control task (i.e., diadochokinetic rate). Language testing was only conducted on individuals whose primary language was English ($N = 11$) because the normative samples for the measures given are based on native English speakers. Two English speakers were unable to complete the full battery at post-test, leaving complete language data sets for 9 people for the Western Aphasia Battery-R and 10 people for the category naming task. Speech motor control data for 17 participants is reported here. All participants completed the entire 36 session hemiparesis protocol.

TABLE 1 | Participant information: age at onset of study (within 5 year range), number of months post-stroke, handedness, race, damage type (cortical/subcortical/mixed), tDCS condition, and which speech/language measures were completed.

Sub #	Age (5 year range)	Post CVA (mos.)	Hand	Race	Damage	tDCS	DDK	Category naming	WAB	DDK severity	Aphasia type
S1	70–75	48	RH	Caucasian	Cortical	Sham	Y	Y	Y	Severe	Transcortical motor
S2	65–70	112	RH	Caucasian	Cortical	Active	Y	Y	Y	Moderate	Anomic
S3	45–50	72	RH	Caucasian	Mixed	Sham	Y	Y	Y	Mild	Broca's
S4	70–75	36	RH	Asian	Cortical	Sham	Y	Y	Y	Mild	Anomic
S5	60–65	8	RH	Caucasian	Mixed	Sham	Y	Y	Y	Mild	Anomic
S6	75–80	12	RH	Caucasian	Mixed	Active	Y	Y	Y	None	Anomic
S7	60–65	48	RH	Caucasian	Cortical	Active	Y	Y	Y	Mild	Conduction
S8	60–65	24	RH	African-American	Mixed	Sham	Y	Y	Y	Mild	Broca's
S9	45–50	228	RH	Caucasian	Subcortical	Active	Y	Y	Y	None	Anomic
S10	45–50	45	RH	Caucasian	Cortical	Active	Y	Y	N	Moderate	n/a
S11	60–65	104	RH	Caucasian	Cortical	Active	Y	N	N	Mild	n/a
S12	75–80	56	LH	Caucasian	Subcortical	Active	Y	N	N	Mild	n/a
S13	75–80	11	RH	African-American	Subcortical	Sham	Y	N	N	None	n/a
S14	75–80	47	RH	Caucasian	Subcortical	Sham	Y	N	N	Mild	n/a
S15	80–85	6	RH	Caucasian	Cortical	Sham	Y	N	N	Mild	n/a
S16	70–75	42	RH	Caucasian	Mixed	Active	Y	N	N	Mild	n/a
S17	45–50	26	RH	Caucasian	Mixed	Active	N	Y	N	n/a	n/a

Diadochokinetic (DDK) severity ratings come from subtest 1 of the Apraxia Battery for Adults, 2nd edition (ABA-2)[2] and aphasia diagnoses come from the Revised Western Aphasia Battery (WAB-R)[4] at pre-test baseline.

Testing Battery

Diadochokinesis

Diadochokinetic rate (DDK) assesses the ability to produce sequential and alternating syllables (e.g., "papapa;" "pataka"). We used the test version from the Apraxia Battery for Adults 2nd version (ABA-2) (2) and followed the scoring protocol outlined in the examiner's manual.

Category Naming

Participants were given one minute to name members of a semantic category (animals; transportation; plants; tools). This frequently used verbal fluency measure requires lexical access and word retrieval (3). Unimpaired speakers typically produce 20+ category members per minute.

Comprehensive Speech-Language Battery

The Western Aphasia Battery-Revised (WAB-R) (4) is a comprehensive aphasia battery, and yields an overall "aphasia quotient" (AQ) indicating aphasia severity (0–100). Scores above 93.8 are within the normal range; changes of 5+ points are considered clinically significant (5).

Procedure

All participants were enrolled in the double-blind repetitive right upper-extremity motor therapy study that included 36 sessions (3x/week) of robotic arm motor therapy (~1 h each) preceded by 20 min of tDCS. In this study, a 2 mA current was delivered by a battery-driven current generator using surface rubber-carbon electrodes (5 × 7 cm; 35 cm^2) surrounded by saline-soaked sponges. The center of the anode was placed 5 cm lateral to the vertex, and the cathode was placed over the right supraorbital region. For participants in the sham tDCS condition, current was ramped up to 2 mA over 30 s and then ramped down to 0 ms (6). The Fugl-Meyer Assessment (FM) (7) scores were obtained pre-test, post-test, and at a 6-month follow-up (not reported here). The FM provided a standardized assessment of upper extremity abilities administered by a licensed occupational therapist or trained research assistant.

Speech-language tasks were administered by an ASHA-certified speech-language pathologist (SLP). Participants were assessed during the week prior to the first treatment session (pre-test baseline), and within 5 days of the last treatment session (post-test). The same SLP administered baseline and post-test evaluations for each participant. Participants did not receive speech-language therapy as part of the treatment.

Data Analysis

To evaluate changes, we performed two analyses for each speech-language measure: a within-subjects paired t-test to evaluate overall change from baseline to post-test; and an independent samples t-test using the difference scores for each participant to evaluate tDCS (active~sham) group differences. Despite the small sample size, we use t-tests to allow for confidence intervals to get a sense of the effect size, and we also report the outcomes of non-parametric Wilcoxon tests throughout the results.

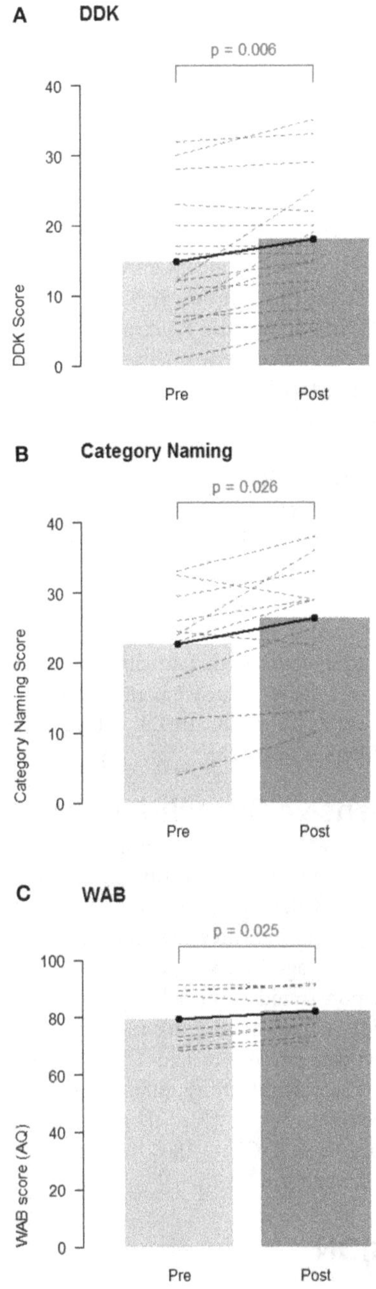

FIGURE 1 | Group changes in performance on speech/language measures. Overall pre-test baseline and post-test changes for **(A)** diadochokinetic rate; **(B)** category naming score; and **(C)** Western Aphasia Battery—Aphasia Quotient (WAB AQ). Barbells represent overall means, and dotted lines represent individual participants.

RESULTS

Demographic and stroke information, as well as tests they completed and tDCS group assignment, are presented in **Table 1**. Consistent with the larger data set and prior published studies, Fugl-Meyer Assessment (FM) (7) scores among these patients significantly increased following the robotic training regimen (mean: 27.3 pre, 35.4 post). Mean pre-to-post increase was 8.1

points [95% confidence interval (CI; 6.4, 9.8); *t*-test: $p < 0.001$; Non parametric Wilcoxon: $p < 0.001$]. As in the full cohort from the robotic arm study, improvement did not differ between tDCS and sham arms in the full set of 17 participants (*t*-test: $p = 0.14$; Non parametric Wilcoxon: $p = 0.13$) or in the subset with WAB data discussed below (*t*-test: $p = 0.28$; Non parametric Wilcoxon: $p = 0.34$).

Diadochokinetic (DDK) Task

A paired *t*-test revealed significant improvement in DDK scores from baseline to post-test [mean: 3.19 points, CI (1.04, 5.34); *t*-test: $p = 0.006$, Non parametric Wilcoxon $p = 0.003$; **Figure 1A**]. There was no difference between participants receiving sham ($N = 8$) and active tDCS [$N = 8$; difference $= -0.38$, CI (-4.10, 4.85), *t*-test: $p = 0.86$].

Category Naming

A paired *t*-test revealed a significant increase in category naming scores from baseline to post-test overall [mean: 3.27 items, CI (0.16, 6.39), *t*-test: $p = 0.026$, Non parametric Wilcoxon $p = 0.036$; **Figure 1B**]. Participants in the sham group ($N = 5$; mean improvement: 6.60 items) improved by significantly more items than participants in the active tDCS group [$N = 6$; mean improvement: 0.50 items; estimated difference $= 6.10$, CI (1.28, 10.92), *t*-test: $p = 0.041$, Non parametric Wilcoxon $= 0.075$].

Comprehensive Speech-Language Battery

A paired *t*-test revealed significant improvement in the WAB-R AQ from baseline to post-test [mean: 2.51 points, CI (0.41, 4.61), *t*-test $p = 0.025$, Non parametric Wilcoxon $= 0.055$, see **Figure 1C**]. This indicates that the participants improved overall in their average WAB-R performance at post-test. One participant demonstrated a clinically significant improvement of at least 5 points (sham condition) and two other participants achieved improvements of 4.6 and 4.9 points (one active and one sham). No significant group differences were seen between participants receiving active ($N = 4$) and sham tDCS [$N = 5$; mean difference: -3.08, CI (-7.90, 1.74), *t*-test $p = 0.15$; Non parametric Wilcoxon $p = 0.19$].

DISCUSSION

In our data, chronic stroke participants with speech and/or language impairment exhibited detectable improvement on speech-language measures following intensive robotic arm rehabilitation preceded by tDCS. Critically, this improvement was observed in the absence of speech-language therapy, suggesting the possibility of synergistic effects across these distinct domains of stroke recovery. It is worth noting that Meinzer et al. (8) reported that tDCS stimulation with this same montage may provide benefits to language processing in older neurotypical adults, suggesting the possibility that gains in language ability could come from the stimulation. However, in our limited data set, there was no effect of tDCS condition in most tasks. While we must be cautious about drawing strong conclusions from this dataset, it is possible that this reflects the fact that there was no explicit speech/language activity paired with the stimulation and that any benefit tDCS may provide in stroke rehabilitation comes from pairing of treatment and stimulation. We also note that recent findings on whether tDCS can affect language processing have been mixed, with recent positive findings reported for tDCS as an adjunct to aphasia therapy (9) and stuttering therapy (10) but null findings also widely reported (11).

In addition, we note that participants receiving sham showed a greater improvement on category naming than those receiving active stimulation, with the difference reaching significance in a *t*-test (but not a non-parametric test). This result leaves open the possibility that active tDCS was actively detrimental to improvement on this task, although it is surprising that this finding would occur for only one measure. We also note that tDCS groups were not matched for speech-language ability as part of the RCT and they were not matched in the study. The small sample size here also precludes us from determining whether other demographic or neurological factors (such as those outlined in **Table 1**) can account for this difference, as any regression analysis that would address this would be problematic due to the number of participants.

The positive overall findings should be treated cautiously in the absence of a control group not receiving robotics. In addition, the finding of an improvement on the WAB was only significant for a *t*-test and not non-parametric tests, and the 95% confidence intervals for that comparison fall below the 5 point threshold used to identify clinically significant improvement on that test. Nevertheless, these findings, in addition to those in Hesse et al. (1) on the subacute population, warrant additional systematic explorations of the benefit of multi-domain therapies for stroke rehabilitation.

AUTHOR CONTRIBUTIONS

AB and CF contributed equally to this manuscript. AB contributed to study concept and design, data analysis and interpretation, drafted, and revised manuscript for intellectual content. CF and DE contributed to study concept and design, data analysis and interpretation, critical revision of manuscript for intellectual content. AR-P contributed to study design. MC, AP-L, GT, HK, FF, JC, and BV contributed to study concept and design. LG and CO contributed to data analysis and interpretation, and critical revision of manuscript for intellectual content.

ACKNOWLEDGMENTS

We thank Gabriella Liscio, Abrielle Gouvin, Amanda Begley, Natasha Sousa, Allison Kornhaas, Gina Gallo, Mara Steinberg Lowe, and Heather Pepper-Lane for assistance with data collection and coding, and Susan Wortman-Jutt for helpful comments during manuscript preparation.

REFERENCES

1. Hesse S, Werner C, Schonhardt EM, Bardeleben A, Jenrich W, Kirker SG. Combined transcranial direct current stimulation and robot-assisted arm training in subacute stroke patients: a pilot study. *Restor Neurol Neurosci.* (2007) 25:9–15.
2. Dabul BL. *Apraxia Battery for Adults.* 2nd ed. Austin, TX: PRO-ED (2000).
3. Cattaneo Z, Pisoni A, Papagno C. Transcranial direct current stimulation over Broca's region improves phonemic and semantic fluency in healthy individuals. *Neuroscience* (2011) 183:64–70. doi: 10.1016/j.neuroscience.2011.03.058
4. Kertesz A. *Western Aphasia Examination – Revised.* San Antonio, TX: Pearson (2006) .
5. Katz RC, Wertz RT. The efficacy of computer-provided reading treatment for chronic aphasic adults. *J Speech Lang Hear Res.* (1997) 40: 493–507.
6. Ambrus GG, Al-Moyed H, Chaieb L, Sarp L, Antal A, Paulus W. The fade-in – short stimulation – fade out approach to sham tDCS – Reliable at 1 mA for naïve and experienced subjects, but not investigators. *Brain Stimul.* (2012) 5:499–504. doi: 10.1016/j.brs.2011.12.001
7. Fugl-Meyer AR, Jaasko L, Leyman I, Olsson S, Steglind S. The post-stroke hemiplegic patient. 1. a method for evaluation of physical performance. *Scand J Rehabil Med.* (1975) 7:13–31.
8. Meinzer M, Lindenberg R, Sieg M, Nachtigall L, Ulm L, Flöel A. Transcranial direct current stimulation of the primary motor cortex improves word-retrieval in older adults. *Front Aging Neurosci.* (2014) 6:253. doi: 10.3389/fnagi.2014.00253
9. Fridriksson J, Rorden C, Elm J, Sen S, George MS, Bonilha L. Transcranial direct current stimulation vs. sham stimulation to treat aphasia after stroke: a randomized clinical trial. *JAMA Neurol.* (2018). doi: 10.1001/jamaneurol.2018.2287. [Epub ahead of print].
10. Chesters J, Möttönen R, Watkins KE. Transcranial direct current stimulation over left inferior frontal cortex improves speech fluency in adults who stutter. *Brain* (2018)141:1161–71. doi: 10.1093/brain/awy011
11. Westwood SJ, Olson A, Miall RC, Nappo R, Romani C. Limits to tDCS effects in language: failures to modulate word production in healthy participants with frontal or temporal tDCS. *Cortex* (2017) 86:64–82. doi: 10.1016/j.cortex.2016.10.016

2

Gait Stability Training in a Virtual Environment Improves Gait and Dynamic Balance Capacity in Incomplete Spinal Cord Injury Patients

Rosanne B. van Dijsseldonk [1,2], Lysanne A. F. de Jong [1], Brenda E. Groen [1,2], Marije Vos-van der Hulst [3], Alexander C. H. Geurts [2,3] and Noel L. W. Keijsers [1,2]*

[1] Department of Research, Sint Maartenskliniek, Nijmegen, Netherlands, [2] Department of Rehabilitation, Cognition and Behavior, Radboud University Medical Center, Donders Institute for Brain, Nijmegen, Netherlands, [3] Department of Rehabilitation, Sint Maartenskliniek, Nijmegen, Netherlands

***Correspondence:**
Rosanne B. van Dijsseldonk
r.vandijsseldonk@maartenskliniek.nl

Many patients with incomplete spinal cord injury (iSCI) have impaired gait and balance capacity, which may impact daily functioning. Reduced walking speed and impaired gait stability are considered important underlying factors for reduced daily functioning. With conventional therapy, patients are limited in training gait stability, but this can be trained on a treadmill in a virtual environment, such as with the Gait Real-time Analysis Interactive Lab (GRAIL). Our objective was to evaluate the effect of 6-weeks GRAIL-training on gait and dynamic balance in ambulatory iSCI patients. In addition, the long-term effect was assessed. Fifteen patients with chronic iSCI participated. The GRAIL training consisted of 12 one-hour training sessions during a 6-week period. Patients performed 2 minute walking tests on the GRAIL in a self-paced mode at the 2nd, and 3rd (baseline measurements) and at the 12th training session. Ten patients performed an additional measurement after 6 months. The primary outcome was walking speed. Secondary outcomes were stride length, stride frequency, step width, and balance confidence. In addition, biomechanical gait stability measures based on the position of the center of mass (CoM) or the extrapolated center of mass (XCoM) relative to the center of pressure (CoP) or the base of support (BoS) were derived: dynamic stability margin (DSM), XCoM-CoP distance in anterior-posterior (AP) and medial-lateral (ML) directions, and CoM-CoP inclination angles in AP and ML directions. The effect of GRAIL-training was tested with a one-way repeated measures ANOVA ($\alpha = 0.05$) and *post-hoc* paired samples t-tests ($\alpha = 0.017$). Walking speed was higher after GRAIL training (1.04 m/s) compared to both baseline measurements (0.85 and 0.93 m/s) ($p < 0.001$). Significant improvements were also found for stride length ($p < 0.001$) and stability measures in AP direction (XCoM-CoP$_{AP}$ ($p < 0.001$) and CoM-CoP$_{AP-angle}$ ($p < 0.001$)). Stride frequency ($p = 0.27$), step width ($p = 0.19$), and stability measures DSM ($p = 0.06$), XCoM-CoP$_{ML}$ ($p = 0.97$), and CoM-CoP$_{ML-angle}$ ($p = 0.69$) did not improve. Balance confidence was increased after

GRAIL training ($p = 0.001$). The effects were remained at 6 months. Increased walking speed, stride length, AP gait stability, and balance confidence suggest that GRAIL-training improves gait and dynamic balance in patients with chronic iSCI. In contrast, stability measures in ML direction did not respond to GRAIL-training.

Keywords: spinal cord injury, virtual reality, gait, balance, stability, ambulatory, rehabilitation, walking

INTRODUCTION

Approximately 60% of the patients with a spinal cord injury (SCI) suffer an incomplete lesion (1). In the chronic phase of an incomplete SCI (iSCI) many patients will encounter deficits at and below the level of the lesion such as muscle weakness, spasticity, and impaired muscle coordination (2). These deficits can impact on functional ambulation (3) and social participation (4). For functional ambulation, walking speed is considered one of the most important parameters (5). Generally, iSCI patients walk at a low preferred walking speed (5) and with a deviant walking pattern (2, 6). One of the underlying causes of the reduced walking performance is impaired balance (7, 8). The high incidence of falls, ranging from 39 to 75% (9, 10), supports the impaired balance in ambulatory patients with iSCI.

Frequently, an important goal of rehabilitation is to improve balance and walking speed. Various interventions and training approaches aiming to improve walking performance in iSCI patients have been introduced and all approaches show some improvement without supremacy of one intervention over others (11). Typical examples of balance and walking training are individual physical therapy and (body-weight-supported) treadmill training. However, these therapies are limited in training patients to react to environmental circumstances without challenging their balance capacity to individual limits.

In recent years, training in a virtual environment has been introduced in rehabilitation (12, 13). In these virtual environments, a simulation of challenging real life situations (such as walking in a forest) can be presented without exposing the user to the direct danger of falling. In this way, patients are given the opportunity to train their gait and balance capacities by exploring their boundaries in a challenging and safe environment (14). Training in virtual environments will provide patients with important prerequisites for motor rehabilitation, such as repetitive practice, feedback about performance, and motivation to endure practice (12). In the virtual environment tasks involving precision stepping, obstacle avoidance, and/or reacting to perturbations, often referred to as "gait adaptability training," can be performed in quick succession. Such training is highly relevant to relearn daily activities such as walking on uneven surfaces or in crowded places, where people need to adapt their walking speed and walking pattern to environmental circumstances (15–18). Previous research shows that gait adaptability training can improve functional ambulation by preventing falls (19) and improving gait stability in elderly, stroke patients, and patients with Parkinson's disease (20–23). In iSCI patients training precision stepping has been shown to improve walking capacity measured with the SCI functional ambulation profile [SCI-FAP, (24)]. More recently, however, Fox and colleagues concluded that the efficacy of gait adaptability training on walking and balance function should be further investigated (25).

Although walking speed is considered to be the most important characteristic of walking performance, balance capacity is a key element of functional ambulation as well (7, 8). Studies that focused on balance in iSCI patients often used the Berg Balance Scale as a primary outcome (8, 26, 27). The Berg Balance Scale is easy to use, but it is known to have a ceiling effect (28) and assesses balance in rather static situations. Measuring gait stability is more complex and often requires additional equipment such as force plates and a motion capture system. Some virtual reality gait training devices, such as the GRAIL (Gait Real-time Analysis Interactive Lab), can be used as both a training and measurement device. The GRAIL consists of an instrumented dual belt treadmill with two embedded force plates and an eight-camera VICON motion capture system (VICON, Oxford, United Kingdom). The self-paced mode of the GRAIL allows patients to vary the treadmill speed during walking, which induces a natural way of walking (29), especially when a visual flow is presented in the virtual environment (30). When reflective markers are adhered to the participants body, the marker data can be captured for objective offline movement analysis. In addition to walking speed, more complex biomechanical measures related to gait stability can be derived. Previous studies showed that these biomechanical gait stability measures were able to distinguish between elderly with and without balance problems (31, 32), between above-knee amputees and control subjects (33), and between more and less affected stroke patients (34). However, the responsiveness of the stability measures to gait training is unknown.

The main objective of this study was to evaluate the effect of 6 weeks GRAIL training on gait and dynamic balance capacity in ambulatory patients with chronic iSCI. In addition, the long-term effect was assessed 6 months after GRAIL training. Walking speed was used as a primary outcome, while other spatio-temporal parameters and gait stability measures were assessed as secondary outcome parameters. We hypothesized that GRAIL training will result in an improved walking speed and gait stability.

MATERIALS AND METHODS

Participants

Patients with iSCI who were referred to GRAIL training by a rehabilitation physician in the Sint Maartenskliniek between June 2016 and December 2017 were eligible to participate in this study. Eligible persons were adults in the chronic phase

(>6 months) with an iSCI [American Spinal Injury Association Impairment Scale (AIS) C or D] who could walk independently for 2 min without assistance [Functional Ambulation Categories (FAC) ≥3]. Patients were excluded if (i) they were not able to walk in the self-paced mode of the GRAIL without using the handrails, (ii) had other neurological or lower limb impairments in addition to the iSCI, (iii) had vision problems, or (iv) had walking and/or balance problems prior to the iSCI. The exclusion criteria (ii), (iii), and (iv) were checked by the researcher through questions. All participants gave written informed consent in accordance with the Declaration of Helsinki. The study was approved by the regional medical ethics committee of Arnhem-Nijmegen (2016–2474) and by the internal review board of the Sint Maartenskliniek.

Equipment

All training sessions and measurements were performed on the GRAIL at the Sint Maartenskliniek in Nijmegen (**Figure 1**). The GRAIL consisted of an instrumented dual belt treadmill with two embedded force plates and an eight-camera VICON motion capture system (VICON, Oxford, United Kingdom). The platform was able to move in several directions to generate mechanical perturbations. In front of the treadmill, virtual reality environments were projected on a 180° semi-cylindrical screen. Reflective markers were adhered to the patients to interact with the virtual environment and to capture kinematic data. The GRAIL system was controlled and the visual information was matched to the treadmill speed with the D-flow software (Motek Forcelink, Amsterdam, the Netherlands, version 3.22.1). To assure safety, patients wore a safety harness without body weight support.

Protocol

Intervention

The GRAIL training consisted of 12 1-h training sessions spread over a 6-week period. Per training session one physical therapist guided the training and a maximum of two physical therapists were responsible for all training sessions given to one patient. All physical therapists were certified GRAIL operators. Each training was individualized, as the physical therapist chose the training applications based on the specific rehabilitation goal and current level of the patient. For instance, patients who had problems maintaining their balance in stance typically performed applications in which they had to shift their weight, whereas patients with gait adaptability problems performed applications in which they had to perform precision stepping or obstacle avoidance. During the GRAIL training multiple applications were performed and after each training session the physical therapist documented the type and level of the performed applications. The applications were categorized in three themes; "gait adaptability," "walking+," "balance in stance" (see **Table 2**). The first GRAIL training session was used for familiarization with the GRAIL system. From the second to the last training session, training intensity, and complexity were gradually and individually increased.

Gait Measurements

To evaluate the effect of GRAIL training on gait and balance, patients performed the 2 minute walking test (2MWT) at the 2nd, 3rd, and last (12th) training sessions (baseline 1, baseline 2, and post measurement, respectively). For familiarization with the task, the 2nd baseline measurement (at the 3rd training session) was added to neutralize early learning (or task adaptation) effects.

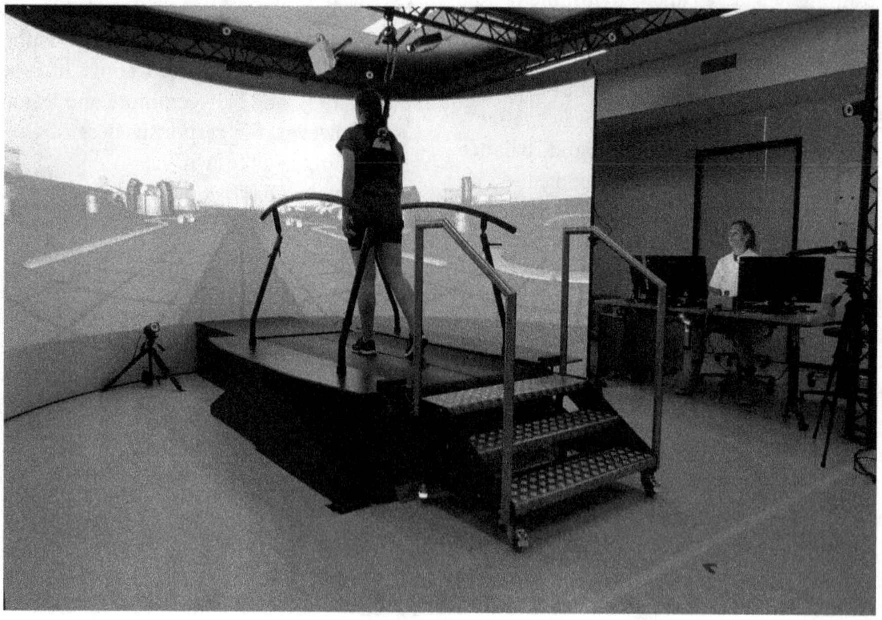

FIGURE 1 | Gait Real-time Analysis Interactive Lab (GRAIL) at the Sint Maartenskliniek. Both persons have given their written and informed consent for publication of the picture.

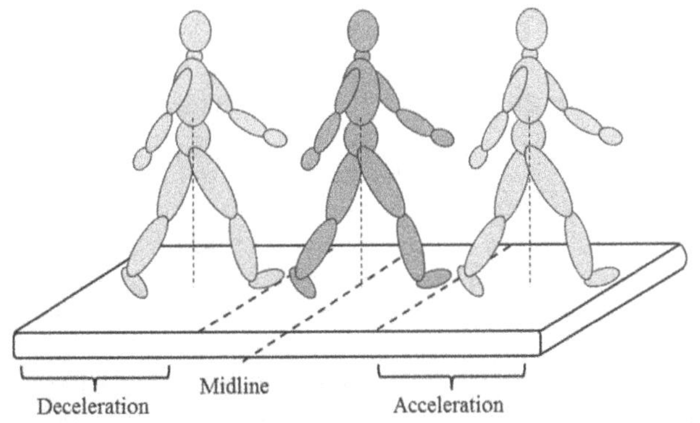

FIGURE 2 | Self-paced mode on the GRAIL.

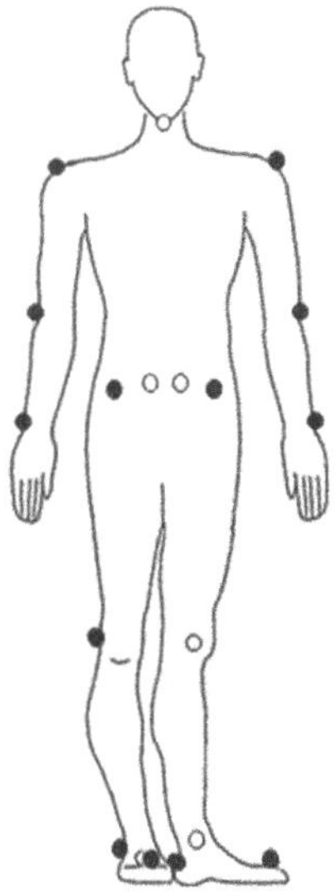

FIGURE 3 | Placement of the reflective markers.

To evaluate the long-term effect of GRAIL training on gait and balance, patients performed one additional 2MWT on the GRAIL 6 months after the last training session (follow-up). Patients performed the 2MWT in the self-paced mode on the GRAIL, which allowed them to walk at a self-selected speed. In the self-paced mode, the speed of the treadmill was automatically controlled using the anterior-posterior (AP) position of the pelvis markers and the AP midline of the treadmill. Walking forward or backward relative to the midline resulted in an acceleration or deceleration of the treadmill, respectively (**Figure 2**). Before measuring the 2MWT, patients received some explanation about the self-paced mode and performed a few practice trials to reach their preferred walking speed in a similar manner as in the study of Plotnik and colleagues (30). During the 2MWT on the GRAIL, patients were instructed to walk as far as possible at a comfortable walking speed in 2 min. Patients received no feedback about their walking speed.

The self-paced mode was set at the lowest sensitivity value of 1.0 (setting ranged between 1 and 5). The maximum acceleration and deceleration of the treadmill was set at 0.25 m/s^2. Before the start of the 2MWT, 19 reflective markers were adhered to the following anatomical landmarks: left and right acromion process, humeral lateral epicondyle, ulnar styloid process, anterior superior iliac spine (ASIS), posterior superior iliac spine (PSIS), femoral lateral epicondyle, lateral malleolus, metatarsal II, calcaneus, and 7th cervical vertebra (**Figure 3**). The data of the reflective markers was sampled at a frequency of 100 Hz and the sample frequency of the force plates was 1,000 Hz. The data of the reflective markers were labeled using VICON Nexus 2.4 and analyzed using MATLAB R2017b. A zero lag second-order Butterworth filter with a cut-off frequency of 10 Hz was used to filter the marker data. A cut-off frequency of 7 Hz was used for the force data. Before the patients walked at their preferred walking speed, the treadmill had to accelerate. To remove the acceleration phase, the first 20 s of the 2MWT were removed before data analysis.

Spatiotemporal parameters

The primary outcome was walking speed defined as the average treadmill speed (m/s). Other spatiotemporal gait parameters (stride length, step width, and stride frequency) were used as secondary outcome parameters. Stride length (cm) was determined as the average AP-distance between the heel markers at two consecutive heel strikes on the same side. Step width (cm) was determined as the average ML-distance between the heel markers at heel strike. Stride frequency (strides/s) was defined as the inverse of the interval between heel strikes of the same foot. Heel strikes were defined as the instant that the calcaneus marker started moving backwards.

Gait stability measures

The stability measures used in the current study were based on the position of the center of mass (CoM) or the extrapolated center of mass (XCoM) relative to the center of pressure (CoP) or the base of support (BoS), during a specific moment of the gait cycle (e.g., double support or heel strike). The position of the CoM depends on sex, body posture, and direction of the limbs. In this study the CoM was calculated using 19 reflective markers according to a method first described by Tisserand et al. (35). The XCoM takes the position and velocity of the CoM into account and is used to formulate requirements for gait stability (36). To calculate the XCoM, the equation of Hof et al was used (36, 37):

$$XCoM = CoM' + \frac{vCoM}{\sqrt{\frac{g}{l}}}$$

CoM' represents the ground projection of the CoM, *vCoM* the velocity of the CoM, $g = 9.81$ m/s^2, and l the maximum height of the CoM (36, 37). The CoP is the centroid of pressure distribution on the plantar surface of the foot and has been used to identify balance control during posture and gait (38). The equation of

Sloot et al was used to calculate the CoP for both force plates (39):

$$CoP_{AP} = \frac{F_{AP} * CoP_V - M_{ML}}{F_V} \quad \& $$
$$CoP_{ML} = \frac{F_{ML} * CoP_V - M_{AP}}{F_V}$$

F represents the force in anterior-posterior ($_{AP}$), medial-lateral ($_{ML}$), and vertical ($_V$) directions, M the moment of force, and CoP_V the vertical distance between the surface of the treadmill belt and the force plates (39). During the double support phase, the weighted average of the CoP in ML and AP directions was calculated based on the CoP of both force plates.

In this study the following five gait stability measures were calculated: the dynamic margin of stability (DSM) (34), the XCoM-CoP distance in AP and ML directions (32, 33), and the CoM-CoP inclination angles in AP and ML directions (31). In general, better gait stability is characterized by a position of the XCoM far in front of the BoS in the AP direction, which suggests that patients are confident in walking at higher speeds with longer steps. In the ML direction, better gait stability is characterized by a position of the XCoM closer to the boundaries of the BoS, often accompanied by walking with a smaller step width. The DSM was calculated as the average of the shortest distance between the front line of the BoS (i.e., the line between the two metatarsal II markers) and the XCoM during double support (34) (See **Figure 4A** for a visual representation). A large positive DSM represents better balance control than a negative DSM (i.e., XCoM within the BoS) or smaller DSM. The distances between the XCoM and CoP were calculated at each heel strike in AP (**Figure 4B**) and ML directions (**Figure 4C**) separately (32, 33). A larger XCoM-CoP_{AP} distance and a smaller XCoM-CoP_{ML} distance reflect better balance control. The CoM-CoP inclination angles were calculated from the angle between the position of the CoM and the vertical line through the CoP (31). The peak inclination angles were defined as the range between the maximum and minimum inclination angles in AP (**Figure 4D**) and ML directions (**Figure 4E**) of each gait cycle. A larger peak inclination angle in the AP direction and a smaller peak inclination angle in the ML direction represent better balance control.

Balance Confidence Assessment

Balance confidence was assessed with the activities specific balance confidence (ABC) (0–100) scale (40, 41) at the second training session (before the first baseline measurement), at the last training session (after the post measurement) and at 6 months after the last training session (after the follow-up measurement).

Statistical Analysis

Effect of GRAIL Training

The spatiotemporal gait parameters (walking speed, stride length, step width, and stride frequency) and gait stability measures

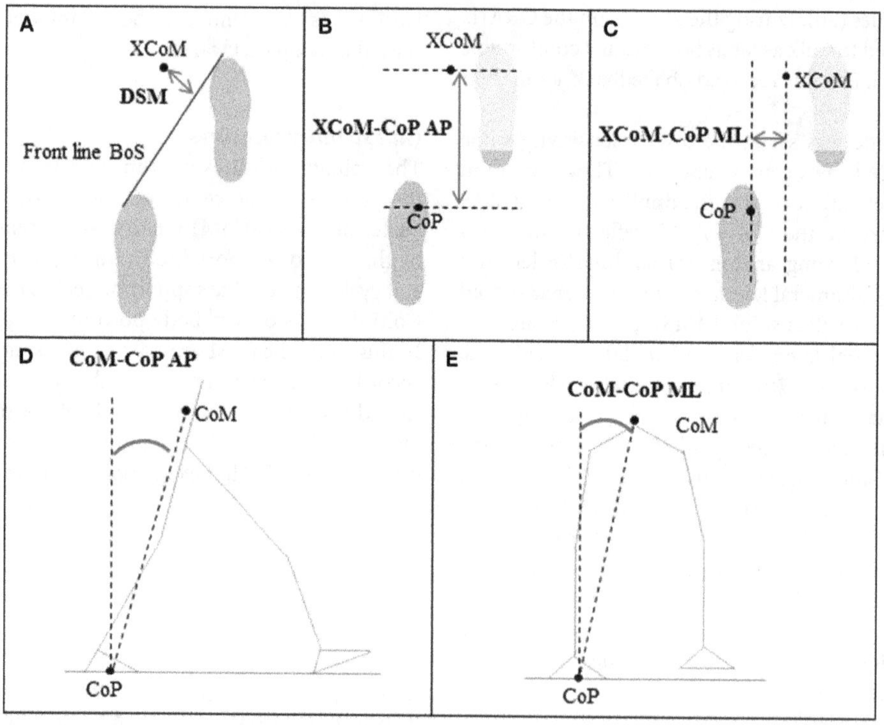

FIGURE 4 | Gait stability measures based on the position of the center of mass (CoM), extrapolated center of mass (XCoM), center of pressure (CoP), and/or base of support (BoS) relative to each other; **(A)** dynamic stability margin (DSM), **(B,C)** XCoM-CoP distance in anterior-posterior (AP) and medial-lateral (ML) direction, **(D,E)** CoM-CoP inclination angles in AP and ML direction.

(DSM, XCoM-CoP$_{AP}$ distance, XCoM-CoP$_{ML}$ distance, CoM-CoP$_{AP-angle}$, and CoM-CoP$_{ML-angle}$) were analyzed using descriptive statistics (mean and standard deviation). Differences in the spatiotemporal gait parameters and gait stability measures between the three measurements (baseline 1, baseline 2, and post measurement) were assessed with a one-way (factor Time) repeated measures ANOVA ($\alpha = 0.05$). If the assumption of sphericity was violated, the degrees of freedom were corrected using Greenhouse-Geisser correction and the Pillai's Trace value (V) was given. In the case of a significant effect of Time, paired samples *t*-tests with Bonferroni correction ($\alpha = 0.017$) were performed to determine which measurements were different from each other. In case the assumption of normality was violated, median, and ranges were calculated and a non-parametric Friedman test ($\alpha = 0.05$) with Wilcoxon signed-rank *post-hoc* test ($\alpha = 0.017$) was performed. The effect of GRAIL training on balance confidence (the scores on the pre and post ABC-scale) was tested with paired samples *t*-test ($\alpha = 0.05$). *F* and *t*-values were given when the repeated measures ANOVA and paired samples *t*-test were used, while X^2_F and *T* were given for the non-parametric Friedman test and Wilcoxon signed-rank test.

Long-Term Effect of GRAIL Training

The long-term effect of GRAIL training was evaluated by testing the differences in spatiotemporal gait parameters (walking speed, stride length, step width, and stride frequency) and gait stability measures (DSM, XCoM-CoP$_{AP}$ distance, XCoM-CoP$_{ML}$ distance, CoM-CoP$_{AP-angle}$, and CoM-CoP$_{ML-angle}$) between the post and follow-up measurements as well as between the baseline 2 and follow-up measurements using paired samples *t*-tests ($\alpha = 0.05$). When the assumption of normality was violated, median, and ranges were calculated and a non-parametric Wilcoxon signed-rank test ($\alpha = 0.05$) was performed. *t*-values were given when the paired samples *t*-test was used, while *T* was given for the non-parametric equivalent, the Wilcoxon signed-rank test.

RESULTS

Participants

In total 20 patients were assessed for eligibility in the study. Three patients were ineligible because they could not walk in the self-paced mode without using the handrails (exclusion criteria). One patient declined to participate. Sixteen patients were included in the study. One dropped out before completing the post measurement, resulting in 15 patients who performed the baseline 1, baseline 2, and post measurements (**Figure 5**). An overview of the patient characteristics is given in **Table 1**.

Content of GRAIL Training

Two patients received 9 and 8 GRAIL training sessions instead of the scheduled 12 training sessions. These patients canceled some training sessions at short notice, which made it impossible to reschedule the sessions within the training period. The other 13 patients received 12 GRAIL training sessions. In total 30 different applications were performed during the GRAIL training. The themes of these applications were categorized in "gait adaptability" (13 applications), "walking^{+}" (8 applications), and "balance in stance" (9 applications). On average, patients performed 3.7 ± 0.9 applications during one training session, of which 1.4 ± 0.4 were gait adaptability applications, 1.3 ± 0.4 walking^{+} applications, and 1.0 ± 0.5 balance in stance applications. The most frequently practiced applications for gait adaptability were "Microbes" (42%), for walking^{+} "Perturbations" (23%), and for balance in stance "Traffic jam" (42%). An explanation of the most frequently practiced applications per theme is depicted in **Table 2**.

Effect of GRAIL Training

Spatiotemporal Parameters

The repeated measures ANOVA revealed significant Time effects of GRAIL training on walking speed [$F_{(2,28)} = 18.53, p < 0.001$]. *Post-hoc* analysis showed that the mean walking speed was significantly higher at post measurement (1.04 ± 0.38 m/s) compared to baseline 1 (0.85 ± 0.41 m/s, $p < 0.001$) and baseline 2 (0.93 ± 0.37 m/s, $p = 0.003$). There was a significant effect of GRAIL training on the stride length, [$F_{(2,28)} = 15.76, p < 0.001$]. Stride length was significantly larger at the post measurement (112 ± 31cm) compared to baseline 1 (94 ± 39 cm, $p < 0.001$) and baseline 2 (101 ± 33 cm, $p = 0.002$). Stride frequency [$V = 0.18, F_{(2,13)} = 1.45, p = 0.27$] and step width [$F_{(2,28)} = 1.76$, $p = 0.19$] were not significantly affected by GRAIL training. The spatiotemporal gait parameters at the three measurements are shown in **Figure 6**.

Gait Stability Measures

The repeated measures ANOVA revealed significant Time effects on XCoM-CoP$_{AP}$ distance [$F_{(2,28)} = 19.48, p < 0.001$] and CoM-CoP$_{AP-angle}$ [$F_{(2,28)} = 15.90$, $p < 0.001$]. The XCoM-CoP$_{AP}$ distance was significantly higher at post measurement (491 ± 175 mm) compared to baseline 1 (404 ± 195 mm, $p < 0.001$) and baseline 2 (441 ± 177 mm, $p = 0.003$). The CoM-CoP$_{AP-angle}$ was significantly higher at post measurement (16.6 ± 5.3°) compared to baseline 1 (14.1 ± 5.5°, $p < 0.001$) and baseline 2 (14.7 ± 4.8°, $p = 0.003$). The Time effect on the DSM nearly reached significance [$V = 0.36$, $F_{(2,13)} = 3.64$, $p = 0.06$], whereas the XCoM-CoP$_{ML}$ distance [$F_{(2,28)} = 0.003$, $p = 0.97$] and CoM-CoP$_{ML-angle}$ [$F_{(2,28)} = 0.38$, $p = 0.69$] were not significantly affected by GRAIL training. **Figure 7** gives an overview of the gait stability measures across time.

Balance Confidence

Patients' balance confidence significantly increased after GRAIL training (76 ± 18), compared to baseline (69 ± 18) [$t_{(13)} = -4.55$, $p = 0.001$]. The balance confidence scores before and after GRAIL training are shown in **Figure 8**.

Long-Term Effect of GRAIL Training

The follow-up measurement was performed by 11 of the 15 patients (**Figure 5**). Two patients did not perform the follow-up measurement due to medical complications, which were

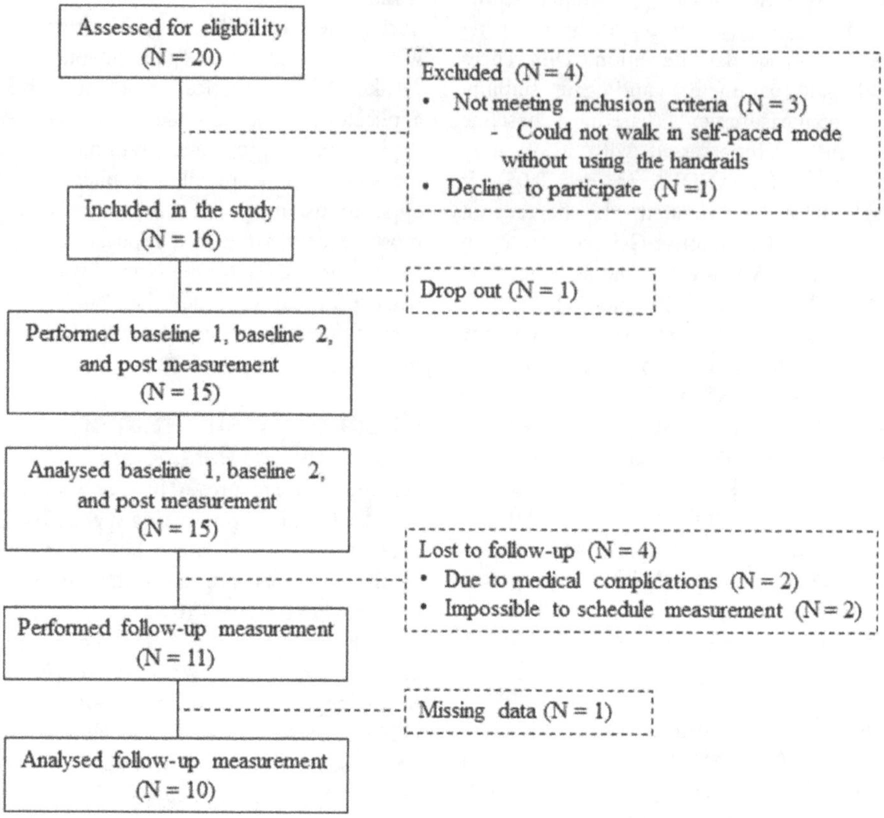

FIGURE 5 | Flow diagram of patients in the study.

TABLE 1 | Patient characteristwics.

	Performed baseline 1, baseline 2 and post measurement (*N* = 15)	Completed follow-up (*N* = 10)
Sex (male/female)	11/4	9/1
Age (years), mean (SD)	59 (12)	59 (12)
Post-injury (months), mean (SD)	42 (48)	42 (46)
AIS*(C/D)	2/13	1/9
BMI**, mean (SD)	27 (2)	26 (2)
FAC***(3/4/5)	1/6/8	1/4/5
More affected side (left/ right/ no difference)	7/3/5	5/1/4

**AIS, American Spinal Injury Association Impairment Scale.*
***BMI, Body-Mass Index.*
****FAC, Functional Ambulatory Category.*

not related to the GRAIL training. Two other patients were lost to follow-up, because it was impossible to schedule their measurements. As a result of a technical error during the follow-up measurement, the data of one additional patient was missing. Therefore, the results of 10 patients were used for the analysis of the long-term effect of GRAIL training (see **Table 1** for patient characteristics).

There was no significant difference in walking speed between post (median 1.13 m/s) and follow-up (median 1.30 m/s) measurement [$T = 20.50$, $p = 0.48$], nor was there a significant difference in stride length [$T = 27$, $p = 0.96$], step width [$t_{(9)} = 0.82$, $p = 0.43$], or stride frequency [$t_{(9)} = -1.04$, $p = 0.33$] between the post measurement and the follow-up measurement. The CoM-$CoP_{ML-angle}$ was significantly smaller in the follow-up (10.3 ± 1.6°) compared to the post measurement (11.4 ± 2.2°), [$t_{(9)} = 2.4$, $p = 0.04$]. The other gait stability measures (DSM, CoM-$CoP_{AP-angle}$ and XCoM-CoP_{AP} and XCoM-CoP_{ML} distances) and balance confidence score were not significantly different at the follow-up measurement compared to the post measurement. An overview of the spatiotemporal gait parameters, gait stability measures and balance confidence are shown in **Table 3**.

Walking speed ($p = 0.03$), stride length ($p = 0.04$), and CoM-$CoP_{AP-angle}$ ($p = 0.03$) were significantly higher in the follow-up measurement compared to the baseline 2 measurement. The other outcome measures (step width, stride frequency, DSM, CoM-$CoP_{ML-angle}$ and XCoM-CoP_{AP} and XCoM-CoP_{ML} distances and balance confidence) were not significantly different at the follow-up measurement compared to the baseline 2 measurement (**Table 3**).

TABLE 2 | Most frequently performed applications on the GRAIL per theme.

Theme	Gait adaptability	Walking+	Balance in stance
Application	"Microbes"	"Perturbations"	"Traffic jam"
Virtual environment	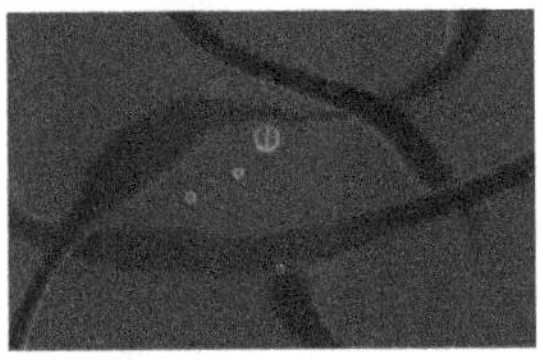	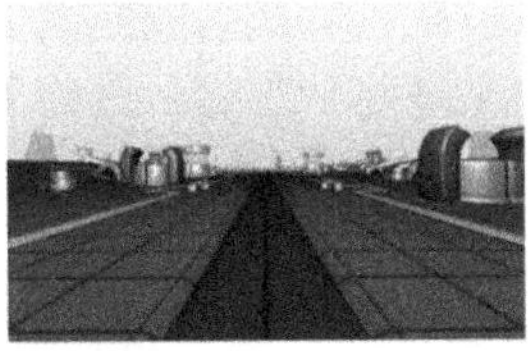	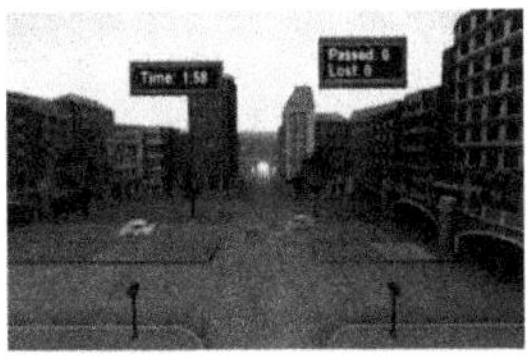
Task	Collecting as many green microbes by changing one's position on the treadmill during gait.	Walking on the treadmill and responding as quickly and accurately as possible to the perturbations.	Letting cars cross the road by lifting the feet in stance.
Training purpose	Accelerate and decelerate, change walking direction, adapt step length, avoid obstacles, and perform foot clearance.	React to: sideward translation of the treadmill, treadmill pitch forward or backward, acceleration or deceleration of one treadmill belt.	Shift weight, perform foot clearance, and initiate steps.

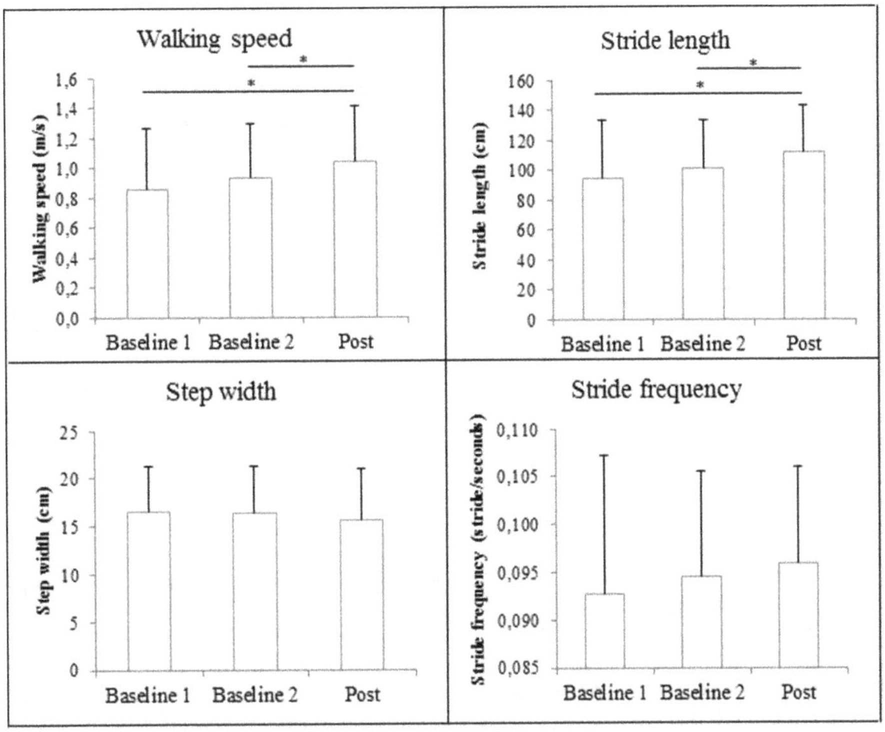

FIGURE 6 | The spatiotemporal gait parameters (means and standard deviations) during the 6 weeks GRAIL training. *Asterisk indicates a *post-hoc* significant difference ($\alpha = 0.017$).

DISCUSSION

The aim of the present study, was to assess the effects of 6 weeks GRAIL training on gait and dynamic balance capacities in chronic iSCI patients. Walking speed was increased after GRAIL training (1.04 m/s) compared to baseline measurements (0.85 and 0.93m/s). Stride length was increased, but stride frequency and step width did not change. In addition, the stability measures in AP direction (XCoM-CoP_{AP} and CoM-$CoP_{AP-angle}$) were improved after GRAIL training, whereas stability measures in ML direction (XCoM-CoP_{ML} and CoM-$CoP_{ML-angle}$) or combining AP and ML directions (DSM) did not change. Patients' confidence in balance was increased after GRAIL training. At the 6 months follow-up measurement,

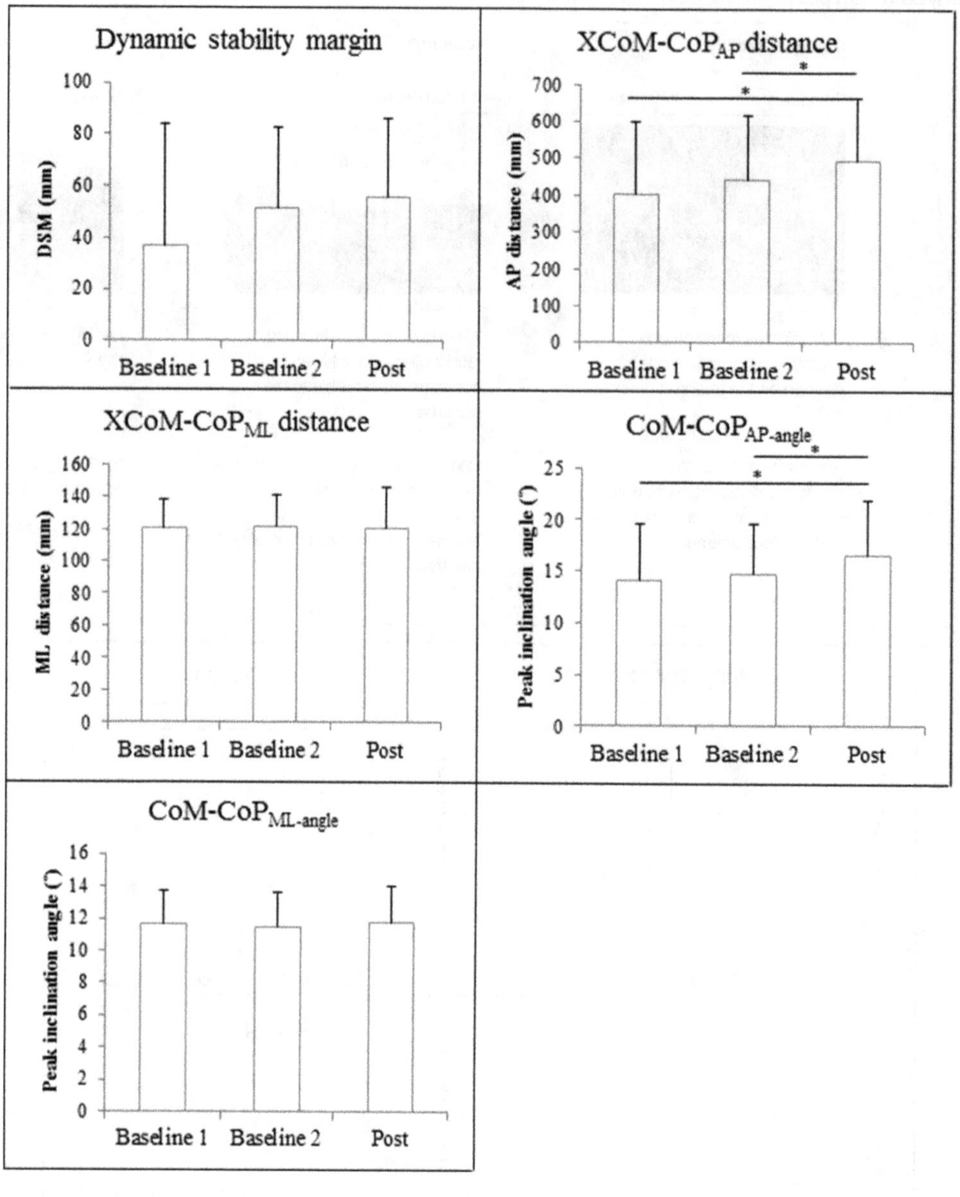

FIGURE 7 | Gait stability (means and standard deviations) during 6 weeks GRAIL training. A visual representation of the gait stability measures is given in **Figure 4**. *Asterisk indicates a *post-hoc* significant difference ($\alpha = 0.017$).

improvements in walking speed, stride length, and the stability measure CoM-CoP$_{AP-angle}$ remained increased compared to baseline.

In patients with iSCI, restoration of ambulation is considered the most important rehabilitation goal (42). Typically interventions in these patients focus on improving locomotion (43). For functional ambulation in daily life, walking speed is considered one of the most important parameters (5). After GRAIL training, walking speed increased by 0.19 m/s compared to baseline 1 and by 0.11 m/s compared to baseline 2. Although previous studies in chronic iSCI patients used more gait training sessions (on average 45; range 24–58) due to a higher training frequency (on average 4 sessions/week; range 3–5), and a longer training duration (on average 12 weeks; range 8–16), these studies showed increases in walking speed ranging from 0.01 to 0.16 m/s (24, 44–48). To our knowledge, only two interventions in chronic iSCI patients resulted in an increase in walking speed in the 0.11 to 0.19 m/s range (44, 47). These interventions consisted of 48 sessions of resistance training combined with aerobic training resulting in an increase of 0.13 m/s (47) and 39 sessions of body-weight-supported treadmill training resulting in an increase of 0.16 m/s (44). Due to the higher number of training session, a larger training effect can be expected. Despite the limited number of GRAIL training sessions in the present study, patients improved their walking speed significantly. This improvement exceeded the reported minimal clinically important difference (MCID) of 0.10 m/s (49) in 10 out of 15 participants, reflecting clinical meaningful effects in these participants. Moreover, the effect on walking speed, stride length, and the stability measure CoM-$CoP_{AP-angle}$ were still present 6 months after the last training session. Therefore, randomized controlled trials (or studies with a randomized cross-over design) are warranted to investigate the intervention effects of GRAIL training compared to other gait training interventions in patients with iSCI.

The increase in walking speed, accompanied by an increase in stride length but with a constant stride frequency, suggests that patients learned to take larger steps because they felt more confident after GRAIL training. Indeed, the statistically significant increase in balance confidence score supports the notion that patients felt more safe after the training. However, only one participants exceeded the reported minimal detectable change (MDC) of 14.87 (50). Therefore, the effect of GRAIL training on balance confidence seems to be relatively small. Nevertheless, the significant increase in balance confidence on a group level could be due to improved gait stability. In the current study, recently developed biomechanical stability measures were used to assess gait stability. In previous studies, these stability measures appeared to be significantly different between more and less impaired stroke patients (34), above-knee amputees and healthy subjects (33), and elderly with and without balance problems (31, 32). To our knowledge, this is the first study to assess these stability measures during gait in a pre- and post-intervention design. The gait stability in AP direction was significantly increased after 6 weeks GRAIL training. Because a high correlation between walking speed and AP gait stability can be expected and because we did not perform a post measurement in which patients walked at baseline speed, it cannot be definitively concluded whether patients walked faster after GRAIL training because of improved gait stability or vice versa. In the present study, the stability measures in the ML direction did not differ between the measurements. Future research should test the clinical value of gait stability measures in different directions in patients with iSCI.

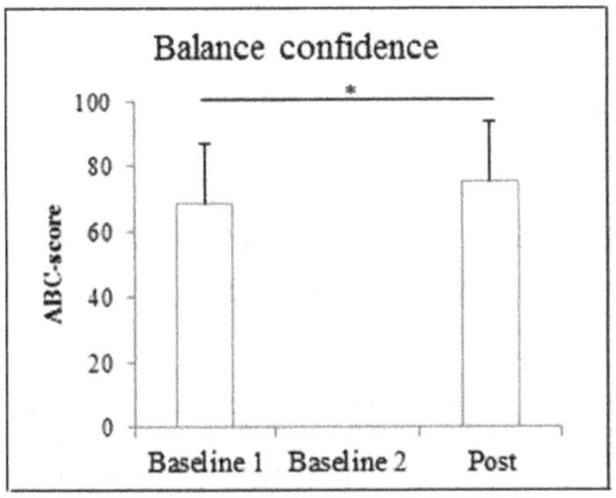

FIGURE 8 | Activities specific balance confidence (ABC) score (means and standard deviations) before and after the 6-weeks GRAIL training. *Asterisk indicates a significant difference (α = 0.05).

Various factors could be responsible for the improved walking speed after GRAIL training. Firstly, patients performed tasks in a complex virtual environment, in which visual and auditory feedback were provided. Patients could make corrections and enhance their motor performance according to the feedback in real time (based on knowledge of performance) as well as at the end of the application (based on knowledge of results) (12). It is well accepted that feedback improves the rate of motor learning (51). Feedback can be particularly beneficial in patients with iSCI in which internal feedback (such as from the proprioceptive system) is disturbed (52). Secondly, different training environments can be quickly alternated during GRAIL training. According to Hedel and colleagues, in well-recovered iSCI patients, such as in the current study, rehabilitation programs should train adaptive locomotion in different environments (52). Thirdly, GRAIL training can be personalized and the intensity and complexity of the applications can be gradually increased. We assume that the effects found in

TABLE 3 | The spatiotemporal gait parameters, gait stability measures and balance confidence in the baseline 2, post and follow-up measurement (*N*=10).

	Baseline 2 measurement (mean ± SD, median [min–max])	Post measurement (mean ± SD, median [min–max])	Follow-up measurement (mean ± SD, median [min–max])	*p* baseline 2 - follow-up	*p* post - follow-up
Walking speed (m/s)	0.89 [0.36–1.45]	1.13 [0.44–1.53]	1.30 [0.34–1.48]	0.03*	0.48
Stride length (cm)	103 [57–144]	118 [68–145]	128 [51–144]	0.04*	0.96
Step width (cm)	14.4 ± 4.7	13.7 ± 5.0	13.0 ± 4.4	0.19	0.43
Stride frequency (stride/s)	0.93 ± 0.13	0.96 ± 0.04	0.97 ± 0.05	0.07	0.33
DSM (mm)	54 ± 36	60 ± 32	57 ± 44	0.70	0.65
XCoM-CoP_{AP} (mm)	431 [161–718]	511 ± 170	525 ± 201 627 [158–696]	0.07	0.62
XCoM-CoP_{ML} (mm)	121 ± 23	118 ± 26	111 ± 22	0.12	0.15
CoM-$CoP_{AP-angle}$ (°)	15.1 ± 4.6	17.4 ± 5.0	17.7 ± 6.0	0.03*	0.77
CoM-$CoP_{ML-angle}$ (°)	10.9 ± 2.3	11.4 ± 2.2	10.3 ± 1.6	0.23	0.04*
ABC-score	70.3 ± 19.0	77.1 ± 19.3	74.5 ± 20.4	0.13	0.09

**Asterisk indicates a significant difference (α = 0.05) in the paired samples t-test (mean ± SD) or Wilcoxon signed-rank test (median [min–max]).*

the current study are partly due to the personalization of the GRAIL training to the patients' individual goals. Therefore, it does not seen appropriate to standardize the GRAIL training for each patient.

Observed improvements could have been caused by a familiarization effect when walking on the GRAIL in the self-paced mode. To neutralize this effect, two baseline measurements were performed, one at the 2nd and the other at the 3rd GRAIL training sessions. Furthermore, a familiarization protocol with self-paced walking on the GRAIL, similar as in the study of Plotnik and colleagues (30), was performed before the first baseline measurement. In the study of Plotnik and colleagues, healthy participants reached their steady walking speed already after ~24 m when visual flow was presented and reached a walking speed comparable with overground walking after merely 7.5 to 17.5 m (30). In the current study, an increase of 0.08 m/s was seen between the baseline 1 and 2 measurements. This increase could be partly due to familiarization with self-paced walking on the GRAIL. Future research should investigate if familiarization with self-paced walking takes more time in patients with impaired gait stability than in healthy subjects. Important to note is that the self-paced walking was not practiced in the subsequent GRAIL training sessions. Nevertheless, patients further increased their walking speed significantly at the post-measurement compared to baseline 2 by 0.11 m/s. Moreover, at 6 months follow-up, this beneficial effect was still present, suggesting a true effect of GRAIL training.

A limitation of the current study is that the follow-up measurement was completed by only 10 patients and that we did not control co-interventions during the period after the GRAIL training. Another limitation is that we do not know how the effect of GRAIL training has affected gait and dynamic balance capacities during overground walking. Although previous studies concluded that self-paced treadmill walking induces natural gait (29) and that gait speed on a treadmill is comparable to overground walking (30), future research should investigate whether the effect of GRAIL training also extends to overground walking, walking in daily life, and to social participation in ambulatory iSCI patients.

CONCLUSION

The increased walking speed, stride length, AP gait stability, and balance confidence suggest that GRAIL training improves gait and dynamic balance capacity in patients with chronic iSCI.

AUTHOR CONTRIBUTIONS

NK, BG, MV, and AG contributed conception and design of the study. MV was responsible for the patient recruitment. LdJ, RvD, and BG performed the measurements. LdJ organized the database. RvD and NK processed the experimental data, performed the analysis, drafted the manuscript, and designed the figures. NK and BG supervised the project. All authors discussed the results and commented on the manuscript.

REFERENCES

1. Nijendijk JHB, Post MWM, Asbeck van FWA. Epidemiology of traumatic spinal cord injuries in the Netherlands in 2010. *Spinal Cord* (2014) 52:258–63. doi: 10.1038/sc.2013.180
2. Barbeau H, Nadeau S, Garneau C. Physical determinants, emerging concepts, and training approaches in gait of individuals with spinal cord injury. *J Neurotrauma* (2006) 23:571–85. doi: 10.1089/neu.2006.23.571
3. Hedel van HJA. Gait speed in relation to categories of functional ambulation after cord spinal injury. *Neurorehabil Neural Repair* (2009) 23:343–50. doi: 10.1177/1545968308324224
4. Lund ML, Nordlund A, Nygård L, Lexell J, Bernspång B. Perceptions of participation and predictors of perceived problems with participation in persons with spinal cord injury. *J Rehabil Med.* (2005) 37:3–8. doi: 10.1080/16501970410031246
5. Lapointe R, Lajoie Y, Serresse O, Barbeau H. Functional community ambulation requirements in incomplete spinal cord injured subjects. *Spinal Cord* (2001) 39:327–35. doi: 10.1038/sj.sc.3101167
6. Pépin A, Norman KE, Barbeau H. Treadmill walking in incomplete spinal-cord-injured subjects: 1. Adaptation to changes in speed. *Spinal Cord* (2003) 41:257–70. doi: 10.1038/sj.sc.3101452
7. Scivoletto G, Romanelli A, Mariotti A, Marinucci D, Tamburella F, Mammone A, et al. Clinical factors that affect walking level and performance in chronic spinal cord lesion patients. *Spine* (2008) 33:259–64. doi: 10.1097/BRS.0b013e3181626ab0
8. Tamburella F, Scivoletto G, Molinari M. Balance training improves static stability and gait in chronic incomplete spinal cord injury subjects: a pilot study. *Eur J Phys Rehabil Med.* (2013) 49:353–64.
9. Brotherton SS, Krause JS, Nietert PJ. Falls in individuals with incomplete spinal cord injury. *Spinal Cord* (2007) 45:37–40. doi: 10.1038/sj.sc.3101909
10. Phonthee S, Saengsuwan J, Siritaratiwat W, Amatachaya S. Incidence and factors associated with falls in independent ambulatory individuals with spinal cord injury: a 6-month prospective study. *Phys Ther.* (2013) 93:1061–72. doi: 10.2522/ptj.20120467
11. Morawietz C, Moffat F. Effects of locomotor training after incomplete spinal cord injury: a systematic review. *Arch Phys Med Rehabil.* (2013) 94:2297–308. doi: 10.1016/j.apmr.2013.06.023
12. Holden MK. Virtual environments for motor rehabilitation : review. *Cyberpsychol Behav.* (2005) 8:187–211. doi: 10.1089/cpb.2005.8.187
13. Papegaaij S, Morang F, Steenbrink F. *Virtual and augmented reality based balance and gait training.* White Paper, (February) (2017).
14. Fung J, Richards CL, Malouin F, McFadyen BJ, Lamontagne A. A treadmill and motion coupled virtual reality system for gait training post-stroke. *Cyberpsychol Behav.* (2006) 9:157–62. doi: 10.1089/cpb.2006.9.157
15. Geerse DJ, Coolen BH, Roerdink M. Walking-adaptability assessments with the interactive walkway: between-systems agreement and sensitivity to task and subject variations. *Gait Posture* (2017) 54:194–201. doi: 10.1016/j.gaitpost.2017.02.021
16. Hak L, Houdijk H, Beek PJ, Van Dieën JH. Steps to take to enhance gait stability: the effect of stride frequency, stride length, and walking speed on local dynamic stability and margins of stability. *PLoS ONE* (2013) 8:e82842. doi: 10.1371/journal.pone.0082842
17. Heeren A, Ooijen M, Geurts A, Day B, Janssen T, Beek P, et al. Step by step: a proof of concept study of C-Mill gait adaptability training in the chronic phase after stroke. *J Rehabil Med.* (2013) 45:616–22. doi: 10.2340/16501977-1180
18. Houdijk H, Oijen van MW, Kraal JJ, Wiggerts HO, Polomski W, Janssen TWJ, et al. Assessing gait adaptability in people with a unilateral amputation on an instrumented treadmill with a projected visual context. *Phys Ther.* (2012) 92:1452–60. doi: 10.2522/ptj.20110362
19. Caetano MJD, Lord SR, Brodie MA, Schoene D, Pelicioni PHS, Sturnieks DL, et al. Executive functioning, concern about falling and quadriceps strength mediate the relationship between impaired gait adaptability and fall risk in older people. *Gait Posture* (2018) 59:188–92. doi: 10.1016/j.gaitpost.2017.10.017

20. Caetano MJD, Lord SR, Schoene D, Pelicioni PHS, Sturnieks DL, Menant JC. Age-related changes in gait adaptability in response to unpredictable obstacles and stepping targets. *Gait Posture* (2016) 46:35–41. doi: 10.1016/j.gaitpost.2016.02.003
21. Corbetta D, Imeri F, Gatti R. Rehabilitation that incorporates virtual reality is more effective than standard rehabilitation for improving walking speed, balance and mobility after stroke: a systematic review. *J Physiother.* (2015) 61:117–24. doi: 10.1016/j.jphys.2015.05.017
22. Galna B, Murphy AT, Morris ME. Obstacle crossing in people with Parkinson's disease: foot clearance and spatiotemporal deficits. *Hum Move Sci.* (2010) 29:843–52. doi: 10.1016/j.humov.2009.09.006
23. Mollaei N, Bicho E, Sousa N, Gago MF. Different protocols for analyzing behavior and adaptability in obstacle crossing in Parkinson's disease. *Clin Inter Aging* (2017) 12:1843–57. doi: 10.2147/CIA.S147428
24. Yang JF, Musselman KE, Livingstone D, Brunton K, Hendricks G, Hill D, et al. Repetitive mass practice or focused precise practice for retraining walking after incomplete spinal cord injury? A pilot randomized clinical trial. Neurorehabil Neural Repair (2014) 28:314–24. doi: 10.1177/1545968313508473
25. Fox EJ, Tester NJ, Butera KA, Howland DR, Spiess MR, Castro-Chapman PL, et al. Retraining walking adaptability following incomplete spinal cord injury. *Spinal Cord Series Cases* (2017) 3:17091. doi: 10.1038/s41394-017-0003-1
26. Villiger M, Bohli D, Kiper D, Pyk P, Spillmann J, Meilick B, et al. Virtual reality-augmented neurorehabilitation improves motor function and reduces neuropathic pain in patients with incomplete spinal cord injury. *Neurorehabil Neural Repair* (2013) 27:675–83. doi: 10.1177/1545968313490999
27. Villiger M, Liviero J, Awai L, Stoop R, Pyk P, Clijsen R, et al. Home-based virtual reality-augmented training improves lower limb muscle strength, balance, and functional mobility following chronic incomplete spinal cord injury. *Front Neurol.* (2017) 8:635. doi: 10.3389/fneur.2017.00635
28. Lemay JF, Nadeau S. Standing balance assessment in ASIA D paraplegic and tetraplegic participants: concurrent validity of the Berg Balance Scale. *Spinal Cord* (2010) 48:245–50. doi: 10.1038/sc.2009.119
29. Sloot LH, van der Krogt MM, Harlaar J. Self-paced versus fixed speed treadmill walking. *Gait Posture* (2014) 39:478–84. doi: 10.1016/j.gaitpost.2013.08.022
30. Plotnik M, Azrad T, Bondi M, Bahat Y, Gimmon Y, Zeilig G, et al. Self-selected gait speed - over ground versus self-paced treadmill walking, a solution for a paradox. (2015) *J Neuroeng Rehabil.* 12:20. doi: 10.1186/s12984-015-0002-z
31. Lee HJ, Chou LS. Detection of gait instability using the center of mass and center of pressure inclination angles. *Arch Phys Med Rehabil.* (2006) 87:569–75. doi: 10.1016/j.apmr.2005.11.033
32. Lugade V, Lin V, Chou LS. Center of mass and base of support interaction during gait. *Gait Posture* (2011) 33:406–11. doi: 10.1016/j.gaitpost.2010.12.013
33. Hof AL, van Bockel RM, Schoppen T, Postema K. Control of lateral balance in walking. Experimental findings in normal subjects and above-knee amputees. *Gait Posture* (2007) 25:250–8. doi: 10.1016/j.gaitpost.2006.04.013
34. Meulen van FB, Weenk D, Buurke JH, Van Beijnum BJF, Veltink PH. Ambulatory assessment of walking balance after stroke using instrumented shoes. (2016) *J Neuroeng Rehabil.* 13:48. doi: 10.1186/s12984-016-0146-5
35. Tisserand R, Robert T, Dumas R, Chèze L. A simplified marker set to define the center of mass for stability analysis in dynamic situations. *Gait Posture* (2016) 48:64–7. doi: 10.1016/j.gaitpost.2016.04.032
36. Hof AL. The "extrapolated center of mass" concept suggests a simple control of balance in walking. *Hum Mov Sci.* (2008) 27:112–25. doi: 10.1016/j.humov.2007.08.003
37. Hof AL, Gazendam MGJ, Sinke WE. The condition for dynamic stability. *J Biomech.* (2005) 38:1–8. doi: 10.1016/j.jbiomech.2004.03.025
38. Lugade V, Kaufman K. Center of pressure trajectory during gait: a comparison of four foot positions. *Gait Posture* (2014) 40:252–4. doi: 10.1016/j.gaitpost.2013.12.023
39. Sloot LH, Houdijk H, Harlaar J. A comprehensive protocol to test instrumented treadmills. *Med Eng Phys.* (2015) 37:610–6. doi: 10.1016/j.medengphy.2015.03.018
40. Arends S, Oude Nijhuis L, Visser J, Stolwijk L, Frenken D, Bloem B. Radboud repository: het meten van valangst bij patiënten met de ziekte van Parkinson. *Tijdschrift Voor Neurol Neurochirurgie* (2007) 108:375–80. Available online at: https://repository.ubn.ru.nl/handle/2066/52512
41. Powell LE, Myers AM. The activities-specific balance confidence (ABC) scale. *J Gerontol A Biol Sci Med Sci.* (1995) 50:M28–34.
42. Ditunno PL, Patrick M, Stineman M, Morganti B, Townson AF, Ditunno JF. Cross-cultural differences in preference for recovery of mobility among spinal cord injury rehabilitation professionals. *Spinal Cord* (2006) 44:567–75. doi: 10.1038/sj.sc.3101876
43. Hedel van HJA, Dietz V. Rehabilitation of locomotion after spinal cord injury. *Restor Neurol Neurosci.* (2010) 28:123–34. doi: 10.3233/RNN-2010-0508
44. Alexeeva N, Sames C, Jacobs PL, Hobday L, DiStasio MM, Mitchell SA, et al. Comparison of training methods to improve walking in persons with chronic spinal cord injury: a randomized clinical trial. *J Spinal Cord Med.* (2011) 34:362–79. doi: 10.1179/2045772311Y.0000000018
45. Field-Fote EC, Lindley SD, Sherman AL. Locomotor training approaches for individuals with spinal cord injury: a preliminary report of walking-related outcomes. *J Neurol Phys Ther.* (2005) 29:127–37. doi: 10.1097/01.NPT.0000282245.31158.09
46. Field-Fote EC, Roach KE. Influence of a locomotor training approach on walking speed and distance in people with chronic spinal cord injury: a randomized clinical trial. *Phys Ther.* (2011) 91:48–60. doi: 10.2522/ptj.20090359
47. Kapadia N, Masani K, Catharine Craven B, Giangregorio LM, Hitzig SL, Richards K, et al. A randomized trial of functional electrical stimulation for walking in incomplete spinal cord injury: effects on walking competency. *J Spinal Cord Med.* (2014) 37:511–24. doi: 10.1179/2045772314Y.0000000263
48. Wirz M, Zemon DH, Rupp R, Scheel A, Colombo G, Dietz V, et al. Effectiveness of automated locomotor training in patients with chronic incomplete spinal cord injury: a multicenter trial. *Arch Phys Med Rehabil.* (2005) 86:672–80. doi: 10.1016/j.apmr.2004.08.004
49. Forrest GF, Hutchinson K, Lorenz DJ, Buehner JJ, VanHiel LR, Sisto SA, et al. Are the 10 meter and 6 minute walk tests redundant in patients with spinal cord injury? *PLoS ONE* (2014) 9:e94108. doi: 10.1371/journal.pone.0094108
50. Shah G, Oates AR, Arora T, Lanovaz JL, Musselman KE. Measuring balance confidence after spinal cord injury: the reliability and validity of the activities-specific balance confidence scale. *J Spinal Cord Med.* (2017) 40:768–76. doi: 10.1080/10790268.2017.1369212
51. Bilodeau EA, Levy CM. Long-term memory as a function of retention time and other conditions of training and recall. *Psychol Rev.* (1964) 71:27–41. doi: 10.1037/h0040397
52. Hedel van HJA, Wirth B, Dietz V. Limits of locomotor ability in subjects with a spinal cord injury. *Spinal Cord* (2005) 43:593–603. doi: 10.1038/sj.sc.3101768

3

Reliability of Wearable-Sensor-Derived Measures of Physical Activity in Wheelchair-Dependent Spinal Cord Injured Patients

Sophie Schneider[1], Werner L. Popp[1,2], Michael Brogioli[1], Urs Albisser[1], László Demkó[1], Isabelle Debecker[3], Inge-Marie Velstra[4], Roger Gassert[2] and Armin Curt[1]*

[1] Spinal Cord Injury Center, Balgrist University Hospital, Zurich, Switzerland, [2] Rehabilitation Engineering Laboratory, Department of Health Sciences and Technology, ETH Zurich, Zurich, Switzerland, [3] REHAB Basel, Clinic for Neurorehabilitation and Paraplegiology, Basel, Switzerland, [4] Clinical Trial Unit, Swiss Paraplegic Center, Nottwil, Switzerland

Correspondence:
Sophie Schneider
sophie.schneider@balgrist.ch

Physical activity (PA) has been shown to have a positive influence on functional recovery in patients after a spinal cord injury (SCI). Hence, it can act as a confounder in clinical intervention studies. Wearable sensors are used to quantify PA in various neurological conditions. However, there is a lack of knowledge about the inter-day reliability of PA measures. The objective of this study was to investigate the single-day reliability of various PA measures in patients with a SCI and to propose recommendations on how many days of PA measurements are required to obtain reliable results. For this, PA of 63 wheelchair-dependent patients with a SCI were measured using wearable sensors. Patients of all age ranges (49.3 ± 16.6 years) and levels of injury (from C1 to L2, ASIA A-D) were included for this study and assessed at three to four different time periods during inpatient rehabilitation (2 weeks, 1 month, 3 months, and if applicable 6 months after injury) and after in-patient rehabilitation in their home-environment (at least 6 months after injury). The metrics of interest were total activity counts, PA intensity levels, metrics of wheeling quantity and metrics of movement quality. Activity counts showed consistently high single-day reliabilities, while measures of PA intensity levels considerably varied depending on the rehabilitation progress. Single-day reliabilities of metrics of movement quantity decreased with rehabilitation progress, while metrics of movement quality increased. To achieve a mean reliability of 0.8, we found that three continuous recording days are required for out-patients, and 2 days for in-patients. Furthermore, the results show similar weekday and weekend wheeling activity for in- and out-patients. To our knowledge, this is the first study to investigate the reliability of an extended set of sensor-based measures of PA in both acute and chronic wheelchair-dependent SCI patients. The results provide recommendations for sensor-based assessments of PA in clinical SCI studies.

Keywords: spinal cord injury, rehabilitation, physical activity, intervention studies, wearable sensors, reliability

INTRODUCTION

Neurological disorders such as Spinal Cord Injury (SCI) are characterized by the different degrees of impairment of motor and sensory function. Earlier studies have investigated the impact of physical activity (PA) on functional recovery and found a positive effect in various neurological diseases (1–3). Past intervention studies in SCI focused on the integration of activity-based therapies with various intensities, duration, and type of PA, into rehabilitation programs to improve functional recovery. The outcome of these studies, however, are contradictory, with some of them showing improved strength or functional ability of the upper limbs (4–7) and performance in daily life (8), whereas others could not show any significant effect on the functional recovery (9, 10). One reason for such divergent results could be the subjective and non-comprehensive assessments of PA performed by the patient outside the controlled interventions. Thus, PA needs to be objectively assessed to better estimate the effects of interventions and the impact of PA on patient recovery in general.

In the past 15 years, accelerometers and inertial measurement units (IMUs) have been introduced to quantify PA more objectively. The use of accelerometers is well established in health sciences, especially in quantifying PA in the able-bodied population (11), elderly (12), children (13), and patients with various neurological conditions such as stroke (14, 15), Parkinson's (16), and multiple sclerosis (17). In SCI, studies have been conducted to develop metrics to capture PA in wheelchair-bound SCI patients (18, 19).

The levels of PA change throughout the rehabilitation process due to neurological recovery and compensation (20, 21), and can differ between individuals (22). Furthermore, they may vary from day to day as well due to environmental factors, but also due to patient characteristics like motivation, or general health status and pain. Therefore, there is a need to quantify how much the PA varies between single days within one patient and how many days are required to account for this variability to obtain a reliable representation of the overall PA level of the subject.

Guidelines on how many days the PA has to be monitored to obtain a reliable representation of the overall PA already exist for healthy adults and children. For healthy adults, a measurement period of 1 week has been suggested (23), while a measurement period of up to 11 days has been suggest for children (24). In older adults, a desired measurement duration of one to 2 days has been reported to achieve good reliabilities for sedentary, low and moderate-to-vigorous physical activity (25). In neurological diseases, e.g., in multiple sclerosis, guidelines suggest 4–6 days for sedentary behavior and 3–7 days for low and moderate-to-vigorous physical activity (26). The existing guidelines, however, cannot easily be translated to the SCI population, and especially not to wheelchair-dependent patients because of the completely different PA patterns such as wheeling instead of walking.

Because of the novelty of PA research in SCI, no comprehensive guidelines on measurement periods exist for this population. Sonenblum et al. (27) proposed a measurement period of 1 week to obtain reliable estimations of PA related solely to wheelchair usage, such as distance wheeled and duration of wheeling episodes. Yet, this conclusion is drawn from a limited number of patients with different neurological conditions, and only in their chronic stages. Since the variability between days might change between the stages and it might also be different for the different metrics of PA, we propose guidelines for the wheelchair-dependent patients on how many days of measurement are required for various measures of PA during the different stages of rehabilitation after the incidence of SCI. The primary aim of this study was to estimate the reliability of several sensor-based metrics of PA at different time points during the rehabilitation progress. The secondary aim was to compare the reliability of PA measures across days of active rehabilitation and on weekends.

METHODS

Patients

In total, 63 patients with SCI were included in this analysis, participating in two observational studies (for information about the protocol see Measurement procedure).

Patients suffering from a traumatic or non-traumatic acute SCI with all NLI and levels of lesion completeness were admitted to this study. Any neurological disease other than SCI, and any orthopedic or psychiatric disorders, were considered as exclusion criteria. Additionally, only wheelchair-dependent patients, defined by a value of < 3 in all the mobility domains (12, 13, and 14) of the Spinal Cord Independence Measure III (SCIM III) (28) were considered for the analysis.

The NLI and completeness of the lesion (AIS) was assessed following the International Standards for Neurological Classification of SCI (ISNCSCI) (29). Patients with an NLI from C1 to Th1 were classified as tetraplegic, while patients with an NLI from Th2 to S2 were classified as paraplegic. Recruitment took place from 2014 until 2017, at the sites of the Swiss Paraplegic Center in Nottwil, the Rehab Basel in Basel and the Balgrist University Hospital in Zurich, Switzerland. All patients signed a written consent before participating in the study in accordance with the Declaration of Helsinki. The study was approved by the ethical committees of the cantons of Zurich (KEK-ZH-Nr. 2013-0202), Lucerne (EK 13018), and Basel (EK 34313) and is registered on clinicaltrials.gov (Identifier: NCT02098122).

Measurement Procedure

For this study, the ReSense modules (30) were used as a measurement device. The ReSense modules are compact IMUs recording 3D acceleration, 3D angular velocity, 3D magnetic field strength, and barometric pressure for more than 24 h continuously. By turning all sensors except the accelerometer off,

Abbreviations: SCI, Spinal Cord Injury; PA, physical activity; IMU, Inertial Measurement Unit; ICC, Intraclass Correlation Coefficient; ***AC***, activity counts; ***LAT***, laterality; MET, metabolic equivalent of task; ***SED***, sedentary activity; ***LPA***, low physical activity; ***MVPA***, moderate-to-vigorous activity; $DIST_{TOT}$, total distance; $DIST_{ACT}$, actively wheeled distance; ***VEL***, mean velocity during active wheeling.

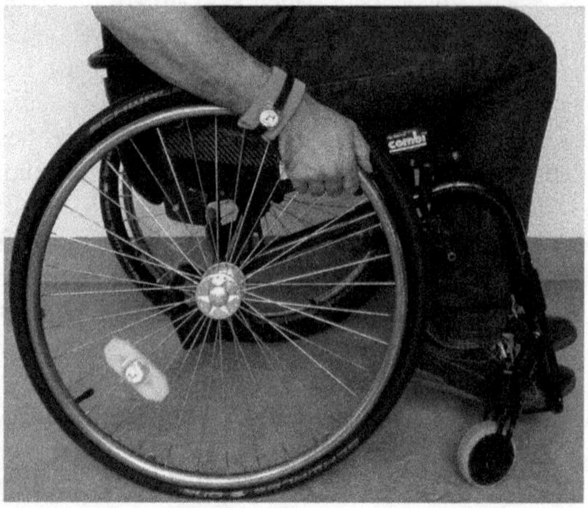

FIGURE 1 | Photograph of one examiner wearing the sensors. One sensor was attached to the right wheel of each wheelchair, one sensor was attached to each wrist.

the battery life can be extended to over 2 weeks. In this study, only the acceleration data were used.

At all time points, patients were equipped with several ReSense modules (**Figure 1**). One sensor measuring acceleration was attached to each wrist with AlphaStrap Blue (North Coast) and Velcro Straps (Velcro) for a duration of three consecutive weekdays to capture upper limb movements. Patients were asked to wear the sensors continuously for about 72 h during day- and nighttime and just take them off for showering or swimming activities. They were told that their amount of activity was being measured and that they should engage in their everyday life actives. Due to the limited battery lifetime, the sensors were exchanged once a day and recharged. Additionally, one module measuring acceleration was mounted on the right wheel of each wheelchair for the duration of seven consecutive days to capture wheeling metrics precisely (18, 31).

Data collection was conducted in the context of two observational studies (**Figure 2**). In the first observational study, patients were measured at five different time points during rehabilitation, each time for 3 consecutive days wearing the wrist sensors, and 7 consecutive days using the wheelchair sensor, respectively. The first four time points were within the clinical rehabilitation facilities ("in-patient"), whereas the last time point took place after discharge ("out-patient"). The in-patient rehabilitation was divided into four distinct stages, which conform to the time windows of the European Multicenter Study about SCI (EMSCI[1]:): very acute (VA), acute 1 (A I), acute 2 (A II), and acute 3 (A III), which are 2 weeks (0–15 days), 1 month (16–40 days), 3 months (70–98 days), and 6 months (150–186 days after injury), respectively. The last time point (out-patient) was defined to be 1 year after injury (chronic stage–C, 300–400 days). It is important to note that at stage A III, some patients were already discharged from the rehabilitation facility and were therefore analyzed within the out-patient group. Dividing the rehabilitation process into different stages has the advantage of stratifying the clinical picture of the patients and enables to analyze the patient data in short time windows in which a minimal functional change can be expected. In the second observational study, different patients were measured once after discharge for 3 consecutive days wearing the wrist sensors, and 7 consecutive days using the wheelchair sensor, respectively, at least 1 year after injury.

Not every patient was measured at every timepoint due to later recruitment or early drop-out and the number of patients of the 3-day measurement can differ from the number of the patients of the 7-day measurement due to technical issues with the sensors (**Table 1**).

Data Analysis And Statistics

The number of included patients varied depending on the specific analysis and time point (**Table 1**). For the analyses focusing on the whole in-patient group, data from stages VA, A I, A II, and partly A III of the 1st observational study were pooled. Similarly, data of the whole out-patient group were pooled from the 2nd observational study, and from stage A III (partly) and C of the 1st observational study.

Preprocessing

The desired sampling rate of the sensor was 50 Hz. However, the exact sampling rate of the ReSense sensors can vary between 49 and 51 Hz. Therefore, the raw data was resampled to 50 Hz using a common set of time points for all the modules that were used together (32). The periods of not wearing the sensors were removed from the data using a semi-automatic algorithm. The algorithm labels periods with 20 min of consecutive zero-counts as potential non-wear times (33). Thereafter, the labeled periods were visually inspected by an expert and manually adapted where necessary.

Sensor-Based Metrics

Sensor-based metrics were divided into 4 major categories: activity counts of overall upper limb movement, PA intensity levels (time spent in sedentary PA, low PA and moderate-to-vigorous PA), metrics of wheeling quantity (total and actively wheeled distance), and metrics of movement quality (upper limb movement laterality and mean wheeling velocity as a proximate of wheeling performance).

Overall upper limb activity

Activity counts (***AC***) were used to enumerate total forearm activity in a generalized way and were calculated by applying the discrete integral over the acceleration magnitude in epochs with the length of 1 min (34) and subsequently averaging the AC values over all epochs. ***AC*** of the right and left wrist were summed up.

PA Intensity levels

Different intensity levels of PA were defined by using AC cut-off values. These cut-off values were derived from previous energy expenditure measures in combination with IMU data (35). The intensity levels were defined by means of the metabolic equivalence of task (MET) adapted for SCI (36), where sedentary

[1]www.emsci.org

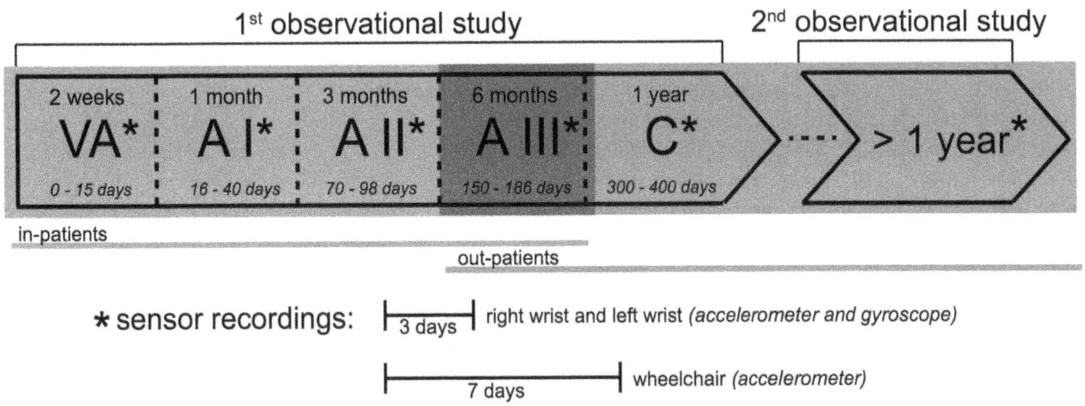

FIGURE 2 | Measurement protocol. This study consists of two observational studies. In the 1st observational study, patients were measured at 5 time points during the rehabilitation process. In the 2nd observational study, a different patient cohort was measured only once, at least 1 year after injury. In stages VA, A I, A II, and partly A III of the 1st observational study, patients were in-patients (red). In the 2nd observational study, as well as partly in A III, and stage C of the 1st observational study, patients were out-patients (blue). At each time point (*), acceleration and angular velocity of the right and left wrists were recorded for 3 days, while the acceleration of the right wheel of the wheelchair was recorded for 7 days. Overall upper limb activity (AC) and PA based on energy expenditure (SED, LPA, and MVPA) were calculated based on the 3 day recordings. All wheeling-related measures ($DIST_{TOT}$, $DIST_{ACT}$, and VEL) were calculated based on the 7 day recordings.

TABLE 1 | Patient demographics for all patients included (third row) as well as split up into patients included included in the 1st and 2nd observational studies for 3-day as well as 7-day measurements (bold values).

		N		Females		Tetraplegics		Age [years]	
		N		N (%)		N (%)		Mean ± sd	
Total patients		63		17 (27)		34 (54)		49.3 ± 16.6	
		3-day	7-day	3-day	7-day	3-day	7-day	3-day	7-day
1st observational study		**41**	**42**	**12 (29)**	**12 (29)**	**26 (63)**	**27 (64)**	**49.4 ± 19.4**	**49.5 ± 19.2**
Very acute (VA)		10	10	2 (20)	2 (20)	7 (70)	7 (70)	43.0 ± 16.5	43.0 ±16.5
Acute 1 (A I)		36	36	11 (31)	11 (31)	22 (61)	23 (64)	48.0 ± 19.4	48.2 ± 19.0
Acute 2 (A II)		21	24	7 (33)	8 (33)	12 (57)	14 (58)	53.2 ± 18.0	52.1 ± 18.5
Acute 3 (A III)	Total	17	20	6 (35)	7 (35)	10 (59)	11 (55)	49.1 ± 19.8	48.1 ± 19.4
	In	14	16	4 (29)	4 (25)	10 (71)	11 (69)	50.1 ± 18.3	48.8 ± 18.8
	Out	3	4	2 (67)	3 (75)	0 (0)	0 (0)	44.0 ± 30.3	45.3 ± 24.9
Chronic (C)		5	4	1 (20)	0 (0)	3 (60)	3 (75)	42.6 ± 18.0	40.8 ± 20.3
2nd observational study		**22**	**19**	**5 (23)**	**5 (26)**	**8 (36)**	**8 (42)**	**49.5 ± 11.5**	**51 ± 11.3**
In-patient*		81	86	24 (30)	25 (29)	51 (63)	55 (64)	49.1 ± 18.5	48.8 ± 18.4
Out-patient*		30	27	8 (27)	8 (30)	11 (37)	11 (41)	47.8 ± 14.5	48.7 ± 14.9

*pooled data set.

Detailed numbers are given for all single stages constituting the 1st observational study: 2 weeks after injury (VA), 4 weeks after injury (A I), 3 months after injury (A II), 6 months after injury (A III), and 1 year after injury (C). In stage A III, in- as well as out-patients are included. For a combined analysis of all in-patients, data of stages VA, A I, A II, and A III (partly) were pooled. Data of stages A III (partly), stage C, as well as the 2nd observational study were pooled for a combined analysis of all out-patients. "Tetraplegics" are defined by a lesion level from C1 to Th1.

activities (***SED***) corresponded to a MET level below 1.5, low physical activity (***LPA***) to a MET value between 1.5 and 3, and moderate-to-vigorous activities (***MVPA***) corresponded to a MET level above 3. SED, LPA, and MVPA are expressed in minutes spent in the respective intensity level per 24 h.

Metrics of wheeling quantity

To calculate wheeling-related metrics, a previously published algorithm (18) was used to (i) detect the phases of wheeling activity by applying heuristic rules, and (ii) to classify these phases into active and passive wheeling by using support vector machine classifiers. The total distance (**$DIST_{TOT}$**) and the distance wheeled actively (**$DIST_{ACT}$**) were extracted from the data and normalized to 24 h.

Metrics of movement quality

Whereas, the three aforementioned categories described how often movements were performed, the following metrics describe how the movements were performed.

Upper limb movement laterality (***LAT***) represents the symmetry of upper limb movements in general. LAT was calculated by computing the AC in epochs of 2 s for the right and left hand, dividing AC of the right hand and left hand and log transforming this ratio. The median value of the absolute log transform was used for the analysis. Details about the calculation can be found in Brogioli et al. (19). Scores for ***LAT*** range from minus to plus infinity quantifying the amount of ***LAT***, with zero for no ***LAT***.

Mean velocity (***VEL***) can be interpreted as a proximate measure for the quality of wheeling. Patients with improved functional ability will be able to wheel on average faster than patients in earlier stages of rehabilitation, or with more severe impairments.

VEL was defined as the mean absolute velocity of active propulsion, and was extracted using the aforementioned wheeling algorithm (18).

Statistics

First, the single-day reliabilities of all sensor-based metrics were calculated. Then the number of days needed for a reliable measurement was identified.

Single-day reliabilities for ***AC***, ***SED***, ***LPA***, ***MVPA***, and ***LAT*** were calculated based on the 3-day measurements, because they require information of the wrist sensors. Single-day reliabilities for $\boldsymbol{DIST_{TOT}}$, $\boldsymbol{DIST_{ACT}}$, and ***VEL*** were calculated based on the 7-day measurements, because they require information of the wheel sensor only.

Single-day reliability was defined as the Intraclass Correlation Coefficient (ICC), which was calculated using a variance portioning approach based on a one-way random effects model, with the random effect being on the subject level (37)

$$\mathrm{ICC} = \frac{\sigma_s^2}{\sigma_s^2 + \sigma_{res}^2}, \quad (1)$$

where σ_s^2 is the between-subject variance and σ_{res}^2 the residual variance. This approach is a well-established method especially in the field of PA research (23, 38, 39).

The confidence intervals for ICC were calculated based on the exact confidence limit equation (40).

According to Koo and Li (41), ICC values higher than 0.9 are considered as excellent, between 0.75 and 0.9 as good, between 0.5 and 0.75 as moderate, and lower than 0.5 as poor reliability.

To calculate the number of days needed for a reliable measurement (N), the Spearman Brown prophecy formula was used (42),

$$\mathrm{N} = \frac{\mathrm{ICC_t} \cdot (1 - \mathrm{ICC_s})}{\mathrm{ICC_s} \cdot (1 - \mathrm{ICC_t})}, \quad (2)$$

where $\mathrm{ICC_t}$ is the desired level of reliability and $\mathrm{ICC_s}$ is the single-day reliability. The desired reliability was set to 0.8, which is considered as an acceptable value according to literature (43).

To assess the relation of the wheeling-related metrics during weekdays and the weekend, equivalence tests were used. For normally distributed data, the Two Sided *T*-test (TOST) approach was used (44). In TOST, an epsilon (ε) has to be defined that corresponds to the level of practical equivalence (LOPE). We chose ε as the mean value of all the standard deviations of the respective metric:

$$\varepsilon = \frac{\sum_{i=1}^{n} \sigma_i^{metric}}{n}, \quad (3)$$

where n is the number of patients, and σ_i^{metric} is the standard deviation of the i-th subject for the metric of interest.

For non-normally distributed data, the TOST procedure was adapted by using the non-parametric Mann-Whitney-Wilcoxon Test instead of the Student's *t*-test.

A sample size calculation was performed according to the method presented in (45). The results of this analysis can be found in **Table S1.**

Preprocessing and calculation of the output metrics was conducted using MATLAB R2017a (MathWorks, Natick, MA, USA). Statistics were computed using R (The R project for Statistical Computing, R Core Team).

RESULTS

Patient Characteristics

The mean age of all patients was 49.3 ± 16.6 years at the time of recruitment. 17 (27%) of the patients were female. ASIA impairment scale (AIS) levels ranged from A to D, (A: 27, B: 9, C: 16, and D: 11 patients at the time of recruitment) and the neurological level of injury (NLI) from C1 to L2 (C1–C4: 17, C5–C8: 17, T1–T5: 6, T6–T12: 19, and L1–L2: 4 patients at the time of recruitment). More detailed information about patient numbers and demographics can be found in **Table 1**.

Single-Day Reliabilities

Single-day reliabilities of metrics of PA varied depending on the time after SCI (i.e., rehabilitation progress) ranging from excellent to poor reliability levels (**Figure 3**). ICC of metrics describing movement quantity (***AC***, ***SED***, ***LPA***, ***MVPA***, $\boldsymbol{DIST_{TOT}}$, and $\boldsymbol{DIST_{ACT}}$) tended to decrease during the rehabilitation progress (**Figures 3A–C**) and decreased e.g., from excellent reliability levels (0.93) for ***LPA*** in stage VA to poor levels (0.44) for ***LPA*** in out-patients. In contrast, measures describing movement quality (***LAT*** and ***VEL***) tended to increase during rehabilitation (**Figure 3D**). Especially, reliability of ***VEL*** improved from a poor level of the ICC (0.19) at stage VA to a moderate level (0.66) for out-patients. Overall upper limb activity (AC) showed excellent ICC levels (ICC > 0.92) during the first three acute stages with a decrease at later stages of rehabilitation to a good level (0.79) and a moderate level (0.65) after discharge (out-patient).

Overall single-day reliabilities were higher in tetraplegic patients than in paraplegic patients for most metrics (**Figure 4**). One exception to this was found in the reliability of MVPA in the out-patients, were the single-day reliability for tetraplegic patients was poor (0.24) and thus lower than the moderate level (0.65) for the paraplegic patients. Furthermore, the single-day reliability of LPA is poor (0.03) in paraplegic out-patients."

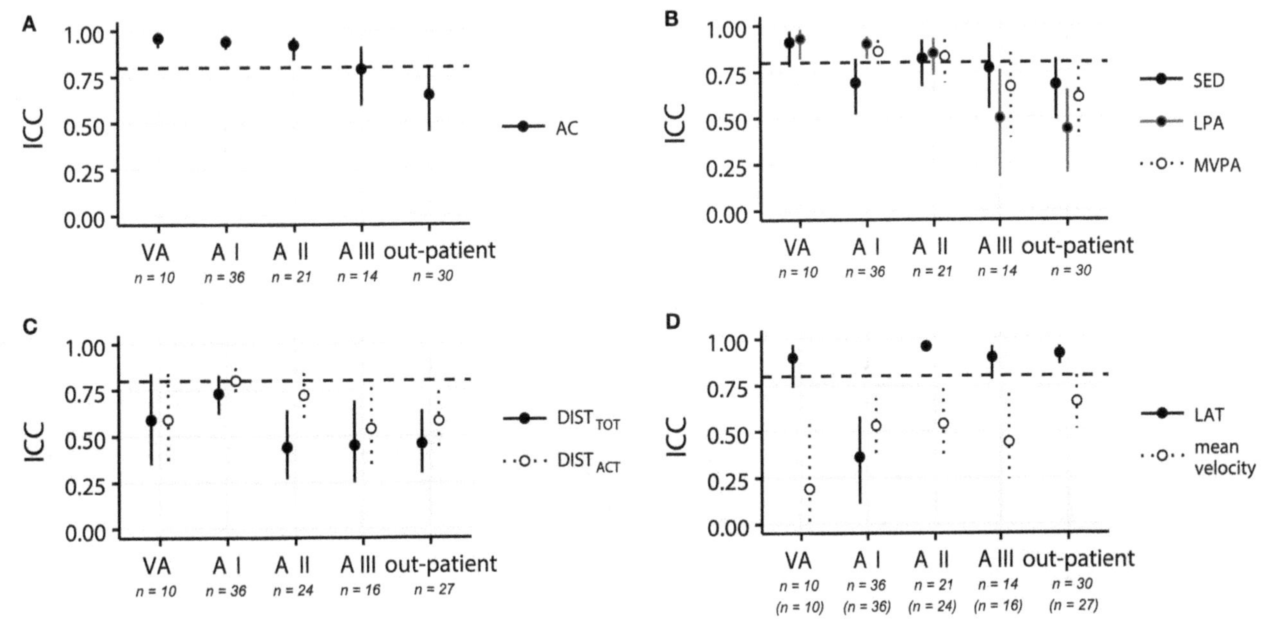

FIGURE 3 | ICC values representing the single-day reliabilities for **(A)** activity counts (AC); **(B)** time spent in sedentary activity (SED), low physical activity (LPA), and moderate-to-vigorous activity (MVPA); **(C)** total distance traveled in a wheelchair ($DIST_{TOT}$) and distance traveled actively in a wheelchair ($DIST_{ACT}$); and **(D)** laterality (LAT) and mean velocity (VEL) for all in-patient rehabilitation stages (very acute (VA–2 weeks after injury), acute I (A I–4 weeks after injury), acute II (A II–3 months after injury) , acute III (A III–6 months after injury), as well as for the out-patients (> 6 months after injury). The horizontal dashed lines depict the ICC level of 0.8, which was chosen as a requirement for a reliable measurement. Solid and dotted lines indicate the confidence intervals. Indicated patient numbers n are the pooled numbers.

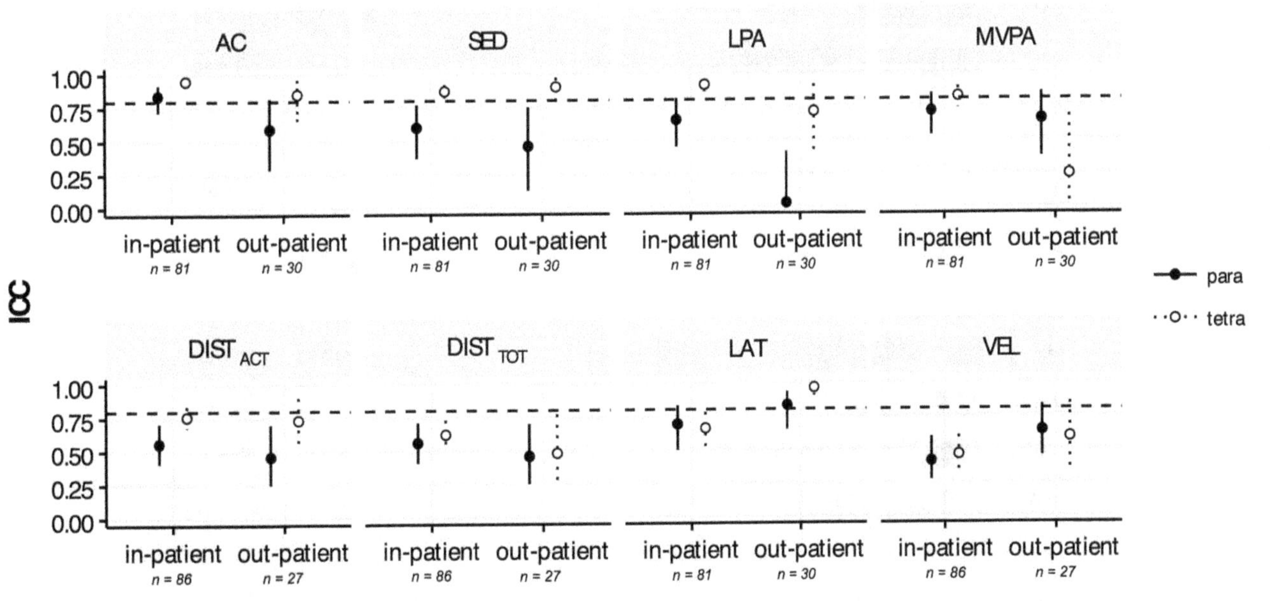

FIGURE 4 | ICC values representing the single-day reliabilities for activity counts (AC), time spent in sedentary activity (SED), low physical activity (LPA), moderate-to-vigorous activity (MVPA), total distance traveled in a wheelchair ($DIST_{TOT}$), distance traveled actively in a wheelchair ($DIST_{ACT}$), laterality (LAT), and mean velocity during active wheeling (VEL) for wheelchair-dependent paraplegic patients (full circle, solid lines) compared to wheelchair-dependent tetraplegic patients (empty circle, dotted lines) for the in-patients (from 2 weeks after injury to 6 months after injury) and out-patients (> 6 months after injury). The dashed horizontal lines depict the ICC level of 0.8, which was chosen as a requirement for a reliable measurement. Solid and dotted lines indicate the confidence intervals. Indicated patient numbers n are the pooled numbers.

Required Number of Days

A mean reliability of 0.8 is reached when monitoring in-patients for 2 days and out-patients for 3 days for all metrics (**Figures 5A,C**). A 7-day measurement is estimated to reach excellent reliabilities for all metrics in both in- and out-patients (**Figures 5B,D**).

Influence of Weekday vs. Weekend

With the chosen LOPEs and a significance level of 0.05, equivalence could be established for $DIST_{TOT}$ as well as $DIST_{ACT}$ between weekdays and the weekend in all in-patients and out-patients, as well as single stages VA and A I (**Table 2**, **Figure 6A**). At stages A II and A III, no equivalence could be shown (**Figure 6A**) for $DIST_{TOT}$ and $DIST_{ACT}$. Results for active distance are very similar to total distance for all stages, and thus not presented.

For ***VEL***, equivalence could be shown in all in-patients and out-patients, as well as at single stages A I, A II, whereas in stage VA and A III no equivalence could be established (**Table 2** and **Figure 6B**).

DISCUSSION

To our knowledge, this study is the first to investigate the reliabilities of a comprehensive set of sensor-based measures of PA in both acute and chronic wheelchair-dependent SCI patients. These findings provide recommendations for the application

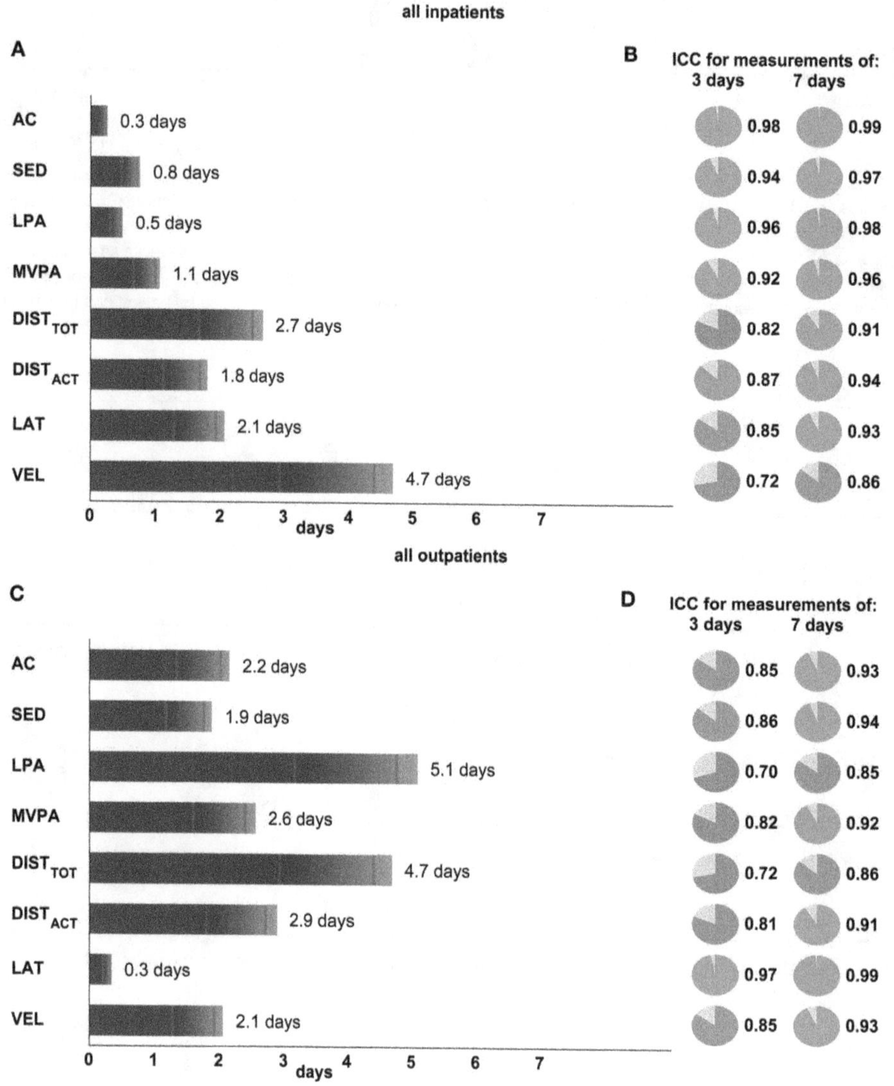

FIGURE 5 | The subfigures on the left side (**A**: in-patients, **C**: out-patients) represent the number of measurement days needed in order to achieve a reliability of 0.8 for different metrics of movement quantity (activity counts – AC, time spent in sedentary activity – SED, in low physical activity – LPA, in moderate-to-vigorous activity – MVPA, total distance wheeled – $DIST_{TOT}$, and distance wheeled actively – $DIST_{ACT}$) as well as metrics of movement quality (laterality – LAT and mean wheeling velocity – VEL). Additionally, the numbers of measurement days needed for a reliability of 0.5 and 0.75 are presented with magenta and blue vertical bars, respectively. The subfigures on the right side (**B**: in-patients, **D**: out-patients) show the reliabilities, which would be achieved when measuring 3 and 7 days, respectively.

TABLE 2 | Descriptive statistics for total distance traveled in a wheelchair (**$DIST_{TOT}$**), distance traveled actively in a wheelchair (**$DIST_{ACT}$**), and mean velocity during active wheeling (**VEL**) performed during weekdays and weekends (mean ± SD and median (IQR) for pooled in-patients and out-patients, as well as all single stages, VA (very acute–2 weeks after injury), A I (acute I–4 weeks after injury), A II (acute II–3 months after injury), A III (acute III–6 months after injury).

	Workday mean (± SD)	Weekend mean (± SD)	Workday median (IQR)	Weekend median (IQR)	Limit of practical equivalence (± LOPE)	Confidence Interval	Equivalence *p*-value
$DIST_{TOT}$ [m]							
In-patients	1910.9 ± 1271.6	1562.3 ± 1312.9	1722.1 (1631.64)	1184.1 (1828.9)	± 750.1	127.8, 538.7	0.001
VA	625.7 ± 499.8	723.2 ± 740.7	467.1 (605.3)	467.3 (409.1)	± 368.6	−338.9, 143.8	0.035
A I	1644.3 ± 1170	1501.1 ± 1321	1576.2 (1133.9)	1040.3 (2078.3)	± 615.1	−148.3, 315.1	<0.001
A II	2264.5 ± 1059.6	1980.9 ± 1502.9	1803.3 (1512.3)	1681.3 (1763.7)	± 744.6	−251.9, 875.6	0.1
A III	2783.7 ± 1346.8	1646.5 ± 1095.4	2742.5 (1724.1)	1551.9 (1550.7)	± 1277.5	817.2, 1618.6	0.399
Out-patients	3365.2 ± 2698.3	2139.9 ± 1367	2462.9 (1367)	1812.4 (621.9)	± 1092.3	31.5, 772.9	0.003
$DIST_{ACT}$ [m]							
In-patients	1686.4 ± 1396	1379 ± 1270.9	1446.8 (1927.7)	1100.2 (1841.7)	± 661.2	130.6, 464.7	<0.001
VA	625.3 ± 499.5	722.9 ± 740.6	467.1 (604.9)	466.8 (408.9)	± 368.6	−338.9, 143.7	0.035
A I	1494.9 ± 1268.1	1370.2 ± 1370.7	1225.8 (1495)	819.8 (2202.4)	± 537.4	−151.8, 264.2	<0.001
A II	1836.8 ± 1427.7	1508.9 ± 1375.6	1690.6 (2562.7)	1160.2 (1466)	± 610.2	−77.6, 712.2	0.108
A III	2555.2 ± 1528.4	1645.7 ± 1094.9	2329.7 (2250)	1551.5 (1546.9)	± 1147	700.9, 1458.9	0.38
Out-patients	2738.7 ± 2605.2	1871.1 ± 1561.7	2443 (2565.7)	1727.8 (1946)	± 672.2	−16.6, 550.3	0.012
VEL [km/h]							
In-patients	1.64 ± 0.43	1.54 ± 0.48	1.54 (0.52)	1.43 (0.77)	± 0.36	0, 0.19	<0.001
VA	1.52 ± 0.32	1.62 ± 0.46	1.47 (0.43)	1.62 (0.66)	± 0.41	−0.42, 0.22	0.055
A I	1.63 ± 0.47	1.56 ± 0.48	1.53 (0.51)	1.48 (0.78)	± 0.35	−0.06, 0.25	0.004
A II	1.68 ± 0.46	1.57 ± 0.55	1.61 (0.49)	1.41 (0.74)	± 0.36	−0.11, 0.26	0.009
A III	1.7 ± 0.37	1.43 ± 0.41	1.67 (0.54)	1.41 (0.58)	± 0.36	0.09, 0.43	0.161
Out-patients	1.53 ± 0.64	1.41 ± 0.51	1.57 (0.81)	1.39 (0.32)	± 0.32	−0.06, 0.17	<0.001

The last three columns contain the calculated limits of practical equivalence (LOPE) used for the equivalence tests, the confidence intervals, and the p-values resulting from the equivalence tests. [a] denotes p-values resulting from the Mann-Whitney-Wilcoxon Test of equivalence for non-normally distributed data, the remaining p-values were calculated using the TOST procedure for normally distributed data.

of sensor-based assessments of PA that enable non-obstructive long term recordings throughout clinical studies in in- and out patients.

Single-Day Reliabilities

Single-day reliabilities of PA metrics depend highly on the clinical condition, i.e., the stage of rehabilitation and the extent of functional impairment. The reliability of measures of movement quantity such as activity counts of upper limb activity, PA intensity levels and wheeling-related metrics decreased during in-patient rehabilitation and in the out-patient setting, while in general was found to be higher for tetraplegic patients. One reason for this might be that in-patients have a more regular daily schedule due to preplanned therapy sessions as observed by therapists at the different rehabilitation centers, resulting in lower variability of daily activities. Reliabilities of metrics of movement quantity are higher in patients with a higher impairment like in tetraplegia and in the early stages of rehabilitation, as the use of the upper limbs for these patients is mostly limited to the very structured therapy sessions, lowering the variability between single days. Additionally, these patients might also reach their upper limits of PA during their daily schedules, resulting in a very low variability between single days.

High reliability levels of upper limb activity in terms of ***AC*** compared to the other quantitative metrics suggest that this measure, although widely used in PA-research, may provide a rather rough approximation of PA levels in SCI patients, lacking the detailed information about PA intensity patterns and specific movements like wheeling.

Metrics based on PA intensity levels show lower single-day reliability levels than ***AC***, suggesting that these metrics capture more detailed information about PA levels which likely vary between single days. Another possible explanation could be that the AC thresholding for this analysis introduces noise into the estimates. Future studies are needed to investigate this in more detail.

The reliability of ***LPA*** in paraplegic out-patients was considerably lower compared to the remaining metrics based on PA intensity levels. Since the reliability is calculated by dividing the between-subject variance by the total variance (Equation 1), for ***LPA*** in paraplegic out-patients, the poor reliability can be explained by a very low variance between the individual patients compared to the variance between the single days. While tetraplegic patients show a much higher between-subject variance, this might be a hint that ***LPA*** could be influenced by the level of impairment of the upper limbs. ***LPA*** is likely to represent activities of daily living, as demonstrated earlier (35).

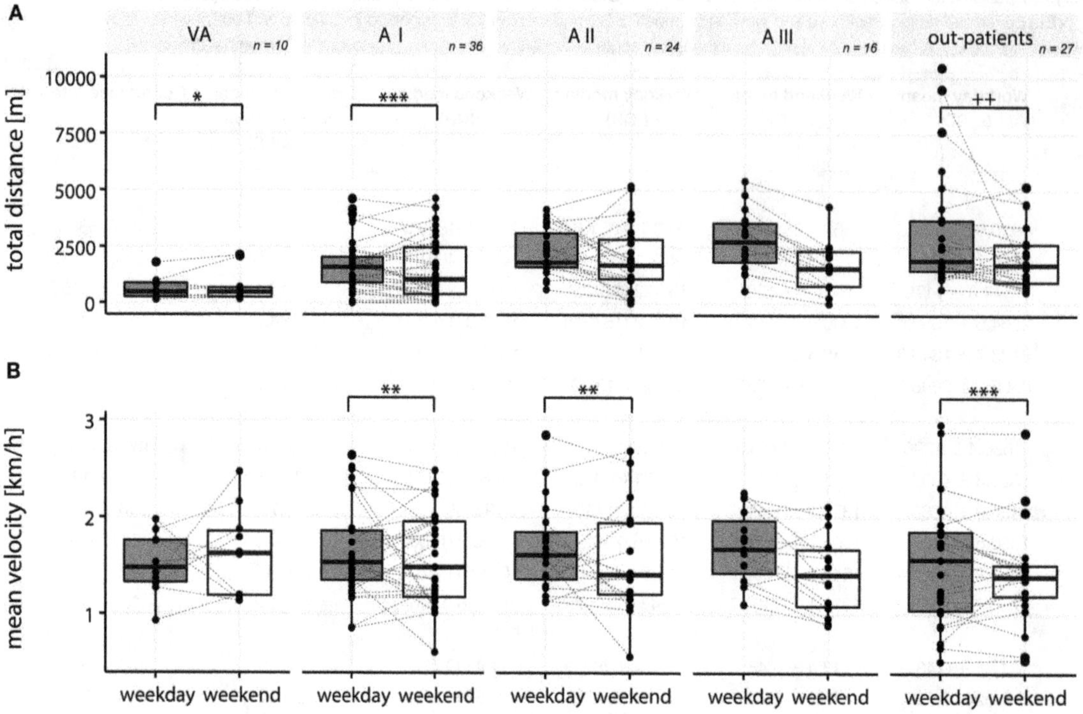

FIGURE 6 | Boxplots for total distance traveled in a wheelchair **(A)** and mean velocity during active wheeling **(B)** during weekdays vs. weekends in all single in-patient stages (VA, AI, AII, AIII), as well as out-patients. */+ denotes p-value of < 0.05, **/++ a *p*-value of < 0.01, ***/+++ a *p*-value of < 0.001, respectively. *P*-values were calculated using the TOST procedure for normally distributed data (*), respectively, the adapted equivalence test based on the Mann-Whitney-Wilcoxon Test for non-normally distributed data (+).

Assuming that a large amount of activities of daily living (not involving mobility), e.g., feeding, showering, and dressing are equally presented in each patient, ***LPA*** should not vary strongly between single patients. This hypothesis is valid for patients that are not impaired in the upper-limbs, i.e., paraplegics, as can be seen in the low variability of ***LPA*** between the patients (***LPA***: SD: 1.1h, Min: 9h, Max: 13h). In contrast, the level of impairment of the upper limbs varies strongly in the tetraplegic group, which might be the reason for a higher variability of ***LPA*** between the patients (***LPA***: SD: 2.8h, Min: 6h, Max: 15 h).

In contrast to the increased reliability in ***LPA*** for tetraplegic outpatients, ***MVPA*** shows a decreased single-day reliability in these patients. A possible reason is that these patients are challenged to even reach moderate-to-vigorous intensities (46, 47) and thus show it only occasionally and not in everyday PA.

In contrast to metrics of movement quantity, single-day reliabilities of metrics of movement quality like ***LAT*** and ***VEL*** increased during the rehabilitation and stayed on a higher level after discharge. During in-patient rehabilitation, patients learn various skills to handle their impairment, e.g., wheeling techniques or compensatory strategies for activities of daily living, which may result in higher variability between single days at the earlier stages of rehabilitation. Moreover, at the beginning of the rehabilitation process arm rehabilitative training is often unilateral (e.g., with ArmeoPower (48) training), leading to a high discrepancy of ***LAT*** between specific therapy sessions and leisure time and thus increasing the variability of ***LAT*** between different days. Furthermore, the therapy schedules may vary strongly between different days at these stages, which can result in more variable measures of movement quality on different days due to dedicated rehabilitation sessions with specific training aims such as improving the function of the more impaired side in tetraplegics leading to a higher variability in measures of movement quality as can be seen for ***LAT*** in the AI stage. After the patients learn certain strategies, they may apply them more consistently during their daily activities, resulting in higher single-day reliabilities at the later stages of rehabilitation. The high reliability of ***LAT*** in the stage VA might be due to the fact that patients are mainly bound to the bed, and not showing much PA in general, which may lead to a higher reliability.

Required Number of Days For Reliable Measures

Based on our data, metrics of movement quality should optimally be measured for 4 days to achieve a mean reliability of 0.8, which is commonly used in the field of PA research (23, 24, 26, 49). In the in-patient setting, we suggest measuring metrics of movement quantity for 2 days to achieve a mean reliability of 0.8, while in the out-patient setting measuring on average for 3 days is required to achieve the same reliability. The findings of high reliability of 2-days recordings increase the applicability of sensor measurements in the clinical routine where, especially in acute patients, wearing sensors for too long may be an additional burden. However, we suggest 4 days to capture all analyzed metrics of movement quantity reliably, and one to 2 days for the measures of movement quality in the out-patient setting.

Measuring for 7 days would yield excellent reliabilities for all metrics in all patients, which might be relevant in research and clinical studies where even the detection of small changes in PA patterns may have an impact on outcomes. However, measurement duration is always in tradeoff with clinical applicability and patient compliance.

Difference Between Weekdays And Weekend

We investigated whether it makes a difference to measure PA on weekends or during the week. For this, only wheeling-related metrics ($DIST_{TOT}$, $DIST_{ACT}$, and ***VEL***) were analyzed, as 7-day recordings were only available from the wheel-mounted sensor. In in-patients as well as in out-patients we could show equivalence of $DIST_{TOT}$ and $DIST_{ACT}$ between weekdays and weekends. This suggests that measurements can be taken on any day of the week, keeping in mind that single days might represent unexpected outliers due to an event not occurring regularly. Nevertheless, the results for the in-patients have to be taken with precautions. Splitting up the in-patients into the single stages, equivalence between weekdays and weekends of $DIST_{TOT}$ and $DIST_{ACT}$ could only be shown at the very early stages of rehabilitation (VA and AI), suggesting that for the stages of A II and A III both weekdays and weekends should be measured in order to obtain a comprehensive picture of the patients' overall PA. During early phases of rehabilitation, patients typically receive individual therapy instead of group therapies and their therapy schedules are less tight as observed by therapist at the different centers. We hypothesize that this could explain the observation of similar amounts of activity on the weekends and during the week. At later stages, however, the therapy schedule of the patients gets tighter during the week, which is why they might use the weekends for recovery. The fact that some patients can leave the rehabilitation facility over the weekend at later stages of rehabilitation might have an additional impact on their different behaviors during weekdays and weekends.

One could hypothesize that in out-patients the wheeling distances differ during weekdays and weekends mainly due to the fact that patients might work during the week and thus show different activity patterns than on the weekends. However, in out-patients, equal wheeling distances ($DIST_{ACT}$ and $DIST_{TOT}$) were found during the week and on the weekends, which might indicate that the patients we measured were not yet, or if then only partially back to work (50) or worked rather from home instead of having a working space away from home.

Equivalence of ***VEL*** could be shown in all in- and out-patients, suggesting that measurements can be taken on any day of the week to reliably capture ***VEL***. However, when examining individual stages of the in-patient rehabilitation, at stage VA as well as at A III, no equivalence could be shown. In the latter stage, patients showed a higher ***VEL*** during the week than on the weekends, which might be due to the integration of sports activities into their therapy schedule, as already shown for ambulatory SCI patients (51). The result found for the stage VA is based on only a limited number of observations as most of these patients do not wheel actively, and thus has to be taken with care.

Comparison to Literature

Our results for the reliabilities of wheeling-related metrics in the out-patients are in line with literature, proposing up to 1 week of measuring wheeling-related PA in wheelchair-dependent chronic SCI patients (27). For ***AC*** as well as PA intensity times (***SED***, ***LPA***, and ***MVPA***), we can only compare our results to those of the able-bodied population. Single-day reliability for ***AC*** was found to be moderate in able-bodied individuals (23), which is consistent with our results in the out-patients. Similarly, single-day reliabilities for ***SED*** and ***MVPA*** are moderate and comparable to our results (23, 25). In contrast to a low single-day reliability found in our study, a good single-day reliability for ***LPA*** has been reported in the able-bodied population (23). This low single-day reliability happens to be distinctive to the wheelchair-dependent SCI population, and thus should not be compared to the able-bodied population.

To the best of our knowledge, this is the first work to analyze the reliability of physical activity metrics in the in-patient setting and thus no comparable data is available.

Choice of Accelerometer Cut-Points

Cut-off points are commonly used to define intensity levels and were established in previous studies for the healthy population (52, 53) and for stroke survivors (54). However, appropriate cut-off values depend on populations and type of wearable sensors used (55). Furthermore, changes in those cut-off values directly influence the metrics of intensity levels (56). Therefore, we defined cut-off values specific for our population of interest and for the wearable sensor used in this study. We calculated our cut-off points based on indirect calorimetry values as commonly done in the field (52–56). Transferring our results to methodologies using different accelerometer cut-off points has to be done carefully, as the influence of the cut-off points on the reliability is unknown, and reliability values might change.

Study Limitations

We would like to emphasize three main limitations of our study. The first one is the moderate sample size particularly in the very acute stage. Sample size is often a problem in SCI research. Especially in very acute stages recruitment of the patients and measuring these is challenging. In reliability studies, low sample size results in larger confidence intervals, making the interpretation of the results more difficult. Nevertheless, our sample size is reasonable if compared to other studies in the SCI population.

A further limitation is recording for only 3 days with the sensors attached to the wrists. Especially in tetraplegic patients, there is a risk of pressure sores caused by wearing the sensor straps for too long. Thus, a longer measurement time would expose the patients to an increased risk of damage to the skin. Furthermore, compliance decreases with increased number of measurement days. This limitation might result in larger confidence intervals.

A sample size calculation was conducted. Assuming an acceptable confidence interval width of 0.2, our sample sizes in the inpatient-setting are sufficient. In the outpatient setting, higher sample sizes would be required to make more precise statements. The problem of large confidence intervals in reliability studies has been addressed previously (45). This issue can be resolved by either increasing the number of subjects or the number of measurement days, and should be considered for further studies.

One limitation in studies using wearable sensors in general are possible behavioral reactions, i.e., subjects could alter their behavior because of the knowledge of being measured. Conflicting statements about the amount of reactivity have been made in literature (57, 58). However, the accuracy of PA measures based on wearable sensors is higher than the accuracy of the conventional questionnaires (59, 60) and thus better suitable to estimate PA levels.

Lastly, PA intensity levels were estimated from activity counts based on a previous study. Dedicated algorithms for the direct estimation of energy expenditure (35, 61) or direct measurements of energy expenditure might lead to slightly altered results, but the latter is very challenging to perform especially with acute patients due to the required equipment and the extensive protocol including standardized food intake and calibration phases.

CONCLUSION

We conclude that single-day reliabilities of metrics to capture PA in acute and chronic wheelchair-dependent SCI patients vary considerably depending on the clinical setting. With increasing functional recovery of the patients, metrics of movement quantity tend to become less reliable, whereas metrics of movement quality become more reliable. Depending on the specific metrics, 2 days are required on average to capture PA reliably in in-patients, whereas 3 days are required for out-patients. Furthermore, we suggest using ***AC*** only as a rather general measure for assessing the overall PA level of patients, and only in combination with more detailed metrics, e.g., PA intensity levels and wheeling-related metrics. This avoids a possible loss of information about the variability of PA during a whole day. Our results are based on a reasonable sample size for this population and thus provide robust recommendations on how to design clinical studies investigating PA as a primary outcome, or as a confounder in intervention studies in order to better evaluate the actual intervention effect.

AUTHOR CONTRIBUTIONS

SS, WP, MB, RG, and AC designed the study. SS, WP, MB, UA, ID, and I-MV collected the experimental data. SS and WP analyzed the data. SS, WP, MB, UA, LD, ID, I-MV, RG, and AC interpreted the results. SS, WP, MB, UA, LD, ID, I-MV, RG, and AC revised the manuscript and approved the final version.

ACKNOWLEDGMENTS

The authors would like to thank the following persons (in alphabetical order) for their valuable help in recruitment, data acquisition, and the interpretation of the results: Karin Akermann, Anne K. Brust, Dr. Angela Frotzler, Fabienne Hasler, Dr. Kerstin Hug, Dr. Margret Hund, Dr. Mike. D. Rinderknecht, and Dr. Michelle L. Starkey.

REFERENCES

1. Lynskey J V, Belanger A, Jung R. Activity-dependent plasticity in spinal cord injury. *J Rehabil Res Dev.* (2008) 45:229–40. doi: 10.1682/JRRD.2007.03.0047
2. Van Peppen RP, Kwakkel G, Wood-Dauphinee S, Hendriks HJ, Van der Wees PJ, Dekker J. The impact of physical therapy on functional outcomes after stroke: what's the evidence? *Clin Rehabil.* (2004) 18:833–62. doi: 10.1191/0269215504cr843oa
3. Damiano DL. Activity, activity, activity: rethinking our physical therapy approach to cerebral palsy. *Phys Ther.* (2006) 86:1534–40. doi: 10.2522/ptj.20050397
4. Beekhuizen KS, Field-Fote EC. Sensory stimulation augments the effects of massed practice training in persons with tetraplegia. *Arch Phys Med Rehabil.* (2008) 89:602–8. doi: 10.1016/j.apmr.2007.11.021
5. Beekhuizen KS, Field-Fote EC. Massed practice versus massed practice with stimulation: effects on upper extremity function and cortical plasticity in individuals with incomplete cervical spinal cord injury. *Neurorehabil Neural Repair.* (2005) 19:33–45. doi: 10.1177/1545968305274517
6. Hodkin EF, Lei Y, Humby J, Glover IS, Choudhury S, Kumar H, et al. Automated FES for upper limb rehabilitation following stroke and spinal cord injury. *IEEE Trans Neural Syst Rehabil Eng.* (2018) 26:1067–74. doi: 10.1109/TNSRE.2018.2816238
7. Francisco GE, Yozbatiran N, Berliner J, O'Malley MK, Pehlivan AU, Kadivar Z, et al. Robot-assisted training of arm and hand movement shows functional improvements for incomplete cervical spinal cord injury. *Am J Phys Med Rehabil.* (2017) 96:S171–7. doi: 10.1097/PHM.0000000000000815
8. Hicks AL, Martin KA, Ditor DS, Latimer AE, Craven C, Bugaresti J, et al. Long-term exercise training in persons with spinal cord injury: effects on strength, arm ergometry performance and psychological well-being. *Spinal Cord* (2003) 41:34–43. doi: 10.1038/sj.sc.3101389
9. Glinsky J, Harvey L, van Es P, Chee S, Gandevia SC. The addition of electrical stimulation to progressive resistance training does not enhance the wrist strength of people with tetraplegia: a randomized controlled trial. *Clin Rehabil.* (2009) 23:696–704. doi: 10.1177/0269215509104171
10. Zariffa J, Kapadia N, Kramer JL, Taylor P, Alizadeh-Meghrazi M, Zivanovic V, et al. Feasibility and efficacy of upper limb robotic rehabilitation in a subacute cervical spinal cord injury population. *Spinal Cord* (2012) 50:220–6. doi: 10.1038/sc.2011.104
11. Godfrey A, Conway R, Meagher D, G OL. Direct measurement of human movement by accelerometry. *Med Eng Phys.* (2008) 30:1364–86. doi: 10.1016/j.medengphy.2008.09.005
12. Najafi B, Aminian K, Paraschiv-Ionescu A, Loew F, Büla CJ, Robert P. Ambulatory system for human motion analysis using a kinematic sensor: monitoring of daily physical activity in the elderly. *IEEE Trans Biomed Eng.* (2003) 50:711–23. doi: 10.1109/TBME.2003.812189
13. Riddoch CJ, Andersen LB, Wedderkopp N, Harro M, Klasson-Heggebø L, Sardinha LB, et al. Physical activity levels and patterns of 9- and 15-yr-old european children. *Med Sci Sport Exerc.* (2004) 36:86–92. doi: 10.1249/01.MSS.0000106174.43932.92
14. Uswatte G, Miltner WH, Foo B, Varma M, Moran S, Taub E. Objective measurement of functional upper-extremity movement using accelerometer recordings transformed with a threshold filter. *Stroke* (2000) 31:662–7. doi: 10.1161/01.STR.31.3.662

15. van der Pas SC, Verbunt JA, Breukelaar DE, van Woerden R, Seelen HA. Assessment of arm activity using triaxial accelerometry in patients with a stroke. *Arch Phys Med Rehabil.* (2011) 92:1437–42. doi: 10.1016/j.apmr.2011.02.021
16. Salarian A, Russmann H, Vingerhoets FJG, Burkhard PR, Aminian K. Ambulatory monitoring of physical activities in patients with Parkinson's disease. *IEEE Trans Biomed Eng.* (2007) 54:2296–9. doi: 10.1109/tbme.2007.896591
17. Motl RW, McAuley E, Snook EM, Gliottoni RC. Physical activity and quality of life in multiple sclerosis: intermediary roles of disability, fatigue, mood, pain, self-efficacy and social support. *Psychol Heal Med.* (2009) 14:111–24. doi: 10.1080/13548500802241902
18. Popp WL, Brogioli M, Leuenberger K, Albisser U, Frotzler A, Curt A, et al. A novel algorithm for detecting active propulsion in wheelchair users following spinal cord injury. *Med Eng Phys.* (2016) 38:267–74. doi: 10.1016/j.medengphy.2015.12.011
19. Brogioli M, Popp WL, Albisser U, Brust AK, Frotzler A, Gassert R, et al. Novel sensor technology to assess independence and limb-use laterality in cervical spinal cord injury. *J Neurotrauma* (2016) 33:1950–7. doi: 10.1089/neu.2015.4362
20. Curt A, Van Hedel HJA, Klaus D, Dietz V. Recovery from a spinal cord injury: significance of compensation, neural plasticity, and repair. *J Neurotrauma* (2008) 25:677–85. doi: 10.1089/neu.2007.0468
21. Anderson KD. Targeting recovery: priorities of the spinal cord-injured population. *J Neurotrauma* (2004) 21:1371–83. doi: 10.1089/neu.2004.21.1371
22. Brogioli M, Schneider S, Popp WL, Albisser U, Brust AK, Velstra I-M, et al. Monitoring upper limb recovery after cervical spinal cord injury: insights beyond assessment scores. *Front Neurol.* (2016) 7:142. doi: 10.3389/fneur.2016.00142
23. Aadland E, Ylvisaker E. Reliability of objectively measured sedentary time and physical activity in adults. *PLoS ONE* (2015) 10:e0133296. doi: 10.1371/journal.pone.0133296
24. Barreira T, Schuna J, Tudor-Locke C, Chaput JP, Church T, Fogelholm M, et al. Reliability of accelerometer-determined physical activity and sedentary behavior in school-aged children: a 12-country study. *Int J Obes Suppl.* (2015) 5:29–35. doi: 10.1038/ijosup.2015.16
25. Falck RS, Landry GJ, Brazendale K, Liu-Ambrose T. Measuring physical activity in older adults using motionwatch 8 actigraphy: how many days are needed? *J Aging Phys Act.* (2017) 25:51–7. doi: 10.1123/japa.2015-0256
26. Klaren RE, Hubbard EA, Zhu W, Motl RW. Reliability of accelerometer scores for measuring sedentary and physical activity behaviors in persons with multiple sclerosis. *Adapt Phys Act Q.* (2016) 33:195–204. doi: 10.1123/APAQ.2015-0007
27. Sonenblum SE, Sprigle S, Lopez RA. Manual wheelchair use: bouts of mobility in everyday life. *Rehabil Res Pract.* (2012) 2012:1–7. doi: 10.1155/2012/753165
28. Catz A, Itzkovich M, Agranov E, Ring H, Tamir A. SCIM–spinal cord independence measure: a new disability scale for patients with spinal cord lesions. *Spinal Cord* (1997) 35:850–6. doi: 10.1038/sj.sc.3100504
29. Kirshblum SC, Burns SP, Biering-Sorensen F, Donovan W, Graves DE, Jha A, et al. International standards for neurological classification of spinal cord injury (revised 2011). *J Spinal Cord Med.* (2011) 34:535–46. doi: 10.1179/204577211X13207446293695
30. Leuenberger K, Gassert R. Low-power sensor module for long-term activity monitoring. *Conf Proc IEEE Eng Med Biol Soc.* (2011) 2011:2237–41. doi: 10.1109/IEMBS.2011.6090424
31. Sonenblum SE, Sprigle S, Harris FH, Maurer CL. Characterization of power wheelchair use in the home and community. *Arch Phys Med Rehabil.* (2008) 89:486–91. doi: 10.1016/j.apmr.2007.09.029
32. Leuenberger KD. *Long-Term Activity and Movement Monitoring in Neurological Patients.* ETH Zurich (2015).
33. Masse CL, Fuemmeler BF, Anderson CB, Matthews CE, Trost SG, Catellier DJ, et al. Accelerometer Data Reduction: A Comparison of Four Reduction Algorithms on Select Outcome Variable. *Med Sci Sport Exerc.* (2005) 37(Suppl. 11):S544–54. doi: 10.1249/01.mss.0000185674.09066.8a
34. Leuenberger K, Gonzenbach R, Wachter S, Luft A., Gassert R. A method to qualitatively assess arm use in stroke survivors in the home environment. *Med Biol Eng Comput.* (2017) 55:141–50. doi: 10.1007/s11517-016-1496-7
35. Popp WL, Richner L, Brogioli M, Wilms B, Spengler, Christina M, et al. Estimation of energy expenditure in wheelchair-bound spinal cord injured individuals using inertial measurement units. *Front Neurol.* (2018) 9:478. doi: 10.3389/fneur.2018.00478
36. Collins EG, Gater D, Kiratli J, Butler J, Hanson K, Edwin Langbein W, et al. Energy cost of physical activities in persons with spinal cord injury. *Med Sci Sport Exerc.* (2010) 42:691–700. doi: 10.1249/MSS.0b013e3181bb902f
37. Martin Bland J, Altman D. Statistical methods for assessing agreement between two methods of clinical measurement. *Lancet* (1986) 327:307–10. doi: 10.1016/S0140-6736(86)90837-8
38. Levin S, Jacobs DR, Ainsworth BE, Richardson MT, Leon AS. Intra-individual variation and estimates of usual physical activity. *Ann Epidemiol.* (1999) 9:481–8. doi: 10.1016/S1047-2797(99)00022-8
39. Trost SG, Pate RR, Freedson PS, Sallis JF, Taylor WC. Using objective physical activity measures with youth: how many days of monitoring are needed? *Med Sci Sports Exerc.* (2000) 32:426–31. doi: 10.1097/00005768-200002000-00025
40. Searle SR. *Linear Models.* New York, NY: John Wiley & Sons, Inc. (1971).
41. Koo TK, Li MY. Cracking the code: providing insight into the fundamentals of research and evidence-based practice a guideline of selecting and reporting intraclass correlation coefficients for reliability research. *J Chiropr Med.* (2016) 15:155–63. doi: 10.1016/j.jcm.2016.02.012
42. McGraw KO, Wong SP. Forming inferences about some intraclass correlation coefficients. *Psychol Methods* (1996) 1:30–46. doi: 10.1037/1082-989X.1.1.30
43. Trost SG, McIver KL, Pate RR. Conducting accelerometer-based activity assessments in field-based research. *Med Sci Sports Exerc.* (2005) 37:S531–43. doi: 10.1249/01.mss.0000185657.86065.98
44. Berger RL, Hsu JC. Bioequivalence trials, intersection–union tests and equivalence confidence set. *Stat Sci.* (1996) 11:283–319.
45. Wolak ME, Fairbairn DJ, Paulsen YR. Guidelines for estimating repeatability. *Methods Ecol Evol.* (2012) 3:129–37. doi: 10.1111/j.2041-210X.2011.00125.x
46. Zbogar D, Eng JJ, Miller WC, Krassioukov A V, Verrier MC. Physical activity outside of structured therapy during inpatient spinal cord injury rehabilitation. *J Neuroeng Rehabil.* (2016) 13:99. doi: 10.1186/s12984-016-0208-8
47. Jörgensen S, Martin Ginis KA, Lexell J. Leisure time physical activity among older adults with long-term spinal cord injury. *Spinal Cord* (2017) 55:848–56. doi: 10.1038/sc.2017.26
48. Keller U, Schölch S, Albisser U, Rudhe C, Curt A, Riener R, et al. Robot-assisted arm assessments in spinal cord injured patients: a consideration of concept study. *PLoS ONE* (2015) 10:e0126948. doi: 10.1371/journal.pone.0126948
49. Tudor-Locke C, Burkett L, Reis JP, Ainsworth BE, Macera CA, Wilson DK. How many days of pedometer monitoring predict weekly physical activity in adults? *Prev Med.* (2005) 40:293–8. doi: 10.1016/j.ypmed.2004.06.003
50. Lidal IB, Huynh TK, Biering-Sørensen F. Return to work following spinal cord injury: a review. *Disabil Rehabil.* (2007) 29:1341–75. doi: 10.1080/09638280701320839
51. Franz M, Richner L, Wirz M, Von Reumont A, Bergner U, Herzog T, et al. Physical therapy is targeted and adjusted over time for the rehabilitation of locomotor function in acute spinal cord injury interventions in physical and sports therapy article. *Spinal Cord* (2018) 56:158–67. doi: 10.1038/s41393-017-0007-5
52. Gorman E, Hanson HM, Yang PH, Khan KM, Liu-Ambrose T, Ashe MC. Accelerometry analysis of physical activity and sedentary behavior in older adults: a systematic review and data analysis. *Eur Rev Aging Phys Act* (2014) 11:35–49. doi: 10.1007/s11556-013-0132-x
53. Kim Y, Beets MW, Welk GJ. Everything you wanted to know about selecting the " right" Actigraph accelerometer cut-points for youth, but...: a systematic review. *J Sci Med Sport* (2012) 15:311–21. doi: 10.1016/j.jsams.2011.12.001
54. Mattlage AE, Redlin SA, Rippee MA, Abraham MG, Rymer MM, Billinger SA. Use of accelerometers to examine sedentary time on an acute stroke unit. *J Neurol Phys Ther.* (2015) 39:166–71. doi: 10.1097/NPT.0000000000000092
55. Lee IM, Shiroma EJ. Using accelerometers to measure physical activity in large-scale epidemiological studies: issues and challenges. *Br J Sports Med.* (2014) 48:197–201. doi: 10.1136/bjsports-2013-093154
56. Loprinzi PD, Lee H, Cardinal BJ, Crespo CJ, Andersen RE, Smit E, et al. The relationship of actigraph accelerometer cut-points for estimating physical activity with selected health outcomes: results from NHANES 2003–06. *Res Q Exerc Sport* (2012) 83:422–30. doi: 10.1080/02701367.2012.10599877
57. Vanhelst J, Béghin L, Drumez E, Coopman S, Gottrand F. . *BMC Med Res Methodol.* (2017) 17:99. doi: 10.1186%2Fs12874-017-0378-5

58. Baumann S, Groß S, Voigt L, Ullrich A, Weymar F, Schwaneberg T, et al. Pitfalls in accelerometer-based measurement of physical activity: the presence of reactivity in an adult population. *Scand J Med Sci Sport* (2018) 28:1056–63. doi: 10.1111/sms.12977
59. Bandmann E. *Physical Activity Questionnaires: A Critical Review of Methods Used in Validity and Reproducibility Studies.* (2008), Swedish School of Sport and Health Sciences
60. Giggins OM, Clay I, Walsh L. Physical activity monitoring in patients with neurological disorders: a review of novel body-worn devices. *Digit Biomarkers* (2017) 1:14–42. doi: 10.1159/000477384
61. Nightingale TE, Rouse PC, Thompson D, Bilzon JLJ. Measurement of physical activity and energy expenditure in wheelchair users: methods, considerations and future directions. *Sport Med Open* (2017) 3:10. doi: 10.1186/s40798-017-0077-0

4

Body Weight Support Combined with Treadmill in the Rehabilitation of Parkinsonian Gait

Eliana Berra[1†], Roberto De Icco[1,2†], Micol Avenali[1,2], Carlotta Dagna[1,2], Silvano Cristina[1], Claudio Pacchetti[1], Mauro Fresia[1], Giorgio Sandrini[1,2] and Cristina Tassorelli[1,2]*

[1] Neurorehabilitation Unit and Parkinson Unit, IRCCS Mondino Foundation, Pavia, Italy, [2] Department of Brain and Behavioral Sciences, University of Pavia, Pavia, Italy

***Correspondence:**
Roberto De Icco
rob.deicco@gmail.com

† These authors have contributed equally to this work

Background: Gait disorders represent disabling symptoms in Parkinson's Disease (PD). The effectiveness of rehabilitation treatment with Body Weight Support Treadmill Training (BWSTT) has been demonstrated in patients with stroke and spinal cord injuries, but limited data is available in PD.

Aims: The aim of the study is to investigate the efficacy of BWSTT in the rehabilitation of gait in PD patients.

Methods: Thirty-six PD inpatients were enrolled and performed rehabilitation treatment for 4-weeks, with daily sessions. Subjects were randomly divided into two groups: both groups underwent daily 40-min sessions of traditional physiokinesitherapy followed by 20-min sessions of overground gait training (Control group) or BWSTT (BWSTT group). The efficacy of BWSTT was evaluated with clinical scales and Computerized Gait Analysis (CGA). Patients were tested at baseline (T0) and at the end of the 4-weeks rehabilitation period (T1).

Results: Both BWSTT and Control groups experienced a significant improvement in clinical scales as FIM and UPDRS and in gait parameters for both interventions. Even if we failed to detect any statistically significant differences between groups in the different clinical and gait parameters, the intragroup analysis captured a specific pattern of qualitative improvement associated to cadence and stride duration for the BWSTT group and to the swing/stance ratio for the Control group. Four patients with chronic pain or anxious symptoms did not tolerate BWSTT.

Conclusions: BWSTT and traditional rehabilitation treatment are both effective in improving clinical motor functions and kinematic gait parameters. BWSTT may represent an option in PD patients with specific symptoms that limit traditional overground gait training, e.g., severe postural instability, balance disorder, orthostatic hypotension. BWSTT is generally well-tolerated, though caution is needed in subjects with chronic pain or with anxious symptoms.

Clinical Trial Registration: www.ClinicalTrials.gov, identifier: NCT03815409

Keywords: body weight support treadmill training, gait rehabilitation, computerized gait analysis, Parkinson's disease, neurorehabilitation

INTRODUCTION

Gait disorders in Parkinson's Disease (PD) are due to dopaminergic nigrostriatal pathways degeneration and represent important components of the disability (1).

In PD, gait is characterized by a significant reduction of stride length (2). Inadequate flexion at the ankle and knee, reduction of heel strike, forward-flexed trunk, reduced arm swing with asymmetric stride times for lower limbs and significant stride-to-stride variability are frequently associated (3–8).

The efficacy of pharmacological treatment with Levodopa is frequently uncomplete (9) and adjuvant rehabilitation treatment is recommended. Body weight supported treadmill training (BWSTT) represents a promising rehabilitative approach for gait impairment in PD (10, 11). Effectiveness of BWSTT on gait, balance and motor function has been demonstrated in different neurological diseases, especially in stroke (12) and spinal cord injury (13). In stroke, authors reported that BWSTT appears as a safe method of training, providing a major sense of security regarding falls and facilitating free leg movements, compared with treadmill alone (12). In addition, stroke patients treated with BWSTT were able to walk for a longer duration and with a minimal increase in heart rates (14). In PD patients, BWSTT has been tested in small controlled studies that have suggested a clinically detectable beneficial effect (10, 11). BWSTT seems also effective in improving balance in PD (15–17), evaluated both with clinical scales (as Berg Balance Scale, BBS) and dynamic posturography (18). In PD, many data in literature show how treadmill training, acting as a sensory cue, improves kinetic and kinematic parameters, studied with computerized gait analysis (CGA), more than physiotherapy alone. Toole and Ganesan highlighted a positive impact of BWSTT on postural instability using instrumental investigations (15, 18). Regarding gait rehabilitation, most of the data recorded with computerized movement analysis derived from BWSTT delivered with robotic devices (19–22). Only a limited number of studies has instead investigated the effect of non-robotic BWSTT on gait kinetic and kinematic data. Ganesan et al. used an instrumental evaluation, but it must be noted that they recorded kinematic gait parameters during a treadmill-assisted walk, which prevents generalization to overground gait (23). Another study (24) showed an improvement in gait speed and cadence after a single session of BWSTT both in PD patients and healthy controls, but did not provide any data on the effect of multiple sessions or on any possible retention of the effect.

In this manuscript we present a revision of the main literature on gait rehabilitation in PD using BWSTT with and without robotic devices, and the findings of a randomized, controlled, parallel-group study conducted on a representative sample of PD subjects to investigate the efficacy of BWSTT using the computerized gait analysis for the precise definition of qualitative and quantitative effects.

Related Works

BWS Delivered Without Robotic Devices

The first report of BWSTT efficacy in gait rehabilitation of PD belongs to Miyai et al. Ten patients with PD were enrolled in a cross-over study and treated for 4 consecutive weeks with BWSTT (20% of unweighting for 12 min followed by another 12-min period of 10% of unweighting) or conventional physical therapy (CPT). The Authors showed that BWSTT was superior to CPT in improving gait disturbances and disability at the end of the rehabilitative period. More specifically BWSTT proved superior to CPT in improving UPDRS scores, gait speed and stride length (10). The same study group in 2002, evaluated the 6-months retention of BWSTT in PD. Twenty-four patients with PD were randomized to receive BWSTT (20% of unweighting for 10 min + 10% of unweighting for 10 min + 0% of unweighting for an additional 10-min period) or CPT 3 times/week for 4 consecutive weeks. All patients were clinically evaluated at baseline and then monthly for 6 months. In this series, gait speed significantly improved in BWSTT respect to CPT only at month 1, while the improvement in the stride length was more marked in BWSTT group with respect to CPT and persisted until month 4 (11).

Toole et al. showed that 6-weeks of BWSTT increased gait speed and stride length, evaluated with clinical tests, and improved balance, measured with Computerized Dynamic Posturography. Of note, in this study no statistical difference in gait was observed when comparing patients treated with treadmill alone with patients treated with treadmill associated with weight-support (15).

In 2008, Fisher et al. speculated on the possible central mechanism responsible for clinical effects of BWSTT. Thirty subjects affected by PD were randomly assigned to three groups: high-intensity group (24 sessions of BWSTT), low-intensity group (24 sessions of CPT), zero-intensity group (8-weeks of education classes). Again, the high-intensity group improved the most at the end of treatment period, in particular in gait speed, step length, stride length, and double support. Of note, in this study a subgroup of patients was also tested with transcranial magnetic stimulation: in the BWSTT group Authors were able to record a lengthening of the cortical silent period, postulating that high-intensity training improved neuronal plasticity in PD, through BDNF and GABA modulation (25).

More recently, Rose et al. studied the efficacy of a high-intensity locomotor training in BWS condition achieved with a positive-pressure antigravity treadmill. When comparing training period (3 sessions/week for 8 weeks) with a control period (no intervention), they found a significant improvement in MDS-UPDRS (total and motor sub-scale) and walking distance (26). Indeed Ganesan et al. randomized 60 PD patients to 3 groups: (1) no specific exercise activity, (2) conventional gait training (30 min sessions, 4 times/week for 1 month), and (3) BWSTT (30 min sessions, 4 times/week for 1 month). At the end of a 4-weeks follow up, both intervention groups showed an improvement in the UPDRS score (total, motor, and sub-scores) and in gait parameters (walking distance, speed, and step length) when compared to non-exercising group; moreover, BWSTT appeared to be significantly superior respect to conventional gait training. At variance from the previous study, this latter one used an instrumental analysis of gait, which unfortunately was performed while the subjects were walking on the treadmill (instrumented 2-min walk test) and not during unassisted overground gait (23).

Lander and Moran studied the spatiotemporal gait effects of BWSTT with an instrumented 6-m device (GAITRite, CIR systems); they studied the effects of a single session of BWSTT in PD and healthy controls and showed an improved gait speed and cadence in both groups. Unfortunately, they did not investigate the effect of repetitive BWSTT sessions (24).

In the future, we hope that BWS might be improved and combined with novel technologies in order to develop new and individualized rehabilitative strategies. In this view, Park et al. combined BWS with a treadmill designed to adapt the walking speed according to the voluntary patient control via a feedback/feedforward control. Moreover, the environment around this BWSTT was enriched by a virtual reality system able to simulate real-life conditions. This approach proved safe and allowed the therapist to treat patients in more realistic overground gait conditions; indeed, the use of virtual obstacles, such as walls or narrow spaces, in the virtual reality setting allowed Authors to study freezing of gait in laboratory (27).

Another example is the combination of BWS with cues rehabilitation; Schlick et al. showed how BWSTT combined with visual cues was more effective in improving step length and gait symmetry when compared to an un-cued condition. It is also noteworthy that this multimodal approach was efficient and well-tolerated in advance PD patient with a V Hoehn and Yahr stage (28).

BWSTT Delivered With Robotic Devices

Ustinova et al. published the first positive case report on the short-term gait rehabilitation efficacy of BWSTT delivered to a PD patient with a robotic device (Lokomat-Hocoma Inc., Volketswil, Switzerland). The intervention consisted in a 2-weeks gait training, delivered 3 times per week, with each session lasting 90–120 min (29).

Lo et al. conducted a pilot study to assess the efficacy of BWSTT delivered with the Lokomat unit in reducing frequency of freezing of gait (FOG) in PD. Authors reported a 20% reduction in the average number of daily episodes of FOG and a 14% improvement in the FOG-questionnaire score (19).

In 2012, Picelli et al. enrolled 41 PD patients in the first randomized controlled study aimed to compare the efficacy of BWSTT delivered with a robot-assisted gait training (RAGT-gait Trainer GT1) to CPT (not focused on gait training) in improving gait in PD. They showed how RAGT was significantly superior respect to CPT in improving the 6-min walking test, the 10-meter walking test, stride length, single/double support ratio, Parkinson's Fatigue Scale and UPDRS score (20).

Carda et al. subsequently designed a randomized controlled study to assess superiority of robotic-gait training with BWS (Lokomat with 50% of unweighting for 15 min followed by 30% unweighting for an additional 15-min period) when compared to treadmill training without BWS. The Authors failed to record any significant differences between groups at the 6-min walking test, the 10-meter walking test and the Time up-and go test, although all the parameters significantly improved in both groups, with a positive effect persisting up to 6 months after rehabilitation (30).

In the paper published by Sale et al., the main aim was the comparison between a new end-effector robotic BWS device (G-EO system device) and treadmill training without weight-support. After 4-weeks of rehabilitation, the statistical analysis showed a significant improvement with the robotic intervention in gait speed, step length and stride length, but the between-group analysis was not statistically significant (21).

In 2013, Picelli et al. designed a comprehensive randomized controlled study aimed to compare robotic BWSTT (RAGT—gait Trainer GT1) with treadmill training without BWS (TT) and CPT. Sixty subjects with mild to moderate PD were enrolled and evaluated before treatment (T0), at the end of a 4-weeks rehabilitative programme (T1) and after 3 months (T2). This study failed to demonstrate the superiority of RAGT in improving gait speed when compared to TT; at variance, both RAGT and TT proved more effective than CPT as regards gait speed and walking capacity. It is worth noting that the improvement in gait speed was considered clinically significant (namely > 0.25 m/s at the 10-meter test) only after the RAGT approach (31).

Finally, Galli et al. compared the effects of BWS delivered with a robotic end effector (G-EO system) with TT not only on the spatio-temporal gait parameters, but also on the range of motion of the most important lower limb joints. The results showed that robotic rehabilitation produced an improvement in the kinematic gait profile at the proximal level (hip and pelvis) when compared to TT without BWS. These results are useful from a clinical point of view because they suggest that rehabilitation with BWS and robotic gait training could be recommended in specific sub-groups of PD patients (for example in those with a deficit of pelvis and hip mobility at baseline) (22).

A CONTROLLED TRIAL COMPARING BWSTT WITH OVERGROUND GAIT TRAINING

Materials and Methods

Subjects

Subjects were enrolled among consecutive PD patients hospitalized in the Neurorehabilitation Unit of the IRCCS Mondino Foundation of Pavia, Italy. Thirty-six patients affected by Idiopathic PD, according to the UK Brain Bank diagnostic criteria were included according to the following inclusion criteria:

- disease stage II–III Hoehn and Yahr (H&Y);
- stable dosage of dopaminomimetic drugs for 3 months before study enrollment.

Exclusion criteria were:

- moderate to severe cognitive impairment (MMSE $\leq$ 21);
- unpredictable motor fluctuations;
- moderate to severe orthopedic diseases or other pathological conditions (e.g., severe postural abnormalities) that might affect gait training.

During the observation period, no change was allowed to the dopaminomimetic drugs.

All participants gave their written informed consent for participation in the study, which was carried out according to the Declaration of Helsinki and was approved by the Ethics Committee. At the time of the approval of the protocol the local Ethics Committee was held at the IRCCS Mondino Foundation.

Demographic and clinical details of the subjects are shown in **Table 1**.

Procedures

Subjects were randomly assigned to two groups: 18 PD patients were assigned to the "BWSTT group" and 18 patients to the "Control group." Before starting treatment, patients of BWSTT group performed a 20-min single session of BWSTT in order to test feasibility and tolerability. Four of them did not tolerate BWSTT: one patient reported an increase in his pre-existing hip pain, two patients with pre-existing spondyloarthrosis complained of low back pain, one patient reported that the procedure induced anxious symptoms. These 4 patients were re-allocated to the Control group, so that the final disposition of patients in the two groups was as follows: 14 patients (8 women and 6 men) in the BWSTT group and 22 patients (10 women and 12 men) in the Control group (**Figure 1**).

Patients in both groups underwent 5 daily rehabilitation sessions per week for 4 consecutive weeks. Both groups underwent daily 40-min sessions of traditional physical therapy (PT) followed by a 20-min session of overground gait training (Control group) or of gait training with BWSTT (BWSTT group).

TABLE 1 | Demographic and clinical characteristics of BWSTT and Control groups.

Demographic and clinical characteristics		BWSTT group ($n = 14$)	Control group ($n = 22$)	p-value
Age (years)		71.9 ± 10.2	71.7 ± 7.5	0.958
Disease duration (years)		11.4 ± 11.4	10.18 ± 4.8	0.652
H&Y stage		2.3 ± 0.6	2.1 ± 0.4	0.479
UPDRS III score		33.4 ± 11.6	34.4 ± 12.0	0.810
FIM score		99.6 ± 12.3	99.6 ± 16.2	0.996
Sex	M	6 (42.9%)	12 (54.5%)	0.733
	F	8 (57.1%)	10 (45.5%)	
Disease onset	Right	2 (14.3%)	10 (45.5%)	0.107
	Left	6 (42.9%)	8 (36.4%)	
	Bilateral	6 (42.9%)	4 (18.2%)	
Patients with freezing (%)		4 (28.6%)	10 (45.5%)	0.485
Therapy	L	3 (21.4%)	4 (18.2%)	0.950
	L-DA	3 (21.4%)	5 (22.7%)	
	L-E	2 (14.3%)	2 (9.1%)	
	L-E-DA	6 (42.9%)	11 (50.0%)	

L, levodopa; DA, dopaminoagonist; E, entacapone.

Traditional Treatment

The traditional PT rehabilitation treatment included passive, active and active-assisted exercises, according to the methods commonly used (Kabat, Bobath) and previously published (32, 33).

Every 40-min treatment session consisted in isotonic and isometric exercises for the major muscles of the limbs and trunk including cardiovascular warm-up exercises (5 min), muscle stretching exercises (10 min), muscle stretching exercises for functional purposes (10 min), balance training exercises (10 min), relaxation exercises (5 min). This protocol was designed in accordance with PD rehabilitation guidelines and evidences in the literature (34).

Treatment With Body Weight Support Treadmill Training (BWSTT)

The sessions were conducted on a treadmill with partial weight unload. Specifically, the patient performed 10-min treadmill walk with a support corresponding to 20% of his/her own weight, followed by a 5-min rest and a second 10-min session on the treadmill with a support corresponding to 10% of his/her own weight. In the initial treadmill session, the starting speed of the treadmill was set to 0.5 km/h, subsequent increments of 0.5 km/h per minute were added to reach the maximum speed that was comfortably tolerated by the patient. This latter was used for the entire training period.

All patients were examined by a neurologist with expertise in movement disorders at the beginning of hospitalization (T0) and at the end of the neurorehabilitation period (+4 weeks, T1). The clinical assessment involved a complete neurological examination and administration of the following clinical scales, validated for the assessment of the disability:

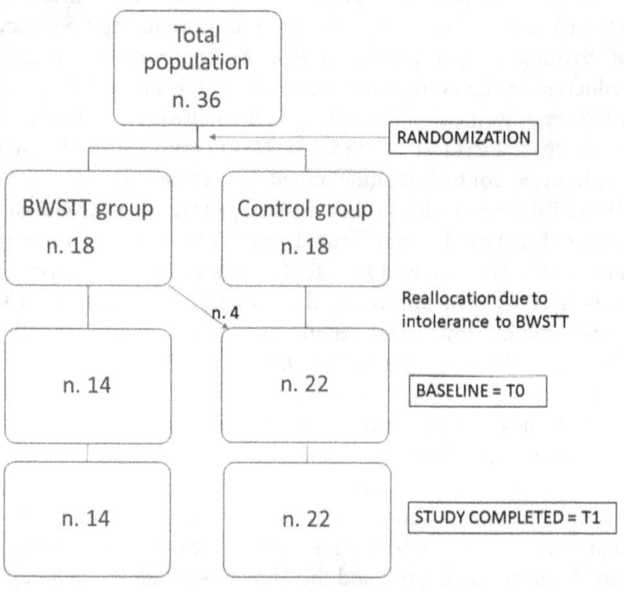

FIGURE 1 | Study flow and patients' disposition.

- for the assessment of PD severity: the Unified Parkinson's Disease Rating Scale, part III (UPDRS-III) (35);
- for the assessment of functional independence: the Functional Independence Measure (FIM) (36).

Computerized Gait Analysis

The instrumental assessment of gait was conducted at T0 and T1 by an experienced laboratory Technician using an Optokinetic Gait Analysis System associated to the software Myolab Clinic (ELITE, BTS Engineering, Milan), composed of six infrared cameras, with a sampling rate of 100 Hz. According to the Davis protocol, 21 spherical reflective markers (15 mm in diameter) were applied along the body. Synchronized data acquisition and data processing were performed by analyzer software (BTS, Milan, Italy). In order to perform kinematic analysis of gait, patients were instructed to walk at their preferred speed along a 10-meter walkway with the initial step on the side of disease onset. For each session, we acquired at least three performances and calculated the mean. In order to obtain the best individual performance, all recordings were conducted in the ON phase. The sessions were recorded at 5-min intervals to allow complete recovery from fatigue.

Data Analysis

After acquisition of the recordings, the video files were analyzed and the spatial-temporal variables were measured during all phases of gait cycle using the software Myolab Clinic (ELITE, BTS Engineering, Milan). We calculated the following variables:

- Speed (m/s);
- Cadence, expressed as the number of steps per minute (step/min);
- Stride duration (s);
- Stride length (m);
- Duration of stance expressed as a percentage of the duration of step (%);
- Duration of swing expressed as a percentage of the duration of step (%);
- Number of strides on a 10-meter distance.

Statistical Analysis

The sample size and power of the study were calculated using the portal "Open Source Epidemiologic Statistics for Public Health" (www.openepi.com). We calculated the sample size with the following parameters: confidence interval (two sided) 95%; power 80%; difference between groups 20% (with a standard deviation between 20 and 25% for each group). The Statistical Package for the Social Sciences (SPSS) for Windows, version 21.0, was used for the calculation.

The distribution of each variable was evaluated using "skewness" and "kurtosis." Moreover, the data were plotted using a "Q-Q plot" that confirmed normal distribution of all tested variables. For qualitative variables we used crosstabs analysis, performing statistical significance with Fisher exact test by case.

Quantitative variables are presented as mean values ± standard deviation. The main analysis regarding clinical scales and gait parameters was performed with the ANOVA (analysis of variance) for repeated measures with two factors: (1) Time (two levels: T0 vs. T1); (2) Group (two levels: BWSTT vs. Control).

We also performed a sub-analysis to asses intra-group variations between T0 and T1 using *t*-test for paired samples; delta percentage variations between groups (BWS vs. controls) were tested using a *t*-test for independent samples. The level of significance was set for convention at a $p < 0.05$, always corrected if necessary.

RESULTS

The demographic and clinical characteristics of the two groups are shown in **Table 1**. No statistically significant differences were found between groups at baseline. Clinical features and gait parameters of each subject at T0 and T1 are presented in **Tables 2–3** for Control and BWSTT groups, respectively.

Clinical Scales

We found a significant effect of factor "Time" for both UPDRS-III score [$F = 102.857$; $df_{(1,34)}$; $p = 0.001$] and FIM score [$F = 63.222$; $df_{(1,34)}$; $p = 0.001$], without any significant interaction for factors "Group" and "Time*Group" (**Table 4**).

In the intra-group sub-analysis, the UPDRS-III score significantly decreased at T1 in both BWSTT group (T0 = 33.4 ± 11.5, T1 = 23.3 ± 9.1; T0 vs. T1 $p = 0.01$) and Control group (T0 = 34.4 ± 12.0, T1 = 26.8 ± 10.6; T0 vs. T1 $p = 0.01$). In line with this result, also FIM significantly improved at T1 in both groups of patients (BWSTT group: T0 = 99.5 ± 12.3, T1 = 107.0 ± 10.4; $p = 0.01$; Control group: T0 = 99.6 ± 16.2, T1 = 110.1 ± 15.5; $p = 0.01$).

Gait Parameters

The main analysis showed a significant effect of factor "Time" for speed [$F = 11{,}306$; $df_{(1,34)}$; $p = 0.002$], cadence [$F = 6.233$; $df_{(1,34)}$; $p = 0.018$), stride duration [$F = 43, 741$; $df_{(1,34)}$; $p = 0.036$] and stride length [$F = 17.700$; $df_{(1,34)}$; $p = 0.001$]. Factor "Group" and the interaction "Time*Group" were not significant for all gait parameters (**Table 4**).

The intragroup sub-analysis showed a significant increase in speed (from 0.6 ± 0.1 to 0.7 ± 0.2 m/s; T0 vs. T1 $p = 0.01$), cadence (from 85.9 ± 16.4 to 90.7 ± 14.1; T0 vs. T1 $p = 0.01$), length of stride (from 0.41 ± 0.1 m to 0.59 ± 0.1 m; T0 vs. T1 $p = 0.04$) and with a reduction in the duration of stride (from 1447.2 ± 283.3 to 1353.3 ± 210.4 ms; T0 vs. T1 $p = 0.01$) and in the number of strides (from 8.2 ± 2.2 to 7.6 ± 1.8 for 10-meters; T0 vs. T1 $p = 0.02$) (**Table 5**) at T1 in the BWSTT group.

In the Control group, at T1 we observed a significant increase in speed (from 0.7 ± 0.2 to 0.8 ± 0.3 m/s; T0 vs. T1 $p = 0.01$) and swing duration (from 35.5 ± 5.7 to 38.7 ± 11.2%; T0 vs. T1 $p = 0.02$), with a consequent reduction of stance duration (from 64.4 ± 5.7 to 61.2 ± 11.1%; T0 vs. T1 $p = 0.02$) (**Table 5**).

When comparing the percent change of the gait parameters induced by the two rehabilitation interventions, no statistically significant differences were found in any gait parameters between Control group and BWSTT group (**Figure 2**).

TABLE 2 | Clinical features and gait parameters (T0 and T1) for each patient in Control group.

ID	Age	Disease duration (years)	Freezing	Disease onset	Therapy	H&Y	UPDRS		FIM		Speed (m/s)		Cadence (step/min)		Stride duration (ms)		Stride length (m)		Stance (%)		Swing (%)		N° strides (10 m)	
							T0	T1	T0	T1	T0	T1	T0	T1	T0	T1	T0	T1	T0	T1	T0	T1	T0	T1
1	70–75	11	Y	Le	L-E-DA	2	28	28	110	110	0.87	1.32	69.6	105.5	1623.2	1137.0	0.70	0.70	67.7	62.0	32.3	38.0	5.0	5.0
2	70–75	7	Y	Le	L-DA	2	40	29	89	95	0.90	0.79	77.2	80.5	1587.2	1389.2	0.59	0.68	66.6	66.4	33.4	33.6	4.0	4.0
3	55–60	6	N	R	L-E-DA	2	39	27	90	104	0.96	1.22	81.3	78.0	1644.2	1538.0	0.66	0.77	67.4	68.3	32.6	31.7	4.0	4.0
4	70–75	6	Y	Le	L	2	44	41	89	94	0.82	0.60	91.5	77.4	1311.0	1551.0	0.50	0.44	76.5	68.8	23.5	31.2	7.0	8.0
5	55–60	5	N	R	L-E	2	11	5	108	126	1.00	1.00	88.6	97.2	1354.0	1377.0	0.62	0.70	65.5	63.0	34.6	37.0	4.0	4.0
6	65–70	14	Y	R	L-E-DA	2	50	43	92	107	0.43	0.49	87.0	83.6	1500.0	1435.7	0.30	0.33	72.6	71.8	27.4	28.1	11.5	10.7
7	70–75	21	Y	Le	L-DA	2	57	44	44	55	0.28	0.50	65.3	74.6	1838.7	1608.3	0.24	0.38	71.1	69.0	28.9	31.0	14.5	9.0
8	60–65	20	N	Le	L-E-DA	2	38	29	105	111	0.77	0.96	79.8	86.7	1561.9	1384.6	0.56	0.62	58.4	47.9	41.5	53.5	6.0	5.5
9	65–70	14	Y	R	L-E-DA	3	50	43	92	107	0.43	0.50	110.8	110.2	1500.0	1435.7	0.30	0.33	62.5	61.9	37.5	38.1	12.0	10.5
10	80–85	7	N	Le	L	2	33	24	96	114	0.58	0.48	70.8	75.3	1699.0	1594.5	0.46	0.35	62.7	67.8	37.3	32.2	8.0	10.0
11	75–80	6	N	R	L-DA	2	57	44	44	55	0.35	0.53	75.1	79.6	1599.0	1508.0	0.26	0.37	61.0	63.7	39.0	36.3	13.5	9.5
12	70–75	10	N	Le	L-DA	2	28	23	105	119	1.16	1.25	115.8	134.7	1036.8	891.3	0.56	0.52	64.6	63.2	35.4	36.8	6.0	6.5
13	70–75	6	N	B	L-E-DA	2	38	29	105	111	0.75	1.07	75.9	94.0	1598.5	1314.0	0.56	0.64	60.4	48.3	39.6	51.8	6.5	5.5
14	75–80	8	Y	B	L-E-DA	3	36	32	109	117	0.82	0.82	81.9	88.3	1467.5	1359.3	0.56	0.52	68.2	69.8	31.8	30.3	6.0	6.5
15	80–85	7	N	R	L	2	29	20	112	121	0.88	1.17	80.8	102.0	1300.5	1178.8	0.61	0.64	65.0	64.8	35.0	35.2	6.0	5.5
16	70–75	10	Y	B	L-E-DA	2	15	10	121	129	0.83	0.95	98.5	94.6	1219.0	1269.5	0.47	0.56	67.5	63.5	32.5	36.5	7.5	6.0
17	75–80	9	N	B	L-E-DA	3	28	22	128	128	0.33	0.31	84.2	86.2	1468.7	1392.3	0.23	0.20	69.6	62.7	30.4	37.3	15.3	19.0
18	75–80	13	Y	R	L-E	2	40	21	100	123	0.88	0.82	85.9	78.8	1401.5	1523.0	0.43	0.58	55.3	58.5	44.7	41.5	6.0	6.0
19	70–75	7	N	R	L-E-DA	2	22	18	92	109	0.77	1.15	92.2	95.7	1304.8	1255.3	0.44	0.67	57.1	64.2	42.9	35.8	7.5	5.0
20	55–60	20	N	Le	L-E-DA	2	33	30	96	105	0.87	0.88	85.0	97.8	1226.3	1240.5	0.48	0.51	61.6	27.3	38.4	72.7	7.5	7.0
21	80–85	8	Y	R	L	2	15	10	105	113	0.50	0.50	99.6	70.9	1109.5	1695.5	0.28	0.39	65.4	68.2	34.6	31.8	12.5	9.0
22	80–85	9	N	R	L-DA	3	34	26	109	116	0.66	0.71	83.1	75.8	1452.5	1485.5	0.48	0.52	63.5	61.8	36.5	38.2	7.5	6.8

Le, left; R, right; B, bilateral, L, levodopa; DA, dopaminoagonist; E, entacapone.

TABLE 3 | Clinical features and gait parameters (T0 and T1) for each patient in BWSTT group.

ID	Age	Disease duration (years)	Freezing	Disease onset	Therapy	H&Y	UPDRS		FIM		Speed (m/s)		Cadence (step/min)		Stride duration (ms)		Stride length (m)		Stance (%)		Swing (%)		N° strides (10 m)	
							T0	T1	T0	T1	T0	T1	T0	T1	T0	T1	T0	T1	T0	T1	T0	T1	T0	T1
23	75–80	12	N	Le	L-E-DA	3	23	14	104	106	0.92	1.00	88.1	96.2	1466.0	1348.8	0.51	0.58	60.5	60.6	39.5	39.4	6.0	6.0
24	65–70	2	N	Le	L-DA	3	46	32	125	111	0.76	0.97	78.5	96.9	1528.5	1238.5	0.54	0.56	60.2	58.7	39.8	41.3	6.5	6.0
25	40–45	9	Y	Le	L-E	2	21	13	109	121	0.75	0.86	71.8	82.1	1675.7	1461.5	0.48	0.58	54.4	54.0	45.6	46.0	6.0	6.0
26	80–85	7	N	R	L-DA	2	28	21	100	111	0.80	0.85	77.7	94.6	1548.8	1275.0	0.53	0.50	70.7	67.2	29.3	32.8	6.0	7.0
27	65–70	23	Y	R	L-E-DA	2	35	22	100	111	0.56	0.73	77.9	77.7	1543.5	1549.8	0.40	0.52	59.3	60.4	40.7	39.6	9.0	6.5
28	70–75	38	N	B	L-E-DA	2	52	28	98	103	1.06	0.90	105.4	107.3	1144.0	1124.3	0.48	0.47	59.7	61.4	40.3	38.6	6.0	7.5
29	70–75	10	N	B	L-E-DA	2	41	31	103	119	0.36	0.52	57.3	77.1	2104.3	1569.0	0.35	0.38	70.1	59.7	29.9	40.3	10.0	9.0
30	75–80	2	N	B	L	2	18	17	104	108	0.57	0.48	81.7	71.9	1470.3	1672.3	0.39	0.48	69.2	72.3	30.8	27.7	9.0	9.5
31	60–65	14	Y	B	L-E-DA	2	33	30	91	105	0.90	1.18	106.9	113.6	1122.5	1056.8	0.47	0.58	64.6	59.0	35.4	41.0	7.5	6.0
32	75–80	1	N	B	L	2	24	21	85	94	0.63	0.67	82.6	88.4	1462.3	1359.3	0.43	0.43	69.6	67.4	30.3	32.6	8.0	8.0
33	75–80	4	N	Le	L	2	36	28	100	102	0.53	0.54	71.9	73.3	1668.5	1638.5	0.41	0.41	53.9	64.4	46.1	35.6	8.5	8.5
34	70–75	1	N	Le	L-E-DA	3	21	9	102	113	0.55	1.03	86.3	98.4	1129.8	1221.0	0.29	0.58	60.3	59.7	39.7	40.3	12.0	6.0
35	85–95	7	N	Le	L-DA	2	37	18	103	114	0.69	0.63	87.8	86.0	1368.5	1397.0	0.44	0.41	64.6	65.9	35.4	34.1	8.0	8.5
36	70–80	30	Y	B	L-E	3	53	43	70	80	0.53	0.55	117.3	113.1	1023.7	1063.3	0.25	0.52	66.8	68.2	33.2	31.8	14.0	13.0

Le, left; R, right; B, bilateral; L, levodopa; DA, dopaminoagonist; E, entacapone.

DISCUSSION

Gait disorders represent common and disabling symptoms in PD. In recent years, multidisciplinary rehabilitation treatment has acquired a key role in improving the motor function (34). Effectiveness of BWSTT in improving gait, balance and motor function evaluated with both clinical scales and instrumental Kinematic Computerized Gait Analysis has been demonstrated in neurological diseases as stroke (12) and spinal cord injuries (13). Previous findings suggested that Treadmill Training (TT) could improve gait parameters in PD patients (16), but data available from the literature on the specific effect of BWSTT in the rehabilitation of gait of PD subjects do not allow conclusive inference. In the literature we can find some reviews on the topic, but the strength of their conclusions is partially limited by methodological bias. In particular, these reviews poorly differentiate between treadmill training used alone, treadmill training plus BWS, or BWS delivered with robotic devices (16, 37), which actually represent quite different modalities of rehabilitation from a methodological point of view.

To the best of our knowledge this is the first controlled study that evaluates the effect of a 4-weeks rehabilitative program with a non-robotic BWSTT using instrumentally-recorded gait parameters in PD patients during overground, spontaneous gait. BWSTT was compared with standard rehabilitation and it induced an improvement in the score of the clinical scales, namely UPDRS and FIM, thus confirming the clinical efficacy reported in previous studies (10, 11, 16, 18). The main analysis of our study showed a significant improvement in multiple parameters of gait at the end of the 4-weeks rehabilitative program in both study groups. In this view, BWSTT did not prove to be more efficient than conventional overground gait training. At the intragroup sub-analysis, however, BWSTT showed a specific profile of improvement upon the kinematic gait parameters recorded with a 6-camera optoelectronic system for CGA. Indeed, at the end of the 4-weeks rehabilitation period only the BWSTT group experienced a significant increase in the stride length, stride duration and cadence, together with a reduction in the number of strides and in the duration of stride. The group receiving standard rehabilitation protocol showed solely a percent reduction in the stance phase of the step with a percent increase in the swing phase.

Different mechanisms may be hypothesized to explain the clinical efficacy of BWSTT on gait and balance. In stroke patients, treadmill training reduces cardiovascular demands and energy expenditure (12, 14). Aerobic training is however not the main driver of the effect, since treadmill training alone resulted in a worse outcome than BWSTT in stroke (12, 14). In the case of PD, a possible role may be played by the impact on BWSTT on baroreflex sensitivity (38), defined as a measure of sensitivity of the cardiac limb of the baroreflex and derived from the change in inter-beat interval for unit change in systolic pressure (39, 40). Indeed, low blood pressure variation and a decrease in baroreflex sensitivity significantly contribute to orthostatic hypotension in PD (41). Ganesan et al. demonstrated that 4-weeks of BWSTT significantly improve baroreflex sensitivity in patients with PD and prevent orthostatic blood pressure fall (38). No conclusive

TABLE 4 | Effect of BWSTT (BWSTT group) and traditional rehabilitation (Control group) on clinical scales and kinematic variables of gait.

Variables	BWSTT group (n = 14)		Control group (n = 22)		ANOVA for repeated measures		
	T0	**T1**	**T0**	**T1**	**Time**	**Group**	**Time*Group**
UPDRS	33.4 ± 11.5	23.3 ± 9.1	34.4 ± 12.0	26.8 ± 10.6	F = 102.857 df (1, 34) **p = 0.001**	F = 0.467 df (1, 34) p = 0.499	F = 2.029 df (1, 34) p = 0.163
FIM	99.5 ± 12.3	107.0 ± 10.4	99.6 ± 16.2	110.1 ± 15.5	F = 63.222 df (1, 34) **p = 0.001**	F = 0.019 df (1, 34) p = 0.892	F = 1.720 df (1, 34) p = 0.198
Speed (m/s)	0.68 ± 0.1	0.78 ± 0.2	0.72 ± 0.2	0.82 ± 0.3	F = 11,306 df (1, 34) **p = 0.002**	F = 0.224 df (1, 34) p = 0.639	F = 0.003 df (1, 34) p = 0.956
Cadence (step/min)	85.9 ± 16.4	90.7 ± 14.1	86.0 ± 16.4	89.0 ± 17.0	F = 6.233 df (1, 34) **p = 0.018**	F = 0.026 df (1, 34) p = 0.872	F = 0.272 df (1, 34) p = 0.606
Stride duration (ms)	1447.2 ± 283.3	1353.3 ± 210.4	1438.0 ± 198, 3	1392.0 ± 251.0	F = 43,741 df (1, 34) **p = 0.036**	F = 0.064 df (1, 34) p = 0.802	F = 0.268 df (1, 34) p = 0.608
Stride length (m)	0.41 ± 0.1	0.49 ± 0.1	0.46 ± 0.1	0.51 ± 0.1	F = 17.700 df (1, 34) **p = 0.001**	F = 0.544 df (1, 34) p = 0.466	F = 0.617 df (1, 34) p = 0.438
Stance (%)	63.0 ± 5.6	62.6 ± 5.0	64.4 ± 5.7	61.2 ± 11.1	F = 1.879 df (1, 34) p = 0.179	F = 0.66 df (1, 34) p = 0.799	F = 1.191 df (1, 34) p = 0.283
Swing (%)	36.9 ± 5.6	37.3 ± 5.0	35.5 ± 5.7	38.7 ± 11.2	F = 1.926 df (1, 34) p = 0.174	F = 0.058 df (1, 34) p = 0.811	F = 1.231 df (1, 34) p = 0.275
N° strides (10 m)	8.2 ± 2.2	7.6 ± 1.8	8.1 ± 3.0	7.6 ± 3.5	F = 3.364 df (1, 34) p = 0.065	F = 0.078 df (1, 34) p = 0.781	F = 0.001 df (1, 34) p = 0.970

ANOVA for repeated measures with two factors: (1) Time (T0 vs. T1) and (2) Group (BWSTT vs. Control). Bold text highlights significant results.

data about gait are available in literature on the comparison between BWSTT and TT in PD. Both treatments seem to improve gait, either when used alone or as an add-on to standard rehabilitation treatment (16). Some Authors have hypothesized a neuromechanical effect of BWSTT, involving central pattern generators (CPGs). CPGs are load and sensory dependent and BWSTT may alter the supraspinal and spinal influences on CPG neuromotor activity (42, 43). Evidence suggests that an abnormal proprioception and dysfunctional sensorimotor integration is frequent in PD. In PD patients, external stimuli are able to modulate the motor pattern. Acoustic, visual and somatosensory cues help the patients to start and maintain a rhythmic motor task (44–46). Each type of cue activates a different pattern of supraspinal motor control. In particular, sensory cues enable the voluntary dorsolateral pre-motor control system, bypassing the supplementary motor area's deficit that alters automatic movement (45). In this frame, it is intuitive that treadmill training, with and without BWS, does represent a symmetrical and repetitive sensory stimulus, capable of increasing the rhythm of motion, and increasing the discharge activity of additional locomotor areas (45). However, in BWSTT, the mechanism could be more complex, leading to an implementation of the activity also on the latter circuit. Studies with near infrared spectroscopy (NIRS) showed, in fact, that treatment with BWSTT induced an increase in activation of the primary and supplementary motor areas in PD patients (47). Other possible explanations of the effectiveness of BWSTT on gait rehabilitation include specific motor learning of the task, improvement in postural reflexes (48), neural plasticity induced by physical activity and dependent activity (neurogenesis, synaptogenesis and molecular adaptation) (49, 50) and the normalization of corticomotor excitability/cortical reorganization, especially in the supplementary motor area in subjects with PD (25). Another possible explanation for the beneficial changes observed following BWSTT is the improvement of balance as suggested by previous reports (18). Unfortunately, our study was not designed to investigate balance.

While the two gait training approaches under investigation showed a different profile of improvement as regards the various gait parameters, the statistical analysis failed to detect significant changes when evaluating the impact of BWSTT and classic overground rehabilitation (in term of percent changes) upon the different gait parameters. As a consequence, it is fair to state that, in terms of efficacy, both treatments may be

TABLE 5 | *Post-hoc* analysis of intragroup changes in gait parameters for BWSTT and Control groups from baseline (T0) to the end of the rehabilitative period (T1).

Variables	BWSTT group ($n = 14$)			Control group ($n = 22$)		
	T0	T1	*p*-value T1 vs. T0	T0	T1	*p*-value T1 vs. T0
Speed (m/s)	0.68 ± 0.1	0.78 ± 0.2	**0.001**	0.72 ± 0.2	0.82 ± 0.3	**0.001**
Cadence (step/min)	85.9 ± 16.4	90.7 ± 14.1	**0.001**	86.0 ± 16.4	89.0 ± 17.0	0.151
Stride duration (ms)	1447.2 ± 283.3	1353.3 ± 210.4	**0.001**	1438.0 ± 198.3	1392.0 ± 251.0	0.143
Stride length (m)	0.41 ± 0.1	0.59 ± 0.1	**0.046**	0.46 ± 0.1	0.51 ± 0.1	0.130
Stance (%)	63.0 ± 5.6	62.6 ± 5.0	0.577	64.4 ± 5.7	61.2 ± 11.1	**0.022**
Swing (%)	36.9 ± 5.6	37.3 ± 5.0	0.575	35.5 ± 5.7	38.7 ± 11.2	**0.022**
N° strides (10 m)	8.2 ± 2.2	7.6 ± 1.8	**0.022**	8.1 ± 3.0	7.6 ± 3.5	0.111

Bold text highlights significant results.

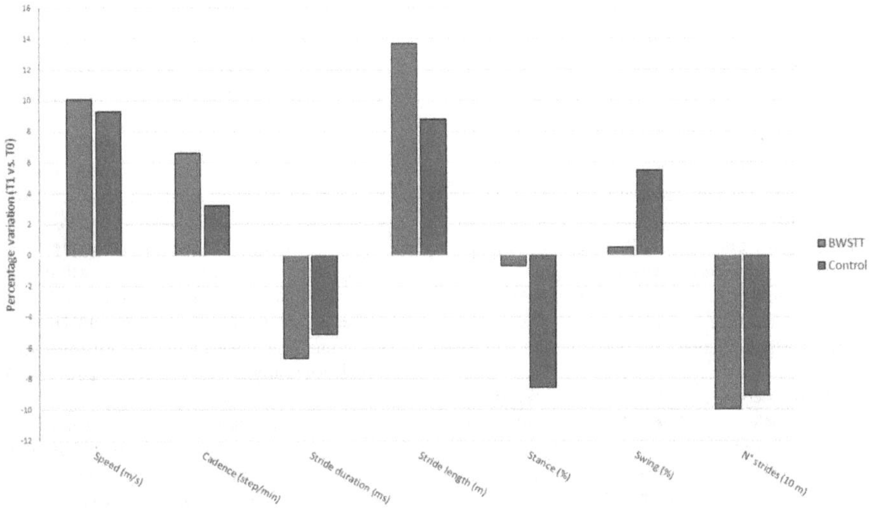

FIGURE 2 | Comparison of delta % changes in gait parameters from baseline (T0) to the end of the rehabilitative period (T1) in BWSTT and Control groups.

proposed for gait rehabilitation in PD patients. What can drive the selection of BWSTT over overground gait training is the safety of the procedure. Indeed, the BWS harness practically prevents falls in patients during the rehabilitative session. This allows physiotherapists to focus more properly on the different segments involved in walking, instead of having to worry about steading the subject. This means that BWSTT may find its ideal indication in the more severely affected PD patients. This impression obviously needs scientific confirmation in specific trials. In this frame, it is important to note that our findings suggest that BWSTT is safe, but may not be well-tolerated by patients with chronic pain and anxious symptoms. Therefore, it is advisable to conduct an initial BWSTT test session in order to assess tolerability before starting treatment.

LIMITATIONS

This study was conducted on a small number of patients who may not be representative of the full extension of the functional disability that is associated to PD. Furthermore, due to the above described tolerance issues, the 2 arms were not perfectly balanced in terms of numerosity. However, though these considerations may limit the transferability of the present data to the general PD population we feel that it is important to report our experience in full because of its useful implication in the real life setting.

In this study we did not evaluate the effect of BWSTT on balance, which may represent one of the components that affect the positive results recorded on the gait performance in our patients. An additional arm, evaluating the effect of treadmill alone, would have increased the possibility to dissect out the role of different components. Further studies are needed to evaluate the effect of BWSTT on orthostatic hypotension and balance.

CONCLUSIONS

In conclusion, our results show that BWSTT and standard traditional rehabilitation treatment are both effective in improving clinical motor functions and kinematic gait parameters in PD. BWSTT showed some interesting peculiarities in its profile of gait improvement. This observation, together with the well-known specific technical features of the procedure suggests that BWSTT treatment may find a preferential indication for gait training in PD patients with moderate or severe postural instability, balance disorders, orthostatic hypotension.

AUTHOR CONTRIBUTIONS

EB designed the protocol and drafted the manuscript. RD designed the protocol, performed the statistical analysis, and revised the manuscript. MA, SC, and CP enrolled patients. CD and MF acquired data for the paper and organized the database. GS and CT provided substantial contributions to the conception of the protocol and critically revised the manuscript.

REFERENCES

1. Morris ME. Movement disorders in people with Parkinson disease: a model for physical therapy. *Phys Ther.* (2000) 80:578–97. doi: 10.1093/ptj/80.6.578
2. Morris ME, Iansek R, Matyas TA, Summers JJ. Stride length regulation in Parkinson's disease. Normalization strategies and underlying mechanisms. *Brain* (1996) 119 (Pt 2):551–68.
3. Knutsson E. An analysis of Parkinsonian gait. *Brain* (1972) 95:475–86. doi: 10.1093/brain/95.3.475
4. Murray MP, Sepic SB, Gardner GM, Downs WJ. Walking patterns of men with Parkinsonism. *Am J Phys Med Rehabil.* (1978) 57:278–94.
5. Bowes SG, Clark PK, Leeman AL, O'Neill CJ, Weller C, Nicholson PW, et al. Determinants of gait in the elderly Parkinsonian on maintenance levodopa/carbidopa therapy. *Br J Clin Pharmacol.* (1990) 30:13–24. doi: 10.1111/j.1365-2125.1990.tb03738.x
6. Blin O, Ferrandez AM, Serratrice G. Quantitative analysis of gait in Parkinson patients: increased variability of stride length. *J Neurol Sci.* (1990) 98:91–7. doi: 10.1016/0022-510X(90)90184-O
7. Ueno E, Yanagisawa N, Takami M. Gait disorders in Parkinsonism. A study with floor reaction forces and EMG. *Adv Neurol.* (1993) 60:414–8.
8. Hausdorff JM, Cudkowicz ME, Firtion R, Wei JY, Goldberger AL. Gait variability and basal ganglia disorders: stride-to-stride variations of gait cycle timing in Parkinson's disease and Huntington's disease. *Mov Dis.* (1998) 13:428–37.
9. Blin O, Ferrandez AM, Pailhous J, Serratrice G. Dopa-sensitive and dopa-resistant gait parameters in Parkinson's disease. *J Neurol Sci.* (1991) 103:51–4.
10. Miyai I, Fujimoto Y, Ueda Y, Yamamoto H, Nozaki S, Saito T, et al. Treadmill training with body weight support: its effect on Parkinson's disease. *Arch Phys Med Rehabil.* (2000) 81:849–52. doi: 10.1053/apmr.2000.4439
11. Miyai I, Fujimoto Y, Yamamoto H, Ueda Y, Saito T, Nozaki S, et al. Long-term effect of body weight-supported treadmill training in Parkinson's disease: a randomized controlled trial. *Arch Phys Med Rehabil.* (2002) 83:1370–3. doi: 10.1053/apmr.2002.34603
12. Mehrholz J, Thomas S, Elsner B. Treadmill training and body weight support for walking after stroke. *Cochrane Database Syst Rev.* (2017) 8:CD002840. doi: 10.1002/14651858.CD002840.pub4
13. Morawietz C, Moffat F. Effects of locomotor training after incomplete spinal cord injury: a systematic review. *Arch Phys Med Rehabil.* (2013) 94:2297–308. doi: 10.1016/j.apmr.2013.06.023
14. Visintin M, Barbeau H. The effects of body weight support on the locomotor pattern of spastic paretic patients. *Can J Neurol Sci.* (1989) 16:315–25. doi: 10.1017/S0317167100029152
15. Toole T, Maitland CG, Warren E, Hubmann MF, Panton L. The effects of loading and unloading treadmill walking on balance, gait, fall risk, and daily function in Parkinsonism. *NeuroRehabilitation* (2005) 20:307–22.
16. Mehrholz J, Kugler J, Storch A, PohlM, Elsner B, Hirsch K. Treadmill training for patients with Parkinson's disease. *Cochrane Database Syst Rev.* (2015) 13:CD007830. doi: 10.1002/14651858.CD007830.pub3
17. Protas EJ, Mitchell K, Williams A, Qureshy H, Caroline K, Lai EC. Gait and step training to reduce falls in Parkinson's disease. *NeuroRehabilitation* (2005) 20:183–90.
18. Ganesan M, Sathyaprabha TN, Gupta A, Pal PK. Effect of partial weight supported treadmill gait training on balance in patients with Parkinson disease. *PM R* (2014) 6:22–33. doi: 10.1016/j.pmrj.2013.08.604
19. Lo AC, Chang VC, Gianfrancesco MA, Friedman JH, Patterson TS, Benedicto DF. Reduction of freezing of gait in Parkinson's disease by repetitive robot-assisted treadmill training: a pilot study. *J Neuroeng Rehabil.* (2010) 7:51. doi: 10.1186/1743-0003-7-51
20. Picelli A, Melotti C, Origano F, Waldner A, Fiaschi A, Santilli V, et al. Robot-assisted gait training in patients with Parkinson disease: a randomized controlled trial. *Neurorehabil Neural Repair.* (2012) 26:353–61. doi: 10.1177/1545968311424417
21. Sale P, De Pandis MF, Le Pera D, Sova I, Cimolin V, Ancillao A, et al. Robot-assisted walking training for individuals with Parkinson's disease: a pilot randomized controlled trial. *BMC Neurol.* (2013) 13:50. doi: 10.1186/1471-2377-13-50
22. Galli M, Cimolin V, De Pandis MF, Le Pera D, Sova I, Albertini G, et al. Robot-assisted gait training versus treadmill training in patients with Parkinson's disease: a kinematic evaluation with gait profile score. *Funct Neurol.* (2016) 31:163–70. doi: 10.11138/fneur/2016.31.3.163
23. Ganesan M, Sathyaprabha TN, Pal PK, Gupta A. Partial body weight-supported treadmill training in patients with Parkinson disease: impact on gait and clinical manifestation. *Arch Phys Med Rehabil.* (2015) 96:1557–65. doi: 10.1016/j.apmr.2015.05.007
24. Lander J, Moran M. Does positive pressure body weight-support alter spatiotemporal gait parameters in healthy and Parkinsonian individuals? *NeuroRehabilitation* (2017) 40:271–6. doi: 10.3233/NRE-161412
25. Fisher B, Wu A, Salem G, Song J, Lin CH, Yip J, et al. The effect of exercise trainining improving motor performance and corticomotor excitability in people with early Parkinson's disease. *Arch Phys Med Rehabil.* (2008) 89:1221–9. doi: 10.1016/j.apmr.2008.01.013
26. Rose MH, Løkkegaard A, Sonne-Holm S, Jensen BR. Improved clinical status, quality of life, and walking capacity in Parkinson's disease after body weight-supported high-intensity locomotor training. *Arch Phys Med Rehabil.* (2013) 94:687–92. doi: 10.1016/j.apmr.2012.11.025
27. Park HS, Yoon JW, Kim J, Iseki K, Hallett M. Development of a VR-based treadmill control interface for gait assessment of patients with Parkinson's disease. *IEEE Int Conf Rehabil Robot.* (2011) 2011: 5975463. doi: 10.1109/icorr.2011.5975463
28. Schlick C, Struppler A, Boetzel K, Plate A, Ilmberger J. Dynamic visual cueing in combination with treadmill training for gait rehabilitation in Parkinson disease. *Am J Phys Med Rehabil.* (2012) 91:75–9. doi: 10.1097/phm.0b013e3182389fe2
29. Ustinova K, Chernikova L, Bilimenko A, Telenkov A, Epstein N. Effect of robotic locomotor training in an individual with Parkinson's disease: a case report. *Disabil Rehabil Assist Technol.* (2011) 6:77–85. doi: 10.3109/17483107.2010.507856
30. Carda S, Invernizzi S, Baricich A, Comi C, Croquelois A, Cisari C. Robotic gait training is not superior to conventional treadmill training in Parkinson disease: a single-blind randomized controlled trial. *Neurorehabil Neural Repair.* (2012) 26:1027–34. doi: 10.1177/1545968312446753
31. Picelli A, Melotti C, Origano F, Neri R, Waldner A, Smania N. Robot-assisted gait training versus equal intensity treadmill training in patients with mild to moderate Parkinson's disease: a randomized controlled trial. *Parkinson Relat Dis.* (2013) 19:605–10. doi: 10.1016/j.parkreldis.2013.02.010
32. Bartolo M, Serrao M, Tassorelli C, Don R, Ranavolo A, Draicchio F, et al. Four-week trunk-specific rehabilitation treatment improves lateral trunk flexion in Parkinson's disease. *Mov Disord.* (2010) 15:325–31. doi: 10.1002/mds.23007
33. Tassorelli C, De Icco R, Alfonsi E, Bartolo M, Serrao M, Avenali M, et al. Botulinum toxin type A potentiates the effect of neuromotor rehabilitation of Pisa syndrome in Parkinson disease: a placebo controlled study. *Parkinson Relat Disord.* (2014) 20:1140–4. doi: 10.1016/j.parkreldis.2014.07.015
34. Mak MK, Wong-Yu IS, Shen X, Chung CL. Long-term effects of exercise and

physical therapy in people with Parkinson disease. *Nat Rev Neurol.* (2017) 13:689–703. doi: 10.1038/nrneurol.2017.128
35. Goetz CG, Fahn S, Martinez-Martin P, Poewe W, Sampaio C, Stebbins GT. Movement disorder society-sponsored revision of the unified Parkinson's disease rating scale (MDS-UPDRS): process, format, and clinimetric testing plan. *Mov Dis.* (2007) 22:41–7. doi: 10.1002/mds.21198
36. Turner-Stokes L, Nyein K, Turner-Stokes T, Gatehouse C. The UK FIM+FAM: development and evaluation. *Clin Rehabil.* (1999) 13:277–87. doi: 10.1191/026921599676896799
37. Herman T, Giladi N, Hausdorff JM. Treadmill training for the treatment of gait disturbances in people with Parkinson's disease: a mini-review. *J Neural Transm.* (2009) 116:307–18. doi: 10.1007/s00702-008-0139-z
38. Ganesan M, Pal P, Gupta A, Sathyaprabha TN. Treadmill gait training improves baroreflex sensitivity in Parkinson's disease. *Clin Auton Res.* (2014) 24:111–8. doi: 10.1007/s10286-014-0236-z
39. Goldstein DS. Arterial baroreflex sensitivity, plasma catecholamines, and pressor responsiveness in essential hypertension. *Circulation* (1983) 68:234–40. doi: 10.1161/01.CIR.68.2.234
40. Kardos A, Watterich G, de Menezes R, Csanady M, Casadei B, Rudas L. Determinants of spontaneous baroreflex sensitivity in a healthy working population. *Hypertension* (2001) 37:911–6. doi: 10.1161/01.HYP.37.3.911
41. Szili-Torok T, Kalman J, Paprika D, Dibo G, Rozsa Z, Rudas L. Depressed baroreflex sensitivity in patients with Alzheimer's and Parkinson's disease. *Neurobiol Aging* (2001) 22:435–8. doi: 10.1016/s0197-4580(01)00210-x
42. Wickelgten I. Teaching the spinal cord to walk. *Science* (1998) 279:319–21. doi: 10.1126/science.279.5349.319
43. McIntosh G, Brown S, Rice R, Thaut M. Rhytmic auditory-motor facilitation of gait patterns in patients with Parkinson's disease. *J Neurol Neurosurg Psychiatr.* (1997) 62:22–6. doi: 10.1136/jnnp.6 2.1.22
44. Majsak MJ, Kaminski T, Gentile AM, Glanagan JR. The reaching movements of patients with Parkinson's disease under self-determined maximal speed and visually cued conditions. *Brain* (1998) 121:755–66.
45. Morris ME, Iansek R, Matyas TA, Summers JJ. Stride length regulation in Parkinson's disease. Normalization strategies and underlying mechanisms. *Brain* (1996) 119:551–68.
46. Platz T, Brown RG, Marsden CD. Training improves the speed of aimed movements in Parkinson's disease. *Brain* (1998) 121:505–14.
47. Hanakawa T, Katsumi Y, Fukuyama H, Honda M, Hayashi T, Kimura J, et al. Mechanism underlying gait disturbance in Parkinson's disease: a single photon emission computed tomography study. *Brain* (1999) 122 (Pt 7):1271–82.
48. Platz T, Brown RG, Marsden CD. Training improves the speed of aimed movements in Parkinson's disease. *Brain* (1998) 121:505–14.
49. Fisher BE, Petzinger GM, Nixon K, Hogg E, Bremmer S, Meshul CK, et al. Exercise-induced behavioral recovery and neuroplasticity in the 1-methyl-4-phenyl-1,2,3,6-tetrahydropyridine-lesioned mouse basal ganglia. *J Neurosci Res.* (2004) 77:378–90. doi: 10.1002/jnr.20162
50. Fox CM, Ramig LO, Ciucci MR, Sapir S, McFarland DH, Farley BG. The science and practice of LSVT/LOUD: neural plasticity-principled approach to treating individuals with Parkinson disease and otherneurological disorders. *Semin Speech Lang.* (2006) 27:283–99. doi: 10.1055/s-2006-955118

5

Action Observation for Neurorehabilitation in Apraxia

Mariella Pazzaglia [1,2]* *and Giulia Galli* [2]

[1] *Department of Psychology, University of Rome "La Sapienza," Rome, Italy,* [2] *IRCCS Fondazione Santa Lucia, Rome, Italy*

***Correspondence:**
Mariella Pazzaglia
mariella.pazzaglia@uniroma1.it

Neurorehabilitation and brain stimulation studies of post-stroke patients suggest that action-observation effects can lead to rapid improvements in the recovery of motor functions and long-term motor cortical reorganization. Apraxia is a clinically important disorder characterized by marked impairment in representing and performing skillful movements [gestures], which limits many daily activities and impedes independent functioning. Recent clinical research has revealed errors of visuo-motor integration in patients with apraxia. This paper presents a rehabilitative perspective focusing on the possibility of action observation as a therapeutic treatment for patients with apraxia. This perspective also outlines impacts on neurorehabilitation and brain repair following the reinforcement of the perceptual-motor coupling. To date, interventions based primarily on action observation in apraxia have not been undertaken.

Keywords: apraxia, action recognition, action execution, mirror activity, neurorehabilitation

INTRODUCTION

Apraxia encompasses a broad spectrum of higher-order purposeful movement disorders (1) and is most often associated with neurological damage to left-hemisphere (2). The accepted definition of apraxia includes deficits in performing, imitating, and recognizing skilled actions involved in the intentional movements, colloquially referred to as gestures (3). Pathological conditions such as apraxia result from an inability to evince the concept of specific actions (4) or to execute related motor programs (5). Classically, apraxia is diagnosed when a patient presents with an inability to execute gestures in response to verbal commands or imitate with different effectors (mouth, hand, or foot) (4), including movements involving the non-paretic limb ipsilateral to the lesion[s]. Although apraxia primarily affects motor activities, studies report that higher impairment levels may be related to visuo-motor integration (6). Recent evidence supports the notion that apraxia influences skilled acts in the environment, interferes with independent functioning, impedes daily activities, and affects the performance of routine self-care (7, 8); that is, persons may have difficulty brushing their teeth (9), eating (7), preparing food (10), and getting dressed (11). As a consequence, patients with apraxia can develop severe anxiety and reductions in the spontaneous use of social gestures (12), leading to isolation and depression (13) and consequent delays in returning to work (14).

Almost 50% of patients with left-hemispheric stroke (15) and ~35% of patients with Alzheimer's disease and corticobasal degeneration (16–18) develop apraxia that persists after illness onset and affects functional abilities. Research to aid in the development and optimization of apraxia neurorehabilitation is crucial. Several approaches for the treatment of apraxia deficits are currently in practice [for a review see (19, 20)], including verbal (21) or pictorial (22) facilitation and the use of physical cues based on repetitive behavioral-training programs with gesture-production exercises. The errorless completion method represents another recent approach (23). Autonomy in activities of daily living tends to be underestimated (24), and rehabilitation studies remain limited due to the nature of disturbances to automatic/voluntary dissociations (i.e., an ability to execute actions only in natural settings). To date, no rehabilitation treatment or therapeutic possibilities based primary on action observation has been studied in apraxia.

THE VALUE OF ACTION OBSERVATION IN TREATING APRAXIA

Language disorders among patients with apraxia who suffer from concomitant aphasia suggest that defects in gesture imitation, rather than gestures in response to verbal commands, are more sensitive indicators of apraxia (25). Goldenberg has proposed that imitation apraxia could be primarily considered a deficit of perceptual analysis (26). Evidence from several studies indicates that perceptual and motor codes are closely associated (27, 28) and that patients with apraxia may be defective both in performing motor acts and in the perceptual code necessary to represent the appropriate gesture. Sunderland and Sluman have shown, for example, that problems orienting a spoon in a bean-spooning task suggest an inability to remember the correct action and to judge the correctness of the perceived action (29).

Although apraxia is commonly considered a motor impairment, deficits in intact gestural perception are not uncommon, occurring in 33% of one sample (30). Such patients, who exhibit deficits in the execution of actions, also commit errors when judging between correctly and incorrectly performed acts (30–32), understanding the meaning of pantomimes (33, 34), discriminating among action-related sounds (35, 36), matching photographs of gestures (26), engaging visuo-motor temporal integration (6), and predicting incoming observed movements (37, 38).

Movement-execution effects in apraxia thus are not purely motor processes and visual representations of given actions may influence the actions' execution by visuo-motor transfer (39). The integrity of gesture representations has important implications for rehabilitation strategies (40). The spatial and temporal use of a body part for the planning of a tool-related action and the imitation of others' actions involve an inherent perceptual component, which can be disturbed following apraxia onset. As a result, modern assessments of apraxia include evaluations of gesture understanding (32, 41).

VISUAL-MOTOR STRATEGIES IN THE REHABILITATION OF PATIENTS WITH LIMB APRAXIA

The notion of common representations for both executed and observed actions is of considerable interest in the applied field of stroke neurorehabilitation (42, 43). Despite the use of state-of-the-art apraxia-evaluation batteries (44) to explore perceptual deficits in the understanding of actions in patients with apraxia, few studies have proposed new rehabilitation programs that include elements of both observation and execution of actions.

Smania et al.'s (45) clinical examinations of 43 left brain-damaged patients with apraxia revealed defective performances in gesture execution and imitation, as well as in the recognition and identification of transitive and intransitive gestures. For their study, approximately half of the patients received training in ecological action production and comprehension; the other half underwent conventional language rehabilitation for the same number of treatment hours. The training, which combined the observation and execution of observed actions, consisted of three progressive phases, each characterized by increasing degrees of difficulty, obtained by phased reductions of facilitation cues as performance improved. After ~30 sessions, therapists recorded significant improvements: approximately 50% improvement in the ADL scale and an average of 40% in the praxis test (22). When only considering apraxia patients with cortical lesions primarily in the fronto-parietal network, the improvement was even greater (45). No significant performance changes were observed in the outcome measures of control patients who did not undergo specific programs of gesture production/observation exercises. Interestingly, authors reported a significant improvement in gesture recognition performance after the apraxia treatment, and a correlation was found between gesture comprehension tests and the ADL questionnaire (ADL-gesture comprehension: $R = 0.37, p = 0.034$) (22). These results suggest that the positive effects of this rehabilitative approach in apraxia require parity in the treatment of both the motor and the perceptual aspects of action processing (45). Of note, beneficial effects persisted for at least 2 months and extended to the daily living activities even of untreated actions, helping patients attain functional independence from their caregivers (22).

Goldenberg and Hagmann (9) developed a particularly successful restorative method in which training comprised two different methods. The first aimed at helping patients to learn and correctly execute complete activities, with therapists providing different support at all clinical steps (e.g., by demonstrating gesture execution and asking patients to imitate them), and reducing the support only when patients were able to perform these steps on their own. The second aimed at directing patients' attention to the functional meaning of objects' individual features and details, critical for various actions. This two-step procedure ensured a double reinforcement of the action's perceptual-motor code: the first online within the simultaneity of the demonstration and the second off-line as a delayed imitation. The combination of these two methods led to significant improvements in trained ADL, but virtually no generalization of training effects was observed between trained and non-trained activities. The therapy's success was preserved among those patients who performed the activities at home but not among those who did not. In a subsequent study (46), the authors developed a slightly different variant to previous approaches in which patients carried out entire activities with a minimum of errors. In this approach, the functional commonalities between different objects were emphasized by providing verbal instructions and visual and gestural support. Effects of these treatments lasted up to 3 months after the treatment ended.

Compensatory treatment indicate that the patients showed large improvements in ADL functioning after rehabilitative programs aiming at teaching visual strategies to overcome the apraxic impairments during execution of everyday activities (47). Patients were taught strategies to compensate internally (e.g., self-verbalization or imagination) or externally (e.g., observation of pictorial cues) the distinct phases of a complex action, while performing the daily activities (47–50).

All described interventions included elements of visuo-motor integration and seemed to indicate that motor and visual relearning in these patients was inextricably intertwined (see **Table 1**).

Perceptual approach has been successfully applied to a different rehabilitative intervention showing how action observation has a positive effect on the performance of a specific motor skill [for a review see (41, 52, 53)]. Patients watch a specific motor act presented in a video clip or in a real demonstration, and simultaneously (or thereafter) performed the same action. A match (or mismatch) between visual signals and the gesture performed drive re-learning about how the limb should move in order to perform the motor act accurately (see **Figure 1** for a hypothetical model on apraxia). Correctly reproducing temporal (56, 57), spatial (58), and body coding (59) helps characterize movements, facilitate the motor patterns that patients have to execute, and stimulate a rapid online correction of movement (58, 60, 61). Observation combined with physical practice in a congruent mode leads to increased motor cortex excitability, and synaptic and cortical map plasticity strengthens the memory trace of the motor act (62). Differently, rehabilitative training based on physical practice alone (300–1,000 daily repetitions) elicits only minimal neural reorganization (63). This combined visual-motor therapy has been shown to improve motor performance in patients that suffered a chronic stroke (64–86), patients with Parkinson's disease (87–92), children with cerebral palsy (93–97) and elderly individuals with reduced cognitive abilities (98). Electrophysiological studies have also reported positive effects of action observation on the recovery of motor functions after acute and chronic stroke (71, 99). This non-invasive, inexpensive, user-friendly approach works more quickly on biological effectors (mouth, limbs, and trunk), promoting better and faster recovery.

A NEURAL SUBSTRATE FOR ACTION OBSERVATION AND EXECUTION IN APRAXIA REHABILITATION

The inextricable link between action perception and execution was first posited in the ideomotor theory, which has been validated through delineation of the brain network, known as the mirror neuron system (MNS). Inspired by single-cell ("mirror neuron") recordings in monkeys (100, 101), many neuroimaging and neurophysiological studies have suggested that the adult human brain is equipped with neural systems and mechanisms that represent both the visual perception and execution of actions in a common format (102). Action deficits among the patients with apraxia may be described at multiple levels. While these levels partially overlap, four levels of hierarchical modeling at which an MNS mechanism can support an observed action (42, 103) are as follows:

(i) *kinematic*: Patients with apraxia frequently present with abnormalities in kinematic movements in the form of motor patterns that are slower, shorter, and less vertical than those of individuals without apraxia (104);
(ii) *motor*: Limb apraxia interferes with the selection and control of the hand-muscle activity (105). Moreover, it interferes with the formation of appropriate hand configurations for using objects (106);
(iii) *goal*: Understanding the immediate purpose of an action is impeded; for example, patients with apraxia are impaired access to mental representation of tool use (33);
(iv) *intention*: Patients present with an altered ability to monitor the early planning phases of their own actions (107).

The cortical areas have been shown to contain mirror neurons that are often described as a part of an integrated sensorimotor information system underpinned by neural activity in the frontal (103), parietal (108), and superior temporal sulcus areas. This system is called the action observation network (AON) (109). In humans, these cortical regions mediate the observation of actions that form a part of the observer's motor repertoire (41). They also contribute to the imitation (110) and comprehension (111) of these movements, and are involved in skill acquisition (112). Lesion symptom mapping studies have reported gestural deficits in patients with apraxia, which are most frequently apparent following lesions in the inferior frontal lobe (30, 113–116), and in supramarginal and angular gyrus (37, 113, 115, 117) of the left hemisphere. However, apraxia has also been observed in patients with damage in posterior middle temporal lobe, anterior temporal lobe (37, 113, 115, 117), occipital, and subcortical regions (6, 118, 119). Despite the damaged neural substrate was not constant across all the studies, it includes the areas that are considered crucial for the AON. Undoubtedly, the mirror neurons just provide a part of the complex information for achieving action comprehension while action recognition and production occur simultaneously by accessing the same neural representations. However, as posited by the influential cognitive neuropsychological models of apraxia (120, 121) and demonstrated by various clinical studies (121–124), the range of possible dissociations between action execution and action understanding that can occur in patients with apraxia is quite multifaceted and cannot be explained by a mere action mirroring mechanism nor by a single lesion locus. Impairments in the visual recognition of action paralleled deficits in performing these actions could depend on both common and distinct neural localization, most of which could be external to mirror regions. Failures in imitating or in recognizing gestures may occur because of damage at any level in the process between perceiving (input lexicon) and performing (output lexicon) an action (120, 121). Indeed, some apraxic patients show deficits in the recognition/discrimination of the gestures, some do not [for a review (125)]. Theoretical and empirical studies suggest that complementary routes to action understanding taking place on the dorso-dorsal and ventro-dorsal stream (126, 127). Lesion in ventral-dorsal stream may impede the top-down activation

TABLE 1 | Apraxia intervention studies.

References	Number of participants		Treatment duration	Type of action	Control	Intervention	Perceptual aspects of training	Improvements in experimental group	No effect
	Experimental group	Control group							
van Heugten et al. (47)	33		30 min for 12 weeks	Everyday activities		Strategy training	Observation of picture sequences Imagination	ADL Barthel Index Apraxia Test Motor functioning	
Goldenberg and Hagmann (9)	15		5 weeks	Three activities from the domains eating, dressing, and grooming		Direct training of the activity: errorless completion of the activity	The patients perform action immediately after observing the therapist's demonstration	10 patients improved on all three trained activities	6 months later, improvement is not maintained without practice
Smania et al. (45)	6	7	35 sessions, three per week	Transitive action Intransitive action Imitation	Aphasia therapy	Gesture recognition Gesture execution	Observation of picture (context, object) Gesture recognition Imitation	Apraxia Test Gesture recognition	Verbal comprehension Oral apraxia
Donkervoort et al. (48)	42	48	8 weeks	Everyday activities	Occupational therapy	Strategy training	Observation of picture sequences Imagination	ADL Barthel Index	Apraxia Test ADL untrained
Goldenberg et al. (46)	6		4 weeks	Four everyday activities		Explorative training vs. Direct training of the activity	The patients perform action immediately after observing the therapist's demonstration	Direct training of activity reduced errors and amount of assistance	Exploration training had no effect on performance
Smania et al. (22)	18	15	30 sessions, three per week	Transitive action Intransitive action Imitation	Aphasia therapy	Gesture recognition Gesture execution	Observation of picture (context, object) Gesture recognition Imitation	Apraxia Test Gesture recognition ADL	Verbal comprehension Oral apraxia
Geusgens et al. (50)	56	57	25 sessions, 8 weeks	Action of daily living	Occupational therapy	Strategy training	Observation of picture sequences	ADL untrained	
Geusgens et al. (49)	29		25 sessions, 8 weeks	Action of daily living		Strategy training	Observation of picture sequences	Apraxia Test ADL trained ADL untrained Barthel Index	Functional Motor Test
Bolognini et al. (51)	6	6	3 sessions, 10 min	Limb gesture imitation	Sham stimulation	Anodal tDCS on the left parietal cortex	Imitation (observation + execution)	Imitation execution	tDCS on the motor cortex

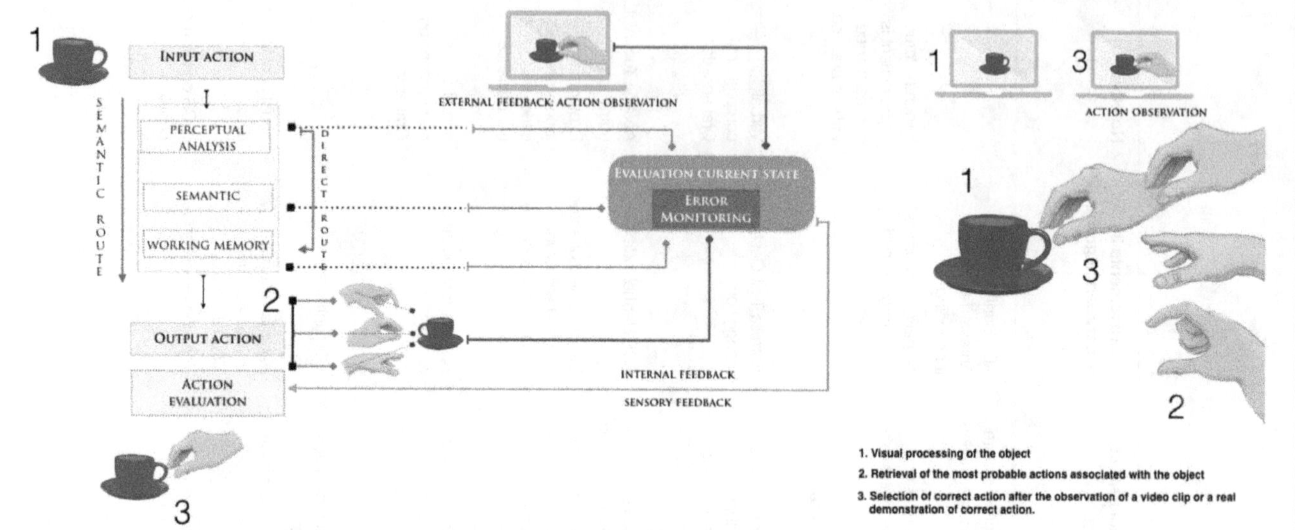

FIGURE 1 | Hypothetical model for performing and recognizing a transitive action [adapted from (54) and (55)]. Failures in performing or recognizing gestures may occur because of damage at any stage in the directional flow between perceiving (input) and performing (output) the action. The observation of a video clip or a real demonstration of action can have a positive effect on the selection and retrieval of the correct movement. In figure the example of grasping a cup of coffee. After the correct visual identification of the object as a cup, patients with apraxia have a difficult retrieval of the correct action associated with that object. When an incorrect movement is performed, a discrepancy occurs between the (correct) action observed on the model and the perception of own (incorrect) performed gesture. Combining motor training and action observation may enhance the relearning of daily actions and strengthen the visuo-motor coupling.

of motor engrams. It may produce disturbances in the on-line selection and integration of distinctive and relevant motor acts that ensure a high recognizability of the gesture (117). This can be responsible for the disordered motor planning, imitation, and motor-memory recall of gesture movements found in patients with apraxia (126, 127). As has been briefly shown, many questions remain, and there may be more than one mechanism leading to apraxia disturb. Given the complexity of the impairment and the separate neural substrates that are typically affected in apraxia, treatments related to action observation to support action execution or relearning of gestures of daily living, can be planned.

NEUROREHABILITATION AND BRAIN REPAIR AFTER APRAXIA

The behavioral success of rehabilitation methods based on the principle of action observation should promote reorganization by adaptive plasticity at the neural level (128, 129). Functional reorganization clearly depends on the residual neural integrity of efferent (motor) and afferent (sensory) information, which leads to improved treatment outcomes among some apraxia patients but not for others. In this perspective, we considered three possible sources of informational content for how neurorehabilitation and brain repair after apraxia works: injury site, elapsed time after apraxia onset, and lesion size.

The first factor to consider is *the location of the infarct*, which can ultimately determine the outcome of rehabilitation treatment. Whereas, lesions of the frontal and parietal cortices in the left hemisphere have been shown to primarily disrupt gesture production in patients with apraxia (2), no clear correlation has been found between lesion location and impairment in visual gesture representation. Apraxic patients with cortical lesions—but not those with subcortical lesions—cannot comprehend the meaning of gestures (130). In rare cases, a lesion in the left occipito-temporal cortex may also critically hamper the ability to recognize gestures in patients with apraxia (120, 131). Patients with parietal lesions have also been reported to exhibit significant impairments in executing gestures but only slight impairments in understanding those performed by others (132). The neural specificity of this disturbed typology may explain why certain patients with apraxia are able to comprehend the meaning of gestures despite being unable to perform them themselves. Accordingly, single-case and group studies report dissociations between action execution and representation and the underpinning damaged neural substrate (121–124). Efficiency and speed of the therapeutic means of action observation depend partly on the different roles that intact and damaged brain regions play in both action production and recognition (125, 133). Neural damage to a functional system can be partial, and studies in monkeys seem to suggest that the frontal and parietal cortices are neurally equipped for such divisions of labor (134).

Several studies have documented that neurorehabilitation techniques involving observation strategies among brain-damaged patients induce long-lasting neural changes in the motor cortex, potentiating activity in the affected areas. In brain-damaged patients, TMS studies have found direct evidence of increased motor-cortex excitability (84), and synaptic and cortical map plasticity have been documented using fMRI (75).

TMS studies have also indicated that action observation alone is able to drive reorganization in the primary motor cortex, strengthening the motor memory of observed actions among young (135) and elderly subjects (mean ages: 34 and 65 years, respectively) (98) and among chronically brain-damaged patients (84). Additionally, a study reported positive effects on gesture imitation of anodal transcranial direct current stimulation (tDCS) on the left parietal compared to sham tDCS, supporting the view that apraxia disorders in Parkinson (136) and in brain left damaged patients (51) can be improved by stimulating distinct structures.

A second factor to consider is the *temporal stage of the illness*. The neural substrates of action production and comprehension could be associated with different physiological mechanisms at different temporal stages of apraxia. Frontal and parietal areas may become temporarily inactive because of cerebral edema and intracranial hypertension, hemodynamic signs of ischemic penumbra, or local inflammatory effects in acute but not chronic stages of apraxia (137). Different studies report that during early periods (including an acute four-week, post-onset phase), impaired gesture recognition may be associated with left frontal–lobe and basal-ganglia lesions (138), whereas in the chronic stages of the illness, these deficits can be associated with left-parietal lesions (32, 37).

In practice, transitory effects such as the inability to mimic actions from visual cues are often observed in apraxia's early stages. If so, an observation intervention in early therapy may be inefficacy.

During later apraxia stages, a close overlap of the networks underlying observation and execution, as indicated by advanced neuroimaging and the lesion locations studies in patients, are helpful in identifying patient in which observative approach is potentially useful. Observation therapy associated with adaptive neurophysiological and neurometabolic changes can be conducted even several years after stroke onset. A session of 4 weeks of active, 18 days-cycle visual/motor training has been found to significantly enhance motor function, with increases in the activity of specific motor areas that possess mirror properties (75). Massed, high-frequency rehabilitative training (300–1,000 daily repetitions) is needed to elicit minimal neural reorganization (63). These increases in cortical activity during both action observation and execution also tend to be present in the hemispheres (139, 140) close to and far from the lesion site.

A third possible factor to consider is that the failure to link perceptual and motor representations in apraxia treatment may be *an effect of infarct size*; larger lesions are more likely to include front parietal injury and may not benefit from observation treatment. Indeed, improvements in imitation (reproduction off-line of the observed gesture) in patients with apraxia are influenced by the size of the parietal lesion (51): the larger the left parietal damage, the smaller the tDCS treatment-related improvement. When a functional system is completely damaged, however, recovery is achieved largely by process of substitution and may depend on the implicit engagement of neural systems to take over the functions of the damaged areas (141).

Whereas, some systems may constitute the sites of gesture performance, others may reduce the impact of deficits (142) by stimulating coupled visual knowledge mechanisms (98). The integrity of both the frontal and parietal cortices might be crucial for re-learning as a result of motor mirroring. Nonetheless, non-injured cortical areas could also trigger additional, independent internal mechanisms that support but are not necessary for guiding the motor system to match vision with motor routines (143, 144). Studies on the neural representations of motor skills based on observations of the motor cortex of macaque monkeys (145) and humans (146) provide empirical support for such an alternative system. These studies suggest that congruent activity during action execution/observation occurs even outside the canonical "mirror area," representing a potential general property of the motor system. Targeting interventions on the basis of specific brain structures intact and damaged that could mediate the effects of training is an important future challenge in cognitive neurorehabilitation.

CONCLUSION

While research on the relationship between observed and executed actions in apraxia neurorehabilitation has a short history, it has already provided insights about the positive effect of a visual-motor training. The observation of actions through a process of visual retrieval may help in the selection of the most probable action, providing a powerful tool for overcoming intentional motor-gestural difficulties (55). Moreover, tailored interventions based on individual's ability to acquire new (or relearn old) motor-memory traces through multisensory [i.e., auditory (35, 147), olfactory (148, 149), and tactile (150–155)] feedback may be the most promising approach for a normal temporal integration action (156, 157). Multisensory stimulation can activate multiple cortical brain structures, inducing cortical reorganization and modulating motor cortical excitability for the stimulated afferents (158, 159). Results are encouraging, but it is important to emphasize that this hypothesis does not imply that all deficits in apraxia can be treated by action observation therapy. Rather, we believe that action observation might be a therapeutic option for improving praxis function among certain specific typologies of patients.

AUTHOR CONTRIBUTIONS

MP: study concept and design, manuscript development, and writing. GG: contributed to the writing of the manuscript.

REFERENCES

1. Leiguarda RC, Marsden CD. Limb apraxias: higher-order disorders of sensorimotor integration. *Brain.* (2000) 123(Pt 5):860–79. doi: 10.1093/brain/123.5.860
2. Haaland KY, Harrington DL, Knight RT. Neural representations of skilled movement. *Brain.* (2000) 123(Pt 11):2306–13. doi: 10.1093/brain/123.11.2306
3. Rothi LJ, Heilman KM. Acquisition and retention of gestures by apraxic patients. *Brain Cogn.* (1984) 3:426–37. doi: 10.1016/0278-2626(84)90032-0

4. Petreska B, Adriani M, Blanke O, Billard AG. Apraxia: a review. *Prog Brain Res.* (2007) 164:61–83. doi: 10.1016/S0079-6123(07)64004-7
5. Wheaton LA, Hallett M. Ideomotor apraxia: a review. *J Neurol Sci.* (2007) 260:1–10. doi: 10.1016/j.jns.2007.04.014
6. Nobusako S, Ishibashi R, Takamura Y, Oda E, Tanigashira Y, Kouno M, et al. Distortion of visuo-motor temporal integration in apraxia: evidence from delayed visual feedback detection tasks and voxel-based lesion-symptom mapping. *Front Neurol.* (2018) 9:709. doi: 10.3389/fneur.2018.00709
7. Foundas AL, Macauley BL, Raymer AM, Maher LM, Heilman KM, Gonzalez Rothi LJ. Ecological implications of limb apraxia: evidence from mealtime behavior. *J Int Neuropsychol Soc.* (1995) 1:62–6. doi: 10.1017/S1355617700000114
8. Hanna-Pladdy B, Heilman KM, Foundas AL. Ecological implications of ideomotor apraxia: evidence from physical activities of daily living. *Neurology.* (2003) 60:487–90. doi: 10.1212/WNL.60.3.487
9. Goldenberg G, Hagmann J. Therapy of activities of daily living in patients with apraxia. *Neuropsychol Rehabil.* (1998) 8:123–41. doi: 10.1080/713755559
10. van Heugten CM, Dekker J, Deelman BG, Stehmann-Saris JC, Kinebanian A. Rehabilitation of stroke patients with apraxia: the role of additional cognitive and motor impairments. *Disabil Rehabil.* (2000) 22:547–54. doi: 10.1080/096382800416797
11. Sunderland A, Walker CM, Walker MF. Action errors and dressing disability after stroke: an ecological approach to neuropsychological assessment and intervention. *Neuropsychol Rehabil.* (2006) 16:666–83. doi: 10.1080/09602010500204385
12. Borod JC, Fitzpatrick PM, Helm-Estabrooks N, Goodglass H. The relationship between limb apraxia and the spontaneous use of communicative gesture in aphasia. *Brain Cogn.* (1989) 10:121–31. doi: 10.1016/0278-2626(89)90079-1
13. Tabaki NE, Vikelis M, Besmertis L, Vemmos K, Stathis P, Mitsikostas DD. Apraxia related with subcortical lesions due to cerebrovascular disease. *Acta Neurol Scand.* (2010) 122:9–14. doi: 10.1111/j.1600-0404.2009.01224.x
14. Saeki S, Ogata H, Okubo T, Takahashi K, Hoshuyama T. Factors influencing return to work after stroke in Japan. *Stroke.* (1993) 24:1182–5. doi: 10.1161/01.STR.24.8.1182
15. Zwinkels A, Geusgens C, van de Sande P, Van Heugten C. Assessment of apraxia: inter-rater reliability of a new apraxia test, association between apraxia and other cognitive deficits and prevalence of apraxia in a rehabilitation setting. *Clin Rehabil.* (2004) 18:819–27. doi: 10.1191/0269215504cr816oa
16. Hodges JR, Bozeat S, Lambon Ralph MA, Patterson K, Spatt J. The role of conceptual knowledge in object use evidence from semantic dementia. *Brain.* (2000) 123:1913–25. doi: 10.1093/brain/123.9.1913
17. Holl AK, Ille R, Wilkinson L, Otti DV, Hödl E, Herranhof B, et al. Impaired ideomotor limb apraxia in cortical and subcortical dementia: a comparison of Alzheimer's and Huntington's disease. *Neurodegener Dis.* (2011) 8:208–15. doi: 10.1159/000322230
18. Nelissen N, Pazzaglia M, Vandenbulcke M, Sunaert S, Fannes K, Dupont P, et al. Gesture discrimination in primary progressive aphasia: the intersection between gesture and language processing pathways. *J Neurosci.* (2010) 30:6334–41. doi: 10.1523/JNEUROSCI.0321-10.2010
19. Cantagallo A, Maini M, Rumiati RI. The cognitive rehabilitation of limb apraxia in patients with stroke. *Neuropsychol Rehabil.* (2012) 22:473–88. doi: 10.1080/09602011.2012.658317
20. Worthington A. Treatments and technologies in the rehabilitation of apraxia and action disorganisation syndrome: a review. *Neurorehabilitation.* (2016) 39:163–74. doi: 10.3233/NRE-161348
21. French B, Thomas LH, Coupe J, McMahon NE, Connell L, Harrison J, et al. Repetitive task training for improving functional ability after stroke. *Cochrane Database Syst Rev.* (2007) 11:CD006073. doi: 10.1002/14651858.CD006073.pub2
22. Smania N, Aglioti SM, Girardi F, Tinazzi M, Fiaschi A, Cosentino A, et al. Rehabilitation of limb apraxia improves daily life activities in patients with stroke. *Neurology.* (2006) 67:2050–2. doi: 10.1212/01.wnl.0000247279.63483.1f
23. Buxbaum LJ, Haaland KY, Hallett M, Wheaton L, Heilman KM, Rodriguez A, et al. Treatment of limb apraxia: moving forward to improved action. *Am J Phys Med Rehabil.* (2008) 87:149–61. doi: 10.1097/PHM.0b013e31815e6727
24. Etcharry-Bouyx F, Le Gall D, Jarry C, Osiurak F. Gestural apraxia. *Rev Neurol.* (2017) 173:430–9. doi: 10.1016/j.neurol.2017.07.005
25. Wang L, Goodglass H. Pantomime, praxis, and aphasia. *Brain Lang.* (1992) 42:402–18. doi: 10.1016/0093-934X(92)90076-Q
26. Goldenberg G. Matching and imitation of hand and finger postures in patients with damage in the left or right hemispheres. *Neuropsychologia.* (1999) 37:559–66. doi: 10.1016/S0028-3932(98)00111-0
27. Hommel B, Musseler J, Aschersleben G, Prinz W. The Theory of Event Coding (TEC): a framework for perception and action planning. *Behav Brain Sci.* (2001) 24:849–78. doi: 10.1017/S0140525X01000103
28. Schutz-Bosbach S, Prinz W. Perceptual resonance: action-induced modulation of perception. *Trends Cogn Sci.* (2007) 11:349–55. doi: 10.1016/j.tics.2007.06.005
29. Sunderland A, Sluman SM. Ideomotor apraxia, visuomotor control and the explicit representation of posture. *Neuropsychologia.* (2000) 38:923–34. doi: 10.1016/S0028-3932(00)00021-X
30. Pazzaglia M, Smania N, Corato E, Aglioti SM. Neural underpinnings of gesture discrimination in patients with limb apraxia. *J Neurosci.* (2008) 28:3030–41. doi: 10.1523/JNEUROSCI.5748-07.2008
31. Heilman KM, Rothi LJ, Valenstein E. Two forms of ideomotor apraxia. *Neurology.* (1982) 32:342–6. doi: 10.1212/WNL.32.4.342
32. Kalenine S, Buxbaum LJ, Coslett HB. Critical brain regions for action recognition: lesion symptom mapping in left hemisphere stroke. *Brain.* (2010) 133:3269–80. doi: 10.1093/brain/awq210
33. Rothi LJ, Heilman KM, Watson RT. Pantomime comprehension and ideomotor apraxia. *J Neurol Neurosurg Psychiatry.* (1985) 48:207–10. doi: 10.1136/jnnp.48.3.207
34. Weiss PH, Rahbari NN, Hesse MD, Fink GR. Deficient sequencing of pantomimes in apraxia. *Neurology.* (2008) 70:834–40. doi: 10.1212/01.wnl.0000297513.78593.dc
35. Pazzaglia M, Pizzamiglio L, Pes E, Aglioti SM. The sound of actions in apraxia. *Curr Biol.* (2008) 18:1766–72. doi: 10.1016/j.cub.2008.09.061
36. Mutha PK, Stapp LH, Sainburg RL, Haaland KY. Motor adaptation deficits in ideomotor apraxia. *J Int Neuropsychol Soc.* (2017) 23:139–49. doi: 10.1017/S135561771600120X
37. Fontana AP, Kilner JM, Rodrigues EC, Joffily M, Nighoghossian N, Vargas CD, et al. Role of the parietal cortex in predicting incoming actions. *NeuroImage.* (2012) 59:556–64. doi: 10.1016/j.neuroimage.2011.07.046
38. Pazzaglia M. Does what you hear predict what you will do and say? *Behav Brain Sci.* (2013) 36:370–1. doi: 10.1017/S0140525X12002804
39. Pazzaglia M. Impact commentaries. Action discrimination: impact of apraxia. *J Neurol Neurosurg Psychiatry.* (2013) 84:477–8. doi: 10.1136/jnnp-2012-304817
40. Buxbaum LJ, Randerath J. Limb apraxia and the left parietal lobe. *Handb Clin Neurol.* (2018) 151:349–63. doi: 10.1016/B978-0-444-63622-5.00017-6
41. Pazzaglia M, Galli G. Translating novel findings of perceptual-motor codes into the neuro-rehabilitation of movement disorders. *Front Behav Neurosci.* 9:222. doi: 10.3389/fnbeh.2015.00222
42. Garrison KA, Winstein CJ, Aziz-Zadeh L. The mirror neuron system: a neural substrate for methods in stroke rehabilitation. *Neurorehabil Neural Repair.* (2010) 24:404–12. doi: 10.1177/1545968309354536
43. Small SL, Buccino G, Solodkin A. The mirror neuron system and treatment of stroke. *Dev Psychobiol.* (2012) 54:293–310. doi: 10.1002/dev.20504
44. Bartolo A, Cubelli R, Della Sala S. Cognitive approach to the assessment of limb apraxia. *Clin Neuropsychol.* (2008) 22:27–45. doi: 10.1080/13854040601139310
45. Smania N, Girardi F, Domenicali C, Lora E, Aglioti S. The rehabilitation of limb apraxia: a study in left-brain-damaged patients. *Arch Phys Med Rehabil.* (2000) 81:379–88. doi: 10.1053/mr.2000.6921
46. Goldenberg G, Daumuller M, Hagmann S. Assessment and therapy of complex activities of daily living in apraxia. *Neuropsychol Rehabil.* (2001) 11:147–69. doi: 10.1080/09602010042000204
47. van Heugten CM, Dekker J, Deelman BG, van Dijk AJ, Stehmann-Saris JC, Kinebanian A. Outcome of strategy training in stroke patients with apraxia: a phase II study. *Clin Rehabil.* (1998) 12:294–303. doi: 10.1191/026921598674468328
48. Donkervoort M, Dekker J, Stehmann-Saris FC, Deeolman BG. Efficacy of strategy training in left hemisphere stroke patients with apraxia:

a randomised clinical trial. *Neuropsychol Rehabil.* (2001) 11:549–66. doi: 10.1080/09602010143000093
49. Geusgens CA, van Heugten CM, Cooijmans JP, Jolles J, van den Heuvel WJ. Transfer effects of a cognitive strategy training for stroke patients with apraxia. *J Clin Exp Neuropsychol.* (2007) 29:831–41. doi: 10.1080/13803390601125971
50. Geusgens C, van Heugten C, Donkervoort M, van den Ende E, Jolles J, van den Heuvel W. Transfer of training effects in stroke patients with apraxia: an exploratory study. *Neuropsychol Rehabil.* (2006) 16:213–29. doi: 10.1080/09602010500172350
51. Bolognini N, Convento S, Banco E, Mattioli F, Tesio L, Vallar G. Improving ideomotor limb apraxia by electrical stimulation of the left posterior parietal cortex. *Brain.* (2015) 138:428–39. doi: 10.1093/brain/awu343
52. Buccino G. Action observation treatment: a novel tool in neurorehabilitation. *Philos Trans R Soc Lond Ser B Biol Sci.* (2014) 369:20130185. doi: 10.1098/rstb.2013.0185
53. Oouchida Y, Suzuki E, Aizu N, Takeuchi N, Izumi SI. Applications of observational learning in neurorehabilitation. *Int J Phys Med Rehabil.* (2013) 1:146. doi: 10.4172/2329-9096.1000146
54. Rothi LJ, Heilman KM. *Apraxia, the Neuropsychology of Action.* Hove: Psychology Press (1997).
55. Pazzaglia M, Galli G. Loss of agency in apraxia. *Front Hum Neurosci.* (2014) 8:751. doi: 10.3389/fnhum.2014.00751
56. Badets A, Blandin Y, Wright DL, Shea CH. Error detection processes during observational learning. *Res Q Exerc Sport.* (2006) 77:177–84. doi: 10.1080/02701367.2006.10599352
57. Badets A, Blandin Y, Shea CH. Intention in motor learning through observation. *Q J Exp Psychol.* (2006) 59:377–86. doi: 10.1080/02724980443000773
58. Heyes CM, Foster CL. Motor learning by observation: evidence from a serial reaction time task. *Q J Exp Psychol.* (2002) 55:593–607. doi: 10.1080/02724980143000389
59. Buchanan JJ, Dean NJ. Specificity in practice benefits learning in novice models and variability in demonstration benefits observational practice. *Psychol Res.* (2010) 74:313–26. doi: 10.1007/s00426-009-0254-y
60. Hecht H, Vogt S, Prinz W. Motor learning enhances perceptual judgment: a case for action-perception transfer. *Psychol Res.* (2001) 65:3–14. doi: 10.1007/s004260000043
61. Casile A, Giese MA. Nonvisual motor training influences biological motion perception. *Curr Biol.* (2006) 16:69–74. doi: 10.1016/j.cub.2005.10.071
62. Rosenkranz K, Williamon A, Rothwell JC. Motorcortical excitability and synaptic plasticity is enhanced in professional musicians. *J Neurosci.* (2007) 27:5200–6. doi: 10.1523/JNEUROSCI.0836-07.2007
63. Kleim JA, Hogg TM, VandenBerg PM, Cooper NR, Bruneau R, Remple M. Cortical synaptogenesis and motor map reorganization occur during late, but not early, phase of motor skill learning. *J Neurosci.* (2004) 24:628–33. doi: 10.1523/JNEUROSCI.3440-03.2004
64. Sale P, Franceschini M. Action observation and mirror neuron network: a tool for motor stroke rehabilitation. *Eur J Phys Rehabil Med.* (2012) 48:313–8.
65. Franceschini M, Ceravolo MG, Agosti M, Cavallini P, Bonassi S, Dall'Armi V, et al. Clinical relevance of action observation in upper-limb stroke rehabilitation: a possible role in recovery of functional dexterity. A randomized clinical trial. *Neurorehabil Neural Repair.* (2012) 26:456–62. doi: 10.1177/1545968311427406
66. Sale P, Ceravolo MG, Franceschini M. Action observation therapy in the subacute phase promotes dexterity recovery in right-hemisphere stroke patients. *Biomed Res Int.* (2014) 2014:457538. doi: 10.1155/2014/457538
67. Park HR, Kim JM, Lee MK, Oh DW. Clinical feasibility of action observation training for walking function of patients with post-stroke hemiparesis: a randomized controlled trial. *Clin Rehabil.* (2014) 28:794–803. doi: 10.1177/0269215514523145
68. Bang DH, Shin WS, Kim SY, Choi JD. The effects of action observational training on walking ability in chronic stroke patients: a double-blind randomized controlled trial. *Clin Rehabil.* (2013) 27:1118–25. doi: 10.1177/0269215513501528
69. Kim SS, Kim TH, Lee BH. Effects of action observational training on cerebral hemodynamic changes of stroke survivors: a fTCD study. *J Phys Ther Sci.* (2014) 26:331–4. doi: 10.1589/jpts.26.331
70. Bonifazi S, Tomaiuolo F, Altoè G, Ceravolo MG, Provinciali L, Marangolo P. Action observation as a useful approach for enhancing recovery of verb production: new evidence from aphasia. *Eur J Phys Rehabil Med.* (2013) 49:473–81.
71. Marangon M, Priftis K, Fedeli M, Masiero S, Tonin P, Piccione F. Lateralization of motor cortex excitability in stroke patients during action observation: a TMS study. *Biomed Res. Int.* (2014) 2014:251041. doi: 10.1155/2014/251041
72. Brunner IC, Skouen JS, Ersland L, Gruner R. Plasticity and response to action observation: a longitudinal FMRI study of potential mirror neurons in patients with subacute stroke. *Neurorehabil Neural Repair.* (2014) 28:874–84. doi: 10.1177/1545968314527350
73. Ertelt D, Binkofski F. Action observation as a tool for neurorehabilitation to moderate motor deficits and aphasia following stroke. *Neural Regener Res.* (2012) 7:2063–74. doi: 10.3969/j.issn.1673-5374.2012.26.008
74. Ertelt D, Hemmelmann C, Dettmers C, Ziegler A, Binkofski F. Observation and execution of upper-limb movements as a tool for rehabilitation of motor deficits in paretic stroke patients: protocol of a randomized clinical trial. *BMC Neurol.* (2012) 12:42. doi: 10.1186/1471-2377-12-42
75. Ertelt D, Small S, Solodkin A, Dettmers C, McNamara A, Binkofski F, et al. Action observation has a positive impact on rehabilitation of motor deficits after stroke. *Neuroimage.* (2007) 36(Suppl. 2):T164–73. doi: 10.1016/j.neuroimage.2007.03.043
76. Franceschini M, Agosti M, Cantagallo A, Sale P, Mancuso M, Buccino G. Mirror neurons: action observation treatment as a tool in stroke rehabilitation. *Eur J Phys Rehabil Med.* (2010) 46:517–23.
77. Kim E, Kim K. Effect of purposeful action observation on upper extremity function in stroke patients. *J Phys Ther Sci.* (2015) 27:2867–9. doi: 10.1589/jpts.27.2867
78. Harmsen WJ, Bussmann JB, Selles RW, Hurkmans HL, Ribbers GM. A mirror therapy-based action observation protocol to improve motor learning after stroke. *Neurorehabil Neural Repair.* (2015) 29:509–16. doi: 10.1177/1545968314558598
79. Dettmers C, Nedelko V, Hassa T, Starrost K, Schoenfeld MA. "Video Therapy": promoting hand function after stroke by action observation training – a pilot randomized controlled trial. *Int J Phys Med Rehabil.* (2014) 2:189. doi: 10.4172/2329-9096.1000189
80. Zhu M-H, Wang J, Gu X-D, Shi M-F, Zeng M, Wang C-Y, et al. Effect of action observation therapy on daily activities and motor recovery in stroke patients. *Int J Nurs Sci.* (2015) 2:279–82. doi: 10.1016/j.ijnss.2015.08.006
81. Kim C, Bang D. Action observation training enhances upper extremity function in subacute stroke survivor with moderate impairment: a double-blind, randomized controlled pilot trial. *J Korean Soc Phys Med.* (2016) 11:133–40. doi: 10.13066/kspm.2016.11.1.133
82. Kuk EJ, Kim JM, Oh DW, Hwang HJ. Effects of action observation therapy on hand dexterity and EEG-based cortical activation patterns in patients with post-stroke hemiparesis. *Top Stroke Rehabil.* (2016) 23:318–25. doi: 10.1080/10749357.2016.1157972
83. Fu J, Zeng M, Shen F, Cui Y, Zhu M, Gu X, et al. Effects of action observation therapy on upper extremity function, daily activities and motion evoked potential in cerebral infarction patients. *Medicine.* (2017) 96:e8080. doi: 10.1097/MD.0000000000008080
84. Celnik P, Webster B, Glasser DM, Cohen LG. Effects of action observation on physical training after stroke. *Stroke.* (2008) 39:1814–20. doi: 10.1161/STROKEAHA.107.508184
85. Cowles T, Clark A, Mares K, Peryer G, Stuck R, Pomeroy V. Observation-to-imitate plus practice could add little to physical therapy benefits within 31 days of stroke: translational randomized controlled trial. *Neurorehabil Neural Repair.* (2013) 27:173–82. doi: 10.1177/1545968312452470
86. Lee D, Roh H, Park J, Lee S, Han S. Drinking behavior training for stroke patients using action observation and practice of upper limb function. *J Phys Ther Sci.* (2013) 25:611–4. doi: 10.1589/jpts.25.611
87. Pelosin E, Bove M, Ruggeri P, Avanzino L, Abbruzzese G. Reduction of bradykinesia of finger movements by a single session of action observation in Parkinson disease. *Neurorehabil Neural Repair.* (2013) 27:552–60. doi: 10.1177/1545968312471905
88. Buccino G, Gatti R, Giusti MC, Negrotti A, Rossi A, Calzetti S, et al. Action observation treatment improves autonomy in daily activities in Parkinson's

disease patients: results from a pilot study. *Mov Disord.* (2011) 26:1963–4. doi: 10.1002/mds.23745
89. Esculier JF, Vaudrin J, Tremblay LE. Corticomotor excitability in Parkinson's disease during observation, imagery and imitation of action: effects of rehabilitation using wii fit and comparison to healthy controls. *J Parkinson's Dis.* (2014) 4:67–75. doi: 10.3233/JPD-130212
90. Pelosin E, Avanzino L, Bove M, Stramesi P, Nieuwboer A, Abbruzzese G. Action observation improves freezing of gait in patients with Parkinson's disease. *Neurorehabil Neural Repair.* (2010) 24:746–52. doi: 10.1177/1545968310368685
91. Castiello U, Ansuini C, Bulgheroni M, Scaravilli T, Nicoletti R. Visuomotor priming effects in Parkinson's disease patients depend on the match between the observed and the executed action. *Neuropsychologia.* (2009) 47:835–42. doi: 10.1016/j.neuropsychologia.2008.12.016
92. Tremblay F, Leonard G, Tremblay L. Corticomotor facilitation associated with observation and imagery of hand actions is impaired in Parkinson's disease. *Exp Brain Res.* (2008) 185:249–57. doi: 10.1007/s00221-007-1150-6
93. Sgandurra G, Ferrari A, Cossu G, Guzzetta A, Fogassi L, Cioni G. Randomized trial of observation and execution of upper extremity actions versus action alone in children with unilateral cerebral palsy. *Neurorehabil Neural Repair.* (2013) 27:808–15. doi: 10.1177/1545968313497101
94. Sgandurra G, Ferrari A, Cossu G, Guzzetta A, Biagi L, Tosetti M, et al. Upper limb children action-observation training (UP-CAT): a randomised controlled trial in hemiplegic cerebral palsy. *BMC Neurol.* (2011) 11:80. doi: 10.1186/1471-2377-11-80
95. Buccino G, Arisi D, Gough P, Aprile D, Ferri C, Serotti L, et al. Improving upper limb motor functions through action observation treatment: a pilot study in children with cerebral palsy. *Dev Med Child Neurol.* (2012) 54:822–8. doi: 10.1111/j.1469-8749.2012.04334.x
96. Kim JY, Kim JM, Ko EY. The effect of the action observation physical training on the upper extremity function in children with cerebral palsy. *J Exerc Rehabil.* (2014) 10:176–83. doi: 10.12965/jer.140114
97. Kim JH, Lee BH. Action observation training for functional activities after stroke: a pilot randomized controlled trial. *Neurorehabilitation.* (2013) 33:565–74. doi: 10.3233/NRE-130991
98. Celnik P, Stefan K, Hummel F, Duque J, Classen J, Cohen LG. Encoding a motor memory in the older adult by action observation. *Neuroimage.* (2006) 29:677–84. doi: 10.1016/j.neuroimage.2005.07.039
99. Liepert J, Greiner J, Dettmers C. Motor excitability changes during action observation in stroke patients. *J Rehabil Med.* (2014) 46:400–5. doi: 10.2340/16501977-1276
100. Fogassi L, Ferrari PF, Gesierich B, Rozzi S, Chersi F, Rizzolatti G. Parietal lobe: from action organization to intention understanding. *Science.* (2005) 308:662–7. doi: 10.1126/science.1106138
101. Gallese V, Fadiga L, Fogassi L, Rizzolatti G. Action recognition in the premotor cortex. *Brain.* (1996) 119 (Pt 2):593–609. doi: 10.1093/brain/119.2.593
102. Rizzolatti G, Craighero L. The mirror-neuron system. *Ann Rev Neurosci.* (2004) 27:169–92. doi: 10.1146/annurev.neuro.27.070203.144230
103. Kilner JM. More than one pathway to action understanding. *Trends Cogn Sci.* (2011) 15:352–7. doi: 10.1016/j.tics.2011.06.005
104. Hermsdorfer J, Li Y, Randerath J, Roby-Brami A, Goldenberg G. Tool use kinematics across different modes of execution. Implications for action representation and apraxia. *Cortex.* (2013) 49:184–99. doi: 10.1016/j.cortex.2011.10.010
105. Leiguarda RC, Merello M, Nouzeilles MI, Balej J, Rivero A, Nogués M. Limb-kinetic apraxia in corticobasal degeneration: clinical and kinematic features. *Mov Disord.* (2003) 18:49–59. doi: 10.1002/mds.10303
106. Sirigu A, Cohen L, Duhamel JR, Pillon B, Dubois B, Agid Y. A selective impairment of hand posture for object utilization in apraxia. *Cortex.* (1995) 31:41–55. doi: 10.1016/S0010-9452(13)80104-9
107. Sirigu A, Duhamel JR, Cohen L, Pillon B, Dubois B, Agid Y. The mental representation of hand movements after parietal cortex damage. *Science.* (1996) 273:1564–8. doi: 10.1126/science.273.5281.1564
108. Grezes J, Decety J. Functional anatomy of execution, mental simulation, observation, and verb generation of actions: a meta-analysis. *Hum Brain Mapp.* (2001) 12:1–19. doi: 10.1002/1097-0193(200101)12:1<1::AID-HBM10>3.0.CO;2-V
109. Grafton ST. Embodied cognition and the simulation of action to understand others. *Ann N Y Acad Sci.* (2009) 1156:97–117. doi: 10.1111/j.1749-6632.2009.04425.x
110. Iacoboni M, Woods RP, Brass M, Bekkering H, Mazziotta JC, Rizzolatti G. Cortical mechanisms of human imitation. *Science.* (1999) 286:2526–8. doi: 10.1126/science.286.5449.2526
111. Flanagan JR, Johansson RS. Action plans used in action observation. *Nature.* (2003) 424:769–71. doi: 10.1038/nature01861
112. Buccino G, Binkofski F, Riggio L. The mirror neuron system and action recognition. *Brain Lang.* (2004) 89:370–6. doi: 10.1016/S0093-934X(03)00356-0
113. Buxbaum LJ, Shapiro AD, Coslett HB. Critical brain regions for tool-related and imitative actions: a componential analysis. *Brain.* (2014) 137:1971–85. doi: 10.1093/brain/awu111
114. Goldenberg G, Hermsdorfer J, Glindemann R, Rorden C, Karnath HO. Pantomime of tool use depends on integrity of left inferior frontal cortex. *Cereb Cortex.* (2007) 17:2769–76. doi: 10.1093/cercor/bhm004
115. Mengotti P, Corradi-Dell'Acqua C, Negri GA, Ukmar M, Pesavento V, Rumiati RI. Selective imitation impairments differentially interact with language processing. *Brain.* (2013). 136:2602–18. doi: 10.1093/brain/awt194
116. Weiss PH, Ubben SD, Kaesberg S, Kalbe E, Kessler J, Liebig T, et al. Where language meets meaningful action: a combined behavior and lesion analysis of aphasia and apraxia. *Brain Struct Funct.* (2016) 221:563–76. doi: 10.1007/s00429-014-0925-3
117. Hoeren M, Kümmerer D, Bormann T, Beume L, Ludwig VM, Vry MS, et al. Neural bases of imitation and pantomime in acute stroke patients: distinct streams for praxis. *Brain.* (2014) 137:2796–810. doi: 10.1093/brain/awu203
118. De Renzi E, Lucchelli F. Ideational apraxia. *Brain.* (1988) 111(Pt 5):1173–85. doi: 10.1093/brain/111.5.1173
119. Bizzozero I, Costato D, Sala SD, Papagno C, Spinnler H, Venneri A. Upper and lower face apraxia: role of the right hemisphere. *Brain.* (2000) 123(Pt 11):2213–30. doi: 10.1093/brain/123.11.2213
120. Rothi LJ, Mack L, Heilman KM. Pantomime agnosia. *J Neurol Neurosurg Psychiatry.* (1986) 49:451–4. doi: 10.1136/jnnp.49.4.451
121. Cubelli R, Marchetti C, Boscolo G, Della Sala S. Cognition in action: testing a model of limb apraxia. *Brain Cogn.* (2000) 44:144–65. doi: 10.1006/brcg.2000.1226
122. Bartolo A, Cubelli R, Della Sala S, Drei S, Marchetti C. Double dissociation between meaningful and meaningless gesture reproduction in apraxia. *Cortex.* (2001) 37:696–9. doi: 10.1016/S0010-9452(08)70617-8
123. Negri GA, Rumiati RI, Zadini A, Ukmar M, Mahon BZ, Caramazza A. What is the role of motor simulation in action and object recognition? Evidence from apraxia. *Cogn Neuropsychol.* (2007) 24:795–816. doi: 10.1080/02643290701707412
124. Aglioti SM, Pazzaglia M. Representing actions through their sound. *Exp Brain Res.* (2010) 206:141–51. doi: 10.1007/s00221-010-2344-x
125. Mahon BZ, Caramazza A. The orchestration of the sensory-motor systems: clues from neuropsychology. *Cogn Neuropsychol.* (2005) 22:480–94. doi: 10.1080/02643290442000446
126. Buxbaum LJ, Kalenine S. Action knowledge, visuomotor activation, and embodiment in the two action systems. *Ann N Y Acad Sci.* (2010) 1191:201–18. doi: 10.1111/j.1749-6632.2010.05447.x
127. Binkofski F, Buxbaum LJ. Two action systems in the human brain. *Brain Lang.* (2013) 127:222–9. doi: 10.1016/j.bandl.2012.07.007
128. Pazzaglia M, Zantedeschi M. Plasticity and awareness of bodily distortion. *Neural Plast.* (2016) 2016:9834340. doi: 10.1155/2016/9834340
129. Buccino G, Molinaro A, Ambrosi C, Arisi D, Mascaro L, Pinardi C, et al. Action observation treatment improves upper limb motor functions in children with cerebral palsy: a combined clinical and brain imaging study. *Neural Plast.* (2018) 2018:4843985. doi: 10.1155/2018/4843985
130. Hanna-Pladdy B, Heilman KM, Foundas AL. Cortical and subcortical contributions to ideomotor apraxia: analysis of task demands and error types. *Brain.* (2001) 124:2513–27. doi: 10.1093/brain/124.12.2513
131. Moro V, Urgesi C, Pernigo S, Lanteri P, Pazzaglia M, Aglioti SM. The neural basis of body form and body action agnosia. *Neuron.* (2008) 60:235–46. doi: 10.1016/j.neuron.2008.09.022
132. Halsband U, Schmitt J, Weyers M, Binkofski F, Grützner G, Freund HJ.

Recognition and imitation of pantomimed motor acts after unilateral parietal and premotor lesions: a perspective on apraxia. *Neuropsychologia.* (2001) 39:200–16. doi: 10.1016/S0028-3932(00)00088-9

133. Hickok G. Eight problems for the mirror neuron theory of action understanding in monkeys and humans. *J Cogn Neurosci.* (2009) 21:1229–43. doi: 10.1162/jocn.2009.21189
134. Fogassi L, Luppino G. Motor functions of the parietal lobe. *Curr Opin Neurobiol.* (2005) 15:626–31. doi: 10.1016/j.conb.2005.10.015
135. Stefan K, Cohen LG, Duque J, Mazzocchio R, Celnik P, Sawaki L, et al. Formation of a motor memory by action observation. *J Neurosci.* (2005) 25:9339–46. doi: 10.1523/JNEUROSCI.2282-05.2005
136. Bianchi M, Cosseddu M, Cotelli M, Manenti R, Brambilla M, Rizzetti MC, et al. Left parietal cortex transcranial direct current stimulation enhances gesture processing in corticobasal syndrome. *Eur J Neurol.* (2015) 22:1317–22. doi: 10.1111/ene.12748
137. Baldwin KA, McCoy SL. Making a case for acute ischemic stroke. *J Pharm Pract.* (2010) 23:387–97. doi: 10.1177/0897190010372325
138. Ferro JM, Martins IP, Mariano G, Caldas AC. CT scan correlates of gesture recognition. *J Neurol Neurosurg Psychiatry.* (1983) 46:943–52. doi: 10.1136/jnnp.46.10.943
139. Catmur C, Gillmeister H, Bird G, Liepelt R, Brass M, Heyes C. Through the looking glass: counter-mirror activation following incompatible sensorimotor learning. *Eur J Neurosci.* (2008) 28:1208–15. doi: 10.1111/j.1460-9568.2008.06419.x
140. Gazzola V, Rizzolatti G, Wicker B, Keysers C. The anthropomorphic brain: the mirror neuron system responds to human and robotic actions. *Neuroimage.* (2007) 35:1674–84. doi: 10.1016/j.neuroimage.2007.02.003
141. Mattar AA, Gribble PL. Motor learning by observing. *Neuron.* (2005) 46:153–60. doi: 10.1016/j.neuron.2005.02.009
142. Buccino G, Solodkin A, Small SL. Functions of the mirror neuron system: implications for neurorehabilitation. *Cogn Behav Neurol.* (2006) 19:55–63. doi: 10.1097/00146965-200603000-00007
143. Dinstein I, Gardner JL, Jazayeri M, Heeger DJ. Executed and observed movements have different distributed representations in human aIPS. *J Neurosci.* (2008) 28:11231–9. doi: 10.1523/JNEUROSCI.3585-08.2008
144. Mahon BZ. Action recognition: is it a motor process? *Curr Biol.* (2008) 18:R1068–9. doi: 10.1016/j.cub.2008.10.001
145. Tkach D, Reimer J, Hatsopoulos NG. Congruent activity during action and action observation in motor cortex. *J Neurosci.* (2007) 27:13241–50. doi: 10.1523/JNEUROSCI.2895-07.2007
146. Brown LE, Wilson ET, Gribble PL. Repetitive transcranial magnetic stimulation to the primary motor cortex interferes with motor learning by observing. *J Cogn Neurosci.* (2009) 21:1013–22. doi: 10.1162/jocn.2009.21079
147. Pazzaglia M, Galli G, Lewis JW, Scivoletto G, Giannini AM, Molinari M. Embodying functionally relevant action sounds in patients with spinal cord injury. *Sci Rep.* (2018) 8:15641. doi: 10.1038/s41598-018-34133-z
148. Pazzaglia M. Body and odors: not just molecules, after all. *Curr Dir Psychol Sci.* (2015) 24:329–33. doi: 10.1177/0963721415575329
149. Aglioti SM, Pazzaglia M. Sounds and scents in (social) action. *Trends Cogn Sci.* (2011) 15:47–55. doi: 10.1016/j.tics.2010.12.003
150. Pazzaglia M, Galli G, Lucci G, Scivoletto G, Molinari M, Haggard P. Phantom limb sensations in the ear of a patient with a brachial plexus lesion. *Cortex.* (2018). doi: 10.1016/j.cortex.2018.08.020. [Epub ahead of print].
151. Pazzaglia M, Haggard P, Scivoletto G, Molinari M, Lenggenhager B. Pain and somatic sensation are transiently normalized by illusory body ownership in a patient with spinal cord injury. *Restor Neurol Neurosci.* (2016) 34:603–13. doi: 10.3233/RNN-150611
152. Costantini M, Bueti D, Pazzaglia M, Aglioti SM. Temporal dynamics of visuo-tactile extinction within and between hemispaces. *Neuropsychology.* (2007) 21:242–50. doi: 10.1037/0894-4105.21.2.242
153. Goldenberg G, Hentze S, Hermsdorfer J. The effect of tactile feedback on pantomime of tool use in apraxia. *Neurology.* (2004) 63:1863–7. doi: 10.1212/01.WNL.0000144283.38174.07
154. Pazzaglia M, Leemhuis E, Giannini AM, Haggard P. The Homuncular Jigsaw: investigations of phantom limb and body awareness following brachial plexus block or avulsion. *J Clin Med.* (2019) 8:E182. doi: 10.3390/jcm8020182
155. Pazzaglia M, Scivoletto G, Giannini AM, Leemhuis E. My hand in my ear: a phantom limb re-induced by the illusion of body ownership in a patient with a brachial plexus lesion. *Psychol Res.* (2019) 83:196–204. doi: 10.1007/s00426-018-1121-5
156. Galli G, Pazzaglia M. Commentary on: "the body social: an enactive approach to the self". A tool for merging bodily and social self in immobile individuals. *Front Psychol.* 6:305. doi: 10.3389/fpsyg.2015.00305
157. Lucci G, Pazzaglia M. Towards multiple interactions of inner and outer sensations in corporeal awareness. *Front Hum Neurosci.* (2015) 9:163. doi: 10.3389/fnhum.2015.00163
158. Cramer SC, Sur M, Dobkin BH, O'Brien C, Sanger TD, Trojanowski JQ, et al. Harnessing neuroplasticity for clinical applications. *Brain.* (2011) 134:1591–609. doi: 10.1093/brain/awr039
159. Law LLF, Fong KNK, Li RKF. Multisensory stimulation to promote upper extremity motor recovery in stroke: a pilot study. *Brit J Occup Ther.* (2018) 81:641–8. doi: 10.1177/0308022618770141

6

Effectiveness of Trigger Point Manual Treatrment on the Frequency, Intensity and Duration of Attacks in Primary Headaches

Luca Falsiroli Maistrello[1], Tommaso Geri[1], Silvia Gianola[2,3], Martina Zaninetti[1,4] and Marco Testa[1]*

[1] Department of Neuroscience, Rehabilitation, Ophthalmology, Genetics, Maternal and Child Health, University of Genova, Genoa, Italy, [2] Unit of Clinical Epidemiology, IRCCS Galeazzi Orthopaedic Institute, Milan, Italy, [3] Center of Biostatistics for Clinical Epidemiology, School of Medicine and Surgery, University of Milano-Bicocca, Monza, Italy, [4] UOC di Recupero e Rieducazione Funzionale, Ospedale Policlinico Borgo Roma, Azienda Ospedaliera Universitaria Integrata di Verona, Verona, Italy

Correspondence:
Tommaso Geri
tommaso.geri@gmail.com

Background: A variety of interventions has been proposed for symptomatology relief in primary headaches. Among these, manual trigger points (TrPs) treatment gains popularity, but its effects have not been investigated yet.

Objective: The aim was to establish the effectiveness of manual TrP compared to minimal active or no active interventions in terms of frequency, intensity, and duration of attacks in adult people with primary headaches.

Methods: We searched MEDLINE, COCHRANE, Web Of Science, and PEDro databases up to November 2017 for randomized controlled trials (RCTs). Two independent reviewers appraised the risk-of-bias (RoB) and the grading of recommendations, assessment, development, and evaluation (GRADE) to evaluate the overall quality of evidence.

Results: Seven RCTs that compared manual treatment vs minimal active intervention were included: 5 focused on tension-type headache (TTH) and 2 on Migraine (MH); 3 out of 7 RCTs had high RoB. Combined TTH and MH results show statistically significant reduction for all outcomes after treatment compared to controls, but the level of evidence was very low. Subgroup analysis showed a statistically significant reduction in attack frequency (no. of attacks per month) after treatment in TTH (MD −3.50; 95% CI from −4.91 to −2.09; 4 RCTs) and in MH (MD −1.92; 95% CI from −3.03 to −0.80; 2 RCTs). Pain intensity (0–100 scale) was reduced in TTH (MD −12.83; 95% CI from −19.49 to −6.17; 4 RCTs) and in MH (MD −13.60; 95% CI from −19.54 to −7.66; 2RCTs). Duration of attacks (hours) was reduced in TTH (MD −0.51; 95% CI from −0.97 to −0.04; 2 RCTs) and in MH (MD −10.68; 95% CI from −14.41 to −6.95; 1 RCT).

Conclusion: Manual TrPs treatment of head and neck muscles may reduce frequency, intensity, and duration of attacks in TTH and MH, but the quality of evidence according to GRADE approach was very low for the presence of few studies, high RoB, and imprecision of results.

Keywords: migraine disorders, tension-type headache, cluster headache, trigger points, myofascial pain syndromes, physical therapy specialty

INTRODUCTION

Headaches are disabling disorders that decrease the health-related quality of life. The mean global annual prevalence of headaches in adults is around 46% (1), while in Europe the gender adjusted 1-year prevalence for any type of headache is 79% (2) with an estimated economic burden of €173 billion yearly among adults aged 18–65 years (3). As in other European countries, headaches in Italy are highly prevalent and associated with significant personal impact and important implications for health policy (4). Therapeutic management option is represented by pharmacological or non-pharmacological interventions (5). Pharmacological treatments are considered the main interventions even though the elevated frequency of attacks increases the risk of drugs' abuse (6). Accordingly, the use of non-pharmacological treatments in the management of primary headaches has the aim of reducing the drugs' consumption, their side effects, and the interaction with the other drugs used for comorbidities (7–9). The recommendation of the European Federation of Neurological Societies guideline indicates that the use of non-pharmacologic therapies, having less side effects than pharmacological therapies (10, 11) may constitute a valid therapeutic option for headaches sufferers, despite their limited scientific basis (12), and the lack of research on the effectiveness of physical therapy treatments.

Tension-type (TTH), migraine (MH), and cluster headache (CH) are considered the three most prevalent primary headaches according to the classification proposed by the International Headache Society (13) that established the clinical criteria useful in the discrimination of headache's attacks. Hence, distinct and specific etiopathological models have been proposed for TTH (14, 15) and MH (16) despite this is a still disputed aspect. In fact, although the IHS classification has been recognized as the most important of the past years (17) some patients with headache may present with overlapping clinical features that makes it difficult to correctly classify them, especially in the case of TTH and MH (18). The concept of a continuum spectrum between these disorders has been proposed to overcome this taxonomic problem (19) and since, its validity has been debated in the past decades (20–22) as the clinical characteristics of patients in both TTH and MH groups come across with more similarities than differences. Patients may share demographic characteristics for specific age groups and respond positively to similar treatments (23); also most triggering factors (e.g., stress) are shared between MH and TTH (24, 25). Moreover, alterations like decreased gray matter in brain areas associated with pain transmission (anterior cingulate, insular cortices, and the dorsal rostral pons) are common in patients with TTH and MH (26, 27). In the so-called continuum model, MH and TTH represent different points on a single continuum of severity, with migraine falling at the more severe end of the symptom spectrum (28–30). Therefore, the different clinical headache expressions are considered the result of the different extent of sensitization occurring at the first- and second-order neurons of the trigeminal nucleus caudalis (TNC) induced by alterations of the trigeminal nerve (30).

Despite the neurophysiologic influence of trigger points (TrPs) on pain mechanisms seems attributable to their action as nociceptive sources (31, 32), the pathophysiology of TrPs on pain still needs to be elucidated (33, 34). Patients with chronic TTH and MH have a greater number of TrPs compared to healthy subjects (35–37); the higher number of TrPs correlates with the severity and the duration of TTH attacks (38), but not in MH attacks (36). Furthermore, even though the pain of MH is predominantly associated with the activation of the trigeminal-vascular system (16), TrPs can be seen as additional stimuli that may contribute to start a migraine attack (37, 39, 40) and the inhibition of TrPs by mean of anesthetic injections led to a decrease in the frequency and severity of migraine attacks (41). The same intervention also promoted the reduction of attacks' frequency and intensity in a case series of patients with CH (42). However, it is unclear whether the TrPs may have a pathogenetic role (14) or constitute a precipitating factor of separate clinical conditions (15). In both cases, the TrPs are involved in the pathophysiology of primary headaches as a peripheral mechanism able to sensitize the TNC (43, 44). Whatever the influence of TrPs on the pathophysiology of TrPS will be, these findings suggest that the TrPs treatment could be useful to prevent or decrease the extent of primary headaches.

Myofascial TrPs treatment is usually pursued with invasive (dry or wet needling) or non-invasive techniques (manual treatment or low-level laser therapy) (32) that, according to the most accepted hypothesis (33), are thought to reduce the ischemia-related nociception activated by the contracture of a small portion of muscle and, consequently, the degree of sensitization of TNC. Among the manual treatment of TrPs several techniques have been proposed that act directly or indirectly on the TrPs. Techniques that are thought to reduce the muscle contraction with mechanical forces (compression, distraction) acting directly

Abbreviations: CTTH, chronic tension type headache; ETTH, episodic tension type headache; FETTH, frequent episodic tension type headache; MH, migraine; CH, cluster headache; TG, treatment group; CG, control group; PG, placebo group; MCIDs, minimal clinical important difference; PIR, post isometric relaxation; CRAC, contract relax antagonist contraction; DT/IDT-MFR, direct/indirect myofascial release; SSTM, specific soft tissue mobilization; PRT, positional release therapy; TNC, trigeminal nucleus caudalis.

on the TrPs site or the surrounding tissues are ischemic compression (45), myofascial release (46), acupressure (47), and specific soft tissues mobilization techniques (48). Indirect techniques, such as muscle energy (49), positional release (50), and strain–counterstrain techniques (51) are thought to reduce muscle contraction for neurophysiological mechanisms regulating the muscle tone.

Several reviews have considered the efficacy of various interventions used in physiotherapy to treat primary headaches, including many manual therapies, multimodal and manipulative approaches, but the results were usually obtained grouping heterogeneous or combined treatment and considering primary headaches as separate entities (5, 9, 52–56). To our knowledge, the effectiveness of neither manual TrPs treatment in case of primary headaches has not been investigated yet nor it has been established considering patients with different primary headaches (MH, TTH) an homogeneous patient group, as proposed by the continuum severity model. The main purpose of this review was to establish the effectiveness of manual treatment of TrPs in reducing frequency, intensity, and duration of primary headaches. We will also investigate additional positive or negative effects of the manual treatment of TrPs and whether there is a manual technique or a treatment dosage to prefer.

METHODS

We conducted this systematic review following the preferred reporting items for systematic reviews and meta-analyses statement (57) and the Cochrane handbook for systematic reviews of interventions (58). The protocol of the review was registered in PROSPERO, an international prospective register of systematic reviews (registration code CRD42016046374) (59).

Eligibility Criteria

Types of Studies

Randomized controlled trials (RCTs) written in English, Italian, or Spanish.

Types of Participants

Participants included in the studies were adult subjects (age >18 years) with primary headaches (TTH, MH, CH) diagnosed using the International Classification of Headache Disorders criteria (13).

Types of Interventions

Any direct or indirect manual treatment targeting the TrPs, such as compression techniques, muscle energy techniques, myofascial techniques, acupressure, soft tissues techniques, or positional release techniques. Studies that proposed different approaches were considered only if the manual TrPs treatment was proposed as the only treatment in one of the intervention groups (60). Studies without manual TrPs treatment or referring to any pharmacological or injection treatment, spinal manipulation, and exercise without manual TrPs treatment were excluded.

Types of Comparators

Acceptable comparators were any type of minimal active intervention (placebo, sham treatment, routine medication, or wait list supported with routine medication) or no active intervention (wait list or no treatment).

Types of Outcomes

We considered as primary outcomes the variation of frequency of the attacks (number of attacks per month), the intensity of attacks [valuated with the 0–100 mm visual analog scale (VAS) or 0–10 numerical pain intensity scale—NPRS or similar scales], and duration of attacks (number of hours per attack). Secondarily, we also considered quality of life, medicine consumption, effects on TrPs, and any adverse event, such as dizziness, bruising, muscle stiffness, and post-treatment pain. Each outcome was considered in the period after the intervention (run-out period).

Search Strategy

The literature search was performed by two independent authors (FML and ZM) on MEDLINE, COCHRANE, Web Of Science, and PEDro databases, without the adoption of limits or filters. Relevant reviews were consulted for additional studies to consider. Last search was done on November 17, 2017. The full search strategy through all databases is reported in Appendix S1 in Supplementary Material.

Study Selection

Two independent authors (FML and ZM) screened the record by title and abstract applying the eligibility criteria. At the end of the screening process, full-text articles were retrieved and assessed for their eligibility in the qualitative and/or quantitative synthesis. Any disagreement was resolved by consensus, otherwise a third author (GT) made the final choice. The inter-reviewers agreement of the eligibility process before consensus was expressed using the Cohen's kappa.

Data Collection

Two authors (FML and ZM) independently collected information from the included trials by an *ad hoc* extraction form. The extracted data were inserted into a pre-formatted table for studies' characteristics, such as author, year, design, country, headache diagnosis, sample size calculation, number of participants recruited, drop-outs, intervention (treatment and control), duration, follow-up, outcomes, and measure unit. Disagreements between reviewers were resolved by consensus or if no agreement could be reached, a third author (GT) was consulted.

Risk of Bias (RoB) Assessment

The internal validity on the included studies was assessed with the Cochrane RoB tool (58). The following domains were appraised: selection bias (random sequence generation and allocation concealment), performance bias (blinding of participants and personnel), detection bias (blinding of outcome assessment), attrition bias (incomplete outcome data), and reporting bias (selective reporting) (58). Each domain could be classified as "high," "low," or "unclear" RoB if the study did not provide sufficient information to judge. Two reviewers (FML and ZM) independently assessed the above-mentioned domains of RoB. Any disagreement was resolved by consensus or if no consensus was obtained a third reviewer (GT) made the final choice. Strength of inter-raters agreement before consensus was expressed using the Cohen's kappa.

Analysis and Synthesis of Results

We evaluated the treatment effects for dichotomized outcomes using the risk ratio (RR), and for continuous outcomes using the pooled mean difference (MD). The variance was expressed with 95% confidence intervals (95% CI). The outcome measures from the individual trials were combined through meta-analysis were possible using random-effects models described by DerSimonian and Laird (61) because a certain degree of heterogeneity of population and treatments would be expected among interventions of trials. If any planned outcome was not reported quantitatively, a comprehensive description was reported. Since similar scales with different ranges were used to measure the intensity of pain (e.g., VAS 0–10 and VAS 0–100), we linearly transformed each scale into a 0–100 scale (correcting the SDs accordingly) in order to directly compare the pain scales. This method proved to be suitable for being able to directly compare different pain scales (62).

For the meta-analyses, we entered the mean values and SDs measured after the intervention (run-out). If SDs were not reported, we calculated it from SEs. All frequencies of attacks were normalized in attacks per month (mean and SD).

The units of randomization and analysis in the included trials were the individual participants. When a trial presented multiple comparisons, in order to overcome a unit-of-analysis error we used a suggested method (63) that consisted in splitting the participants of the intervention (64) or the comparison groups (65) in two or more groups with smaller sample size, but equal means and SDs in order to avoid the loss of data that could have occurred when only a single pair of interventions is chosen or a treatment group (TG) is deleted.

We analyzed heterogeneity by means of the I^2 statistic and the Chi^2 test. A *P*-value of less than 0.1 indicated a statistically significant heterogeneity for the Chi^2 test (66). The percentage of I^2 represented the degree of heterogeneity: percentages of 25, 50, and 75% indicated a low, moderate, and high degree of heterogeneity, respectively (66). If a study did not provide usable summary measures for an outcome it was included in the review, but excluded from the meta-analysis, e.g., Lawler and Cameron (67). For included studies, the number of lost to follow-up in each group and reasons for attrition were recorded. For missing data, similarity of group was evaluated, then the corresponding authors of included studies were contacted (e.g., emailing or writing to corresponding author/s) and if no information were provided, we conducted analyses using only available data (i.e., we did not impute missing data) (63).

We pooled studies through a subgroup analysis according to the type of specific headache. Furthermore, sensitivity analyses for RoB assessment were planned in case of sufficient numbers of studies in each pairwise comparison.

The software used was Cochrane Review Manager Version 5.3 (68).

Level of Evidence

To evaluate the overall quality of evidence, we used the grading of recommendations assessment, development and evaluation approach (GRADE), for the main outcome based on the methodological quality of included trials (69). The highest quality rating is for evidence based on RCTs with a low RoB. However, it is possible for authors to downgrade this level of evidence to moderate, low, or even very low. The quality of evidence depends on the presence of five factors: study limitation (RoB), indirectness of evidence, unexplained heterogeneity or inconsistency of results, imprecision of results, and high probability of publication bias (70). For the RoB factor, the evidence was arbitrary downgraded by one level when two criteria were judged as high or unclear, and by two levels when more than two criteria displayed high or unclear risk. The software used was GRADEPro GDT (71).

Two authors (FML and ZM) independently assessed the quality of evidence and the RoB. In case of doubt, another reviewer (GT) was consulted for the final choice. Strength of inter-raters agreement before consensus was expressed using the Cohen's kappa.

RESULTS

Study Selection

We identified 914 records through databases searching and 8 from additional references (52, 53, 72, 73). After removal of duplicates, a total of 390 records were selected for screening. We excluded 356 records after reading title and abstract. Of the 34 remaining articles assessed, only seven were considered eligible (**Figure 1**) (60, 64, 65, 67, 74–76). The inter-reviewer agreement regarding study eligibility was moderate with a kappa of 0.69.

General Study Characteristics

All studies were RCTs; five trials concerned TTH (60, 64, 65, 74, 75) and two MH (67, 76). No studies were found concerning CH (**Table 1**).

The pooled population was of 316 subjects (mean age 39.0 ± 11.6 years) with a significant majority of female subjects (251 F, $P < 0.05$). A mean of 45.1 (±9.2) patients were randomized in each trial. One RCT concerned chronic TTH (75, 77), one concerned episodic TTH (65), two considered both frequent-episodic TTH and chronic TTH (60, 64), one RCT concerned MH with and without Aura (67), and two RCTs concerned undefined/unclassified TTH (74) and MH (76).

The TTH subgroup consisted of 225 subjects (71% of the whole population; mean age 38.9 ± 9.8 years) with a significant majority of female subjects (188 F, $P < 0.05$). One hundred and twenty-six subjects had chronic TTH (60, 64, 74, 75, 77), 55 had frequent-episodic TTH (60, 64), and 47 had episodic TTH (65).

The MH subgroup consisted of 91 subjects (29% of the whole population; mean age 39.3 ± 13.5 years) with a not significant

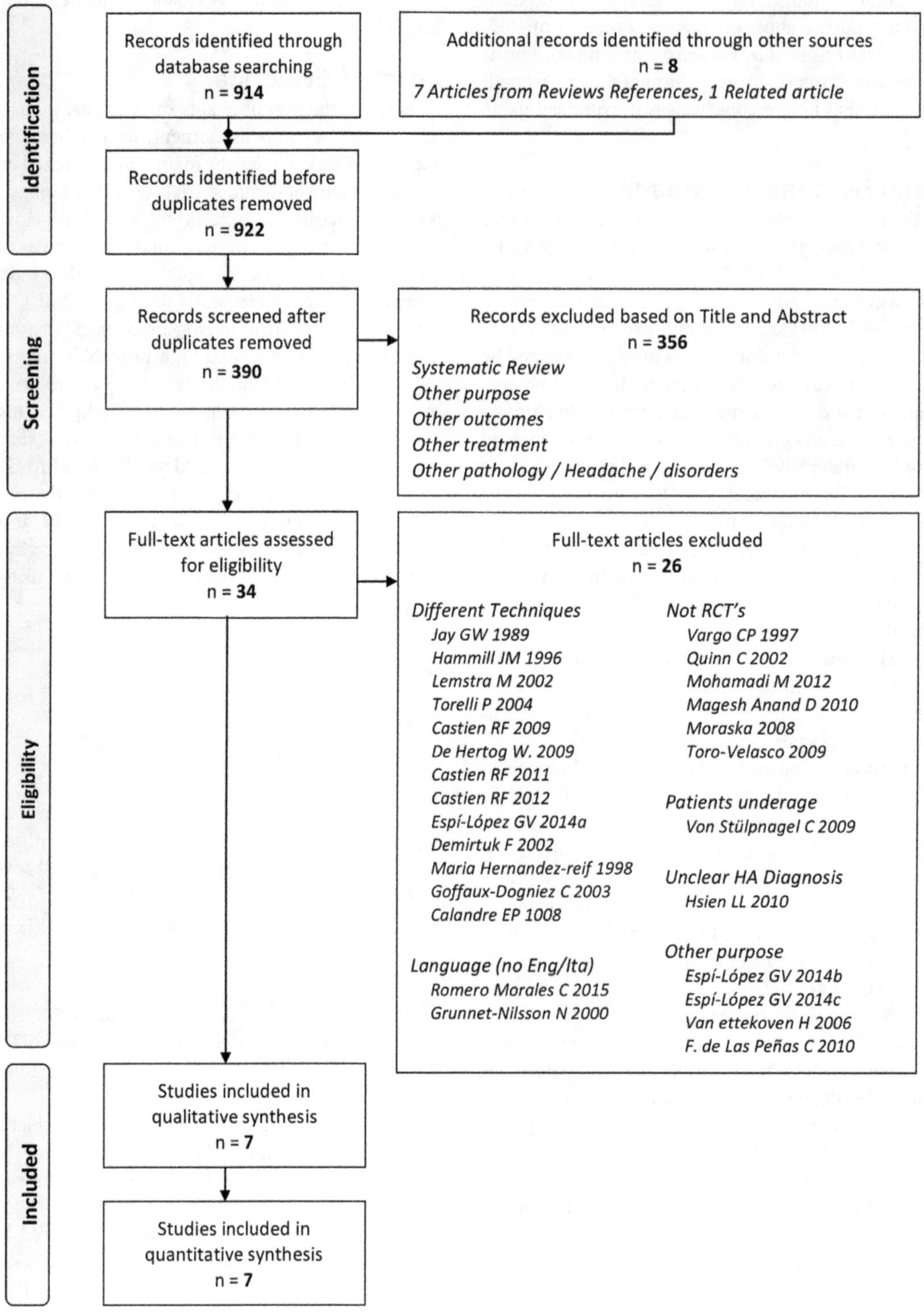

FIGURE 1 | Studies selection flow diagram.

majority of female subjects (63 F, $P = 0.41$). Sixty subjects had MH without Aura (67, 76) and 31 had MH with Aura (67, 76).

Headaches were diagnosed using the International Classification of Headache Disorders criteria (13). In five trials (60, 64, 65, 74, 76), the diagnosis was done by a neurologist while in two trials the diagnosis was made either on the score of the Headache History Inventory (67) or by a general practitioner (75).

TABLE 1 | Characteristics of included studies.

Reference, Design, Country	HA diagnosis, No. of subjects recruited, drop-out, sample size calculation (primary outcome), trial arms, and No. of participants	Intervention treatment/ control	Duration/follow-up	Outcomes/measure units
Ajimsha (65), RCT, India	CTTH/ETTH (diagnosis by neurologist) $N = 63$ (36 F, CTTH = 9, ETTH = 47) Drop-out: 7 Sample size calculation: no Trial arm: N (mean age ± SD) TG1: 22 (43.7 ± 5.6) TG2: 22 (44.7 ± 5.2) CG: 12 (43.0 ± 5.4)	All groups: two 60′ sessions per week for 12 weeks. TG1: treatment with DT-MFR protocol. TG2: treatment with IDT-MFR protocol. CG: slow soft stroking with finger pads all over the head in the same area of MFR techniques.	Duration 16 weeks: – 4 weeks baseline – 12 weeks treatment Run-out: – 4 weeks post treatment	Self reported daily headache diary – Frequency: no. of days with HA per 4 weeks – Intensity and duration: not assessed
Berggreen (75), RCT, Denmark	CTTH (diagnosis by general practitioner) $N = 43$ (43 F) Drop-out: 4 Sample size calculation: yes (pain) Trial arm: N (mean age ± SD) TG: 19 (38.8 ± 13.7) CG: 16 (42.3 ± 10.2)	TG: one session of TrPs treatment with ischemic compression per week for 10 weeks. CG: no treatment	Duration 14 weeks: – 4 weeks baseline – 10 weeks treatment Run out: – 4 weeks post treatment	Self reported daily headache diary – Intensity: 100 mm VAS – Frequency and duration: not assessed Other outcomes: – Inconvenience of the pain: 100 mm VAS – Medicine consumption – Number of TrPs – Multidimensional pain: MPQ Mc gill pain questionnaire; – Quality of life: SF36
Ferragut-Garcías (60), RCT, Balearic Islands	CTTH/FETTH (diagnosis by neurologist) $N = 100$ (78 F, CTTH = 41, FETTH = 56) Drop-out: 3 Sample size calculation: yes (HIT-6) Trial arm: N (mean age ± SD) TG1: 23 (38.1 ± 10.9) TG2: 25 (39.4 ± 11.0) TG3: 25 (40.8 ± 12.1) PG: 24 (40.5 ± 12.0)	All groups: Six 15′ sessions: 2 in the first week, 2 in the second week, and 1 each in the third and the fourth week. TG1: 3′ of soft tissue techniques in each pair of craniocervical region muscles. TG2[a]: neural mobilization techniques TG3[a]: treatment 1 and 2 combined PG: sham massage	Duration 6 weeks: – 2 weeks baseline – 4 weeks treatment Run out: – 2 weeks post treatment Follow-up: – 4 weeks after treatment	Self reported daily headache diary – Frequency of attack: no. of days with HA in 2 weeks – Intensity: 0–10 mm VAS – Duration: not assessed Other outcomes: – Pressure pain treshold – Quality of life: headache impact test-6 HIT-6
Ghanbari (74), RCT, Iran	CTTH (diagnosis by neurologist) $N = 30$ (28 F) No drop-out. Sample size calculation: estimated from previous study; primary outcome not spec. Trial arm: N (mean age ± SD) TG: 15 (37.7 ± 8.6) CG: 15 (36.3 ± 7.5)	TG: five sessions (from 60′ to 100′) of positional release therapy (PRT) in 2 weeks. CG: routine medications with NSAIDs as abortive drugs and TCAs as prophilactic drugs	Duration 4 weeks: – 2 weeks baseline – 2 weeks treatment Run-out: – 2 weeks post treatment	Self reported daily headache diary – Frequency of attack: no. of days with HA in 2 weeks – Intensity: 10 point NPI – Duration: number of hours per attack. Other outcomes: – Tablet count: no. of pain rescue tablet used – TrPs sensitivity measured by digital force gage and numeric pain intensity
Ghanbari (76), RCT, Iran	MH (diagnosis by neurologist) $N = 44$ (24 F) No drop-out Sample size calculation: no Trial arm: N (mean age) TG: 22 (38.7) CG: 22 (35.9)	TG: five 90′ sessions of PRT in 2 weeks + routine medications with NSAIDs, nortriptyline, propranolol, and depakine. CG: routine medications with NSAIDs, nortriptyline, propranolol and depakine	Duration 4 weeks: – 2 weeks baseline – 2 weeks treatment Run out: – 4 weeks post treatment Follow-up: – 2 and 4 months post treatment	Self reported daily headache diary – Frequency of attack: no. of days with HA – Intensity: 0–5 pain scale – Duration: number of hours per attack. Other outcomes: – Tablet count: no. of pain rescue tablet used – TrPs sensitivity measured by digital force gage – Cervical range of motion by clinical goniometer (flexion, extension, rotation, lateral flection)
Lawler (67), RCT, New Zealand	MH (diagnosis by questionnaire) $N = 48$ (40 F) Drop-out: 4 Sample size calculation: no Trial arm: N (mean age ± SD) GT: 23 (41.3 ± 13.5) GC: 21 (41.3 ± 13.5)	GT: one 45′ sessions every week for 6 weeks. Trigger-point treatment of the back, shoulders, neck, and head with myofascial release (3 min), deep ischemic compression, and cross-fiber work CG: no treatment	Duration 13 weeks: – 4 wk baseline – 6 wk treatment. Run out: – 3 wk post treatment	Self reported daily headache diary – Frequency of attack: no. of days with HA – Intensity: 0–5 pain scale – Duration: not assessed. Other outcomes: – Drugs consumption – Effect after treatment on heart rate, state anxiety, and salivary cortisol. – Stress and coping: perceived stress scale. – State anxiety: STAI-sf state anxiety scale

(Continued)

TABLE 1 | Continued

Reference, Design, Country	HA diagnosis, No. of subjects recruited, drop-out, sample size calculation (primary outcome), trial arms, and No. of participants	Intervention treatment/ control	Duration/follow-up	Outcomes/measure units
Moraska (64), RCT, USA	CTTH/FETTH (diagnosis by neurologist) N = 62 (48 F, CTTH = 30, FETTH = 26) Drop-out: 6 Sample size calculation: yes (frequency) Trial arm: N (mean age ± SD) TG: 17 (32.1 ± 12.0) PG: 19 (34.7 ± 11.1) CG: 20 (33.4 ± 9.0)	All groups: two 45′ session per week for 6 weeks. TG: manual TrPs treatment composed by 15′ of myofascial release, 20′ of trigger point release massage TRP, 10′ PIR PG: detuned ultrasound in specified head and neck muscle areas CG: no treatment	Duration 10 weeks: – 4 wk baseline – 6 wk treatment Run out: – 4 wk post treatment	Self reported daily headache diary – Frequency of attack: no. of days with HA in 4 weeks – Intensity: 100 mm VAS – Duration: number of hours per attack. Other outcomes: – Use of pain medication – Perceived clinical change – Pressure pain treshold – Quality of life: headache disability inventory and headache impact test-6 HIT-6

RCT, randomized controlled trial; F, female; wk, weeks; CTTH, chronic tension type headache; ETTH, episodic tension type headache; FETTH, frequent episodic tension type headache; MH, migraine; TG, treatment group; CG, control group; PG, placebo group; VAS, visual analog scale; NPI, numeric pain index; HA, headache; wk, weeks; TrPs, trigger points.

[a]Results from these groups were not included into quantitative analysis.

TABLE 2 | Classification of the different TrPs manual treatment techniques.

Reference	Headache	Compression techniques	Muscle energy techniques	Myofascial techniques	Soft tissues techniques	Positional release techniques
		Ischemic compression Pressure release TRP Trigger Point Release Massage	**PIR CRAC**	**Myofascial release DT/IDT-MFR**	**SSTM Deep transverse friction**	**PRT**
Ajimsha (65)	TTH			X		
Berggreen (75)	TTH	X				
Ferragut-Garcías (60)	TTH	X				
Ghanbari (74)	TTH					X
Moraska (64)	TTH	X	X	X		
Ghanbari (76)	MH					X
Lawler (67)	MH	X		X	X	

TTH, tension type headache; MH, migraine; PIR, post isometric relaxation; CRAC, contract relax antagonist contraction; DT/IDT-MFR, direct/indirect myofascial release; SSTM, specific soft tissue mobilization; PRT, positional release therapy.

All the selected studies compared manual treatment versus minimal active treatment: placebo (64), sham massage (60, 65), routine medication supported with pharmacological prophilactic treatment (74), and wait list supported with routine medication (64, 67, 75, 76).

Treatment and Sessions

The duration of intervention and the number of treatments ranged from 5 sessions in 2 weeks to 24 sessions in 12 weeks with an average number of 2 sessions per week; the run-out/follow-up period varied from a minimum of 2 weeks to a maximum of 4 months after the end of treatment. The duration of the single session ranged from 15 to 100′.

The treatments proposed across all studies were heterogeneous: ischemic compression, myofascial release, muscle energy, soft tissue treatment, and positional release (**Table 2**).

Stretching was often used as warm-up and cool-down technique. The muscles mainly treated were the upper trapezius, the sternocleidomastoid, and the suboccipitals; secondarily, other neck or head muscles were treated (**Table 3**).

RoB Within Studies

None of the studies had a low RoB for all methodological items, while 3 out of 7 studies had more than one high RoB domain (64, 65, 67). Three RCTs had low risk in allocation concealment (60, 64, 75). As we expected for manual interventions, the blinding of participants and providers was always unachievable while blinding of assessors was adequately reported only in 2 out of 7 studies (60, 65). One RCT had high risk for incomplete outcome data because some patients did not maintain headache diaries as advised (65). One RCT had high risk in selective reporting because primary data about intensity were not provided (67) (**Figures 2** and **3**). The agreement between reviewers for individual domains of the Cochrane RoB tool was moderate (k = 0.72). Consensus was always achieved between the pair of initial reviewers.

Synthesis of the Results

For primary outcome (frequency, intensity, and duration), the original measures extracted in each trial are reported in **Table 4**.

The summary of findings for each outcome in TTH and MH and the quality of assessment are reported in **Table 5**.

TABLE 3 | Muscles and/or muscle groups treated in the trials.

Reference	Headache	Upper trapezius	Suboccipital	Sternocleidomastoid	Masseter	Temporalis	Pterygoid medial/lateral	Anterior neck muscles	Facial	Splenius Capitis	Splenius Cervicis	Occipital	Posterior Cervical	Cervical Multifidus	Rotators-Interspinalis	Levator Scapulae	Semispinalis Capitis
Ajimsha (65)	TTH	X	X	X									X				
Berggreen (75)	TTH	X	X	X	X	X	X	X	X	X	X	X	X				
Ferragut-Garcías (60)	TTH	X	X	X	X	X											
Ghanbari (74)	TTH	X	X	X										X	X		
Moraska (64)	TTH	X	X	X													
Ghanbari (76)	MH	X	X	X										X	X		
Lawler (67)	MH	X	X	X	X	X										X	

TTH, tension type headache; MH, migraine.

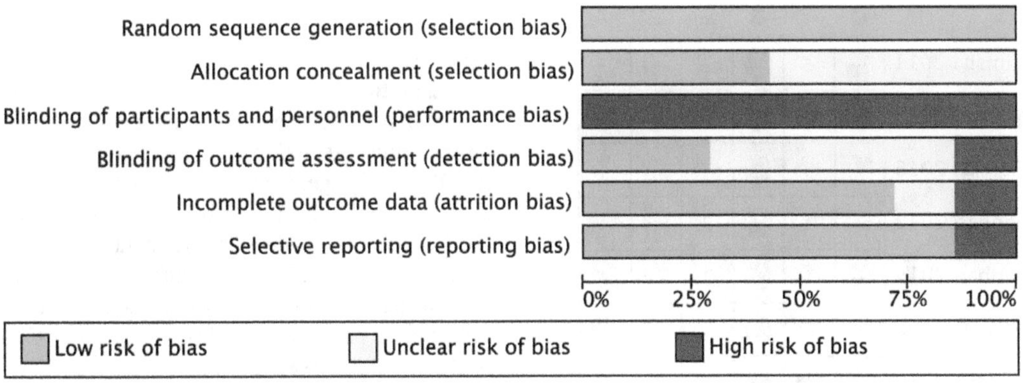

FIGURE 2 | Risk of bias (RoB) graph: review authors' judgments about each RoB item presented as percentages across all included studies.

The comparisons of interventions listed by outcome for both TTH and MH are reported in Appendix S2 in Supplementary Material.

Meta-analyses of the pooled results with separated analyses of TTH and MH as subgroups are shown for frequency (**Figure 4**), intensity (**Figure 5**), and duration (**Figure 6**). Sensitivity analyses for RoB assessment were not conducted due to the insufficient numbers of studies in each pairwise comparison.

TrPs Manual Treatment vs Minimal Active Intervention on TTH and MH Combined

Frequency

A total of six trials (277 subjects) assessed the frequency of attacks as number of attacks per month; three trials had high RoB (64, 65, 67) and three had low RoB (60, 74, 76). The analysis of combined results indicated a statistically significant reduction in frequency of attacks per month after treatment favored the experimental group compared to control, with a mean reduction of 3.05 attacks/month (MD −3.05; 95% CI from −4.11 to −2.00; $P < 0.01$; $I^2 = 64\%$; see **Figure 4**).

Intensity

A total of six trials (256 subjects) assessed the intensity of pain using different scales (0–100) VAS (64, 75), 0–10 VAS/NPI (numeric pain index) (60, 74), 0–5 pain scale (76); only five trials were included into the quantitative analysis for this outcome due to missing original data from one study (67), although we tried to contact the authors. We found one trial with high RoB (64), while four trials had low RoB (60, 74–76). Analysis of combined results (referred to a normalized 0–100 scale) showed a significant reduction of intensity of attacks in the experimental group (MD −12.93; 95% CI from −18.70 to −7.16; $P < 0.001$; $I^2 = 90\%$; see **Figure 5**).

Duration

A total of three trials (130 subjects) assessed the duration of attacks; one had high RoB (64) and two had low RoB (74, 76). A mean reduction of 1.69 h per attack (MD −1.69; 95% CI from −2.93 to −0.46; $P < 0.01$; $I^2 = 91\%$; see **Figure 6**) favored the experimental group compared to control. A greater reduction was found in the trial concerning MH that compared the routine medication supported with the intervention versus routine medication alone

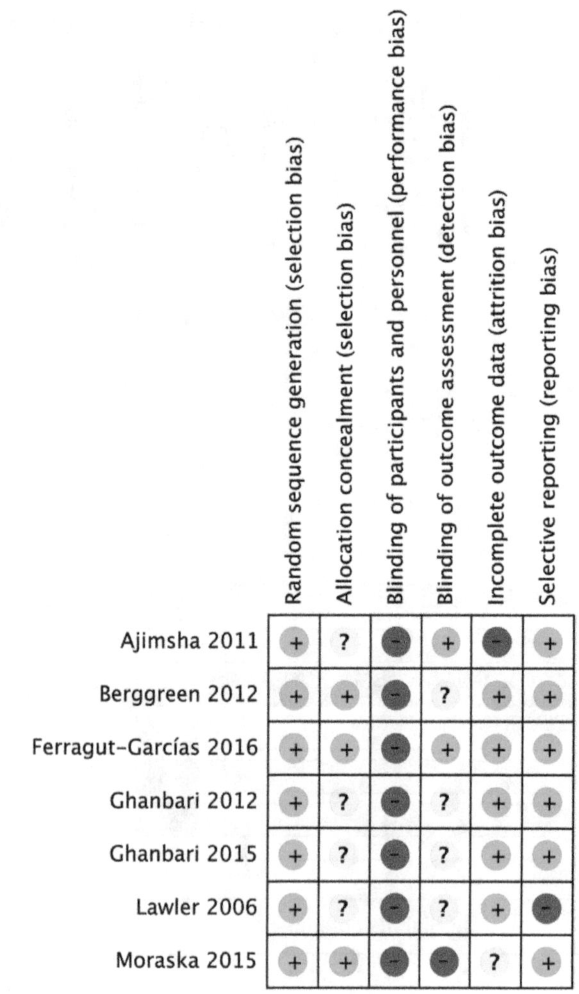

FIGURE 3 | Risk of bias (RoB) summary: review authors' judgments about each RoB item for each included study.

with a mean reduction of 10.68 h per attacks (MD −10.68; 95% CI from −14.41 to −6.95; $P < 0.001$; see **Figure 6**).

Subgroup Analysis: Treatment Effects on TTH

Frequency

Four trials (189 subjects) of which two had high RoB (64, 65) and two had low risk (60, 74) which assessed the frequency of attacks. Analysis of combined results indicated a statistically significant reduction in frequency of attacks after treatment in the intervention group compared to control with a mean reduction of 3.50 attacks/month (MD −3.50; 95% CI from −4.91 to −2.09; $P < 0.001$; I^2 72%, see **Figure 4**).

Intensity

Four trials (168 subjects), three with low RoB (60, 74, 75) and one with high RoB (64) assessed intensity of pain using different scales [0–100 VAS (64, 75), 0–10 VAS/NPI (60, 74)]. The combined results (referred to a normalized 0–100 scale) indicated a statistically significant reduction in intensity of attacks after treatment in the intervention group compared to control group (CG) (MD −12.83; 95% CI from −19.49 to −6.17; $P < 0.001$; $I^2 = 92\%$, see **Figure 5**).

Duration

Two trials (86 subjects), one with high RoB (64) and one with low RoB (74) assessed the duration of attacks measured in hours. Analysis of combined results indicated a small reduction in duration of attacks after treatment in the intervention group compared CG with a mean reduction of 0.51 h per attacks (MD −0.51; 95% CI from −0.97 to −0.04; $P = 0.03$; $I^2 = 54\%$; see **Figure 6**).

Subgroup Analysis: Treatment Effects on MH

Frequency

Two trials (88 subjects), one with high RoB (67) and one with low RoB (76) assessed the frequency of attacks. A statistically significant reduction in frequency of attacks after treatment was observed in the intervention group with a mean reduction of 1.92 attacks/month (MD −1.92; 95% CI from −3.03 to −0.80; $P < 0.001$; $I^2 = 0\%$; see **Figure 4**).

Intensity

The same two trials (88 subjects) assessed the intensity of pain (0–5 pain scale). Lawler and Cameron (67) reported no significant group × time interaction effect revealed by the repeated measures ANOVA of changes from baseline to follow-up [$F_{(1, 42)} = 0.82$, ns; $d = 0.11$]; although we tried to contact the authors, we could not include these values in the meta-analysis as original data were unavailable (67). The results of the second trial (referred to a normalized 0–100 scale) indicated a statistically significant reduction in pain intensity (MD −13.60; 95% CI from −19.54 to −7.66; $P < 0.001$; see **Figure 5**).

Duration

Only one trial (44 subjects) with low RoB (76) reported a statistically significant reduction in duration of attacks after treatment in the intervention with a mean reduction of 10.68 h per attacks (MD −10.68; 95% CI from −14.41 to −6.95; $P < 0.001$; see **Figure 6**).

Additional Treatment Effects on TTH and MH

Number of Active TrPs

Number of Active TrPs in TTH, one RCT reported a significant decrease in the number of active TrPs in patients treated with ischemic compression (75).

Pressure Pain Threshold (PTT) and TrPs Sensitivity

Pressure pain threshold and TrPs sensitivity in TTH, two RCTs reported the increase of the PPT in treated muscles only in patients manually treated ($P < 0.01$) (60, 64); one RCT reported a significant reduction for sensitivity of TrPs only in the TG after intervention ($P < 0.01$) and at follow-up ($P = 0.015$) in TTH (74). The same results on TrPs sensitivity were reported in one RCT regarding MH (76).

Tablet Count and Medicine Consumption

Tablet count and medicine consumption in TTH, one RCT reported a significant reduction in tablet count after treatment

TABLE 4 | Original values extracted from trials regarding frequency, intensity, and duration in TTH and MH measured at baseline, after treatment, and at follow-up.

Outcome	Study	Headache	Comparator	Scale	Group	Randomized	Drop out	Available	Baseline	Post treatment/run-out	Follow-up
Frequency of attacks	Ferragut-Garcías (60)	TTH	Sham massage	Attacks × 4 weeks[a]	Treatment	25	2	23	**17.2 ± 4.6**	**9.4 ± 2.8**	**9.6 ± 3.4**
					Control (sham massage)	25	1	24	**14.4 ± 5.4**	**13.8 ± 5.0**	**13.6 ± 4.6**
	Moraska (64)	TTH	(1) Placebo	Attacks × 4 weeks[a]	Treatment	20	3	17	**14.88 ± 0.92**	**10.44 ± 1.3**	
			(2) Wait list		Placebo (detuned US)	21	2	19	**15.24 ± 0.84**	**11.84 ± 1.31**	
					Control (wait list)	21	1	20	**14.76 ± 0.84**	**12.86 ± 1.27**	
	Ajimsha (65)	TTH	Sham massage	Attacks × 4 weeks	Treatment 1	25	3	22	12.0 ± 2.8	4.9 ± 1.7	
					Treatment 2	25	3	22	12.4 ± 2.8	5.7 ± 1.3	
					Control	13	1	12	12.0 ± 2.5	10.4 ± 2.7	
	Ghanbari (74)	TTH	Routine medication	Attacks × 4 weeks[a]	Treatment	15	0	15	**24.88 ± 4.44**	**15.32 ± 8.90**	
					Control	15	0	15	**22.26 ± 3.98**	**20.40 ± 4.80**	
	Lawler (67)	MH	Wait list	Attacks × 4 weeks[a]	Treatment	24	1	23	**6.08 ± 5.00**	**4.28 ± 5.36**	
					Control	24	3	21	**7.04 ± 4.96**	**6.88 ± 5.32**	
	Ghanbari (76)	MH	Routine medication	Attacks × 4 weeks[a]	Treatment	22	0	22	**8.00 ± 2.54**	**4.26 ± 1.64**	**4.62 ± 1.98**
					Control	22	0	22	**7.9 ± 1.98**	**6.08 ± 2.34**	**5.62 ± 1.90**
Intensity of attacks	Ferragut-Garcías (60)	TTH	Sham massage	0–10 VAS[b]	Treatment	25	2	23	**44 ± 11**	**28 ± 8**	**28 ± 10**
					Control	25	1	24	**56 ± 11**	**54 ± 10**	**54 ± 11**
	Moraska (64)	TTH	(1) placebo	0–100 VAS	Treatment	20	3	17	31.4 ± 2.69	22.8 ± 3.03	
			(2) Wait list		Placebo (detuned US)	21	2	19	33.3 ± 2.52	31.5 ± 2.80	
					Control (wait list)	21	1	20	31.2 ± 2.46	29.0 ± 2.74	
	Berggreen (75)	TTH	Wait list	0–100 VAS	Treatment	20	1	19	28.0 ± 15.9	16.2 ± 11.8	
					Control	19	3	16	26.6 ± 12.6	24.9 ± 14.5	
	Ghanbari (74)	TTH	Routine medication	0–10 NPI[b]	Treatment	15	0	15	**58.0 ± 17.5**	**46.9 ± 24.9**	
					Control	15	0	15	**60.3 ± 9.9**	**63.6 ± 11.4**	
	Lawler (67)	MH	Wait list	0–5 pain scale	Treatment	24	1	23	No data[a]	No data[a]	
					Control	24	3	21	No data[a]	No data[a]	
	Ghanbari (76)	MH	Routine medication	0–5 pain scale[b]	Treatment	22	0	22	**66.8 ± 17.4**	**42.2 ± 11.6**	**39.0 ± 15**
					Control	22	0	22	**70.0 ± 14.2**	**55.8 ± 8.2**	**55.2 ± 14.8**
Duration of attacks	Moraska (64)	TTH	(1) Placebo	Hours × attack	Treatment	20	3	17	3.15 ± 0.43	2.65 ± 0.47	
			(2) WAIT list		Placebo (Detuned US)	21	2	19	2.86 ± 0.40	3.01 ± 0.44	
					Control (wait list)	21	1	20	3.02 ± 0.39	3.12 ± 0.43	
	Ghanbari (74)	TTH	Routine medication	Hours × attack	Treatment	15	0	15	6.42 ± 5.70	2.19 ± 2.28	
					Control	15	0	15	5.37 ± 3.47	5.02 ± 3.93	
	Ghanbari (76)	MH	Routine medication	Hours × attack	Treatment	22	0	22	35.59 ± 13.3	8.54 ± 3.76	8.95 ± 5.12
					Control	22	0	22	35.36 ± 8.85	19.22 ± 8.09	18.0 ± 9.27

[a]*Values indicated in bold have been normalized as attacks per month.*
[b]*Values indicated in bold have been normalized to a 0–100 numeric pain scale.*
UC, usual care; RM, routine medication; US, ultrasound; TTH, tension type headache; MH, migraine; VAS, visual analog scale; NPI, numeric pain index.

TABLE 5 | Summary of findings and quality of assessment.

Quality assessment							Summary of findings					Importance
							No. of patients		Effect			
No. of studies	Study design	Risk of bias	Inconsistency	Indirectness	Imprecision	Other considerations	Manual TrPs treatment	Other treatment	Relative (95% CI)	Absolute (95% CI)	Quality	
Frequency (attacks/month)—TTH and MH pooled												
6	Randomized trials	Serious[a,b,c,d]	Serious[e]	Not serious	Serious[f]	None	144	133	–	MD **3.05 lower** (4.11 lower to 2.00 lower)	⊕◯◯◯ Very low	Critical
Frequency (attacks/month)—TTH												
4	Randomized trials	Serious[a,b]	Serious[e]	Not serious	Serious[f]	None	99	90	–	MD **3.50 lower** (4.91 lower to 2.09 lower)	⊕◯◯◯ Very low	Critical
Frequency (attacks/month)—MH												
2	Randomized trials	Serious[a]	Not serious	Not serious	Serious[f]	None	45	43	–	MD **1.92 lower** (3.03 lower to 0.80 lower)	⊕⊕◯◯ Low	Critical
Intensity (0–100 scale)—TTH and MH pooled												
6	Randomized trials	Very serious[a,b,c,d]	Very serious[g]	Not serious	Serious[f]	None	96	116	–	MD **12.93 lower** (18.70 lower to 7.16 lower)	⊕◯◯◯ Very low	Important
Intensity (0–100 scale)—TTH												
4	Randomized trials	Very serious[a,d,f,h]	Very serious[g]	Not serious	Serious[f]	None	74	94	–	MD **12.83 lower** (19.49 lower to 6.17 lower)	⊕◯◯◯ Very low	Important
Intensity (0–100 scale)—MH												
2[i]	Randomized trials	Very serious[a,d]	Not serious	Not serious	Very serious[f,j]	None	22	22	–	MD **13.60 lower** (19.54 lower to 7.66 lower)	⊕◯◯◯ Very low	Important
Duration (hours)—TTH and MH pooled												
3	Randomized trials	Serious[a]	Very serious[g]	Not serious	Serious[f]	None	54	76	–	MD **1.69 lower** (2.93 lower to 0.46 lower)	⊕◯◯◯ Very low	Important
Duration (hours)—TTH												
2	Randomized trials	Serious[a]	Serious[e]	Not serious	Serious[f]	None	32	54	–	MD **0.51 lower** (0.97 lower to 0.04 lower)	⊕◯◯◯ Very low	Important
Duration (hours)—MH												
1	Randomized trials	Serious[a]	Not serious	Not serious	Very serious[f,j]	None	22	22	–	MD **10.68 lower** (14.41 lower to 6.95 lower)	⊕◯◯◯ Very low	Important

[a] *Lack of blinding of participants and personnel.*
[b] *Lack of blinding of outcome assessment.*
[c] *Unclear allocation concealment.*
[d] *Selective reporting (reporting bias).*
[e] *Moderate heterogeneity (50 < I^2 < 75%).*
[f] *Less than 400 subjects.*
[g] *High heterogeneity (I^2 > 75%).*
[h] *Incomplete outcome data (attrition bias).*
[i] *One trial excluded from quantitative analysis due to reporting bias.*
[j] *Only one trial.*
TTH, tension type headache; MH, migraine; TrPs, trigger points; MD, mean difference; CI, confidence interval.

Study or Subgroup	Manual TrPs Treatment Mean	SD	Total	Control Mean	SD	Total	Weight	Mean Difference IV, Random, 95% CI
1.1.1 TTH								
Ajimsha 2011 (1)	5.7	1.3	22	10.4	2.7	6	11.4%	-4.70 [-6.93, -2.47]
Ajimsha 2011 (2)	4.9	1.71	22	10.4	2.7	6	11.1%	-5.50 [-7.78, -3.22]
Ferragut-Garcías 2016 (3)	9.4	2.8	23	13.8	5	24	11.0%	-4.40 [-6.70, -2.10]
Ghanbari 2012 (4)	15.32	8.9	15	20.4	4.8	15	3.6%	-5.08 [-10.20, 0.04]
Moraska 2015 (5)	10.44	1.3	8	11.84	1.31	19	18.6%	-1.40 [-2.48, -0.32]
Moraska 2015 (6)	10.44	1.3	9	12.86	1.27	20	19.0%	-2.42 [-3.44, -1.40]
Subtotal (95% CI)			**99**			**90**	**74.7%**	**-3.50 [-4.91, -2.09]**
Heterogeneity: Tau² = 1.93; Chi² = 17.73, df = 5 (P = 0.003); I² = 72%								
Test for overall effect: Z = 4.87 (P < 0.00001)								
1.1.2 MH								
Ghanbari 2015 (7)	4.26	1.64	22	6.08	2.34	22	17.8%	-1.82 [-3.01, -0.63]
Lawler 2006 (8)	4.28	5.36	23	6.88	5.32	21	7.5%	-2.60 [-5.76, 0.56]
Subtotal (95% CI)			**45**			**43**	**25.3%**	**-1.92 [-3.03, -0.80]**
Heterogeneity: Tau² = 0.00; Chi² = 0.20, df = 1 (P = 0.65); I² = 0%								
Test for overall effect: Z = 3.36 (P = 0.0008)								
Total (95% CI)			**144**			**133**	**100.0%**	**-3.05 [-4.11, -2.00]**
Heterogeneity: Tau² = 1.26; Chi² = 19.30, df = 7 (P = 0.007); I² = 64%								
Test for overall effect: Z = 5.67 (P < 0.00001)								
Test for subgroup differences: Chi² = 2.98, df = 1 (P = 0.08), I² = 66.5%								

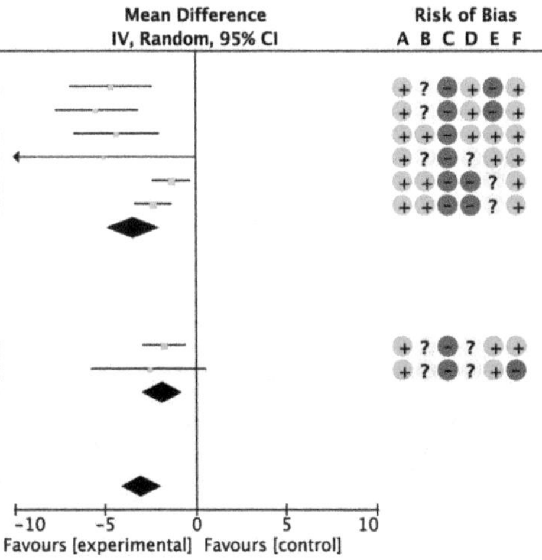

Footnotes
(1) 24 sessions in 12 weeks; Indirect Technique VS Sham massage
(2) 24 sessions in 12 weeks; Direct Technique VS Sham massage
(3) 6 sessions in 4 weeks; Pressure release VS Sham massage
(4) 5 sessions in 2 weeks; Positional release therapy VS Routine medication
(5) 12 sessions in 6 weeks; Trigger point release massage VS Detuned US
(6) 12 sessions in 6 weeks; Trigger point release massage VS Wait list
(7) 5 sessions in 2 weeks; Manual treatment + Routine Medication VS Routine Medication
(8) 6 sessions in 6 weeks; Release massage VS Wait List

Risk of bias legend
(A) Random sequence generation (selection bias)
(B) Allocation concealment (selection bias)
(C) Blinding of participants and personnel (performance bias)
(D) Blinding of outcome assessment (detection bias)
(E) Incomplete outcome data (attrition bias)
(F) Selective reporting (reporting bias)

FIGURE 4 | Forest plot of comparison for frequency (no. of attacks per month) compared with minimal active intervention in TTH (top) and MH (bottom). Abbreviations: TTH, tension-type headache; MH, Migraine; CI, confidence interval.

Study or Subgroup	Experimental Mean	SD	Total	Control Mean	SD	Total	Weight	Mean Difference IV, Random, 95% CI
1.2.1 TTH								
Berggreen 2012 (1)	16.2	11.8	19	24.9	14.5	16	14.1%	-8.70 [-17.57, 0.17]
Ferragut-Garcías 2016 (2)	28	8	23	54	10	24	18.1%	-26.00 [-31.17, -20.83]
Ghanbari 2012 (3)	46.9	24.9	15	63.6	11.4	15	9.5%	-16.70 [-30.56, -2.84]
Moraska 2015 (4)	22.8	3.03	9	29	2.74	20	20.5%	-6.20 [-8.52, -3.88]
Moraska 2015 (5)	22.8	3.03	8	31.5	2.8	19	20.4%	-8.70 [-11.15, -6.25]
Subtotal (95% CI)			**74**			**94**	**82.7%**	**-12.83 [-19.49, -6.17]**
Heterogeneity: Tau² = 45.89; Chi² = 48.36, df = 4 (P < 0.00001); I² = 92%								
Test for overall effect: Z = 3.78 (P = 0.0002)								
1.2.2 MH								
Ghanbari 2015 (6)	42.2	11.6	22	55.8	8.2	22	17.3%	-13.60 [-19.54, -7.66]
Lawler 2006 (7)	0	0	23	0	0	21		Not estimable
Subtotal (95% CI)			**45**			**43**	**17.3%**	**-13.60 [-19.54, -7.66]**
Heterogeneity: Not applicable								
Test for overall effect: Z = 4.49 (P < 0.00001)								
Total (95% CI)			**119**			**137**	**100.0%**	**-12.93 [-18.70, -7.16]**
Heterogeneity: Tau² = 40.88; Chi² = 50.29, df = 5 (P < 0.00001); I² = 90%								
Test for overall effect: Z = 4.39 (P < 0.0001)								
Test for subgroup differences: Chi² = 0.03, df = 1 (P = 0.87), I² = 0%								

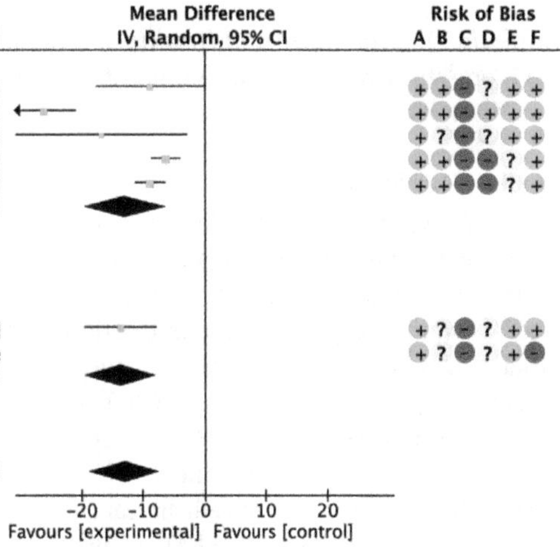

Footnotes
(1) 10 sessions in 10 weeks; VS wait list
(2) 6 sessions in 4 weeks; Pressure release VS Sham Massage
(3) 5 sessions in 2 weeks; Positional release therapy VS Routine Medication
(4) 12 sessions in 6 weeks; Trigger point release massage VS Wait list
(5) 12 sessions in 6 weeks; Trigger point release massage VS Detuned US
(6) 5 sessions in 2 weeks; Manual treatment + Routine Medication VS Routine Medication
(7) 6 sessions in 6 weeks; Release massage VS Wait List. Original data not avaiable.

Risk of bias legend
(A) Random sequence generation (selection bias)
(B) Allocation concealment (selection bias)
(C) Blinding of participants and personnel (performance bias)
(D) Blinding of outcome assessment (detection bias)
(E) Incomplete outcome data (attrition bias)
(F) Selective reporting (reporting bias)

FIGURE 5 | Forest plot of comparison for pain intensity (0–100 scale) compared with minimal active intervention in TTH (top) and MH (bottom). Abbreviations: TTH, tension-type headache; CI, confidence interval; MH, Migraine.

phase ($P < 0.01$), but the result persisted only in manual TG after 2 weeks follow-up ($p < 0.01$) (74). A second study reported a not significant reduction of drug's use only in the TG ($P = 0.46$) (75) while in a third study, no significant TG differences have been measured (64). In MH, one RCT reported a significant reduction in tablet count in both treatment (receiving manual PRT

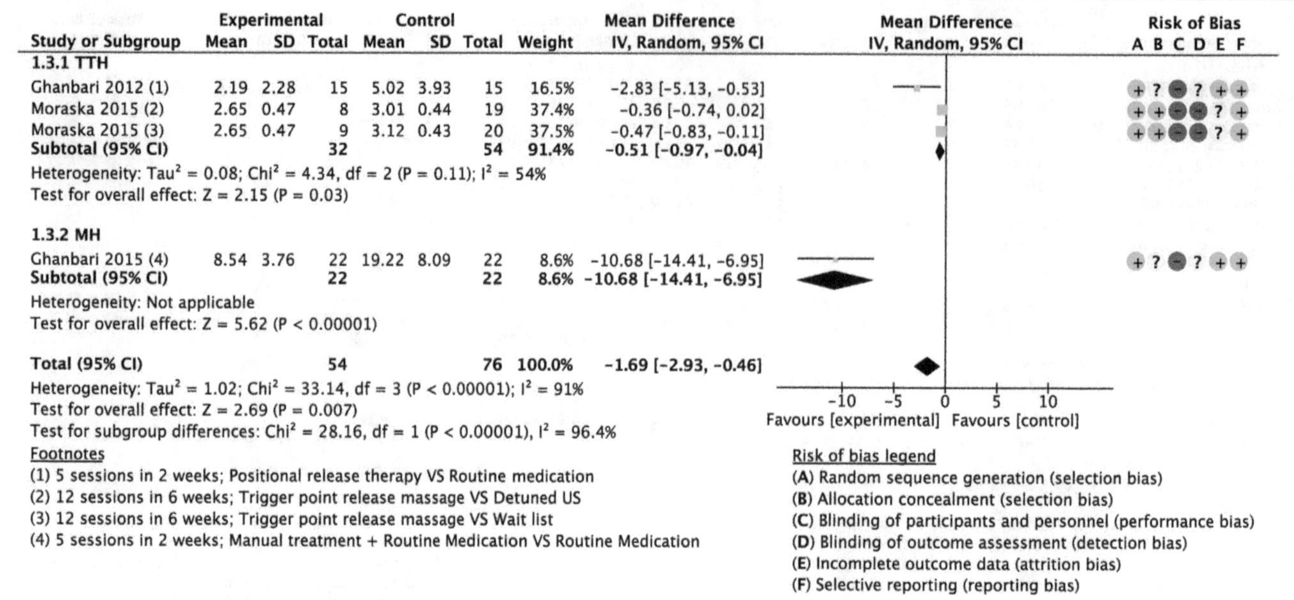

FIGURE 6 | Forest plot of comparison for attacks duration (hours) compared with minimal active intervention in TTH (top) and MH (bottom). Abbreviations: TTH, tension-type headache; MH, Migraine; CI, confidence interval.

and medical therapy) and CG (receiving only medical therapy); differences between groups at various follow-up were always significant ($P < 0.001$) (76).

McGill Pain Questionnaire and Quality of Life (SF36)

In TTH, one study reported not significant differences between manual TG and control (75).

Headache Disability Inventory (HDI), Headache Impact Test-6 (HIT-6), and Perceived Clinical Change

In TTH, one study reported a significant decrease in HDI scores only in manual TG ($P < 0.001$) (64). Other two studies reported a significant group × time interaction in HIT-6 scores; Moraska et al. (64) detected effects over time for both manual treatment and placebo group (*P*'s < 0.01) but not in the CG ($P = 0.52$); Ferragut-Garcias et al. (60) detected effects over time for all manual TGs (*P*'s < 0.001) and CG ($P < 0.05$) compared to baseline. Regarding the perceived clinical change, greater pain reduction was observed for manual TG compared to placebo or CGs ($P < 0.01$) (64).

Quality and Quantity of Sleep and Stress and Coping (PSS)

Quality and quantity of sleep and stress and coping in MH the TG displayed a significant improvement of sleep quality, but not of the total amount of sleeping hours (67); in the same study, TG displayed no significant change in stress and coping levels during both treatment and at follow-up [state trait anxiety inventory scale (STAI) and perceived stress scale (PSS)]; otherwise a significant deterioration of these outcomes was found only in the CG (67).

Cervical ROM

In MH, one study reported a significant increase of cervical rotation in both experimental and CGs, but flexion, extension, and side bend increased only in experimental group after 4 months of follow-up (all *P*'s < 0.001) (76).

DISCUSSION

The present manuscript aimed at establishing the effectiveness of the TrPs manual treatment in reducing the frequency, intensity, and duration of attacks of primary headaches in adults. In order to explore this goal the authors' agreement in performing articles selection and RoB assessment was moderate (Cohen's k ranged from 0.69 to 0.72), supporting the methodological validity of the research.

The quality of the level of evidence ranged from low to very low in favor of manual TrPs treatment compared to minimal active intervention in the reduction of the frequency, intensity, and duration of the attacks in the patients with TTH and MH measured in the run-out period after intervention. Further findings having very low quality of the evidence were a greater reduction of frequency of attacks in patients with TTH and of the duration of attacks in the MH subgroup, while the intensity of attacks was similarly reduced in both subgroups.

The different extent of efficacy of the TrP treatment on the primary headaches considered either as separated entities or according to the continuum model needs to be substantiated in light of the most accepted hypotheses on the TrP induced pain. The integrated TrP hypothesis (33) proposed that a muscle overload causes ischemia and hypoxia in the muscle tissue leading to a cascade of biochemical events that finally ends in sarcomere contraction (e.g., a TrP) and produces nociceptive pain and tenderness of (pericranial) muscles. In contrast, the neuritis model (34, 78) hypothesized an inflammation of a peripheral nerve that produced a TrP as the result of ectopic impulses coming from the site of inflammation, while muscle pain and tenderness are described in terms of secondary hyperalgesia arising from the inflamed nerve. Considering primary headaches as separated entities, in case of TTH it has been proposed that the transformation from infrequent to chronic TTH is the result of the sensitization of the TNC (14, 43, 79) due to the presence of TrP according to the integrated TrP hypothesis. Thus, this mechanism is likely to explain the greater reduction of frequency and intensity of attacks for patients with TTH found in the present manuscript, but it is contradicted to some extent by the lack of reduction of duration of attacks as the de-sensitization of the TNC would also reduce the length of an attack likewise. In case of MH, it has been proposed according to the integrated TrP hypothesis that the nociceptive inputs arising from active TrPs may excite the TNC, activate the already sensitized trigemino-vascular system (16) and, consequently, promote a migraine attack (44). This mechanism may explain why frequency decreases to a little extent also in the MH group even though the reduction of intensity and duration of attacks seems paradoxical as the pain is driven by the trigemino-vascular system and not by the presence of TrPs which, constituting a precipitating factors, should influence only the frequency of the attacks. Furthermore, considering the vascular genesis proposed for TTH (15), the integrated TrP hypothesis is supported by the reduction of frequency of attacks with subtle effects on the reduction of duration of attacks, even though we should not expect a reduction of intensity of headache pain as previously described for MH.

The neuritis model better supports our results in terms of pooled groups and analyzed as subgroups. In fact, as MH may be the result of the central sensitization of the TNC due to inflammation of peripheral nerves it is possible that a TrPs treatment reduces frequency, intensity, and duration of MH attacks. Furthermore, supposing that the duration of attacks is driven by the central sensitization of the TNC according to the continuum model (30), the neuritis model may also explain why in TTH the duration of attacks is not reduced as TTH represents a mild form of migraine in which attacks are less intense and last less. However, the mechanisms of action of TrPs treatment with a neuritis model perspective remains unclear as TrPs are seen as the result of ectopic stimuli arising from the nerves and a link between muscular treatment and resolution of nerve inflammation has not been established yet apart from a reduction of mechanical forces on the nerves (80). Therefore, despite the proven effectiveness of the TrPs treatment on primary headaches, there is still the need to understand properly on which basis the manual TrPs treatment might work. For example, in one study (64) that delivered a sham treatment (detuned ultrasound) to the CG, an improvement was observed and this phenomenon pose several questions on which are the mechanisms underpinning the effectiveness of unblinded interventions, such as a placebo effect (81), as it may also activate cortical mechanisms of pain inhibition.

Our findings are in contrast with the result of a previous meta-analysis of Luedtke et al. (56) that reported no effect of physiotherapy (based mainly on exercises, modalities, relaxation techniques, and education) versus various comparators (any type of placebo intervention, any other active intervention as well as waiting list or standard care) in terms of intensity, frequency, and duration outcomes on primary headaches (56); however, authors included only one study adopting the TrP therapy, also present in the present manuscript (74), and did not consider primary headaches as an homogeneous group. It is, therefore, possible that the lack of specificity of treatments different from the TrPs therapy did not aim at the sensitization of the TNC and this may explain the different results. Finally, our results are consistent with two reviews reporting that a combination of massage therapy and exercise has the same efficacy of prophylactic treatment in patient with CTTH (52) and with MH (53).

At this time, we were unable to identify the most effective technique among those proposed as the treatments were delivered with a great variability in terms of techniques used (compression techniques, myofascial release, muscle energy, soft tissues, and positional release techniques) and their dosage (time of individual session, length of the treatment session, and the number of treatment per week); often the treatment protocols involved the use of more than a single technique. Furthermore, as the results were presented for MH and TTH merging episodic and chronic conditions, it was impossible to establish whether the effectiveness of TrPs manual treatment may differ among conditions with different frequency of attacks. Despite these considerations, both in TTH and MH, the muscles treated were mainly the sternocleidomastoideus, the upper trapezius, and the sub-occipitals and this could represent an important clinical indication for the operators.

Regarding pain reduction, although we have normalized the different scales to a single 0–100 scale, standardized unidimensional pain scales should be used in future studies to determine whether the obtained reduction has a clinical relevance and not merely a statistical significance.

Despite planned, we were not able to report on the additional negative effects of the manual treatment of TrPs as the included studies did not report them. The additional positive effects were reported sparsely in the retrieved studies, therefore, and they were grouped in three macro categories called medicine consumption, quality of life, and effects on TrPs. The evidences on reduction of medicine consumption were controversial: in patients with TTH one study reported a reduction (74, 76) and others no difference in the number of tablets taken (64, 75), while in MH the manual TrPs treatment may support the pharmacological treatment (75). The same doubts were present on the quality of life category, as there were no differences in questionnaires measuring general health (75) in patient with TTH and anxiety and stress in patients with MH (67). An effect was found for questionnaires like the HDI and the HIT-6 (60, 64). Furthermore, despite a similar amount of sleeping hours, the quality of sleep improved in patients with MH (67). For the category effects on TrPs, a reduction of the number of active TrPs (75) and an increased pressure pain threshold were found in the muscles manually treated (64, 74).

Our findings must be interpreted with caution for the weakness of the level of the evidence mainly due to the high RoB within studies and imprecision in results. Moreover, as the majority of the included studies had short-term follow-up, the long-term effect of TrPs manual treatment still needs to be established.

Performance and detection bias mainly constituted the judgment of high RoB across our trials downgrading the level of evidence. Performance bias refers to systematic differences between groups in the care that is provided, or in exposure to factors other than the interventions of interest. Detection bias refers to systematic differences between groups in how outcomes are determined (82). Blinding may reduce the risk that knowledge of which intervention was received, rather than the intervention itself, affects outcomes: it is a cornerstone of treatment evaluation (83). Lack of blinding in RCTs has been shown to be associated with more exaggerated estimated intervention effects (84, 85). As expected, blinding of participants and providers was not present in all of our studies. In fact, blinding is more difficult to obtain in trials assessing non-pharmacological treatments, such as manual therapy. Therefore, researchers and readers must be aware of existing methods of blinding to be able to appraise the feasibility of blinding in a trial (83). For example, in manual therapy, patients could be blind to the active placebo therapy (83). However, if blinding is not possible researchers could standardize the treatment of the groups (apart from the intervention), consider an expertise-based trial design, use objective, and reliable outcomes if possible, and consider duplicate assessment (86). Nevertheless, when performance bias could not be avoided, at least blinding of assessors must be performed to ensure unbiased ascertainment of outcomes (87), mostly in subjective outcomes (84). Furthermore, considering the chronicity of primary headaches, the use of single case research design (SCR) to demonstrate treatment efficacy may also have a role (88). SCR has been considered as a possible method for the scientific evaluation of manual therapies (89) and several reports argue for this (90–92).

The second important reason for downgrading the level of evidence was imprecision in results mainly due to an unwarranted paucity of participants included in the comparisons (mean of 45 subjects) that avoid to reach the optimal information size. Considering the high prevalence of headache and the largely adopted manual treatments, physical therapists and researchers should demonstrate that manual therapy represents a valid option (for example, no risk of toxicity or overuse of medications) in the spectrum of headache therapies. Only if they invest more efforts to enhance powered and well-designed RCTs, the interventions can be universally accepted by the evidence-based medicine. Therefore, we call for a launch of further well-designed trials. Particularly, we encourage clinicians, researchers, and all stakeholders to promote multicenter trials focused in manual therapy treatment for TTH and/or MG. Multicenter trials should be based on a powered sample size calculation needed to reach the clinical relevance of the manual treatment versus the minimal intervention. The RoB should be minimized at least through the blinding of assessment. Moreover, a trial sequential analysis could be proposed in order to aim at the firm evidence, confirming or confuting our preliminary results.

LIMITATIONS

The present review has some limitations that need to be addressed. Because we did not attempt to identify unpublished RCTs and our inclusion criteria were limited to only three languages, a publication bias could have occurred. The high variability of the delivered treatments prevented us from the identification of the most effective technique among those proposed. Even if epidemiological studies have determined that women are more likely to suffer from TTH and that female gender constitutes a risk factor for this disease (93), the higher prevalence of women in the TTH subgroup could make the results less applicable to the general population.

CONCLUSION

There was very low evidence that manual TrPs treatment of the head and neck muscles may constitute a useful treatment to reduce frequency, intensity, and duration of attack in patients with TTH and MH. The included studies did not report any additional negative effects, while positive effects regarding reduction of medicine consumption were controversial.

AUTHOR CONTRIBUTIONS

FML prepared the draft, planned the overall design, performed the search and quality/methodological assessment of the included studies. GT had the original idea of the study, planned the design, prepared the draft, and revised the drafted manuscript. ZM performed the search and quality/methodological assessment of the included studies. GS revised the methodological part and the synthesis of results. TM revised the final manuscript. All five authors have read and approved the final manuscript before submission.

REFERENCES

1. Stovner L, Hagen K, Jensen R, Katsarava Z, Lipton R, Scher A, et al. The global burden of headache: a documentation of headache prevalence and disability worldwide. *Cephalalgia* (2007) 27:193–210. doi:10.1111/j.1468-2982.2007.01288.x
2. Steiner TJ, Stovner LJ, Katsarava Z, Lainez JM, Lampl C, Lanteri-Minet M, et al. The impact of headache in Europe: principal results of the Eurolight project. *J Headache Pain* (2014) 15:31. doi:10.1186/1129-2377-15-31
3. Linde M, Gustavsson A, Stovner LJ, Steiner TJ, Barre J, Katsarava Z, et al. The cost of headache disorders in Europe: the Eurolight project. *Eur J Neurol* (2012) 19:703–11. doi:10.1111/j.1468-1331.2011.03612.x
4. Allena M, Steiner TJ, Sances G, Carugno B, Balsamo F, Nappi G, et al. Impact of headache disorders in Italy and the public-health and policy implications: a population-based study within the Eurolight project. *J Headache Pain* (2015) 16:100. doi:10.1186/s10194-015-0584-7
5. Fernandez-de-Las-Penas C, Cuadrado ML. Physical therapy for headaches. *Cephalalgia* (2016) 36:1134–42. doi:10.1177/0333102415596445
6. Grande RB, Aaseth K, Gulbrandsen P, Lundqvist C, Russell MB. Prevalence of primary chronic headache in a population-based sample of 30- to 44-year-old persons. The Akershus study of chronic headache. *Neuroepidemiology* (2008) 30:76–83. doi:10.1159/000116244
7. Kristoffersen ES, Grande RB, Aaseth K, Lundqvist C, Russell MB. Management of primary chronic headache in the general population: the Akershus study of chronic headache. *J Headache Pain* (2012) 13:113–20. doi:10.1007/s10194-011-0391-8
8. Aaseth K, Grande RB, Kvaerner KJ, Gulbrandsen P, Lundqvist C, Russell MB. Prevalence of secondary chronic headaches in a population-based sample of 30–44-year-old persons. The Akershus study of chronic headache. *Cephalalgia* (2008) 28:705–13. doi:10.1111/j.1468-2982.2008.01577.x

9. Bronfort G, Nilsson N, Haas M, Evans R, Goldsmith CH, Assendelft WJ, et al. Non-invasive physical treatments for chronic/recurrent headache. *Cochrane Database Syst Rev* (2004) 3:CD001878. doi:10.1002/14651858.CD001878.pub2
10. Carnes D, Mars TS, Mullinger B, Froud R, Underwood M. Adverse events and manual therapy: a systematic review. *Man Ther* (2010) 15:355–63. doi:10.1016/j.math.2009.12.006
11. Jensen R. Diagnosis, epidemiology, and impact of tension-type headache. *Curr Pain Headache Rep* (2003) 7:455–9. doi:10.1007/s11916-003-0061-x
12. Bendtsen L, Evers S, Linde M, Mitsikostas DD, Sandrini G, Schoenen J. EFNS guideline on the treatment of tension-type headache – report of an EFNS task force. *Eur J Neurol* (2010) 17:1318–25. doi:10.1111/j.1468-1331.2010.03070.x
13. Headache Classification Committee of the International Headache Society. The international classification of headache disorders, 3rd edition (beta version). *Cephalalgia* (2013) 33:629–808. doi:10.1177/0333102413485658
14. Bendtsen L, Ashina S, Moore A, Steiner TJ. Muscles and their role in episodic tension-type headache: implications for treatment. *Eur J Pain* (2016) 20:166–75. doi:10.1002/ejp.748
15. Chen Y. Advances in the pathophysiology of tension-type headache: from stress to central sensitization. *Curr Pain Headache Rep* (2009) 13:484–94. doi:10.1007/s11916-009-0078-x
16. Noseda R, Burstein R. Migraine pathophysiology: anatomy of the trigeminovascular pathway and associated neurological symptoms, cortical spreading depression, sensitization, and modulation of pain. *Pain* (2013) 154(Suppl 1): S44–53. doi:10.1016/j.pain.2013.07.021
17. Olesen J. The international classification of headache disorders. *Headache* (2008) 48:691–3. doi:10.1111/j.1526-4610.2008.01121.x
18. Lipton RB, Bigal ME, Diamond M, Freitag F, Reed ML, Stewart WF, et al. Migraine prevalence, disease burden, and the need for preventive therapy. *Neurology* (2007) 68:343–9. doi:10.1212/01.wnl.0000252808.97649.21
19. Featherstone HJ. Migraine and muscle contraction headaches: a continuum. *Headache* (1985) 25:194–8. doi:10.1111/j.1526-4610.1985.hed2504194.x
20. Bakal DA, Demjen S, Kaganov J. The continuous nature of headache susceptibility. *Soc Sci Med* (1984) 19:1305–11. doi:10.1016/0277-9536(84)90017-0
21. Nelson CF. The tension headache, migraine headache continuum: a hypothesis. *J Manipulative Physiol Ther* (1994) 17:156–67.
22. Marcus DA. Migraine and tension-type headaches: the questionable validity of current classification systems. *Clin J Pain* (1992) 8:28–36; discussion 37–28. doi:10.1097/00002508-199203000-00006
23. Vargas BB. Tension-type headache and migraine: two points on a continuum? *Curr Pain Headache Rep* (2008) 12:433–6. doi:10.1007/s11916-008-0073-7
24. Spierings EL, Ranke AH, Honkoop PC. Precipitating and aggravating factors of migraine versus tension-type headache. *Headache* (2001) 41:554–8. doi:10.1046/j.1526-4610.2001.041006554.x
25. Pellegrino ABW, Davis-Martin RE, Houle TT, Turner DP, Smitherman TA. Perceived triggers of primary headache disorders: a meta-analysis. *Cephalalgia* (2017). doi:10.1177/0333102417727535
26. Schmidt-Wilcke T, Leinisch E, Straube A, Kampfe N, Draganski B, Diener HC, et al. Gray matter decrease in patients with chronic tension type headache. *Neurology* (2005) 65:1483–6. doi:10.1212/01.wnl.0000183067.94400.80
27. Schmidt-Wilcke T, Luerding R, Weigand T, Jurgens T, Schuierer G, Leinisch E, et al. Striatal grey matter increase in patients suffering from fibromyalgia – a voxel-based morphometry study. *Pain* (2007) 132(Suppl 1):S109–16. doi:10.1016/j.pain.2007.05.010
28. Turner DP, Smitherman TA, Black AK, Penzien DB, Porter JA, Lofland KR, et al. Are migraine and tension-type headache diagnostic types or points on a severity continuum? An exploration of the latent taxometric structure of headache. *Pain* (2015) 156:1200–7. doi:10.1097/j.pain.0000000000000157
29. Peres MF, Goncalves AL, Krymchantowski A. Migraine, tension-type headache, and transformed migraine. *Curr Pain Headache Rep* (2007) 11:449–53. doi:10.1007/s11916-007-0232-2
30. Cady RK. The convergence hypothesis. *Headache* (2007) 47(Suppl 1):S44–51. doi:10.1111/j.1526-4610.2007.00676.x
31. Ge HY, Arendt-Nielsen L. Latent myofascial trigger points. *Curr Pain Headache Rep* (2011) 15:386–92. doi:10.1007/s11916-011-0210-6
32. Celik D, Mutlu EK. Clinical implication of latent myofascial trigger point. *Curr Pain Headache Rep* (2013) 17:353. doi:10.1007/s11916-013-0353-8
33. Gerwin RD, Dommerholt J, Shah JP. An expansion of Simons' integrated hypothesis of trigger point formation. *Curr Pain Headache Rep* (2004) 8:468–75. doi:10.1007/s11916-004-0069-x
34. Quintner JL, Bove GM, Cohen ML. A critical evaluation of the trigger point phenomenon. *Rheumatology (Oxford)* (2015) 54:392–9. doi:10.1093/rheumatology/keu471
35. Couppe C, Torelli P, Fuglsang-Frederiksen A, Andersen KV, Jensen R. Myofascial trigger points are very prevalent in patients with chronic tension-type headache: a double-blinded controlled study. *Clin J Pain* (2007) 23:23–7. doi:10.1097/01.ajp.0000210946.34676.7d
36. Ferracini GN, Florencio LL, Dach F, Chaves TC, Palacios-Cena M, Fernandez-de-Las-Penas C, et al. Myofascial trigger points and migraine-related disability in women with episodic and chronic migraine. *Clin J Pain* (2017) 33:109–15. doi:10.1097/AJP.0000000000000387
37. Fernandez-de-Las-Penas C, Cuadrado ML, Pareja JA. Myofascial trigger points, neck mobility and forward head posture in unilateral migraine. *Cephalalgia* (2006) 26:1061–70. doi:10.1111/j.1468-2982.2006.01162.x
38. Fernandez-de-Las-Penas C, Alonso-Blanco C, Cuadrado ML, Gerwin RD, Pareja JA. Myofascial trigger points and their relationship to headache clinical parameters in chronic tension-type headache. *Headache* (2006) 46:1264–72. doi:10.1111/j.1526-4610.2006.00440.x
39. Calandre EP, Hidalgo J, Garcia-Leiva JM, Rico-Villademoros F. Trigger point evaluation in migraine patients: an indication of peripheral sensitization linked to migraine predisposition? *Eur J Neurol* (2006) 13:244–9. doi:10.1111/j.1468-1331.2006.01181.x
40. Noudeh YJ, Vatankhah N, Baradaran HR. Reduction of current migraine headache pain following neck massage and spinal manipulation. *Int J Ther Massage Bodywork* (2012) 5:5–13.
41. Garcia-Leiva JM, Hidalgo J, Rico-Villademoros F, Moreno V, Calandre EP. Effectiveness of ropivacaine trigger points inactivation in the prophylactic management of patients with severe migraine. *Pain Med* (2007) 8:65–70. doi:10.1111/j.1526-4637.2007.00251.x
42. Calandre EP, Hidalgo J, Garcia-Leiva JM, Rico-Villademoros F, Delgado-Rodriguez A. Myofascial trigger points in cluster headache patients: a case series. *Head Face Med* (2008) 4:32. doi:10.1186/1746-160X-4-32
43. Fernandez-de-las-Penas C, Cuadrado ML, Arendt-Nielsen L, Simons DG, Pareja JA. Myofascial trigger points and sensitization: an updated pain model for tension-type headache. *Cephalalgia* (2007) 27:383–93. doi:10.1111/j.1468-2982.2007.01295.x
44. Giamberardino MA, Tafuri E, Savini A, Fabrizio A, Affaitati G, Lerza R, et al. Contribution of myofascial trigger points to migraine symptoms. *J Pain* (2007) 8:869–78. doi:10.1016/j.jpain.2007.06.002
45. Cagnie B, Castelein B, Pollie F, Steelant L, Verhoeyen H, Cools A. Evidence for the use of ischemic compression and dry needling in the management of trigger points of the upper trapezius in patients with neck pain: a systematic review. *Am J Phys Med Rehabil* (2015) 94:573–83. doi:10.1097/PHM.0000000000000266
46. Ajimsha MS, Al-Mudahka NR, Al-Madzhar JA. Effectiveness of myofascial release: systematic review of randomized controlled trials. *J Bodyw Mov Ther* (2015) 19:102–12. doi:10.1016/j.jbmt.2014.06.001
47. Hsieh LL, Liou HH, Lee LH, Chen TH, Yen AM. Effect of acupressure and trigger points in treating headache: a randomized controlled trial. *Am J Chin Med* (2010) 38:1–14. doi:10.1142/S0192415X10007634
48. Kojidi MM, Okhovatian F, Rahimi A, Baghban AA, Azimi H. Comparison between the effects of passive and active soft tissue therapies on latent trigger points of upper trapezius muscle in women: single-blind, randomized clinical trial. *J Chiropr Med* (2016) 15:235–42. doi:10.1016/j.jcm.2016.08.010
49. Yeganeh Lari A, Okhovatian F, Naimi S, Baghban AA. The effect of the combination of dry needling and MET on latent trigger point upper trapezius in females. *Man Ther* (2016) 21:204–9. doi:10.1016/j.math.2015.08.004
50. Mohammadi Kojidi M, Okhovatian F, Rahimi A, Baghban AA, Azimi H. The influence of positional release therapy on the myofascial trigger points of the upper trapezius muscle in computer users. *J Bodyw Mov Ther* (2016) 20:767–73. doi:10.1016/j.jbmt.2016.04.006
51. Wong CK, Abraham T, Karimi P, Ow-Wing C. Strain counterstrain technique to decrease tender point palpation pain compared to control conditions: a systematic review with meta-analysis. *J Bodyw Mov Ther* (2014) 18:165–73. doi:10.1016/j.jbmt.2013.09.010
52. Chaibi A, Russell MB. Manual therapies for primary chronic headaches: a systematic review of randomized controlled trials. *J Headache Pain* (2014) 15:67. doi:10.1186/1129-2377-15-67

53. Chaibi A, Tuchin PJ, Russell MB. Manual therapies for migraine: a systematic review. *J Headache Pain* (2011) 12:127–33. doi:10.1007/s10194-011-0296-6
54. Lenssinck ML, Damen L, Verhagen AP, Berger MY, Passchier J, Koes BW. The effectiveness of physiotherapy and manipulation in patients with tension-type headache: a systematic review. *Pain* (2004) 112:381–8. doi:10.1016/j.pain.2004.09.026
55. Posadzki P, Ernst E. Spinal manipulations for tension-type headaches: a systematic review of randomized controlled trials. *Complement Ther Med* (2012) 20:232–9. doi:10.1016/j.ctim.2011.12.001
56. Luedtke K, Allers A, Schulte LH, May A. Efficacy of interventions used by physiotherapists for patients with headache and migraine-systematic review and meta-analysis. *Cephalalgia* (2016) 36:474–92. doi:10.1177/0333102415597889
57. Moher D, Liberati A, Tetzlaff J, Altman DG. Preferred reporting items for systematic reviews and meta-analyses: the PRISMA statement. *J Clin Epidemiol* (2009) 62:1006–12. doi:10.1016/j.jclinepi.2009.06.005
58. Higgins JPT, Green S, editors. *Cochrane Handbook for Systematic Reviews of Interventions. Version 5.1.0.* The Cochrane Collaboration (2011). Available from: http://handbook.cochrane.org
59. Geri T, Falsiroli Maistrello L, Gianola S, Zaninetti M, Testa M. *Effectiveness of Trigger Point Manual Treatment on the Frequency, Intensity and Duration of Attack in Primary Headaches: A Systematic Review and Meta-Analysis of Randomized Controlled Trials* (2016). CRD42016046374. PROSPERO. Available from: http://www.crd.york.ac.uk/PROSPERO/display_record.php?ID=CRD42016046374
60. Ferragut-Garcias A, Plaza-Manzano G, Rodriguez-Blanco C, Velasco-Roldan O, Pecos-Martin D, Oliva-Pascual-Vaca J, et al. Effectiveness of a treatment involving soft tissue techniques and/or neural mobilization techniques in the management of tension-type headache: a randomized controlled trial. *Arch Phys Med Rehabil* (2016) 98(2):211–9.e2. doi:10.1016/j.apmr.2016.08.466
61. DerSimonian R, Laird N. Meta-analysis in clinical trials. *Control Clin Trials* (1986) 7:177–88. doi:10.1016/0197-2456(86)90046-2
62. Herr K, Spratt KF, Garand L, Li L. Evaluation of the Iowa pain thermometer and other selected pain intensity scales in younger and older adult cohorts using controlled clinical pain: a preliminary study. *Pain Med* (2007) 8:585–600. doi:10.1111/j.1526-4637.2007.00316.x
63. Higgins JPT, Deeks JJ, Altman DG. Chapter 16: Special topics in statistics. In: Higgins JPT, Green S, editors. *Cochrane Handbook for Systematic Reviews of Interventions. Version 5.1.0.* The Cochrane Collaboration (2011). Available from: http://handbook-5-1.cochrane.org/ [Updated: March 2011].
64. Moraska AF, Stenerson L, Butryn N, Krutsch JP, Schmiege SJ, Mann JD. Myofascial trigger point-focused head and neck massage for recurrent tension-type headache: a randomized, placebo-controlled clinical trial. *Clin J Pain* (2015) 31:159–68. doi:10.1097/AJP.0000000000000091
65. Ajimsha MS. Effectiveness of direct vs indirect technique myofascial release in the management of tension-type headache. *J Bodyw Mov Ther* (2011) 15:431–5. doi:10.1016/j.jbmt.2011.01.021
66. Higgins JP, Thompson SG, Deeks JJ, Altman DG. Measuring inconsistency in meta-analyses. *BMJ* (2003) 327:557–60. doi:10.1136/bmj.327.7414.557
67. Lawler SP, Cameron LD. A randomized, controlled trial of massage therapy as a treatment for migraine. *Ann Behav Med* (2006) 32:50–9. doi:10.1207/s15324796abm3201_6
68. The Cochrane Collaboration. *Review Manager (RevMan) [Computer program]. Version 5.3.* Copenhagen: The Nordic Cochrane Center (2014). Available from: http://community.cochrane.org/tools/review-production-tools/revman-5/about-revman-5 (Accessed: January 29, 2017).
69. Schunemann HJ, Oxman AD, Brozek J, Glasziou P, Bossuyt P, Chang S, et al. GRADE: assessing the quality of evidence for diagnostic recommendations. *Evid Based Med* (2008) 13:162–3. doi:10.1136/ebm.13.6.162-a
70. Guyatt GH, Oxman AD, Vist GE, Kunz R, Falck-Ytter Y, Alonso-Coello P, et al. GRADE: an emerging consensus on rating quality of evidence and strength of recommendations. *BMJ* (2008) 336:924–6. doi:10.1136/bmj.39489.470347.AD
71. GRADEpro Guideline Development Tool. *GRADEpro GDT.* McMaster University (Developed by Evidence Prime, Inc.) (2015). Available from: https://gradepro.org/cite.html (Accessed: June 06, 2017).
72. Fernandez-de-Las-Penas C, Alonso-Blanco C, Cuadrado ML, Miangolarra JC, Barriga FJ, Pareja JA. Are manual therapies effective in reducing pain from tension-type headache? A systematic review. *Clin J Pain* (2006) 22:278–85. doi:10.1097/01.ajp.0000173017.64741.86
73. Lozano Lopez C, Mesa Jimenez J, de la Hoz Aizpurua JL, Pareja Grande J, Fernandez de Las Penas C. Efficacy of manual therapy in the treatment of tension-type headache. A systematic review from 2000–2013. *Neurologia* (2014) 31(6):357–69. doi:10.1016/j.nrl.2014.01.002
74. Ghanbari A, Rahimijaberi A, Mohamadi M, Abbasi L, Sarvestani FK. The effect of trigger point management by positional release therapy on tension type headache. *NeuroRehabilitation* (2012) 30:333–9. doi:10.3233/NRE-2012-0764
75. Berggreen S, Wiik E, Lund H. Treatment of myofascial trigger points in female patients with chronic tension-type headache – a randomized controlled trial. *Adv Physiother* (2012) 14:10–7. doi:10.3109/14038196.2011.647333
76. Ghanbari A, Askarzadeh S, Petramfar P, Mohamadi M. Migraine responds better to a combination of medical therapy and trigger point management than routine medical therapy alone. *NeuroRehabilitation* (2015) 37:157–63. doi:10.3233/NRE-151248
77. Toro-Velasco C, Arroyo-Morales M, Fernandez-de-Las-Penas C, Cleland JA, Barrero-Hernandez FJ. Short-term effects of manual therapy on heart rate variability, mood state, and pressure pain sensitivity in patients with chronic tension-type headache: a pilot study. *J Manipulative Physiol Ther* (2009) 32:527–35. doi:10.1016/j.jmpt.2009.08.011
78. Quintner JL, Cohen ML. Referred pain of peripheral nerve origin: an alternative to the "myofascial pain" construct. *Clin J Pain* (1994) 10:243–51. doi:10.1097/00002508-199409000-00012
79. Ashina S, Bendtsen L, Ashina M. Pathophysiology of tension-type headache. *Curr Pain Headache Rep* (2005) 9:415–22. doi:10.1007/s11916-005-0021-8
80. Dilley A, Odeyinde S, Greening J, Lynn B. Longitudinal sliding of the median nerve in patients with non-specific arm pain. *Man Ther* (2008) 13:536–43. doi:10.1016/j.math.2007.07.004
81. Rossettini G, Testa M. Manual therapy RCTs: should we control placebo in placebo control? *Eur J Phys Rehabil Med* (2017). doi:10.23736/S1973-9087.17.05024-9
82. Altman DG, Schulz KF, Moher D, Egger M, Davidoff F, Elbourne D, et al. The revised CONSORT statement for reporting randomized trials: explanation and elaboration. *Ann Intern Med* (2001) 134:663–94. doi:10.7326/0003-4819-134-8-200104170-00012
83. Boutron I, Guittet L, Estellat C, Moher D, Hrobjartsson A, Ravaud P. Reporting methods of blinding in randomized trials assessing nonpharmacological treatments. *PLoS Med* (2007) 4:e61. doi:10.1371/journal.pmed.0040061
84. Wood L, Egger M, Gluud LL, Schulz KF, Juni P, Altman DG, et al. Empirical evidence of bias in treatment effect estimates in controlled trials with different interventions and outcomes: meta-epidemiological study. *BMJ* (2008) 336:601–5. doi:10.1136/bmj.39465.451748.AD
85. Pildal J, Hrobjartsson A, Jorgensen KJ, Hilden J, Altman DG, Gotzsche PC. Impact of allocation concealment on conclusions drawn from meta-analyses of randomized trials. *Int J Epidemiol* (2007) 36:847–57. doi:10.1093/ije/dym087
86. Karanicolas PJ, Farrokhyar F, Bhandari M. Practical tips for surgical research: blinding: who, what, when, why, how? *Can J Surg* (2010) 53:345–8.
87. Boutron I, Moher D, Altman DG, Schulz KF, Ravaud P; CONSORT Group. Extending the CONSORT statement to randomized trials of nonpharmacologic treatment: explanation and elaboration. *Ann Intern Med* (2008) 148:295–309. doi:10.7326/0003-4819-148-4-200802190-00008
88. Rvachew S, Matthews T. Demonstrating treatment efficacy using the single subject randomization design: a tutorial and demonstration. *J Commun Disord* (2017) 67:1–13. doi:10.1016/j.jcomdis.2017.04.003
89. Wolery M, Harris SR. Interpreting results of single-subject research designs. *Phys Ther* (1982) 62:445–52. doi:10.1093/ptj/62.4.445
90. Maricar N, Shacklady C, McLoughlin L. Effect of Maitland mobilization and exercises for the treatment of shoulder adhesive capsulitis: a single-case design. *Physiother Theory Pract* (2009) 25:203–17. doi:10.1080/09593980902776654
91. Puentedura EJ, Brooksby CL, Wallmann HW, Landers MR. Rehabilitation following lumbosacral percutaneous nucleoplasty: a case report. *J Orthop Sports Phys Ther* (2010) 40:214–24. doi:10.2519/jospt.2010.3115
92. Treleaven J. A tailored sensorimotor approach for management of whiplash associated disorders. A single case study. *Man Ther* (2010) 15:206–9. doi:10.1016/j.math.2009.05.001
93. Lyngberg AC, Rasmussen BK, Jorgensen T, Jensen R. Has the prevalence of migraine and tension-type headache changed over a 12-year period? A Danish population survey. *Eur J Epidemiol* (2005) 20:243–9. doi:10.1007/s10654-004-6519-2

7

Patient-Active Control of a Powered Exoskeleton Targeting Upper Limb Rehabilitation Training

Qingcong Wu[1*], *Xingsong Wang*[2], *Bai Chen*[1] *and Hongtao Wu*[1]

[1] *College of Mechanical and Electrical Engineering, Nanjing University of Aeronautics and Astronautics, Nanjing, China,*
[2] *College of Mechanical Engineering, Southeast University, Nanjing, China*

***Correspondence:**
Qingcong Wu
wuqc@nuaa.edu.cn

Robot-assisted therapy affords effective advantages to the rehabilitation training of patients with motion impairment problems. To meet the challenge of integrating the active participation of a patient in robotic training, this study presents an admittance-based patient-active control scheme for real-time intention-driven control of a powered upper limb exoskeleton. A comprehensive overview is proposed to introduce the major mechanical structure and the real-time control system of the developed therapeutic robot, which provides seven actuated degrees of freedom and achieves the natural ranges of human arm movement. Moreover, the dynamic characteristics of the human-exoskeleton system are studied via a Lagrangian method. The patient-active control strategy consisting of an admittance module and a virtual environment module is developed to regulate the robot configurations and interaction forces during rehabilitation training. An audiovisual game-like interface is integrated into the therapeutic system to encourage the voluntary efforts of the patient and recover the neural plasticity of the brain. Further experimental investigation, involving a position tracking experiment, a free arm training experiment, and a virtual airplane-game operation experiment, is conducted with three healthy subjects and eight hemiplegic patients with different motor abilities. Experimental results validate the feasibility of the proposed scheme in providing patient-active rehabilitation training.

Keywords: upper limb exoskeleton, robot-assisted, rehabilitation training, patient-active control, intention-driven, virtual environment

INTRODUCTION

Stroke is a severe neurological disease caused by the blockages or rupture of cerebral blood vessels, leading to significant physical disability and cognitive impairment (1, 2). The recent statistics from the World Health Organization indicate that worldwide 15 million people annually suffer from the effect of stroke, and more than 5 million stroke patients survive and, however, require a prolonged physical therapy to recover motor function. Recent trends predict increased stroke incidence at younger ages in the upcoming years (3, 4). Approximately four-fifths of all survived stroke patients suffer from the problems of hemiparesis or hemiplegia and, as a result, have difficulties in performing activities of daily living (ADL). Stroke causes tremendous mental and economic pressure on the patients and their families (5). Medical research has proved that, owing to the neural plasticity of the human brain, appropriate rehabilitation trainings are beneficial for stroke survivors to recover musculoskeletal motor abilities. Repetitive and task-oriented functional activities have substantial positive effects on improving motor coordination and avoiding muscle atrophy (6, 7). Traditional stroke rehabilitation therapy involves many medical disciplines, such as orthopedics, physical medicine, and neurophysiology (8, 9). Physiotherapists and medical personnel are required to provide for months one-on-one interactions to patients that are labor intensive, time consuming, patient-passive, and costly. Besides, the effectiveness of traditional therapeutic trainings is limited by the personal experiences and skills of therapists (10, 11).

In recent decades, robot-assisted rehabilitation therapies have attracted increasing attention because of their unique advantages and promising applications (12, 13). Compared with the traditional manual repetitive therapy, the use of robotic technologies helps improve the performance and efficiency of therapeutic training (14). Robot-assisted therapy can deliver high-intensive, long-endurance, and goal-directed rehabilitation treatments and reduce expense. Besides, the physical parameters and the training performance of patients can be monitored and evaluated via built-in sensing systems that facilitate the improvement of the rehabilitation strategy (15, 16). Many therapeutic robots have been developed to improve the motor functions of the upper extremity of disabled stroke patients exhibiting permanent sensorimotor arm impairments (17). The existing robots used for upper limb training can be basically classified into two types: end-point robots and exoskeleton robots. End-point robots work by applying external forces to the distal end of impaired limbs, and some examples are MIME (18), HipBot (19), GENTLE/s (20), and TA-WREX (21). Comparatively, exoskeleton robots have complex structures similar to anatomy of the human skeleton; some examples of such robots are NMES (22), HES (23), NEUROExos (24), CAREX-7 (25), IntelliArm (26), BONES (27), and RUPERT (28). The joints of the exoskeleton need to be aligned with the human anatomical joints for effective transfer of interactive forces.

The control strategies applied in therapeutic robots are important to ensure the effectiveness of rehabilitation training. So far, according to the training requirement of patients with different impairment severities, many control schemes have been developed to perform therapy and accelerate recovery. Early rehabilitation robot systems implemented patient-passive control algorithms to imitate the manual therapeutic actions of therapists. These training schemes are suitable for patients with severe paralysis to passively execute repetitive reaching tasks along predefined trajectories. Primary clinical results indicate that patient-passive training contributes to motivating muscle contraction and preventing deterioration of arm functions. The control of the human–robot interaction system is a great challenge due to its highly nonlinear characteristics. Many control algorithms have been proposed to enhance the tracking accuracy of passive training, such as the robust adaptive neural controller (29), fuzzy adaptive backstepping controller (30), neural proportional–integral–derivative (PID) controller (31), fuzzy sliding mode controller (32), and neuron PI controller (33).

The major disadvantage of patient-passive training is that the active participation of patients is neglected during therapeutic treatment (34). Several studies suggest that, for the patients who have regained parts of motor functions, the rehabilitation treatment integrated with the voluntary efforts of patients facilitates the recovery of lost motor ability (35). The patient-active control, normally referred as patient-cooperative control and assist-as-needed control, is capable of regulating the human–robot interaction depending on the motion intention and the disability level of patients. Keller et al. proposed an exoskeleton for pediatric arm rehabilitation. A multimodal patient-cooperative control strategy was developed to assist upper limb movements with an audiovisual game-like interface (36). Duschauwicke et al. proposed an impedance-based control approach for patient-cooperative robot-aided gait rehabilitation. The affected limb was constrained with a virtual tunnel around the desired spatial path (37). Ye et al. proposed an adaptive electromyography (EMG) signals-based control strategy for an exoskeleton to provide efficient motion guidance and training assistance (38). Oldewurtel et al. developed a hybrid admittance–impedance controller to maximize the contribution of patients during rehabilitation training (39). Banala et al. developed a force-field assist-as-need controller for intensive gait rehabilitation training (40). However, there are two limitations in the existing patient-cooperative control strategies. Firstly, the rehabilitation training process is not completely patient-active, as the patient needs to perform training tasks along a certain predefined trajectory. Secondly, existing control strategies are executed in self-designed virtual scenarios that are generally too simple, rough, and uninteresting. Besides, applying a certain control strategy to different virtual reality scenarios is difficult.

Taking the above issues into consideration, the main contribution of this paper is to develop a control strategy for an upper limb exoskeleton to assist disabled patients in performing active rehabilitation training in a virtual scenario based on their own active motion intentions. Firstly, the overall structure design and the real-time control system of the exoskeleton system are briefly introduced. A dynamic model of the human–robot interaction system is then established using the Lagrangian approach. After that, an admittance-based patient-active controller combined with an audiovisual therapy interface is proposed to induce the active participation of patients during training. Existing commercial virtual games without a specific predetermined training trajectory can be integrated into the controller via a virtual keyboard unit. Finally, three types of experiments, namely the position tracking experiment without interaction force, the free arm movement experiment, and the virtual airplane-game operation experiment, are conducted with healthy and disabled subjects. The experimental results demonstrate the feasibility of the proposed exoskeleton and control strategy.

MATERIALS AND METHODS

Exoskeleton Robot Design

The architecture of the proposed exoskeleton is shown in **Figure 1**. This wearable force-feedback exoskeleton robot has seven actuated degrees of freedom (DOFs) and two passive DOFs covering the natural range of movement (ROM) of humans in ADL. The robot has been designed with an open-chain structure to mimic the anatomy of the human

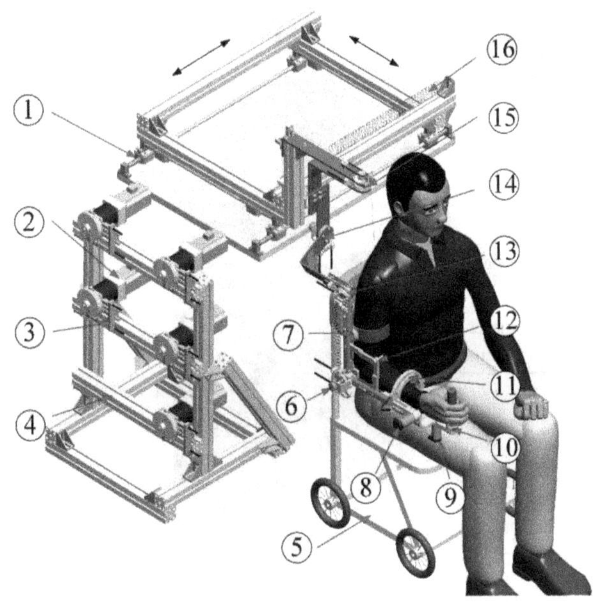

FIGURE 1 | Architecture of upper limb rehabilitation exoskeleton (1-Self-aligning platform; 2-AC servo motor; 3-Bowden cable components; 4-Support frame; 5-Wheelchair; 6-Elbow flexion/extension; 7-Proximal force/torque sensor; 8-Wrist flexion/extension; 9-Wrist ulnal/radial deviation; 10-Distal force/torque sensor; 11-Forearm pronation/supination; 12-Auxiliary links; 13-Shoulder flexion/extension; 14-Shoulder abduction/adduction; 15-Shoulder internal/external; 16-Free-length spring).

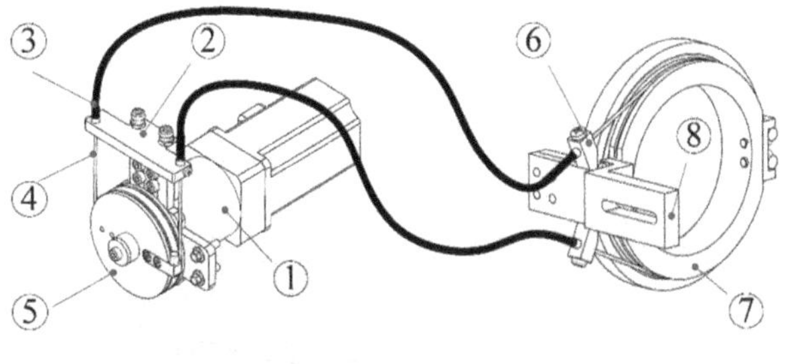

FIGURE 2 | Schematic of the Bowden-cable actuation system (1-Servo motor and planetary gear reducer; 2-Pretension device; 3-Outer sheath; 4-Inner cable; 5- Proximal pulley; 6-Cable supports; 7-Distal pulley; 8-Exoskeleton link).

right arm and provide controllable assistance torque to each robot joint. There are three actuated DOFs at the shoulder for internal/external rotation, abduction/adduction, and flexion/extension; two DOFs at the elbow for flexion/extension and pronation/supination; and two DOFs at the wrist for flexion/extension and ulnal/radial deviation. Besides, since the center of rotation of the glenohumeral joint varies with the shoulder girdle movement, the robot is mounted on a self-aligning platform with two passive translational DOFs to compensate the human–robot misalignment and to guarantee interaction comfort.

The lengths of the upper arm and the forearm as well as the shoulder height of the exoskeleton can be adjusted to satisfy the dimensions of patients with body heights in the range of 1.6 m to 1.9 m. The revolute robot joints at the shoulder and the elbow are actuated by the flexible Bowden-cable actuation systems located on the remote support frame (41). The schematic of the Bowden-cable actuator is depicted in **Figure 2**. It mainly consists of a servo AC motor (SGMAV-04A, YASKAWA) combined with a planetary gear reducer (Yantong, transmission ratio: 40) used to produce a maximum torque of 35 Nm, two bendable Bowden-cable transmission units used to transmit driving torque from the proximal pulley to the distal pulley, and a pretension device used to adjust cable pretension and eliminate the slacking problem resulting from cable elasticity. In addition, the wrist joints of the exoskeleton are actuated by two high-precision coreless DC servo motors (JG-37, ASLONG).

A passive gravity-compensation mechanism made up of two zero free-length springs and two auxiliary parallel links is integrated into the exoskeleton to balance the gravity of the entire system [detailed description can be found in (42)]. The configuration of the exoskeleton is measured by using a rotary potentiometer (WDJ22A-10K) encapsulated in each robot joint. Two six-axis force/torque (F/T) sensors (NANO-25, ATI) are located at the upper arm and the end-effector to acquire the interaction forces between the robot and the operator. The custom Velcro fasteners attached to the upper arm and the forearm of the exoskeleton facilitate the connection and separation between the human arm and the robot. For safety, the available ROM of each actuated joint is limited via a mechanical stop to avoid collisions and excessive motion. Two dead-man buttons are available to both the patient and physiotherapists to immediately shut down the motor power in the case of an emergency.

Electrical Control System

The closed-loop real-time control system of the therapeutic exoskeleton is built in the MATLAB/Real-Time-Workshop (RTW) environment with a hierarchical architecture, as shown in **Figure 3**. Two industrial personal computers (IPC-610H, Advantech Inc.) are used as the host and target computers. The host computer is capable of transforming the Simulink control model to the executable codes, while the target computer takes charge of implementing the embedded targeted codes and regulating the operation of the robot system. The analog feedback signals from the potentiometers and F/T sensors are amplified by power amplifiers (LKM-66, FMS) and acquired via three industrial analog-to-digital converters (PCL-818, Advantech Inc.). The control algorithm running in the target computer is converted into analog output signals by two industrial digital-to-analog cards (PCL-726, Advantech Inc.) The output analog signals are transmitted to the servo drivers to control servo motors with a sampling rate of 1 kHz.

Dynamics Modeling

It is important to analyze the dynamic characteristics of the exoskeleton equipped on the right arm of the operator to improve the control system performance. The overall dynamic model

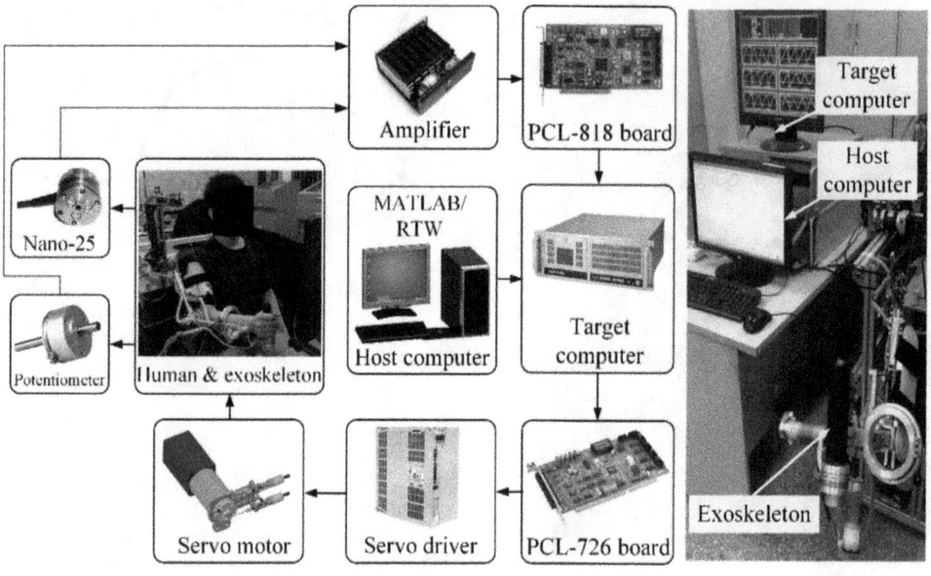

FIGURE 3 | The MATLAB/Real-Time-Workshop/xPC control system. **(A)** Hardware architecture diagram. **(B)** Experimental setup.

of the exoskeleton with human–robot interaction forces can be established based on the Lagrangian approach as follows:

$$\mathbf{M}(\boldsymbol{\theta})\ddot{\boldsymbol{\theta}} + \mathbf{V}(\boldsymbol{\theta}, \dot{\boldsymbol{\theta}}) + \boldsymbol{\tau}_{\mathrm{f}}(\boldsymbol{\theta}, \dot{\boldsymbol{\theta}}) + \mathbf{D}_{\mathrm{u}} - \mathbf{J}_1^T(\boldsymbol{\theta})\boldsymbol{\Gamma}_1 - \mathbf{J}_2^T(\boldsymbol{\theta})\boldsymbol{\Gamma}_2 = \boldsymbol{\tau}, \tag{1}$$

where $\boldsymbol{\theta}, \dot{\boldsymbol{\theta}}$, and $\ddot{\boldsymbol{\theta}}$ denote the vectors of generalized positions, velocities, and accelerations of actuated joints. $\mathbf{M}(\boldsymbol{\theta})$ represents the symmetric positive-defined system inertia matrix. $\mathbf{V}(\boldsymbol{\theta}, \dot{\boldsymbol{\theta}})$ denotes the vector of centrifugal and Coriolis torque. $\boldsymbol{\tau}_{\mathrm{f}}(\boldsymbol{\theta}, \dot{\boldsymbol{\theta}})$ is the friction vector of the robot system. $\mathbf{D}_{\mathrm{u}}$ represents the lumped effects of uncertainties. $\boldsymbol{\Gamma}_1$ and Γ_2 represent the Cartesian interaction forces acting on the upper arm and the end-effector of the exoskeleton, respectively. Jacobian matrixes, $\mathbf{J}_1(\boldsymbol{\theta})$ and $\mathbf{J}_2(\boldsymbol{\theta})$, provide the mapping from the interaction forces to the torques at robot joints, and they can be derived from the kinematics model of the exoskeleton (43). The vector τ is the output driving torques of servo motors.

It should be pointed out that the vector of gravitational torque is eliminated in Equation (1), as the proposed exoskeleton robot is kept in a static balanced state during the operation (42). Note that since the movement range of the passive self-aligning platform is fairly limited and small during rehabilitation training, the platform is assumed to be stationary while developing the system dynamic model. The experimental results obtained in our previous work have verified the rationality of this assumption.

The friction existing in the exoskeleton system can be basically subdivided into three parts: the friction from Bowden-cable transmission systems $\boldsymbol{\tau}_b(\boldsymbol{\theta}, \dot{\boldsymbol{\theta}})$, the friction from the reducers of motors $\boldsymbol{\tau}_r(\boldsymbol{\theta}, \dot{\boldsymbol{\theta}})$, and the friction from robot joints $\boldsymbol{\tau}_j(\boldsymbol{\theta}, \dot{\boldsymbol{\theta}})$. Thus, we have

$$\boldsymbol{\tau}_{\mathrm{f}}(\boldsymbol{\theta}, \dot{\boldsymbol{\theta}}) = \boldsymbol{\tau}_{\mathrm{b}}(\boldsymbol{\theta}, \dot{\boldsymbol{\theta}}) + \boldsymbol{\tau}_{\mathrm{r}}(\boldsymbol{\theta}, \dot{\boldsymbol{\theta}}) + \boldsymbol{\tau}_{\mathrm{j}}(\boldsymbol{\theta}, \dot{\boldsymbol{\theta}}). \tag{2}$$

The friction of the Bowden-cable transmission can be derived from the torque transmission model presented in our previous research (41). The relation between the motor-driving torque acting on the ith proximal pulley, i.e., $\tau_{in,i}$, and the output torque acting on the ith robot joint, i.e., $\tau_{out,i}$, can be described using the following equation:

$$\tau_{in,i} = \frac{r_1}{r_2}\tau_{out,i} + \mathrm{sign}(\dot{\theta}_i)2T_i r_1 \lambda_i \mu_i \tag{3}$$

where T_i and λ_i are the cable pretension and the bending angle of the ith Bowden-cable unit. The term μ_i represents the Coulomb friction coefficient. r_1 and r_2 denote the radiuses of the proximal pulley and the distal pulley. Note that the values of r_1 and r_2 of the presented exoskeleton are equal to 25 mm. Thus, Equation (3) can be refined as

$$\tau_{in,i} - \tau_{out,i} = \tau_{b,i} = \mathrm{sign}(\dot{\theta}_i)2T_i r_1 \lambda_i \mu_i, \tag{4}$$

where $\tau_{b,i}$ is the friction torque from the ith Bowden-cable transmission unit.

According to the existing research results (44), the friction of the motor reducers and robot joints can be simplified as a Coulomb-viscous model as follows:

$$\tau_{r,i} + \tau_{j,i} = b_i \dot{\theta}_i + \mathrm{sign}(\dot{\theta}_i)\tau_{c,i}, \tag{5}$$

where $\tau_{r,i}$ and $\tau_{j,i}$ represent the friction torques from the ith reducer and robot joint. b_i is the coefficient of viscosity. $\tau_{c,i}$ denotes the Coulomb friction torque.

Therefore, by inserting Equations (4, 5) into Equation (2), the ith element of the integrated system friction vector can be obtained and expressed as

$$\tau_{f,i} = b_i\dot{\theta}_i + \text{sign}(\dot{\theta}_i)\left[2T_i r_1 \lambda_i \mu_i + \tau_{c,i}\right] = b_i\dot{\theta}_i + \text{sign}(\dot{\theta}_i)\tau_{e,i}. \quad (6)$$

Here, $\tau_{e,i}$ represents the equivalent parameter for the Coulomb friction torque.

Patient-Active Admittance Control

Robot-assisted rehabilitation training with games played in virtual reality environments has positive effects on inducing active patient participation and encouraging the neural plasticity of the brain (36). Thus, in our research, a patient-active training strategy is developed by integrating an admittance control module and a virtual environment module. The overall block diagram describing the major components of the proposed control scheme is depicted in **Figure 4**. The exoskeleton system is equipped with a graphical guidance interface running on a commercial computer with different virtual games. During rehabilitation training, the operator was seated on a chair with the upper arm connected to the exoskeleton via a custom-made cuff and the palm grasping the end-effector. Instructions were presented on the screen placed in front of the therapeutic robot. The visual and acoustical feedbacks from the virtual environment provide effective guidance for the operator to enhance the awareness of training performance and execute the required training tasks. The system can provide quantitatively evaluated reports for proposed exercises. The statistical training results facilitate therapists to modulate the exercise difficulty levels and training intensity based on the practical recovery status of patients and therapeutic goals.

The real-time information about robot configuration and human–robot interaction, which are acquired from F/T sensors, position sensors, as well as the switches and pushbuttons mounted at the end-effector, are transmitted into a virtual keyboard unit to handle the virtual game process. The virtual keyboard unit was developed in the Microsoft Visual C++ programming environment and used as the interface between the operator and the virtual environment, allowing patient-active training during rehabilitation. In other words, the disabled patient can play the virtual game by actively manipulating the exoskeleton, and this is beneficial to the recovery of motor function and mental confidence. Communication between the RTW control system and the virtual environment was established via the transmission control protocol/internet protocol (TCP/IP).

The admittance control module is developed to regulate the robot configurations and human–robot interaction forces at the end-effector while executing patient-active training. The fed-back forces from the end-effector, $\mathbf{F}_e(t)$, measured by the distal F/T sensor are transformed into the actual forces in basic Cartesian space, $\mathbf{F}(t)$, through coordinate conversion. The force errors, $\Delta\mathbf{F}(t)$, between the desired interaction forces, $\mathbf{F}_d(t)$, and the actual interaction forces at the end-effector are transmitted into an admittance filter to compute the value of position regulation, $\Delta\mathbf{P}(t)$. The desired impedance characteristic describing the relationship between interaction force and end-effector position can be expressed as

$$\Delta\mathbf{F}(t) = \mathbf{M}_d\Delta\ddot{\mathbf{P}}(t) + \mathbf{B}_d\Delta\dot{\mathbf{P}}(t) + \mathbf{K}_d\Delta\mathbf{P}(t), \quad (7)$$

where

$$\begin{cases} \Delta\mathbf{F}(t) = \mathbf{F}(t) - \mathbf{F}_d(t) \\ \Delta\mathbf{P}(t) = \mathbf{P}_c(t) - \mathbf{P}_d(t) \end{cases}$$

Here $\mathbf{P}_d$ (t) denotes the desired inertial training position of the end-effector predefined according to the virtual game scenes; $\mathbf{P}_c$ (t) denotes the corresponding control position of the end-effector in Cartesian space; $\mathbf{M}_d$, $\mathbf{B}_d$, and $\mathbf{K}_d$ are the objective inertia, damping, and stiffness of the admittance filter.

Thus, in the frequency domain, Equation (7) can be represented as

$$\frac{\Delta\mathbf{F}(s)}{\mathbf{M}_d s^2 + \mathbf{B}_d s + \mathbf{K}_d} = \Delta\mathbf{P}(s). \quad (8)$$

The resultant control position, $\mathbf{P}_c$ (t), which depends on the distal interaction forces and admittance parameters, can be converted to the angular position in joint coordinates, $\boldsymbol{\theta}_c$ (t), via the inverse kinematics of the robot. A detailed description of the analytical inverse kinematic resolution of the proposed redundant exoskeleton has been analyzed in (43).

Thus, from Equations (7, 8), we have

$$\text{Inv}\left(\mathbf{P}_d(t) + \Delta\mathbf{P}(t)\right) = \text{Inv}\left(\mathbf{P}_c(t)\right) = \boldsymbol{\theta}_c(t), \quad (9)$$

where Inv $(\cdot)$ denotes the inverse kinematic calculation. The inner position controller is implemented to move the robot to the desired position expressed by $\boldsymbol{\theta}_c$ (t). The position control was realized by using a fuzzy sliding mode control (FSMC) scheme developed based on the system dynamics model, and it was proposed in our previous research (45).

According to Equation (1), since the inertia matrix is symmetric and positive definite, the dynamic model is refined as

$$\ddot{\boldsymbol{\theta}} = \mathbf{M}(\boldsymbol{\theta})^{-1}\left[\boldsymbol{\tau} - \mathbf{V}(\boldsymbol{\theta},\dot{\boldsymbol{\theta}}) - \boldsymbol{\tau}_f(\boldsymbol{\theta},\dot{\boldsymbol{\theta}}) - \mathbf{D}_u + \mathbf{J}_1^T(\boldsymbol{\theta})\boldsymbol{\Gamma}_1 + \mathbf{J}_2^T(\boldsymbol{\theta})\boldsymbol{\Gamma}_2\right]. \quad (10)$$

The switching function of sliding surface $\mathbf{S}(t)$ can be defined as

$$\mathbf{S}(t) = \boldsymbol{\lambda}\boldsymbol{e}(t) + \boldsymbol{\eta}\dot{\boldsymbol{e}}(t), \quad (11)$$

where $\mathbf{e}(t) = \boldsymbol{\theta}_c(t) - \boldsymbol{\theta}(t)$ denotes the position tracking error. $\dot{\mathbf{e}}(t) = \dot{\boldsymbol{\theta}}_c(t) - \dot{\boldsymbol{\theta}}(t)$ denotes the velocity tracking error. λ and η represent the positive diagonal matrixes of proportional gain and derivative gain.

Combining Equations (10, 11), the deviation of the sliding variable can be calculated as

$$\dot{\mathbf{S}}(t) = \boldsymbol{\lambda}\dot{\boldsymbol{e}}(t) + \boldsymbol{\eta}\ddot{\boldsymbol{\theta}}_c(t) - \boldsymbol{\eta}\mathbf{M}(\boldsymbol{\theta})^{-1}\left[\boldsymbol{\tau} - \mathbf{V}(\boldsymbol{\theta},\dot{\boldsymbol{\theta}}) - \boldsymbol{\tau}_f(\boldsymbol{\theta},\dot{\boldsymbol{\theta}}) - \mathbf{D}_u + \mathbf{J}_1^T(\boldsymbol{\theta})\boldsymbol{\Gamma}_1 + \mathbf{J}_2^T(\boldsymbol{\theta})\boldsymbol{\Gamma}_2\right], \quad (12)$$

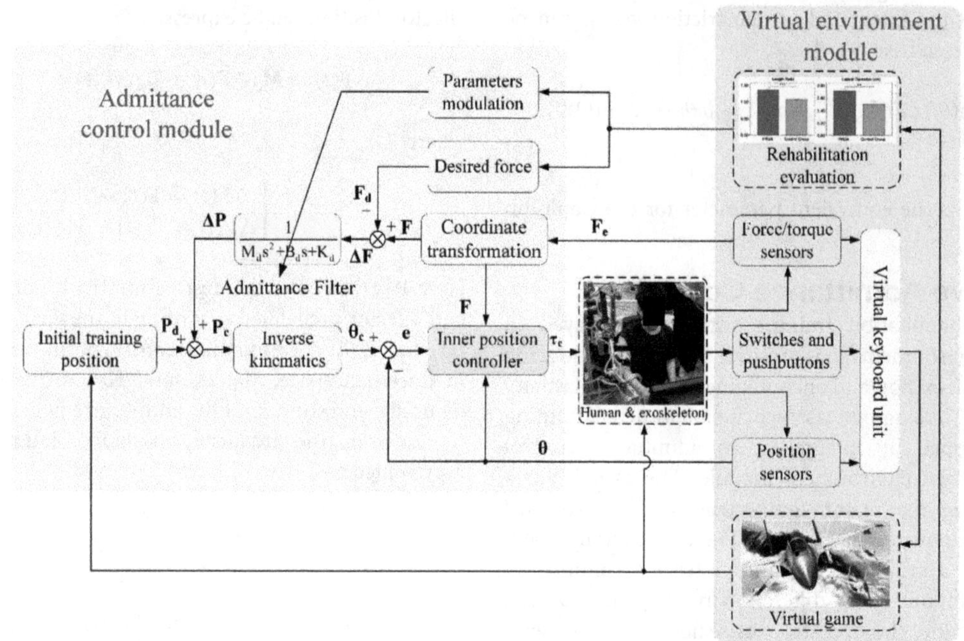

FIGURE 4 | Overall block diagram of the proposed admittance-based patient-active control strategy.

And then, the control law can be designed as

$$\mathbf{u}(t) = \mathbf{M}(\boldsymbol{\theta})\boldsymbol{\eta}^{-1}\boldsymbol{\lambda}\dot{e}(t) + \mathbf{M}(\boldsymbol{\theta})\ddot{\boldsymbol{\theta}}_c(t) + \mathbf{V}(\boldsymbol{\theta}, \dot{\boldsymbol{\theta}}) + \boldsymbol{\tau}_f(\boldsymbol{\theta}, \dot{\boldsymbol{\theta}}) - \mathbf{J}_1^T(\boldsymbol{\theta})\boldsymbol{\Gamma}_1 - \mathbf{J}_2^T(\boldsymbol{\theta})\boldsymbol{\Gamma}_2 + \varepsilon\mathbf{M}(\boldsymbol{\theta})\boldsymbol{\eta}^{-1}\mathrm{sgn}(\mathbf{S}), \tag{13}$$

where sgn (·) means the sign function. ε represents a positive switching gain computed by a fuzzy controller (45).

For the purpose of demonstrating the stability of the proposed patient-active control algorithm, a positive definite Lyapunov function candidate is defined as

$$\mathbf{V} = \frac{1}{2}\mathbf{S}^{\mathrm{T}}(t)\mathbf{S}(t). \tag{14}$$

Differentiating Equation (14) with respect to time t and combining Equations (10) with Equation (13) yields Equation (15) as follows.

$$\begin{aligned}
\dot{\mathbf{V}} &= \mathbf{S}^{\mathrm{T}}(t)\dot{\mathbf{S}}(t) \\
&= \mathbf{S}^{\mathrm{T}}(t)\Big[\boldsymbol{\lambda}\dot{\mathbf{e}}(t) + \boldsymbol{\eta}\ddot{\boldsymbol{\theta}}_c(t) - \boldsymbol{\eta}\mathbf{M}(\boldsymbol{\theta})^{-1}[\mathbf{u}(t) - \mathbf{V}(\boldsymbol{\theta}, \dot{\boldsymbol{\theta}}) \\
&\quad - \boldsymbol{\tau}_f(\boldsymbol{\theta}, \dot{\boldsymbol{\theta}}) - \mathbf{D}_u + \mathbf{J}_1^T(\boldsymbol{\theta})\boldsymbol{\Gamma}_1 + \mathbf{J}_2^T(\boldsymbol{\theta})\boldsymbol{\Gamma}_2]\Big] \\
&= \mathbf{S}^{\mathrm{T}}(t)\Big[\boldsymbol{\lambda}\dot{\mathbf{e}}(t) + \boldsymbol{\eta}\ddot{\boldsymbol{\theta}}_c(t) - \boldsymbol{\eta}\mathbf{M}(\boldsymbol{\theta})^{-1}[\mathbf{M}(\boldsymbol{\theta})\boldsymbol{\eta}^{-1}\boldsymbol{\lambda}\dot{\mathbf{e}}(t) \\
&\quad + \mathbf{M}(\boldsymbol{\theta})\ddot{\boldsymbol{\theta}}_c(t) - \mathbf{D}_u + \boldsymbol{\varepsilon}\mathbf{M}(\boldsymbol{\theta})\boldsymbol{\eta}^{-1}\mathrm{sgn}(\mathbf{S})]\Big] \\
&= \mathbf{S}^{\mathrm{T}}(t)[-\boldsymbol{\eta}\mathbf{M}(\boldsymbol{\theta})^{-1}(\varepsilon\mathbf{M}(\boldsymbol{\theta})\boldsymbol{\eta}^{-1}\mathrm{sgn}(\mathbf{S}) - \mathbf{D}_u)] \\
&= \mathbf{S}^{\mathrm{T}}(t)\boldsymbol{\eta}\mathbf{M}(\boldsymbol{\theta})^{-1}\mathbf{D}_u - \varepsilon\mathbf{S}^{\mathrm{T}}(t)\mathrm{sgn}(\mathbf{S}) \\
&= \mathbf{S}^{\mathrm{T}}(t)\boldsymbol{\eta}\mathbf{M}(\boldsymbol{\theta})^{-1}\mathbf{D}_u - \varepsilon\sum_{i=1}^{6}|S_i|
\end{aligned} \tag{15}$$

Here, the lumped effects of uncertainties $\mathbf{D}_u$ are supposed to satisfy the following assumption.

Assumption 1: The boundary of the uncertainty term can be given as (46)

$$|\mathbf{D}_\mathbf{u}| < \gamma. \tag{16}$$

If the positive switching gain is selected as

$$\varepsilon > \left|\boldsymbol{\eta}\mathbf{M}(\boldsymbol{\theta})^{-1}\mathbf{D}_u\right|, \tag{17}$$

then (16) can be rewritten as

$$\dot{\mathbf{V}} = \mathbf{S}^{\mathrm{T}}(t)\boldsymbol{\eta}\mathbf{M}(\boldsymbol{\theta})^{-1}\mathbf{D}_u - \varepsilon\sum_{i=1}^{6}|S_i| < \varepsilon\left|\mathbf{S}^{\mathrm{T}}(t)\right| - \varepsilon\sum_{i=1}^{6}|S_i| < 0 \tag{18}$$

Here, it can be observed that $\dot{V}(t)$ is negative definite. Thus, the proposed controller satisfies the Lyapunov stability criteria, and the position tracking error gradually converges to the sliding surface $S(t) = 0$ in finite time.

RESULTS

Upon completing the hardware design, dynamic modeling, and controller development, three typical experiments were conducted on the exoskeleton to validate the feasibility of the proposed patient-active admittance control strategy. In the first case, the position tracking experiment without the operator and external interactions was carried out to analyze the control performance of the inner fuzzy sliding mode position controller. In the second case, the free arm movement training experiment with different admittance parameters was conducted with three healthy subjects. In the third case, the virtual airplane-game operation training with graphical guidance was carried out with two healthy subjects and eight stroke patients with different Fugl-Meyer assessment (FMA) scores (47). The ethical approval of the implemented experimental approaches have been obtained from the Human Subjects Ethics Subcommittee of the Nanjing University of Aeronautics and Astronautics. The participants of this research were recruited from the local districts through advertisement. The research on the developed patient-active control strategy had been conducted since February 2017. The upper limb rehabilitation exoskeleton system was designed by Qingcong Wu and Xingsong Wang.

Position Tracking Experiments

According to the control diagram illustrated in **Figure 4**, the proposed admittance-based patient-active control scheme will be converted into a position controller to track the predefined training trajectory, if the desired force and the actual human–robot interaction force are equal to zero. Actually, the inner position controller is one of the kernel algorithms of the patient-active control method, as it is responsible for modulating the exoskeleton configuration based on the position regulation value output from the admittance filter. Therefore, it is necessary to demonstrate the feasibility of the proposed FSMC-based inner position control strategy.

The position tracking experiment without the participation of the subject was carried out to evaluate the position control performance. The desired position trajectory of the end-effector, which is defined in the base robot coordinate frame of the exoskeleton and parallel to the coronal plane, is shown in **Figure 5A**. There are four waypoints (A, B, C, and D) defined in the available workspace of the exoskeleton, and the initial location of the end-effector is set to Point A. The overall trajectory can be divided into four continuous subtrajectories. Firstly, the end-effector is controlled to move horizontally from point A to point B in 4 s. It also takes 4 s to move from point B to point C. The third subtrajectory is designed to follow the path from point C to point D in 4 s. Finally, the end-effector is returned from point D to point A in the last 4 s. It should be pointed out that, to guarantee the smoothness of the trajectory and avoid undesirable impact phenomena, the subtrajectory between two points is determined based on the minimum jerk cost principle (48). The terminal motion states of the former subtrajectory, including the positions, velocities, and accelerations, are the same as the initial motion states of the next subtrajectory.

The experimental performance of the proposed FSMC algorithm was compared to that of a conventional PID controller. The selected control parameters of the PID controller (i.e., proportional gain, integral gain, and derivative gain) were estimated via the Ziegler–Nichols method and carefully optimized by trial and error. The control parameters of the FSMC algorithm were optimally adjusted by intensive tests to improve control accuracy and ensure system stability. The results of trajectory tracking experiments with different control

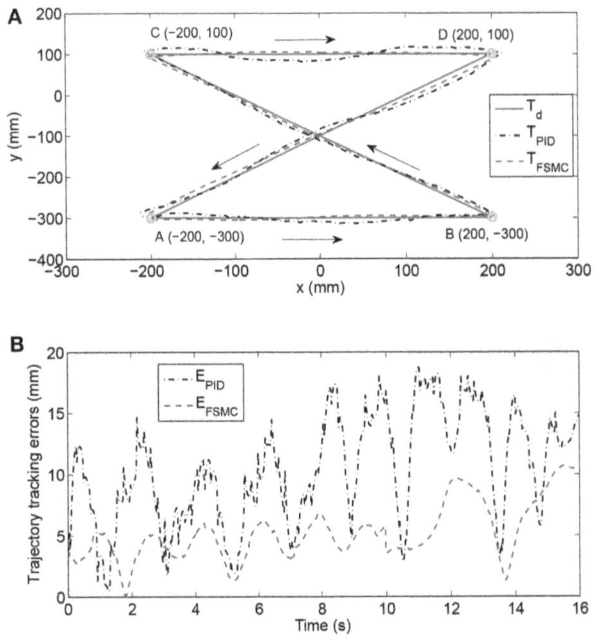

FIGURE 5 | Experimental results of position tracking tests with different control schemes. **(A)** The comparison among desired trajectory, the trajectory with PID controller, and the trajectory with fuzzy sliding mode controller (FSMC). **(B)** Time histories of position tracking errors.

strategies are compared in **Figure 5A**. In addition, the time histories of position tracking errors, which are defined as the absolute distance between the desired and actual coordinates of the end-effector, are illustrated in **Figure 5B**. As can be observed, the tracking performance of the FSMC scheme has turned out to be far more effective than that of the PID controller. More specifically, the average output-tracking error declines from 10.42 mm (PID) to 5.21 mm (FSMC), while the root-mean-square error (RMSE) declines from 11.56 mm (PID) to 5.78 mm (FSMC) during the experiments. The peak-to-peak error is smaller (10.15 mm) with the FSMC strategy in comparison with that with the PID algorithm (18.75 mm). Therefore, the obtained results of position tracking experiments confirm the validity of the inner position controller.

Free Arm Training Experiment

The fundamental purpose of developing the patient-active control framework is to encourage the voluntary efforts and active participations of patients during rehabilitation training. The basic function of the admittance control module, as the core component of the patient-active controller, is to modulate the configuration of the exoskeleton according to the detected real-time human–robot interaction force and the desired mechanical admittance characteristic. Hence, the second experiment was conducted to evaluate the feasibility of the admittance controller in free arm operation training.

In this experiment, three healthy neurologically intact volunteers with various anthropometric parameters and ages

TABLE 1 | Admittance parameters of different working conditions.

Conditions	M_d (Ns^2/mm)	B_d (Ns/mm)	K_d (N/mm)
E1	diag [0.060, 0.060, 0.060]	diag [0.060, 0.060, 0.060]	diag [0.060, 0.060, 0.060]
E2	diag [0.025, 0.025, 0.025]	diag [0.025, 0.025, 0.025]	diag [0.025, 0.025, 0.025]
E3	diag [0.015, 0.015, 0.015]	diag [0.015, 0.015, 0.015]	diag [0.015, 0.015, 0.015]

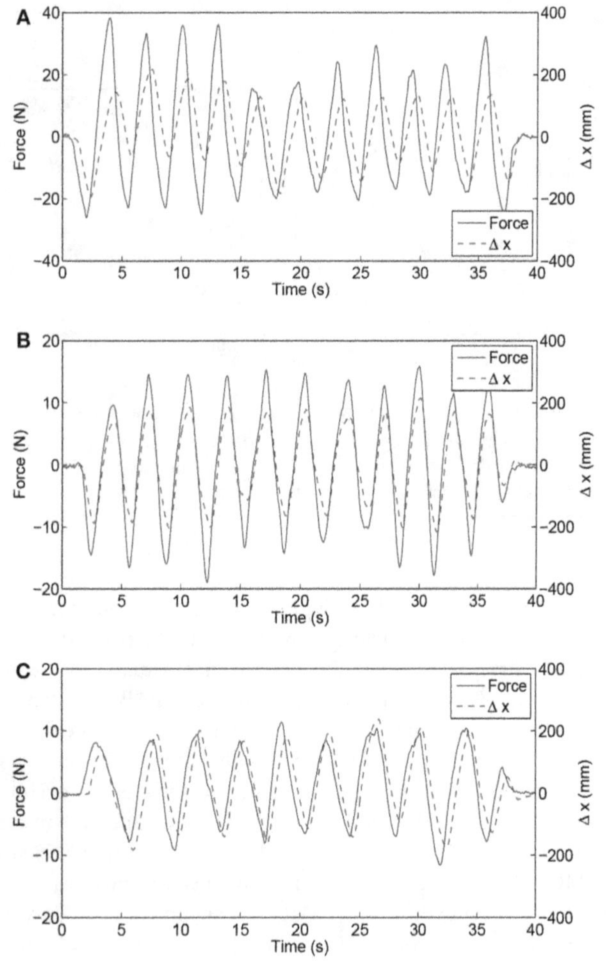

FIGURE 6 | Experimental results of free arm training tests conducted with healthy subject H1 with different admittance parameters. **(A)** Results under condition E1. **(B)** Results under condition E2. **(C)** Results under condition E3.

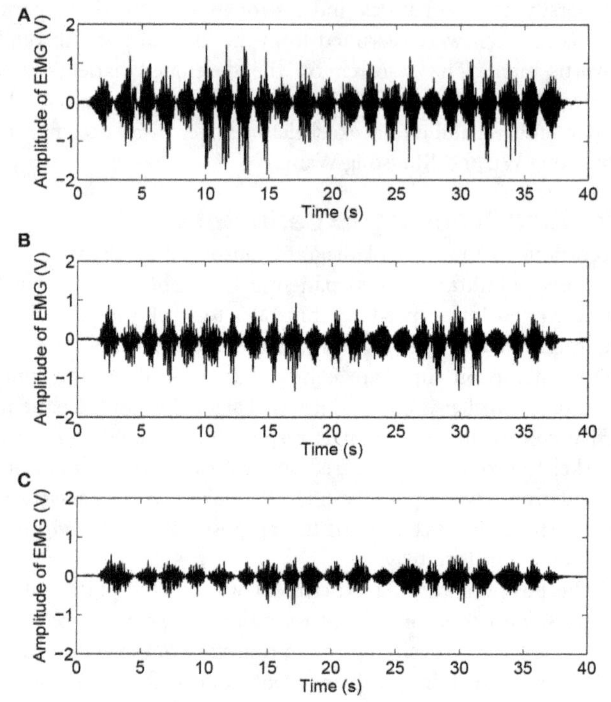

FIGURE 7 | Time histories of EMG activity levels of bicipital muscle during free arm training tests conducted with healthy subject H1 for different admittance parameters. **(A)** EMG signals under condition E1. **(B)** EMG signals under condition E2. **(C)** EMG signals under condition E3.

(subject H1: male, height/1.7 m, weight/62.5 kg, age/29 years; subject H2: male, height/1.76 m, weight/66.2 kg, age/22 years; subject H3: female, height/1.62 m, weight/51.8 kg, age/46 years) were asked to undergo free arm movement trainings with different admittance parameters. The volunteers were comfortably positioned in the therapeutic system with their right arms wearing the exoskeleton. The limb lengths and the joint axes of the upper arm and the forearm of the exoskeleton were adjusted in accordance with the anthropometric parameters of wearers. Next, the subjects grasped the end-effector of the exoskeleton and actively performed horizontal reciprocating movements along the x-axis of the base coordinate system. The relation between the interaction force, measured by the distal F/T sensor of the end-effector, and the position deviation $\mathbf{\Delta x}$, calculated from the positions of the robot's joints and inverse kinematics, reflects the corresponding training difficulty and intensity. The range of position deviation was generally restricted within the interval of [−400, 400 mm].

To compare and investigate the training performance with different admittance parameters, three different groups of parameters (E1, E2, and E3) were implemented to the admittance filter during the free arm movement experiments, as shown in **Table 1**. The subjects were required to repeat the aforementioned training task six times for each condition.

Existing study results indicate that the EMG signals provide information on the scale of muscular power and activation patterns (49). Besides, the results from our previous tests show that the EMG signal strength from the bicipital muscle and the brachioradialis muscle were larger than those from the brachialis muscle and the triceps muscle during free arm operation. Therefore, to analyze and compare the training intensity with different admittance parameters, the surface EMG signals from the bicipital and brachioradialis muscles of the wearers were acquired during the free arm training process. The measurement system mainly consists of active bipolar surface electrodes and sensors (Sunlephant-6 EMG System, Sichiray) used to obtain original signals, an integrated processing unit (SHIELD-EKG, Olimex) used for signal acquisition, amplification, and filtering, and a data analysis system running the Microsoft Visual Studio environment used for offline analysis. Before data acquisition, the exposed skin areas over the bicipital muscle and the brachioradialis muscle were cleaned with an alcohol pad to decrease contact resistance. The surface electrodes, with an effective area of 10 × 10 mm for each unit, were attached to the skin via double-faced adhesive tape. The EMG signals were sampled at 1 kHz with 12-bit resolution and filtered by using a third-order Butterworth high-pass filter with a cut-off frequency of 20 Hz. The processed signals were wirelessly transmitted to the data analysis system via a Bluetooth network.

As shown in **Figure 6**, the experimental results of subject H1 (single trial) present the relationships between the interaction force and position variation with different admittance parameters. It can be clearly observed that during the patient-active operation experiments, the changing tendency of position deviation is basically consistent with that of the interaction force. The active forces, from the subject and applied to the end-effector, lead to a corresponding modulation of robot configuration and, as a result, realize the active participation in rehabilitation training. Furthermore, increases in admittance parameters cause larger interaction forces for the same free arm training task. **Figure 7** compares the EMG activity levels of subject H1 under different experimental conditions. The RMS approach is used for the feature extraction of raw EMG signals in this research. The RMS EMG value of the bicipital muscle under experimental condition E1 (0.466 V) turned out to be larger than those under condition E2 (0.281 V) and condition E3 (0.165 V).

Moreover, the experimental results (six trials) of the RMS EMG values from the bicipital muscle of different subjects and admittance parameters are compared in **Figure 8**. It can be concluded that the increase in the admittance parameters of the proposed patient-active control scheme leads to the increase of EMG activity levels. However, the specific surface EMG activity levels vary from person to person during the same experiment. The statistical results for the bicipital muscle and brachioradialis muscle are compared in **Table 2**. The experimental results indicate that by modulating the admittance filter, motion resistance and training intensity during

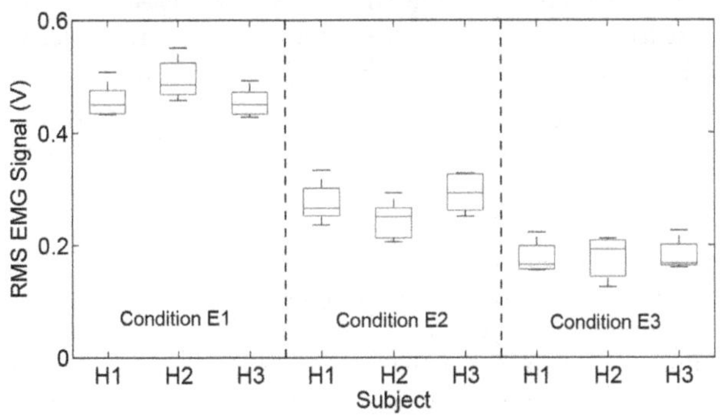

FIGURE 8 | Comparison results of RMS EMG values of bicipital muscles for different subjects and admittance parameters.

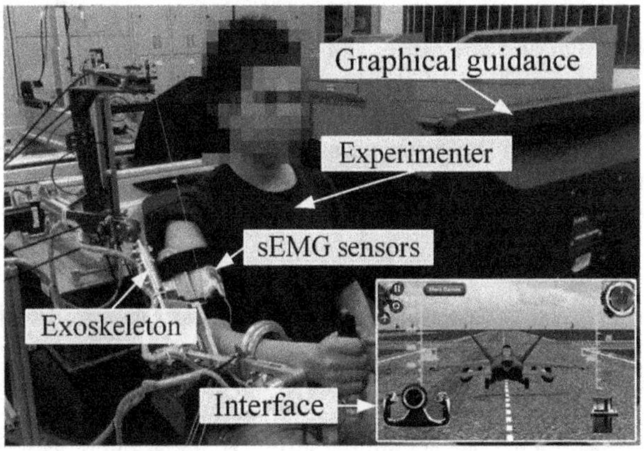

FIGURE 9 | Experimental scenarios of a healthy volunteer conducting virtual airplane-game operation experiment.

TABLE 2 | Comparison of statistical results of RMS EMG values of bicipital muscle and brachioradialis muscle under different experimental conditions.

Con	RMS EMG values of different subjects (V)											
	H1				H2				H3			
	Biceps		Brachioradialis		Biceps		Brachioradialis		Biceps		Brachioradialis	
	Max	Med	Max	Med	Max	Med	Max	Med	Max	Med	Max	Med
E1	0.51	0.45	0.46	0.40	0.55	0.48	0.50	0.43	0.49	0.46	0.42	0.37
E2	0.33	0.27	0.30	0.24	0.29	0.25	0.35	0.25	0.32	0.30	0.28	0.21
E3	0.22	0.16	0.21	0.15	0.21	0.19	0.26	0.20	0.22	0.17	0.19	0.15

Con, condition; Max, maximum value; Med, median value.

TABLE 3 | Characteristics of the subjects participating in experiments.

Sub	Gender	Age (years)	Height (m)	Weight (kg)	FMA score (upper limb)	FMA score (shoulder)	FMA score (wrist)	FMA score (hand)	Status
H1	Male	26–30	1.70	62.5	66 (full)	16	10	22	Healthy
H2	Male	21–25	1.76	66.2	66 (full)	16	10	22	Healthy
P1	Male	61–65	1.73	66.2	60	15	8	21	Slight paralysis
P2	Female	36–40	1.56	47.2	58	14	8	20	Slight paralysis
P3	Female	46–50	1.71	62.6	51	12	7	18	Moderate paralysis
P4	Male	56–60	1.70	66.5	49	13	6	18	Moderate paralysis
P5	Male	66–70	1.82	75.3	41	11	5	16	Moderate paralysis
P6	Male	41–45	1.76	62.0	38	10	6	15	Moderate paralysis
P7	Male	46–50	1.79	64.7	16	5	3	4	Severe paralysis
P8	Female	51–55	1.70	61.5	8	2	2	2	Severe paralysis

patient-active rehabilitation therapy can be rationally adjusted to meet the capabilities and requirements of different patients.

Virtual Airplane-Game Operation Experiment

The purpose of the third experiment was to evaluate the practical feasibility by applying the proposed admittance-based patient-active controller to rehabilitation training in a virtual reality environment. **Figure 9** presents the experimental scenarios in which a healthy volunteer wearing an exoskeleton actively plays the virtual airplane-game with visual and acoustical feedback instructions. There were ten volunteers (two healthy subjects and eight post-stroke chronic patients) with various FMA scores participating in the virtual airplane-game operation experiment. The detailed anthropometry parameters and the motor ability of each subject are presented in **Table 3**.

During the trial, the participants were required to actively manipulate the exoskeleton system and control the virtual airplane prototype displayed on the screen to accomplish the requested actions along the predesigned trajectory, including the taking-off operation, landing operation, and free-flight operation. To modulate the sensitivity of game control and improve the maneuverability of virtual training, the predefined thresholds of position variation (100 mm) and interaction force (10 N) were integrated into the virtual keyboard program. Only if the position variation and detected force exceed the respective threshold simultaneously, the virtual keyboard unit will trigger the corresponding keys to regulate the game process. In this way, the virtual keyboard acts as the interface that maps the human–robot interaction force and the robot configuration to the operations in the airplane game.

In this experiment, the admittance parameters were set as follows: $\mathbf{M}_d$ = diag [0.03, 0.04, 0.06] Ns^2/mm, $\mathbf{B}_d$ = diag [0.05, 0.04, 0.08] Ns/mm, $\mathbf{K}_d$ = diag [0.05, 0.06, 0.08] N/mm. All the subjects were required to make their best efforts to complete the airplane operation task six times. **Figure 10** presents the experimental results of virtual airplane-game operations performed by healthy subject H1 in a single trial. More specifically, **Figures 10A,B** present the comparisons of interaction forces and position deviations in different directions of the base coordinate system. Further, the resultant interaction forces and combined position deviations are compared in **Figure 10C**. It can be seen that the variation tendencies of human–robot interaction forces are consistent with those of position deviations. The time history of the amplitude of EMG signals is depicted in **Figure 10D**, and the calculated RMS EMG value of the bicipital muscle is ~0.407 V. The subject wearing the exoskeleton system was able to actively handle the motion of the virtual airplane during rehabilitation training. Thus, experimental results substantiate the feasibility of the proposed control strategy.

The execution time required to finish the airplane operation task reflects the difficulty of the game for a specific participant. The execution times for the subjects with different FMA scores were recorded and compared (**Figure 11**). The average execution time for each subject was obtained (H1: 25.6 s; H2: 23.9 s, P1: 42.7 s; P2: 56.8 s; P3: 88.6 s; P4: 93.2 s; P5: 145.3 s; P6: 173.5 s). It should be pointed out that subjects P7 and P8 with severe paralysis were not able to complete the required training task and hence their data were excluded from the statistical data. The experimental results show that, with the proposed exoskeleton system and patient-active control strategy, a subject with adequate motor function capacity is able to actively handle the motion of virtual airplane and complete the requested training task in the virtual environment. The required execution time increases with decreasing motor function capacity of patients. The active participation of patients can be encouraged. However, the developed patient-active control scheme is not suitable for severely paralyzed patients, who require passive repetition training with the assistance of an exoskeleton.

DISCUSSION

From the results of three different experiments—the position tracking experiment, the free arm training experiment, and the virtual airplane-game operation experiment—it can be observed that the proposed FSMC-based admittance control strategy is capable of providing patient-active mode training during rehabilitation. More specifically, from the results of position tracking tests, it can be seen that the inner FSMC

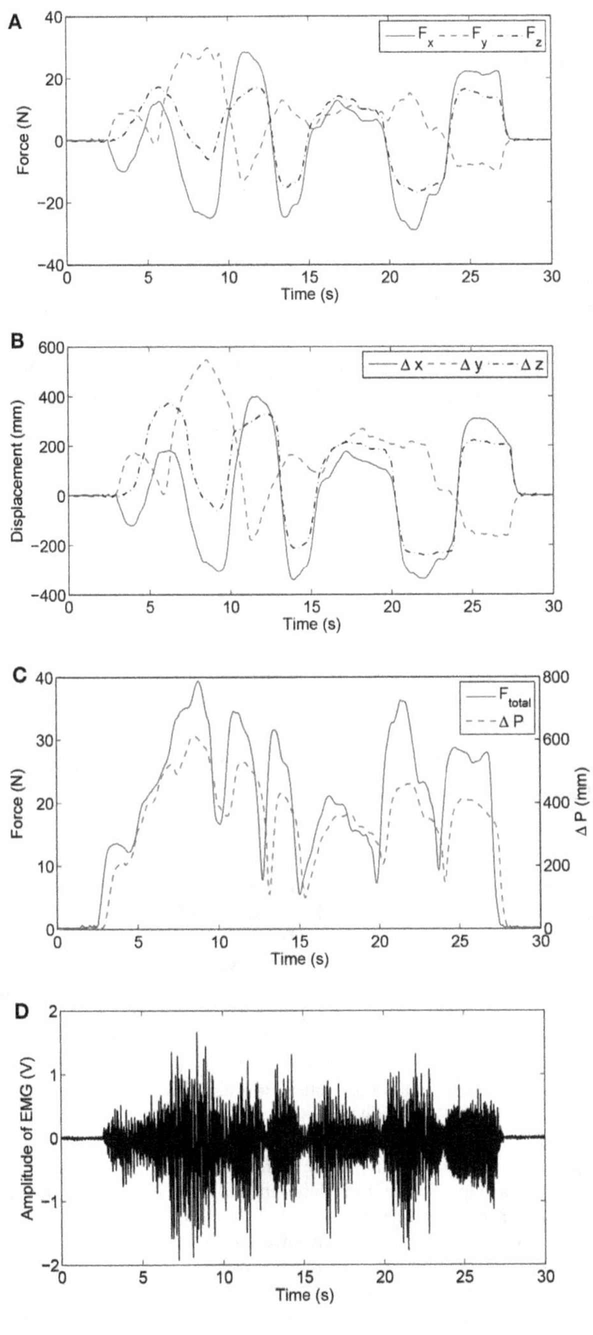

FIGURE 10 | Experimental results of virtual airplane-game operation training executed by healthy subject H1. **(A)** Interaction forces in different directions. **(B)** Position deviations in different directions. **(C)** Comparisons of the resultant interaction force and combined position deviation. **(D)** Time history of EMG activity levels of bicipital muscle.

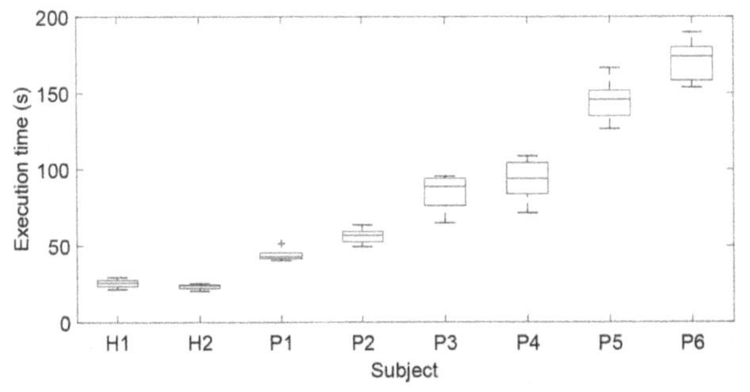

FIGURE 11 | Comparison results of execution times for subjects with different FMA scores required to complete the virtual airplane-game operation task.

position controller is capable of achieving smaller tracking errors and better control performance when compared with the conventional PID controller, and can ensure the modulation accuracy of robot configuration based on the output value of the admittance filter. From the results of the free arm training experiment conducted with three healthy participants with different admittance parameters, it can be observed that the developed FSMC-based admittance controller can assist the patient actively undergo the free arm movement trainings with desired training difficulty and intensity. Moreover, it is able to encourage the voluntary efforts and active participations of patients during rehabilitation training. The increase of the admittance parameters of patient-active controller leads to the increase of motion resistance and the EMG activity levels of the bicipital muscle. According to the results of virtual airplane-game operation experiment conducted with two healthy volunteers and eight post-stroke chronic patients with various FMA scores, it can be found that, with the developed admittance-based patient-active control strategy, the volunteer wearing the exoskeleton system is able to actively handle the motion of virtual airplane during rehabilitation training. The rehabilitation training integrated with commercial virtual games without a specific predefined trajectory has valid impact on enhancing the interestingness of physical therapy and, furthermore, contributes to neurological rehabilitation and psychotherapy. The experimental results for different disabled patients indicate that the required execution time of the same operation task increases with the decrease of motor functions of patients. Besides, the feasibility in encouraging active participation has been proved from the statements of volunteers. In the actual performance, the protocol for each patient should be selected based on several factors, such as the detailed FMA scores of patient, the desired rehabilitation training programs, the quantitatively statistical training reports from the evaluation system, and the experience of physiotherapists.

Limitations

There are several limitations in the proposed exoskeleton and control strategy. Firstly, the proposed patient-active controller can be used with patients with good cognitive function, fair sitting balance, and good upper limb motor performance; it cannot be applied to severely paralyzed subjects without any motor functions. The resistance from the exoskeleton needs to be overcome during patient-active training. Secondly, the proposed exoskeleton can be used only for patients with right-sided weakness, thus limiting the range of applicability. An extension of this research will be to improve the control strategy to be suitable for severely paralyzed patients. The mechanical structure will be further optimized to realize the switch between right arm training and left arm training. The effectiveness of the proposed rehabilitation exoskeleton system and control strategy will be tested and demonstrated via a more substantial trial in future works. Besides, the perceived value and motivation of patient will be qualitatively evaluated by using electroencephalography (EEG) sensor. A rational rehabilitation evaluation system will be developed to estimate recovery progress. The controller parameters, such as the admittance filter, should be optimized based on the evaluation of patients to improve treatment efficiency. In addition, the therapeutic training of the human hand will be integrated into the rehabilitation system.

CONCLUSION

This paper dealt with the development and validation of an upper limb exoskeleton and a patient-active admittance control strategy, which can be applied to assist the patients with affected arm motor functions in performing active training in virtual environments. Firstly, the major hardware of the wearable exoskeleton system, including the gravity-balanced mechanical structure with $7 + 2$ DOFs and the MATLAB/RTW real-time control system, was briefly introduced. Then, the system dynamic model was established using the Lagrangian method. To encourage the active participation of patients during rehabilitation training, a patient-active controller was proposed based on the dynamic model. A patient wearing the exoskeleton can undergo active rehabilitation training with the guidance of a graphical interface, and the training trajectory is not constrained to a specific predetermined trajectory. Different kinds of existing commercial virtual games, which are far more realistic and interesting than the simple self-designed ones, can be integrated into the proposed control strategy via a virtual keyboard unit. The feasibilities of the proposed therapeutic system and control strategy were verified via three pilot tests. A position tracking experiment was carried out to evaluate the performance of the inner fuzzy sliding mode position control strategy. A free arm training experiment was conducted with three healthy subjects to study the functionality of the admittance module during free arm operation. To verify the practical feasibility of applying the patient-active control strategy to the training within virtual environments, a virtual airplane-game operation experiment was conducted with ten volunteers with different FMA scores.

AUTHOR CONTRIBUTIONS

QW and XW participated in the design of this study. QW and BC carried out the experiments and analyzed the experimental data. HW contributed in the exoskeleton development and maintenance. QW wrote and modified the manuscript. All authors read and approved the manuscript.

REFERENCES

1. Writing Group M, Mozaffarian D, Benjamin EJ, Go AS, Arnett DK, Blaha MJ, et al. Executive summary: heart disease and stroke statistics – 2016 update: a report from the American Heart Association. *Circulation* (2016) 133:447–54. doi: 10.1161/cir.0000000000000366
2. Langhorne P, Bernhardt J, Kwakkel G. Stroke rehabilitation. *Lancet* (2011) 377:1693–702. doi: 10.1016/S0140-6736(11)60325-5
3. Vanbellingen T, Filius SJ, Nyffeler T, van Wegen EEH. Usability of videogame-based dexterity training in the early rehabilitation phase of stroke patients: a pilot study. *Front Neurol.* (2017) 8:654. doi: 10.3389/fneur.2017.00654
4. Dobkin B. Rehabilitation after stroke. *N Engl J Med.* (2005) 352:1677–84. doi: 10.1056/NEJMcp043511
5. Niu J, Yang Q, Wang X, Song R. Sliding mode tracking control of a wire-driven upper-limb rehabilitation robot with nonlinear disturbance observer. *Front Neurol.* (2017) 8:646. doi: 10.3389/fneur.2017.00646
6. Huang FC, Patton JL. Augmented dynamics and motor exploration as training for stroke. *IEEE Trans. Biomed. Eng* (2013) 60:838–44. doi: 10.1109/TBME.2012.2192116
7. Winstein CJ, Stein J, Arena R, Bates B, Cherney LR, Cramer SC, et al. Guidelines for adult stroke rehabilitation and recovery. *Stroke* (2016) 47:e98–169. doi: 10.1161/STR.0000000000000098
8. Morris DM, Taub E. Constraint-induced therapy approach to restoring function after neurological injury. *Top Stroke Rehabil.* (2001) 8:16–30. doi: 10.1310/bljx-m89n-ptpy-jdkw
9. Pollock A, Farmer SE, Brady MC, Langhorne P, Mead GE, Mehrholz J, et al. Interventions for improving upper limb function after stroke. *Cochrane Database Syst Rev.* (2014) 11:CD010820. doi: 10.1002/14651858.CD010820.pub2
10. Meng W, Liu Q, Zhou ZD, Ai QS, Sheng B, Xie SQ. Recent development of mechanisms and control strategies for robot-assisted lower limb rehabilitation. *Mechatronics* (2015) 31:132–45. doi: 10.1016/j.mechatronics.2015.04.005
11. Harris JE, Eng JJ. Strength training improves upper-limb function in individuals with stroke. *Stroke* (2010) 41:136–40. doi: 10.1161/STROKEAHA.109.567438
12. Wu QC, Wang XS, Du FP, Zhang XB. Design and control of a powered hip exoskeleton for walking assistance. *Int J Adv Robot Syst.* (2015) 12:1–12. doi: 10.5772/59991
13. Wagner TH, Lo AC, Peduzzi P, Bravata DM, Huang GD, Krebs HI, et al. An economic analysis of robot-assisted therapy for long-term upperlimb impairment after stroke. *Stroke* (2011) 42:2630–2. doi: 10.1161/STROKEAHA.110.606442
14. Wilkins KB, Owen M, Ingo C, Carmona C, Dewald JPA, Yao J. Neural plasticity in moderate to severe chronic stroke following a device-assisted task-specific arm/hand intervention. *Front Neurol.* (2017) 8:284. doi: 10.3389/fneur.2017.00284
15. Lu Z, Tong KY, Shin H, Li S, Zhou P. Advanced myoelectric control for robotic hand-assisted training: outcome from a stroke patient. *Front Neurol.* (2017) 8:107. doi: 10.3389/fneur.2017.00107
16. Wu QC, Wang XS, Chen B, Wu HT. Development of a minimal-intervention-based admittance control strategy for upper extremity rehabilitation exoskeleton. *IEEE Trans Syst Man Cy-S* (2018) 48:1005-16. doi: 10.1109/TSMC.2017.2771227
17. Qian Q, Hu X, Lai Q, Ng SC, Zheng Y, Poon W. Early stroke rehabilitation of the upper limb assisted with an electromyography-driven neuromuscular electrical stimulation-robotic arm. *Front Neurol.* (2017) 8:447. doi: 10.3389/fneur.2017.00447
18. Burgar CG, Lum PS, Scremin AME, Garber SL, Van der Loos HFM, Kenney D, et al. Robot-assisted upper-limb therapy in acute rehabilitation setting following stroke: department of veterans affairs multisite clinical trial. *J Rehabil Res Dev.* (2011) 48:445–58. doi: 10.1682/JRRD.2010.04.0062
19. Guzmán-Valdivia CH, Blanco-Ortega A, Oliver-Salazar MA, Gomez-Becerra FA, Carrera-Escobedo JL. HipBot – the design, development and control of a therapeutic robot for hip rehabilitation. *Mechatronics* (2015) 30:55–64. doi: 10.1016/j.mechatronics.2015.06.007

20. Rui L, Amirabdollahian F, Topping M, Driessen B, Harwin W. Upper limb robot mediated stroke therapy-GENTLE/s approach. *Auton Robots* (2003) 15:35–51. doi: 10.1023/A:1024436732030
21. Jones CL, Kamper DG. Involuntary neuromuscular coupling between the thumb and finger of stroke survivors during dynamic movement. *Front Neurol.* (2018) 9:84. doi: 10.3389/fneur.2018.00084
22. Nam C, Rong W, Li W, Xie Y, Hu X, Zheng Y. The effects of upper-limb training assisted with an electromyography-driven neuromuscular electrical stimulation robotic hand on chronic stroke. *Front Neurol.* (2017) 8:679. doi: 10.3389/fneur.2017.00679
23. Conti R, Meli E, Ridolfi A. A novel kinematic architecture for portable hand exoskeletons. *Mechatronics* (2016) 35:192–207. doi: 10.1016/j.mechatronics.2016.03.002
24. Lenzi T, De Rossi SMM, Vitiello N, Carrozza MC. Intention-based EMG control for powered exoskeletons. *IEEE Trans Biomed Eng.* (2012) 59:2180–90. doi: 10.1109/TBME.2012.2198821
25. Cui X, Chen W, Jin X, Agrawal SK. Design of a 7-DOF cable-driven arm exoskeleton (CAREX-7) and a controller for dexterous motion training or assistance. *IEEE-ASME Trans Mech.* (2017) 22:161–72. doi: 10.1109/TMECH.2016.2618888
26. Ren YP, Kang SH, Park HS, Wu YN, Zhang LQ. Developing a multi-joint upper limb exoskeleton robot for diagnosis, therapy, and outcome evaluation in neurorehabilitation. *IEEE Trans Neural Syst Rehabil Eng.* (2013) 21:490–9. doi: 10.1109/TNSRE.2012.2225073
27. Klein J, Spencer S, Allington J, Bobrow JE, Reinkensmeyer DJ. Optimization of a parallel shoulder mechanism to achieve a high-force, low-mass, robotic-arm exoskeleton. *IEEE Trans Robot.* (2010) 26:710–5. doi: 10.1109/TRO.2010.2052170
28. Huang J, Tu XK, He JP. Design and evaluation of the RUPERT wearable upper extremity exoskeleton robot for clinical and in-home therapies. *IEEE Trans Syst Man Cybern Syst.* (2016) 46:926–35. doi: 10.1109/TSMC.2015.2497205
29. Mefoued S. A robust adaptive neural control scheme to drive an actuated orthosis for assistance of knee movements. *Neurocomputing* (2014) 140:27–40. doi: 10.1016/j.neucom.2014.03.038
30. Li ZJ, Su CY, Li GL, Su H. Fuzzy approximation-based adaptive backstepping control of an exoskeleton for human upper limbs. *IEEE Trans Fuzzy Syst.* (2015) 23:555–66. doi: 10.1109/TFUZZ.2014.2317511
31. Yu W, Rosen J. Neural PID control of robot manipulators with application to an upper limb exoskeleton. *IEEE Trans Cybernetics* (2013) 43:673–84. doi: 10.1109/TSMCB.2012.2214381
32. Liu Q, Liu D, Meng W, Zhou ZD, Ai QS. Fuzzy sliding mode control of a multi-DOF parallel robot in rehabilitation environment. *Int J Hum Robot.* (2014) 11:1450004. doi: 10.1142/S0219843614500042
33. Jiang XZ, Huang XH, Xiong CH, Sun RL, Xiong YL. Position control of a rehabilitation robotic joint based on neuron proportion-integral and feedforward control. *J Comput Nonlin Dyn.* (2012) 7:024502. doi: 10.1115/1.4005436
34. Hu XL, Tong KY, Song R, Zheng XJ, Leung WW. A comparison between electromyography-driven robot and passive motion device on wrist rehabilitation for chronic stroke. *Neurorehabil Neural Repair* (2009) 23:837–46. doi: 10.1177/1545968309338191
35. Kim B, Deshpande AD. An upper-body rehabilitation exoskeleton Harmony with an anatomical shoulder mechanism: Design, modeling, control, and performance evaluation. *Int J Robot Res.* (2017) 36:414–35. doi: 10.1177/0278364917706743
36. Keller U, van Hedel HJA, Klamroth-Marganska V, Riener R. ChARMin: the first actuated exoskeleton robot for pediatric arm rehabilitation. *IEEE-ASME Trans Mech.* (2016) 21:2201–13. doi: 10.1109/TMECH.2016.2559799
37. Duschauwicke A, Von ZJ, Caprez A, Lunenburger L, Riener R. Path control: a method for patient-cooperative robot-aided gait rehabilitation. *IEEE Trans Neural Syst Rehabil Eng.* (2010) 18:38–48. doi: 10.1109/TNSRE.2009.2033061
38. Ye WJ, Li ZJ, Yang CG, Chen F, Su CY. Motion detection enhanced control of an upper limb exoskeleton robot for rehabilitation training. *Int J Hum Robot.* (2017) 14:1650031. doi: 10.1142/S0219843616500316
39. Oldewurtel F, Mihelj M, Nef T, Riener R. Patient-cooperative control strategies for coordinated functional arm movements. In: *IEEE Conf Euro Cont Conf.* Kos, Greece (2007). p. 2527–34.
40. Banala SK, Kim SH, Agrawal SK, Scholz JP. Robot assisted gait training with active leg exoskeleton (ALEX). *IEEE Trans Neural Syst Rehabil Eng.* (2009) 17:2–8. doi: 10.1109/BIOROB.2008.4762885
41. Wu QC, Wang XS, Chen L, Du FP. Transmission model and compensation control of double-tendon-sheath actuation system. *IEEE Trans Ind Electron.* (2015) 62:1599–609. doi: 10.1109/TIE.2014.2360062
42. Wu QC, Wang XS, Du FP. Development and analysis of a gravity-balanced exoskeleton for active rehabilitation training of upper limb. *Proc Inst Mech Eng C J Mech Eng Sci.* (2016) 230:3777–90. doi: 10.1177/0954406215616415
43. Wu QC, Wang XS, Du FP. Analytical inverse kinematic resolution of a redundant exoskeleton for upper-limb rehabilitation. *Int J Hum Robot.* (2016) 13:1550042. doi: 10.1142/S0219843615500425
44. Ju MS, Lin CC, Lin DH, Hwang IS, Chen SM. A rehabilitation robot with force-position hybrid fuzzy controller: hybrid fuzzy control of rehabilitation robot. *IEEE Trans Neural Syst Rehabil Eng.* (2005) 13:349–58. doi: 10.1109/TNSRE.2005.847354
45. Wu QC, Wang XS, Du FP, Xi RR. Modeling and position control of a therapeutic exoskeleton targeting upper extremity rehabilitation. *Proc Inst Mech Eng C J Mech Eng Sci.* (2017) 231:4360–73. doi: 10.1177/0954406216668204
46. Amer AF, Sallam EA, Elawady WM. Adaptive fuzzy sliding mode control using supervisory fuzzy control for 3 DOF planar robot manipulators. *Appl Soft Comput J.* (2011) 11:4943–53. doi: 10.1016/j.asoc.2011.06.005
47. Gladstone DJ, Danells CJ, Black SE. The Fugl-Meyer assessment of motor recovery after stroke: a critical review of its measurement properties. *Neurorehabil Neural Repair* (2002) 16:232–40. doi: 10.1177/154596802401105171
48. Lo HS. *Exoskeleton Robot for Upper Limb Rehabilitation: Design Analysis and Control.* Ph.D. dissertation, Dept. Mech. Eng., Auckland Univ., Auckland (2014).
49. Kong K, Jeon D. Design and control of an exoskeleton for the elderly and patients. *IEEE-ASME Trans Mech.* (2006) 11:428–32. doi: 10.1109/TMECH.2006.878550

8

Perturbation-Based Balance Training to Improve Step Quality in the Chronic Phase after Stroke

Hanneke J. R. van Duijnhoven [1†], Jolanda M. B. Roelofs [1†], Jasper J. den Boer [1], Frits C. Lem [2], Rifka Hofman [3], Geert E. A. van Bon [1], Alexander C. H. Geurts [1,4†] and Vivian Weerdesteyn [1,4†]*

[1] Department of Rehabilitation, Donders Institute for Brain, Cognition and Behaviour, Radboud University Medical Center, Nijmegen, Netherlands, [2] Department of Rehabilitation, Sint Maartenskliniek, Nijmegen, Netherlands, [3] Rehabilitation Medical Centre Klimmendaal, Arnhem, Netherlands, [4] Research, Sint Maartenskliniek, Nijmegen, Netherlands

***Correspondence:**
Hanneke J. R. van Duijnhoven
hanneke.vanduijnhoven@radboudumc.nl

† These authors have contributed equally to this work

Introduction: People with stroke often have impaired stepping responses following balance perturbations, which increases their risk of falling. Computer-controlled movable platforms are promising tools for delivering perturbation-based balance training under safe and standardized circumstances.

Purpose: This proof-of-concept study aimed to identify whether a 5-week perturbation-based balance training program on a movable platform improves reactive step quality in people with chronic stroke.

Materials and Methods: Twenty people with chronic stroke received a 5-week perturbation-based balance training (10 sessions, 45 min) on a movable platform. As the primary outcome, backward, and forward reactive step quality (i.e., leg angle at stepping-foot contact) was assessed with a lean-and-release (i.e., non-trained) task at pre-intervention, immediately post-intervention, and 6 weeks after intervention (follow-up). Additionally, reactive step quality was assessed on the movable platform in multiple directions, as well as, the percentage side steps upon sideward perturbations. To ensure that changes in the primary outcome could not solely be attributed to learning effects on the task due to repeated testing, 10 randomly selected participants received an additional pre-intervention assessment, 6 weeks prior to training. Clinical assesments included the 6-item Activity-specific Balance Confidence (6-ABC) scale, Berg Balance Scale (BBS), Trunk Impairment Scale (TIS), 10-Meter Walking Test (10-MWT), and Timed Up and Go-test (TUG).

Results: After lean-and-release, we observed 4.3° and 2.8° greater leg angles at post compared to pre-intervention in the backward and forward direction, respectively. Leg angles also significantly improved in all perturbation directions on the movable platform. In addition, participants took 39% more paretic and 46% more non-paretic side steps. These effects were retained at follow-up. Post-intervention, BBS and TIS scores had improved. At follow-up, TIS and 6-ABC scores had significantly improved compared to pre-intervention. No significant changes were observed between the two pre-intervention assessments (n=10).

Conclusion: A 5-week perturbation-based balance training on a movable platform appears to improve reactive step quality in people with chronic stroke. Importantly, improvements were retained after 6 weeks. Further controlled studies in larger patient samples are needed to verify these results and to establish whether this translates to fewer falls in daily life.

Keywords: paresis, neurological rehabilitation, postural balance, exercise therapy, physical therapy modalities

INTRODUCTION

Falls are among the most common complications after stroke (1). Post-stroke fall incidence rates vary between 1.4 and 5.0 falls each person-year (2). Falls are associated with worsening of functional outcomes post stroke (3). A vicious circle of falling, fear of falling, and inactivity can lead to further functional decline (2).

Impaired balance and gait capacities are the most important risk factors for falls after stroke (4, 5). Improving these capacities is, therefore, an important goal in rehabilitation. However, a Cochrane review on interventions for preventing falls after stroke did not show beneficial effects of exercise training aimed at improving balance and gait on fall rates (6). This is in contrast with the overwhelming evidence from the healthy elderly population, in which group- and home-based exercise programs do reduce fall rates and fall risk (7). The question arises whether the types of exercise training previously used in the stroke population are indeed suitable.

One important aspect that has yet received only limited attention in previous training programs for people with stroke is the role of reactive stepping responses while standing and walking (8–11). Following balance perturbations, fast and accurate stepping is an essential strategy to prevent falling (12, 13). People with stroke have an impaired capacity to execute such reactive stepping responses, particularly with the paretic leg (14–19). In fact, impaired stepping responses have been related to falling in people after stroke (20) and have shown to be predictive of fall risk after discharge from inpatient rehabilitation (21). Therefore, improving these reactive stepping responses following balance perturbations seems to be an important target for balance training after stroke.

Recent systematic literature reviews showed that perturbation-based balance training is effective to reduce fall risk in both healthy older adults and in people with Parkinson's disease (22, 23). In addition, a prospective cohort study showed lower fall rates for a group of participants in the subacute phase after stroke who received perturbation-based balance training during inpatient rehabilitation, when compared to a matched historical control group (11). Very recently, a first study on this type of training in the chronic phase after stroke has been published (24). In this study, the experimental group received therapist-induced balance perturbations and demonstrated improved reactive balance control when tested under the trained circumstances. Yet, no significant reduction in fall rate was observed compared to the control group. These observations call for further research on the generalizability of perturbation-based balance training to non-trained circumstances in people with chronic stroke. In addition, it may be that the effects of perturbation-based balance training can be enhanced by further increasing the intensity and unpredictability of the perturbations, thus providing a greater challenge for this group.

For delivering challenging perturbation-based balance training under safe and standardized circumstances, computer-controlled movable platforms [e.g., the Radboud Falls Simulator (RFS) (25)] are helpful. We here report the results of a proof-of-principle study to evaluate the effects of a 5-week training program on a movable platform, aimed at improving reactive step quality in multiple perturbation directions, and at enhancing side stepping upon sideward perturbations with the paretic and non-paretic leg. As a primary outcome, reactive step quality in the backward and forward directions was assessed with a lean-and-release (i.e., non-trained) task at pre-intervention, immediately post-intervention, and at 6 weeks follow-up. In addition, reactive step quality was assessed on the movable platform in multiple directions, as well as, the percentage side steps taken upon sideward perturbations. In the present study, we focused on community-dwelling people in the chronic phase after stroke, as in this phase no further neurological recovery should be expected (26). In addition, during the chronic phase, people are frequently exposed to balance perturbations in daily life. We hypothesized that our participants would show improved reactive step quality and enhanced side stepping after completion of a 5-week perturbation-based balance training program.

METHODS

Participants

From the outpatient rehabilitation population of our university hospital, a total of 20 persons in the chronic phase (>6 months) after stroke were included. Participant characteristics are given in

TABLE 1 | Characteristics of study participants (n = 20).

Sex (men/women, % men)	12/8, 60%
Age (years)*	60.1 (8.1)
Months since stroke*	50 (39.4)
Stroke type (ischemic/hemorrhagic, % ischemic)	12/8, 60%
Affected body side (left/right, % left)	12/8, 60%
Fall history (number of falls in previous year)*	1.6 (1.8)
MMSE (range: 0–30)*	27.8 (1.9)
QVT lateral malleolus affected side (range: 0–8)*	4.2 (2.2)
MI-LE (range: 0–100)*	63.3 (19.8)
FMA-LE (range: 0–100%)*	64.9 (17.7)
FAC (4/5, % FAC 4)	4/16, 20%

*MMSE, mini mental state examination; QVT, quantitative vibration threshold; MI-LE, Motricity Index lower extremity; FMA-LE, Fugl-Meyer assessment lower extremity; FAC, Functional Ambulation Categories. *Values are presented in means (SD).*

Table 1. They had to be able to stand and walk "independently" as defined by a Functional Ambulation Categories (FAC) score of 4 or 5 (27). Exclusion criteria were (1) other neurological or musculoskeletal conditions affecting balance; (2) health conditions in which physical exercise was contra-indicated; (3) use of psychotropic drugs or other medication negatively affecting balance; (4) severe cognitive problems [Mini Mental State Examination (MMSE) <24] (28); (5) persistent unilateral spatial neglect [Behavioral Inattention Test-Star Cancellation Test <44) (29)]; and (6) behavioral problems interfering with compliance to the study protocol. The study protocol was approved by the Medical Ethical Board of the region Arnhem-Nijmegen and all participants gave written informed consent in accordance with the Declaration of Helsinki. This study was registered in the Netherlands Trial Register (NTR number 3804, http://www.trialregister.nl/trialreg/admin/rctview.asp?TC=3804).

Design and Study Protocol

We conducted a proof-of-principle study in which the participants received a 5-week perturbation-based balance training. Forty persons were invited for an intake visit to determine eligibility (**Figure 1**), and (after inclusion, $n = 20$) to determine participants' demographic and clinical characteristics [sex, age, months since stroke, type of stroke, affected body side, history of falls, quantitative vibration threshold (QVT) (30), Motricity Index lower extremity (MI-LE) (31), and Fugl-Meyer Assessment lower extremity (FMA-LE) (32)]. In addition, at the intake visit, initial training intensity was determined on the platform for each participant in each perturbation direction (see section Intervention). Thereafter, all assessments of reactive stepping, as well as, all clinical tests (see section Outcomes) were performed by each participant at pre-intervention, post-intervention (6 weeks after pre-intervention), and follow-up (12 weeks after pre-intervention). Yet, 10 participants (50%) who were randomly selected based on block randomization with stratification for severity of paresis (Motricity Index—Leg <64% vs. Motricity Index—Leg ≥64%), received an additional pre-intervention assessment of reactive stepping 6 weeks prior to the final pre-intervention assessment (see **Figure 1**). By comparing the results of both pre-intervention assessments in this subgroup, we were able to account for potential effects of repeated testing on reactive stepping. In the week after the (final) pre-intervention assessment, all participants started the 5-week perturbation-based balance training. More information about the study protocol as well as the raw data supporting the conclusions of this manuscript will be made available by the authors, without undue reservation, to any qualified researcher upon request.

Intervention

The 5-week perturbation-based balance training program was delivered on the RFS [120 × 180 cm; Baat Medical, Enschede, The Netherlands (25)]. This movable platform can evoke reactive stepping responses by support-surface translations at magnitudes up to 4.5 m/s^2 in any given horizontal direction. In designing our new training program we aimed to achieve a high intensity (i.e., number of perturbations), large variation (i.e., directions of perturbations), and high challenge (i.e., high perturbation magnitudes) of reactive stepping exercises, yet under safe circumstances. The use of this computerized technology allowed us to set these perturbation parameters in a highly standardized manner.

The selection of exercises in our program was inspired by the existing literature on reactive stepping responses in people with stroke and in healthy elderly (33–36). After a balance perturbation, people with stroke show a low step quality in all directions, with a tendency to use multiple steps (36), a slow execution of steps (36), and a preference to use the non-paretic leg (34, 35). Generally, the paretic leg shows difficulties both in executing a stepping response and in support limb control while stepping with the non-paretic side (17). For sideward perturbations, side stepping has proven to be a more efficient and effective strategy than using cross-over steps (37, 38), yet people with stroke and healthy elderly tend to prefer cross-over steps during recovery responses from sideward perturbations (18, 38). Therefore, the aim of the training program was to improve step quality after balance perturbations in eight different directions (forward, backward, both sideward, and four diagonal directions) by promoting the use of a single step, prevail side steps over cross-over steps, and enhance the speed of stepping. Reactive stepping was practiced both with the paretic and with the non-paretic leg. To achieve optimal results we used several previously reported and well known techniques like verbal feedback, blockage of the preferred leg, and stepping toward a target (39).

Participants received 45 min of training, two times a week, 5 weeks in a row, under supervision of a trained physiotherapist. During each session, participants received a total of 60–80 perturbations. During all exercises, participants were secured by a safety harness attached to a sliding rail on the ceiling. The level of difficulty was gradually increased across sessions based on a standardized protocol, yet based on an individualized initial training intensity in each perturbation direction, as determined during the intake visit. Initial training intensity was defined as the maximal intensity at which participants were able to restore their balance without taking a step, plus 0.25 m/s^2. We progressed the difficulty of the training program by: (1) increasing the intensity

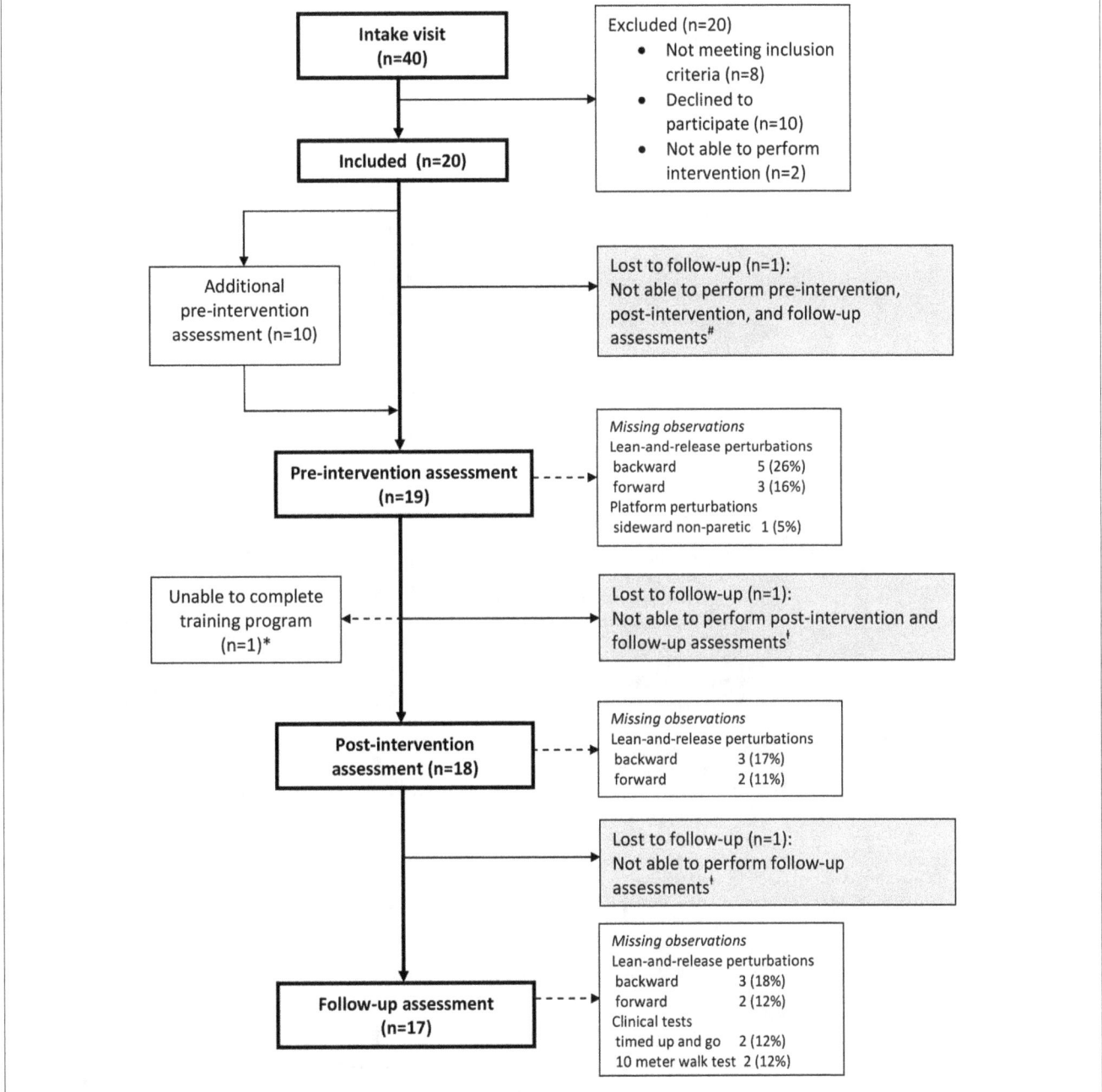

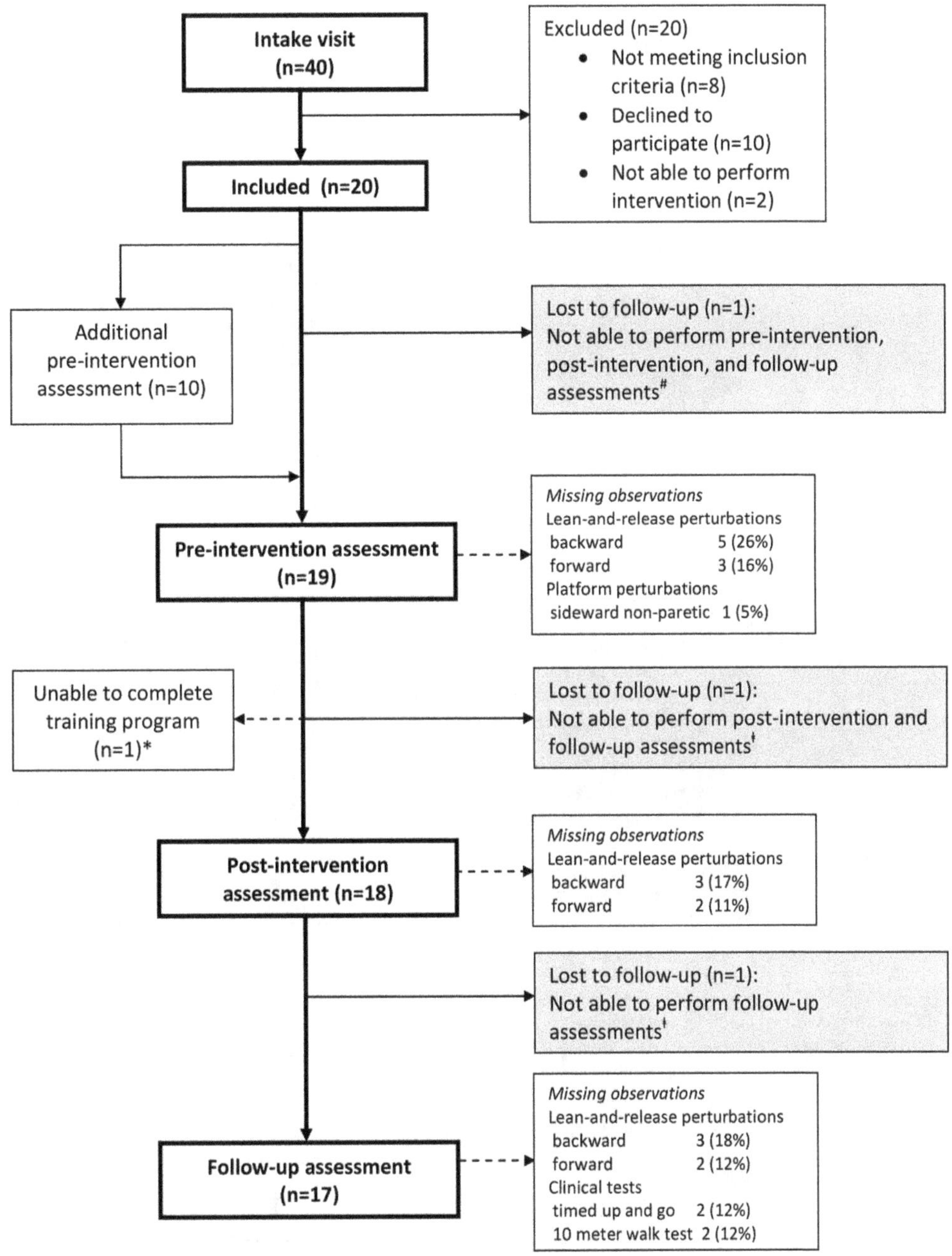

FIGURE 1 | Flow of participants. *One participant was able to complete only 3 out of 10 training sessions due to low back pain. Observations were included in all analyses according to the intention-to-treat principle. #Lost to follow-up due to hip fracture after a fall, unrelated to the intervention. ‡Lost to follow-up due to illness, unrelated to the study.

of the perturbation; (2) increasing the unpredictability of the start and the direction of the perturbations across sessions; and (3) by adding dual tasks starting from training session 6 (see **Tables 2, 3** for details on the content of the training program).

The 10 participants who performed two pre-intervention assessments were allowed to continue usual care during the 6 weeks in between these assessments, including any kind of physical therapy (if applicable). All participants were asked to refrain from additional balance exercises at home during the training period, but were free to receive (or continue) usual care during the follow-up.

Reactive Stepping Assessment

During pre, post, and follow-up assessments, reactive stepping was recorded following two types of balance perturbations: lean-and-release perturbations (backward and forward directions) and platform perturbations (backward, forward, sideward paretic, sideward non-paretic directions). During all recordings,

TABLE 2 | Content of the perturbation-based balance training program.

Session	Intensity of the perturbation	Predictability of the perturbation	Direction#	Additional training conditions
1	Initial*	Direction indicated and countdown to perturbation onset	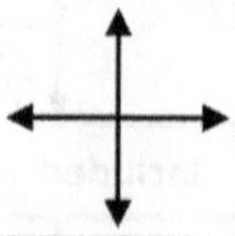	
2	Initial	Direction indicated	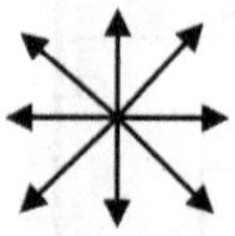	
3	125% of initial	Direction indicated	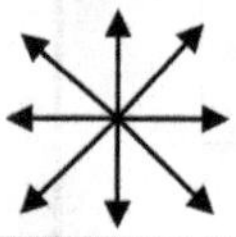	
4	125% of initial	Random direction within blocks that contained perturbations in two directions [see graph: diagonal steps with paretic leg (blue) and non-paretic leg (red)]	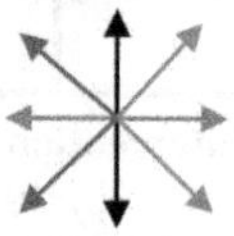	
5	150% of initial	Random direction within blocks that contained perturbations in two directions [see graph: diagonal steps with paretic leg (blue) and non-paretic leg (red)]	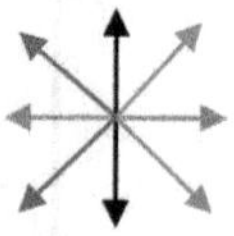	
6	150% of initial	Random direction within blocks that contained perturbations in two directions [see graph: diagonal steps with either leg forward (purple) or backward (green)]	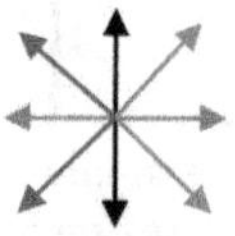	Cognitive dual task (visual Stroop task)
7	175% of initial	Random direction within blocks that contained perturbations in two directions (see graph for colored combinations)	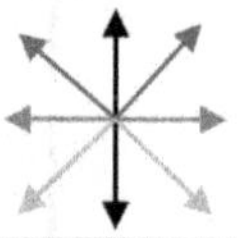	Motor dual task (marching in place)
8	175% of initial	All directions in random order	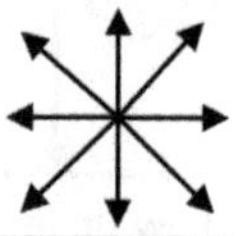	Cognitive dual task (visual Stroop task)
9	200% of initial	All directions in random order	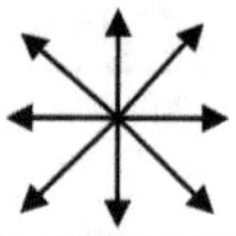	Motor dual task (marching in place)
10	200% of initial	All directions in random order	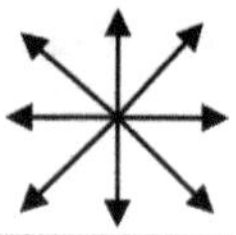	Combined cognitive and motor dual task

**The initial training intensity was the maximal intensity at which participants restored their balance without taking a step, plus 0.25 m/s^2.*
#The arrows in the graph depict the perturbation direction (forward, backward, paretic, non-paretic, and four diagonal directions).

participants wore their own shoes and stood at a fixed foot position with a distance of 4.5 cm between the medial sides of both feet. They wore a safety harness (attached to a sliding rail on the ceiling) to prevent them from falling, but which did not provide body (weight) support.

The lean-and-release task is a frequently used experimental paradigm for studying reactive stepping responses (21, 35, 40). Importantly, this type of perturbation was not trained and was, therefore, selected as the primary outcome. Using different types of perturbation for training and assessment is in line with a previous study on perturbation-based balance training (33). Participants were instructed to lean into the tether at an inclincation angle of 10° and, upon its unexpected release, to recover their balance by taking a single step. They were free to select which leg they used for stepping. After several practice trials, 10 outcome trials were recorded, five trials in the backward and five trials in the forward direction.

During the platform perturbation trials, participants received unpredictable and sudden horizontal translations in the forward, backward, sideward paretic, and sideward non-paretic directions. They were instructed to recover their balance with a single step. Perturbations consisted of an acceleration (300 ms), constant velocity (500 ms), and deceleration phase (300 ms). During the first assessment, the perturbation intensity was gradually increased with increments of 0.25 m/s^2 until the participants reached the maximum intensity at which they were able to recover their balance with one step (multiple stepping threshold, maximal 4.5 m/s^2). During the subsequent assessments, we used a fixed protocol with random perturbations in each direction, until the individual multiple stepping threshold (as determined during the first assessment) was reached. During all assessments, we ultimately recorded six outcome trials, three trials at the multiple stepping threshold and another three trials at one level (+0.125 m/s^2) above this intensity.

In addition to these formal assessments, we also monitored progress of participants' reactive step quality on the platform across training sessions (sessions 1, 4, 7, and 10). Due to time limitations or technical problems, we managed to do this in full for 14 of the 20 participants. These participants received additional platform perturbations after the training session, alternating in the forward and backward directions, at the maximum of their capacity (i.e., 0.125 m/s^2 above their individual multiple stepping threshold).

Reactive stepping responses were recorded at 100 Hz using an 8-camera 3D motion capture system (Vicon Motion Systems, Oxford, UK). Reflective markers were placed on anatomical landmarks according to the Vicon Plug-in-Gait model (41). An additional reflective marker was placed on the translating platform to correct marker positions for platform movement. Marker trajectory data were filtered with a second order, 5 Hz low-pass, zero-lag Butterworth filter.

From these data, we assessed the quality of the reactive step. This step quality is typically determined by how far the stepping foot is placed away from the centre of mass (CoM) into the direction of the induced loss of balance (15, 42–45). We expressed this foot-to-CoM relationship as the leg angle at first stepping-foot contact (**Figure 2**). In previous studies, the leg angle at stepping foot contact accurately distinguished between falls and successful recovery in healthy young subjects (43) and between single and multiple reactive steps in older women (42) and stroke survivors (19). The leg angle was defined as the angle between the vertical and the line connecting the mid-pelvis to the second metatarsal (backward and forward perturbations) or to the lateral malleolus (sideward perturbations) of the stepping foot. Larger positive leg angles correspond to better step quality.

Outcomes

The primary outcome was reactive step quality (i.e., leg angle at first stepping-foot contact) following lean-and-release perturbations in the backward and forward directions. The

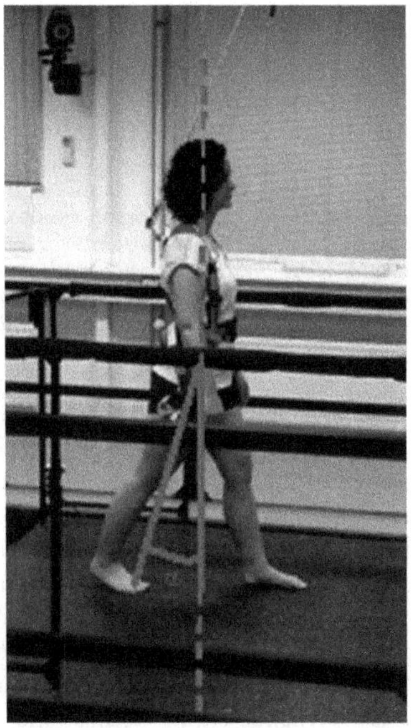

FIGURE 2 | Definition of the leg angle. Reactive step quality was expressed as the leg angle (α) at stepping-foot contact. This figure shows the leg angle for a backward step.

TABLE 3 | Training intensities per session (m/s^2) [Values are presented in means (SD)].

Session	Forward perturbations	Backward perturbations	Perturbations toward paretic side	Perturbations toward non-paretic side
1 and 2	1.02 (0.21)	0.83 (0.18)	1.06 (0.22)	1.10 (0.20)
3 and 4	1.28 (0.24)	1.05 (0.23)	1.35 (0.28)	1.41 (0.24)
5 and 6	1.53 (0.30)	1.28 (0.26)	1.61 (0.31)	1.67 (0.29)
7 and 8	1.80 (0.34)	1.49 (0.31)	1.88 (0.39)	1.94 (0.35)
9 and 10	2.04 (0.41)	1.67 (0.36)	2.14 (0.44)	2.21 (0.40)
Multiple stepping threshold	3.03 (1.36)	2.21 (0.88)	1.78 (0.90)	1.68 (0.96)

TABLE 4 | Primary and secondary outcome measures.

	Pre-intervention Mean (SE) (*n* = 20)	Post-intervention Mean (SE) (*n* = 20)	Follow-up Mean (SE) (*n* = 20)	Main effect of time (*p*-value) (*n* = 20)	First pre-intervention Mean (SE) (*n* = 10)	Final pre-intervention Mean (SE) (*n* = 10)	Main effect of time (*p*-value) (*n* = 10)
PRIMARY OUTCOMES							
Lean-and-release perturbations							
Backward leg angle (°)	0.3 (1.2)	4.6 (1.3)	4.0 (1.2)	0.001	−1.6 (1.7)	−0.8 (1.2)	0.589
Forward leg angle (°)	22.4 (0.8)	25.2 (0.5)	25.1 (0.7)	<0.001	23.0 (1.1)	23.0 (1.2)	0.987
SECONDARY OUTCOMES							
Platform Perturbations							
Backward leg angle (°)	−2.0 (1.4)	2.1 (1.1)	2.5 (0.8)	0.001	−3.5 (1.7)	−3.2 (1.5)	0.730
Forward leg angle (°)	21.1 (0.8)	23.6 (0.5)	23.3 (0.7)	0.001	20.1 (1.5)	20.4 (0.8)	0.699
Paretic side step (%)	19 (8)	59 (11)	58 (11)	0.001	29 (15)	30 (15)	0.907
Non-paretic side step (%)	37 (10)	84 (6)	80 (7)	<0.001	21 (14)	38 (16)	0.374
Paretic side step leg angle (°)*	17.6 (1.5)	19.8 (1.3)	19.4 (1.2)	0.012			
Non-paretic side step leg angle (°)*	17.6 (0.7)	18.8 (0.6)	19.7 (0.5)	0.001			
Clinical Scales							
BBS	52.4 (0.9)	53.3 (0.7)	52.7 (0.8)	0.047			
TIS	16.1 (0.6)	17.9 (0.7)	16.7 (0.6)	<0.001			
6-ABC	41.5 (5.7)	45.1 (4.8)	49.4 (5.6)	0.014			
Comfortable walking speed (km/h)	3.5 (0.2)	3.7 (0.2)	3.6 (0.2)	0.127			
TUG (s)	10.4 (0.8)	10.8 (0.8)	10.0 (0.8)	0.307			

Estimated marginal means (standard errors) for leg angles, percentage side steps, and clinical scales at pre-intervention, post-intervention, and follow-up for the total study sample (n = 20) and mean values (standard errors) for leg angles and percentage side steps at the first and final pre-intervention assessment (n = 10).

**Only three participants who received two pre-intervention assessments (n = 10) took a paretic side step at both assessments, whereas none of the participants took a non-paretic side step at both assessments. Therefore, sideward leg angles were not compared between pre-intervention assessments. BBS, Berg Balance Scale (range: 0–56); TIS, Trunk Impairment Scale (range: 0–23); 6-ABC, 6-item short version of the Activity-specific Balance Confidence scale (range: 0–100%); TUG, Timed Up and Go test.*

reactive step quality in four directions and the proportion of side steps upon sideward perturbations on the platform were used as secondary outcome measures. In addition, several clinical tests were performed, namely: (1) the 6-item short version of the Activity-specific Balance Confidence scale (6-ABC; range: 0–100%) to assess the balance confidence for performing daily-life activities (46); (2) the Berg Balance Scale (BBS; range: 0–56) to test balance performance during activities of varying difficulty (47); (3) the Trunk Impairment Scale (TIS; range: 0–23) to evaluate static and dynamic sitting balance and coordination of trunk movement (48); (4) the 10-Meter Walking Test at comfortable walking speed (10-MWT); and (5) the Timed Up and Go test (TUG) to quantify functional mobility (49). To determine the ability of participants to recover balance according to the instructions (i.e., with a single step), we also calculated the success rate for the lean-and-release and platform perturbations.

Statistical Analysis

We first verified by means of Generalized Estimated Equations modeling (GEE, autoregressive correlation structure) that potentially confounding variables [i.e., initial inclination angles for lean-and-release perturbations, the stepping leg (paretic/non-paretic), the maximal percentage of body weight supported by the harness system, and the angle of the trunk with the vertical at first stepping-foot contact] were not different between pre-intervention, post-intervention, and follow-up for the primary outcome assessments. As these analyses yielded no significant effects of time, we did not include these variables in further analyses.

To study changes in the primary and secondary outcomes (i.e., leg angles, percentages side steps, clinical scales) following training, we conducted a GEE analysis with time (pre-intervention, post-intervention, and follow-up) as within-subject factor. Furthermore, for the subgroup of participants who received two pre-intervention assessments, we determined the effects of repeated testing on reactive stepping by means of paired *t*-tests. Statistical analyses were performed with SPSS (version 22.0). $P < 0.05$ was considered statistically significant.

RESULTS

The inclusion flow diagram (**Figure 1**) shows the numbers (and reasons) of participants who were lost to follow-up, as well as, any missing observations at the assessments. No intervention-related adverse events were reported. **Table 4** shows a detailed overview of all outcome measures at pre-intervention, post-intervention, and follow-up ($n = 20$), together with the reactive stepping data for the two pre-intervention assessments ($n = 10$). Participants were not always able to regain balance with a single step. **Table 5** shows the percentage of successful lean-and-release and platform perturbation trials at pre-intervention, post-intervention, and follow-up.

Lean-and-Release Perturbations

Backward and forward leg angles at post-intervention were significantly larger compared to pre-intervention (backward: $\Delta_{pre-post} = 4.3 \pm 1.3°$, $p = 0.001$; forward: $\Delta_{pre-post} = 2.8 \pm 0.7°$, $p < 0.001$; **Figure 3** and **Table 4**). These larger leg angles were retained six weeks after training at follow-up (backward: $\Delta_{pre-fu} = 3.8 \pm 1.2°$, $p = 0.001$; forward: $\Delta_{pre-fu} = 2.7 \pm 0.6°$, $p < 0.001$). For both directions, leg angles were not different between the two pre-intervention assessments.

Platform Perturbations

For backward and forward platform perturbations, leg angles at post-intervention were significantly larger compared to pre-intervention (backward: $\Delta_{pre-post} = 4.1 \pm 1.2°$, $p = 0.001$; forward: $\Delta_{pre-post} = 2.5 \pm 0.8°$, $p = 0.001$; **Table 4**). This difference in leg angle was retained at follow-up (backward: $\Delta_{pre-fu} = 4.5 \pm 1.2°$, $p < 0.001$; forward: $\Delta_{pre-fu} = 2.2 \pm 0.6°$, $p < 0.001$). For sideward perturbations, the percentage of paretic and non-paretic side steps increased from pre- to post-intervention (paretic: $\Delta_{pre-post} = 39 \pm 12\%$, $p = 0.001$, **Figure 4A**; non-paretic: $\Delta_{pre-post} = 46 \pm 9\%$, $p < 0.001$, **Figure 4B**). This effect was also retained at follow-up (paretic: $\Delta_{pre-fu} = 38 \pm 11\%$, $p = 0.001$; non-paretic: $\Delta_{pre-fu} = 43 \pm 9\%$, $p < 0.001$). Furthermore, the number of participants who took at least one side step had increased after training. Before the start of the intervention, six and ten participants took one or more side steps with the paretic and non-paretic leg, respectively, which numbers increased to 12 and 17 at the post-intervention assessment. For side steps toward the paretic side, leg angles increased from pre- to post-intervention ($\Delta_{pre-post} = 2.3 \pm 0.8°$, $p = 0.004$), which effect was retained at follow-up ($\Delta_{pre-fu} = 1.9 \pm 0.7°$, $p = 0.006$). For side steps toward the non-paretic side, leg angles at post-intervention were not significantly larger compared to pre-intervention, although a trend toward larger leg angles was visible ($\Delta_{pre-post} = 1.2 \pm 0.7°$, $p = 0.075$). Six weeks after training, at follow-up, non-paretic leg angles were significantly larger compared to pre-intervention ($\Delta_{pre-fu} = 2.1 \pm 0.6°$, $p = 0.001$).

TABLE 5 | Percentage (SD) of trials recovered with a single step.

	Pre-intervention	Post-intervention	Follow-up
LEAN-AND-RELEASE PERTURBATIONS			
Backward	64 (44)	73 (42)	80 (39)
Forward	73 (41)	82 (33)	81 (35)
PLATFORM PERTURBATIONS			
Backward	38 (24)	81 (23)	85 (25)
Forward	56 (35)	92 (18)	93 (14)
Toward paretic side*	28 (21)	66 (41)	69 (37)
Toward non-paretic side*	36 (32)	92 (12)	80 (25)

N.B. This concerns both side steps and cross-over steps.

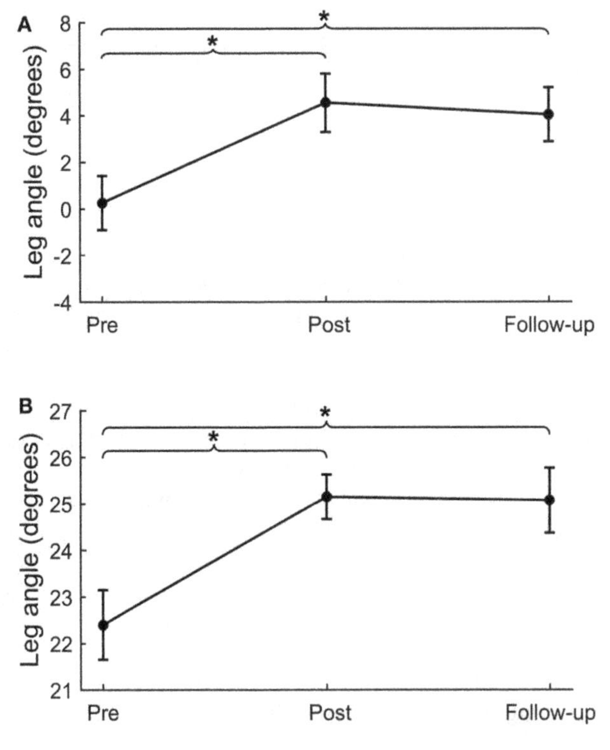

FIGURE 3 | Lean-and-release perturbations. Step quality (i.e., leg angle) for lean-and-release perturbations in the backward **(A)** and forward **(B)** directions. *$p < 0.01$.

Clinical Tests

Participants had a slightly higher BBS score at post compared to pre-intervention ($\Delta_{pre-post} = 0.9 \pm 0.4$, $p = 0.021$), however, this effect was not retained at follow-up ($\Delta_{pre-fu} = 0.4 \pm 0.6$, $p = 0.493$). Yet, TIS scores at post-intervention and at follow-up were significantly higher compared to pre-intervention ($\Delta_{pre-post} = 1.8 \pm 0.5$, $p < 0.001$; $\Delta_{pre-fu} = 0.7 \pm 0.3$, $p = 0.022$). The difference in 6-ABC scores between pre- and post-intervention did not reach statistical significance ($\Delta_{pre-post} = 3.7 \pm 3.1$, $p = 0.240$), however, at follow-up, participants rated their balance confidence significantly higher compared to pre-intervention ($\Delta_{pre-fu} = 7.9 \pm 2.9$, $p = 0.007$). For comfortable walking speed and TUG no significant differences were found between pre-intervention, post-intervention, or follow-up.

Progress of Step Quality

During the intervention period, backward leg angles increased from training session 1-7 ($\Delta_{s1-s7} = 3.4 \pm 4.8°$, $p = 0.041$), but did not further increase at subsequent sessions. The forward leg angle increased from session 1-4 ($\Delta_{s1-s4} = 1.8 \pm 2.6°$, $p = 0.033$), but did not further increase at subsequent sessions (**Figure 5**).

DISCUSSION

This proof-of-principle study investigated whether a 5-week perturbation-based multidirectional balance training program was able to improve reactive stepping in 20 persons in the chronic phase after stroke. In accordance with our hypotheses, we found that after completion of the training program reactive step quality had improved in the backward, forward, and both

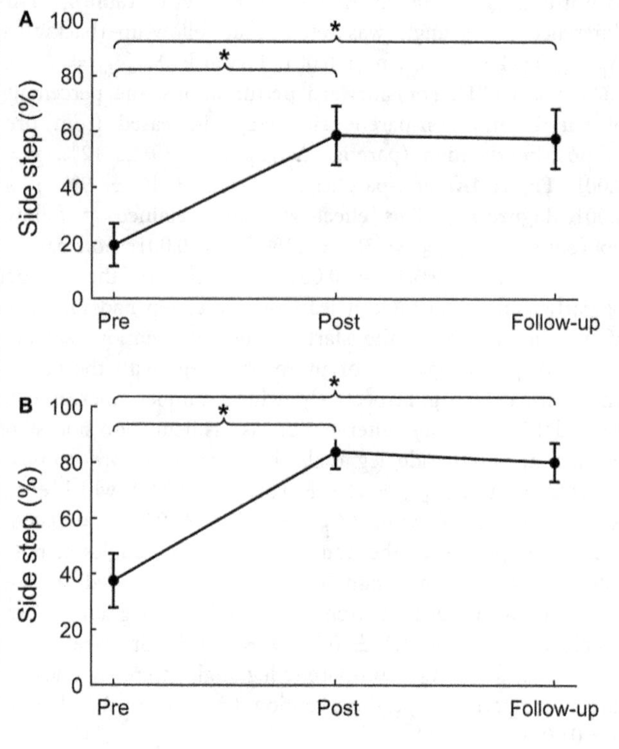

FIGURE 4 | Sideward platform perturbations. Percentage of side steps for platform perturbations in the sideward paretic **(A)** and sideward non-paretic **(B)** directions. *$p < 0.01$.

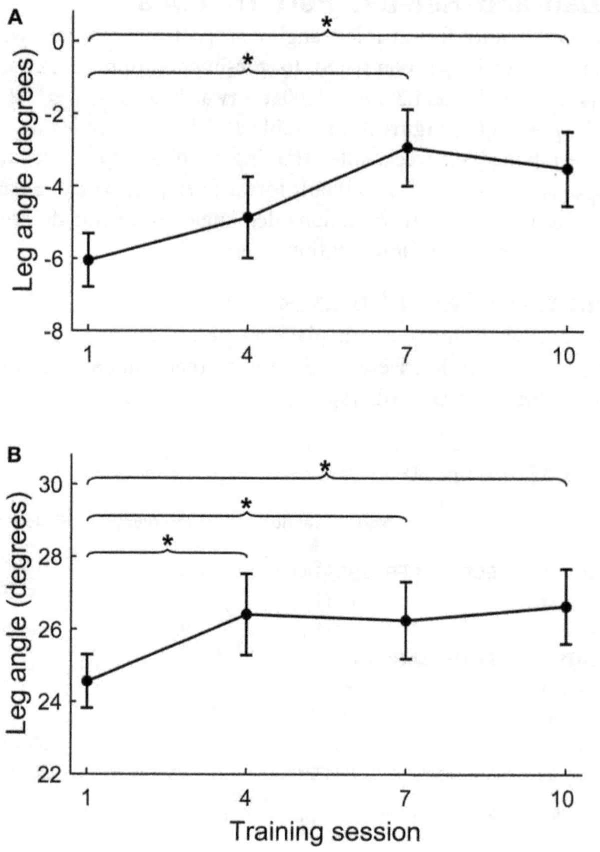

FIGURE 5 | Course of leg angle improvement across training sessions. Course of improvement in step quality (i.e., leg angle) across training sessions 1, 4, 7, and 10 for backward **(A)** and forward **(B)** platform perturbations. For practical reasons, we placed the reflective markers during the training sessions on the feet and L4 vertebra, instead of on the feet and both spina iliaca as was done during the formal assessments. Therefore, leg angles from the training sessions and assessments are not directly comparable. *$p < 0.05$.

sideward directions. In addition, both paretic and non-paretic side steps were more frequently used for recovering balance upon sideward perturbations. Both types of effect were retained at follow-up. Several clinical scales showed significant immediate (BBS, TIS) and/or delayed (TIS, 6-ABC) training effects as well, albeit relatively small sized compared to the assessments of reactive stepping.

The hypothesis that our perturbation-based balance training would improve step quality in people with chronic stroke was corroborated by an increase in leg angle at first stepping-foot contact following lean-and-release perturbations of 4.3 (backward) and 2.8 degrees (forward) between pre- and post-intervention. This parameter has previously been shown to be a valid indicator of reactive step quality, as it accurately distinguished between successful (no fall) and unsuccessful (fall) recovery following large balance perturbations (43) and between single and multiple stepping in elderly individuals and people with stroke (19, 42). At post-intervention, the leg angles during the platform perturbations showed similar improvements as those observed during lean-and-release perturbations (4.1 and 2.5 degrees in the backward and forward directions, respectively). As the lean-and-release perturbations were not included in the training program, we conclude that generalization of the training effects to non-trained tasks has occurred, which implies "real" training effects. Importantly, these improvements were retained for both types of perturbations after a period of 6 weeks during which no further practice of reactive stepping took place. Although these results are promising, it remains unknown for how long the observed improvements in reactive stepping are retained after this follow-up period of 6 weeks.

The notion that perturbation-based balance training can improve reactive stepping is in accordance with a previous study in community-dwelling older adults (33). After 6 weeks (18 sessions of 30 min) of perturbation training, these elderly persons more frequently used single stepping responses and had less foot collisions during sideward perturbations. Since foot collisions mostly occur during cross-over steps, the reduction in collisions is in line with our observation of more side steps being taken after the training. Only one case study in a sub-acute stroke patient (9) has previously been published on training-induced improvements in reactive step quality. This study demonstrated increased effectiveness of reactive stepping responses and increased use of the paretic leg for stepping after targeted perturbation training. As the training was provided in the sub-acute phase, it remained unknown whether improved reactive stepping was caused by spontaneous neurological recovery, by training-induced functional recovery, or by a combination of both. Although, generally, neurological (motor) recovery cannot be expected beyond 3 months after stroke (50), functional recovery can still be reached in the chronic phase (51). In this study, we indeed found that targeted balance training resulted in (further) functional recovery in a relatively high functioning group of chronic stroke patients. During training, participants were "forced" to step with both the paretic and non-paretic leg in response to challenging perturbations. This type of training may unmask latent motor capacity, especially of the proximal leg and trunk muscles, that may have decayed as a result of stroke. This process may be based on the same mechanisms that underlie the effects of constrained induced movement therapy of the upper limb, but the exact neurophysiological mechanisms are a relevant topic for further research. As there are no established methods for measuring reactive step quality in people with stroke, the clinical relevance of the presently observed improvements remains to be identified. Nevertheless, in young adults an increase in leg angle of just 1 degree resulted in a three-fold greater odds of successfully recovering from a large backward perturbation (43). Hence, we conclude that the presently observed improvements in step quality are substantial, and most likely clinically relevant.

Although our training period of 5 weeks appears sufficiently long to achieve gains in reactive stepping, we raise the question whether there might have been further room for improvement. In the first training session, we conservatively chose a perturbation intensity only slightly above the individual stepping thresholds. Perturbation intensity was gradually increased each week according to a pre-defined protocol. Yet, it turned out that in the anteroposterior directions, the average perturbation intensities in the final training sessions were still below the participants' multiple stepping thresholds, as measured during the first balance assessment (see **Table 3**). In addition, we monitored progress in forward and backward step quality (across sessions 1, 4, 7, and 10) and observed a plateau from session 4 onwards for forward and from session 7 onwards for backward step quality (see **Figure 5**). These observations indicate that we have been rather conservative in progressing the level of difficulty across training sessions. Hence, for future application of the training protocol, we suggest to further challenge the participants by including greater increments in perturbation intensities.

The improvements that we observed in reactive stepping were accompanied by a perceived increase in balance confidence (as shown by the higher scores on the 6-ABC at follow-up). Yet, we found only minor and transient gains on the BBS as a clinical balance test, which were not considered clinically relevant. In the remaining clinical outcomes, we found no significant changes, except for a modest improvement in TIS scores at post-intervention and follow-up. These observations are in line with a recent study on perturbation-based balance training in people in the sub-acute phase after stroke, which resulted in a reduction in fall risk and fall rates compared to a historical cohort, yet without between-group differences on clinical test outcomes (11). One reason for this apparent discrepancy may be that the clinical tests included in our study do not capture (improvements in) reactive stepping, being the primary aim of our perturbation-based training program. Indeed, Innes et al. (52) found a wide range in BBS scores across stroke participants, which did not correspond to their level of reactive stepping capacity. Another explanation may be that our participants already had near-maximum BBS scores (median: 54, range: 42–56) at pre-intervention, leaving little room for further improvement. Yet, they did have impairments in reactive stepping, as their multiple stepping thresholds (i.e., the maximum perturbation intensity that could be sustained with a single step) were substantially lower than in healthy peers. For example, backward multiple stepping thresholds in our participants were 2.2 vs. 3.5 m/s^2 in healthy peers (18). Hence, it seems that for our group of community ambulators after stroke (comfortable walking speed >0.8 m/s in 16 of the 19 participants), the ceiling effect in BBS scores results in an underestimation of their balance impairments. Therefore, in future studies on perturbation-based training, we recommend to consider alternative clinical balance tests that do include an assessment of reactive balance control. The mini-BEST, for instance, includes reactive stepping tests and also has a smaller ceiling effect than the BBS (53), which may further add to its suitability for community ambulators.

In this study, the use of the RFS had the advantage of delivering a training program that was standardized, safe, challenging and of high intensity. Yet, it should be mentioned that this type of technology is not yet widely available and future developments should be targeted at designing cheaper and more easy-to-use training devices for perturbation-based balance training. Another limitation of our study is that the leg angle at first stepping-foot contact did not provide insight into which part of the stepping response specifically responded to the perturbation-based balance training. Such insight could further enhance our understanding of functional balance recovery after stroke and, thereby, help optimize rehabilitation strategies for this patient group. Although the fact that we did not include a control group is an obvious limitation, a subgroup of 10 participants showed no differences in reactive stepping between the first and final pre-intervention assessments (before the start of the training). This result supports the notion that the observed improvements in reactive stepping after training are attributable to the perturbation-based balance training. Another limitation is the predictability of perturbation direction during the lean-and-release task. In the backward and forward platform perturbations, however, we found similar improvements in leg angles after training compared to the lean-and-release task. As perturbation direction during the platform perturbations was randomized across four different directions (backward, forward, sideward paretic, and sideward non-paretic), it appears that improvements in reactive stepping are not solely attributable to anticipation of participants.

Although we found improvements in reactive step quality after perturbation-based balance training, we did not evaluate whether our training program also contributed to fewer falls in daily life. Previous research showed, however, that impaired quality of reactive steps is related to increased fall rates during inpatient stroke rehabilitation (20), and that perturbation-based training in the sub-acute phase can reduce fall risk (11). These findings suggest that perturbation-based balance training may be an effective intervention for reducing fall rates, not only in the sub-acute phase but also in the chronic phase after stroke (10). Our chronic stroke participants were able to apply the learned stepping responses in non-trained circumstances and, importantly, retained their improvements in reactive stepping over a 6-week period without further practice. Therefore, perturbation-based balance training appears promising for improving the ability to recover from balance perturbations outside the laboratory or clinical setting (for example while experiencing trips or slips in daily life). Yet, further controlled studies in larger patient samples are needed to verify our results and to establish whether an improved step quality indeed translates to fewer falls in daily life.

AUTHOR CONTRIBUTIONS

HvD, AG, and VW: study conception and design. HvD, JdB, FL, and AG: eligibility assessment. HvD, JR, GvB, and RH: data collection. HvD, JR, AG, and VW: analysis and interpretation. AG and VW: funding and supervision. HvD, JR, and VW: drafting of the manuscript. HvD, JR, JdB, FL, GvB, RH, AG, and VW: critical revision.

REFERENCES

1. Langhorne P, Stott DJ, Robertson L, MacDonald J, Jones L, McAlpine C, et al. Medical complications after stroke: a multicenter study. *Stroke* (2000) 31:1223–9. doi: 10.1161/01.STR.31.6.1223
2. Weerdesteyn V, de Niet M, van Duijnhoven HJ, Geurts AC. Falls in individuals with stroke. *J Rehabil Res Dev.* (2008) 45:1195–214. doi: 10.1682/JRRD.2007.09.0145
3. Rohweder G, Ellekjaer H, Salvesen O, Naalsund E, Indredavik B. Functional outcome after common poststroke complications occurring in the first 90 days. *Stroke* (2015) 46:65–70. doi: 10.1161/STROKEAHA.114.006667
4. Weerdesteyn V, Laing AC, Robinovitch SN. Automated postural responses are modified in a functional manner by instruction. *Exp Brain Res.* (2008) 186:571–80. doi: 10.1007/s00221-007-1260-1
5. Minet LR, Peterson E, von Koch L, Ytterberg C. Occurrence and predictors of falls in people with stroke: six-year prospective study. *Stroke* (2015) 46:2688–90. doi: 10.1161/STROKEAHA.115.010496
6. Verheyden G, Weerdesteyn V, Pickering R, Kunkel D, Lennon S, Geurts A, et al. Interventions for preventing falls in people after stroke. *Cochrane Database Syst Rev.* (2013) 5:CD008728. doi: 10.1002/14651858.CD008728.pub2
7. Gillespie L, Robertson M, Gillespie W, Sherrington C, Gates S, Clemson L, et al. Interventions for preventing falls in older people living in the community. *Cochrane Database Syst Rev.* (2012) 2:CD007146. doi: 10.1002/14651858.CD007146.pub3
8. Marigold DS, Inglis T, Eng JJ, Harris JE, Dawson AS, Gylfadottir S. Exercise leads to faster postural reflexes, improved balance and mobility, and fewer falls in older persons with chronic stroke. *J Am Geriatr Soc.* (2005) 53:416–23. doi: 10.1111/j.1532-5415.2005.53158.x
9. Mansfield A, Inness EL, Komar J, Biasin L, Brunton K, Lakhani B, et al. Training rapid stepping responses in an individual with stroke. *Phys Ther.* (2011) 91:958–69. doi: 10.2522/ptj.20100212
10. Mansfield A, Aqui A, Centen A, Danells CJ, DePaul VG, Knorr S, et al. Perturbation training to promote safe independent mobility post-stroke: study protocol for a randomized controlled trial. *BMC Neurol.* (2015) 15:87. doi: 10.1186/s12883-015-0347-8
11. Mansfield A, Schinkel-Ivy A, Danells CJ, Aqui A, Aryan R, Biasin L, et al. Does perturbation training prevent falls after discharge from stroke rehabilitation? A prospective cohort study with historical control. *J Stroke Cerebrovasc Dis.* (2017) 26:2174–80. doi: 10.1016/j.jstrokecerebrovasdis.2017.04.041
12. Maki B, McIlroy W. The role of limb movements in maintaining upright stance:the "Change-in-Support" strategy. *Phys Ther.* (1997) 77:488–507. doi: 10.1093/ptj/77.5.488
13. Runge CF, Shupert CL, Horak FB, Zajac FE. Ankle and hip postural strategies defined by joint torques. *Gait Post.* (1999) 10:161–70. doi: 10.1016/S0966-6362(99)00032-6
14. Geurts AC, de Haart M, van Nes IJ, Duysens J. A review of standing balance recovery from stroke. *Gait Post.* (2005) 22:267–81. doi: 10.1016/j.gaitpost.2004.10.002
15. Honeycutt CF, Nevisipour M, Grabiner MD. Characteristics and adaptive strategies linked with falls in stroke survivors from analysis of laboratory-induced falls. *J Biomech.* (2016) 49:3313–9. doi: 10.1016/j.jbiomech.2016.08.019
16. Inness EL, Mansfield A, Bayley M, McIlroy WE. Reactive stepping after stroke: determinants of time to foot off in the paretic and nonparetic limb. *J Neurol Phys Ther.* (2016) 40:196–202. doi: 10.1097/NPT.0000000000000132
17. Kajrolkar T, Bhatt T. Falls-risk post-stroke: examining contributions from paretic versus non paretic limbs to unexpected forward gait slips. *J Biomech.* (2016) 49:2702–8. doi: 10.1016/j.jbiomech.2016.06.005
18. de Kam D, Roelofs JMB, Bruijnes A, Geurts ACH, Weerdesteyn V. The next step in understanding impaired reactive balance control in people with stroke: the role of defective early automatic postural responses. *Neurorehabil Neural Repair.* (2017) 31:708–16. doi: 10.1177/1545968317718267
19. de Kam D, Roelofs JMB, Geurts ACH, Weerdesteyn V. Body configuration at first stepping-foot contact predicts backward balance recovery capacity in people with chronic stroke. *PLoS ONE* (2018) 13:e0192961. doi: 10.1371/journal.pone.0192961
20. Mansfield A, Inness EL, Wong JS, Fraser JE, McIlroy WE. Is impaired control of reactive stepping related to falls during inpatient stroke rehabilitation? *Neurorehabil Neural Repair.* (2013) 27:526–33. doi: 10.1177/1545968313478486
21. Mansfield A, Wong JS, McIlroy WE, Biasin L, Brunton K, Bayley M, et al. Do measures of reactive balance control predict falls in people with stroke returning to the community? *Physiotherapy* (2015) 101:373–80. doi: 10.1016/j.physio.2015.01.009
22. Mansfield A, Wong JS, Bryce J, Knorr S, Patterson KK. Does perturbation-based balance training prevent falls? Systematic review and meta-analysis of preliminary randomized controlled trials. *Phys Ther.* (2015) 95:700–9. doi: 10.2522/ptj.20140090
23. Gerards MHG, McCrum C, Mansfield A, Meijer K. Perturbation-based balance training for falls reduction among older adults: current evidence and implications for clinical practice. *Geriatr Gerontol Int.* (2017) 17:2294–303. doi: 10.1111/ggi.13082
24. Mansfield A, Aqui A, Danells CJ, Knorr S, Centen A, DePaul VG, et al. Does perturbation-based balance training prevent falls among individuals with chronic stroke? A randomised controlled trial. *BMJ Open* (2018) 8:e021510. doi: 10.1136/bmjopen-2018-021510
25. Nonnekes J, de Kam D, Geurts AC, Weerdesteyn V, Bloem BR. Unraveling the mechanisms underlying postural instability in Parkinson's disease using dynamic posturography. *Expert Rev Neurother.* (2013) 13:1303–8. doi: 10.1586/14737175.2013.839231
26. Kwakkel G, Kollen BJ. Predicting activities after stroke: what is clinically relevant? *Int J Stroke* (2013) 8:25–32. doi: 10.1111/j.1747-4949.2012.00967.x
27. Holden MK, Gill KM, Magliozzi MR, Nathan J, Piehl-Baker L. Clinical gait assessment in the neurologically impaired. Reliability and meaningfulness. *Phys Ther.* (1984) 64:35–40. doi: 10.1093/ptj/64.1.35
28. Folstein MF, Folstein SE, McHugh PR. "Mini-mental state." A practical method for grading the cognitive state of patients for the clinician. *J Psychiatr Res.* (1975) 12:189–98. doi: 10.1016/0022-3956(75)90026-6

29. Wilson B, Cockburn J, Halligan P. Development of a behavioral test of visuospatial neglect. *Arch Phys Med Rehabil.* (1987) 68:98–102.
30. Pestronk A, Florence J, Levine T, Al-Lozi MT, Lopate G, Miller T, et al. Sensory exam with a quantitative tuning fork: rapid, sensitive and predictive of SNAP amplitude. *Neurology* (2004) 62:461–4. doi: 10.1212/01.WNL.0000106939.41855.36
31. Collin C, Wade D. Assessing motor impairment after stroke: a pilot reliability study. *J Neurol Neurosurg Psychiatr.* (1990) 53:576–9. doi: 10.1136/jnnp.53.7.576
32. Gladstone DJ, Danells CJ, Black SE. The fugl-meyer assessment of motor recovery after stroke: a critical review of its measurement properties. *Neurorehabil Neural Repair.* (2002) 16:232–40. doi: 10.1177/154596802401105171
33. Mansfield A, Peters AL, Liu BA, Maki BE. Effect of a perturbation-based balance training program on compensatory stepping and grasping reactions in older adults: a randomized controlled trial. *Phys Ther.* (2010) 90:476–91. doi: 10.2522/ptj.20090070
34. Lakhani B, Mansfield A, Inness EL, McIlroy WE. Characterizing the determinants of limb preference for compensatory stepping in healthy young adults. *Gait Post.* (2011) 33:200–4. doi: 10.1016/j.gaitpost.2010.11.005
35. Mansfield A, Inness EL, Lakhani B, McIlroy WE. Determinants of limb preference for initiating compensatory stepping poststroke. *Arch Phys Med Rehabil.* (2012) 93:1179–84. doi: 10.1016/j.apmr.2012.02.006
36. Lakhani B, Mansfield A, Inness EL, McIlroy WE. Compensatory stepping responses in individuals with stroke: a pilot study. *Physiother Theory Pract.* (2011) 27:299–309. doi: 10.3109/09593985.2010.501848
37. Maki BE, McIlroy WE, Perry SD. Influence of lateral destabilization on compensatory stepping responses. *J Biomechanics* (1996) 29:343–53. doi: 10.1016/0021-9290(95)00053-4
38. Maki BE, Edmondstone MA, McIlroy WE. Age-related differences in laterally directed compensatory stepping behavior. *J Gerontol.* (2000) 55A:M270–7. doi: 10.1093/gerona/55.5.M270
39. Mansfield A, Peters AL, Liu BA, Maki BE. A perturbation-based balance training program for older adults: study protocol for a randomised controlled trial. *BMC Geriatr.* (2007) 7:12. doi: 10.1186/1471-2318-7-12
40. Do MC, Breniere Y, Brenguier P. A biomechanical study of balance recovery during the fall forward. *J Biomech.* (1982) 15:933–9. doi: 10.1016/0021-9290(82)90011-2
41. Davis R, Ounpuu S, Tyburski D, Gage J. A gait analysis data collection and reduction technique. *Hum Mov Sci.* (1991) 10:575–87. doi: 10.1016/0167-9457(91)90046-Z
42. Hsiao E, Robinovitch S. Elderly subjects' ability to recover balance with a single backward step associates with body configuration at step contact. *J Gerontol.* (2001) 56A:M42–7. doi: 10.1093/gerona/56.1.m42
43. Weerdesteyn V, Laing AC, Robinovitch SN. The body configuration at step contact critically determines the successfulness of balance recovery in response to large backward perturbations. *Gait Post.* (2012) 35:462–6. doi: 10.1016/j.gaitpost.2011.11.008
44. Kajrolkar T, Yang F, Pai YC, Bhatt T. Dynamic stability and compensatory stepping responses during anterior gait-slip perturbations in people with chronic hemiparetic stroke. *J Biomech.* (2014) 47:2751–8. doi: 10.1016/j.jbiomech.2014.04.051
45. De Kam D. *Postural Instability in People with Chronic Stroke and Parkinson's Disease: Dynamic Perspectives.* Doctoral dissertation (2017) Radboud University.
46. Peretz C, Herman T, Hausdorff JM, Giladi N. Assessing fear of falling: can a short version of the activities-specific balance confidence scale be useful? *Mov Disord.* (2006) 21:2101–5. doi: 10.1002/mds.21113
47. Berg KO, Wood-Dauphinee SL, Williams JI, Maki B. Measuring balance in the elderly: validation of an instrument. *Can J Public Health* (1992) 83 (Suppl. 2):S7–11.
48. Verheyden G, Nieuwboer A, Mertin J, Preger R, Kiekens C, De Weerdt W. The Trunk Impairment Scale: a new tool to measure motor impairment of the trunk after stroke. *Clin Rehabil.* (2004) 18:326–34. doi: 10.1191/0269215504cr733oa
49. Podsiadlo D, Richardson S. The timed "Up & Go": a test of basic functional mobility for frail elderly persons. *J Am Geriatr Soc.* (1991) 39:142–8. doi: 10.1111/j.1532-5415.1991.tb01616.x
50. Kwakkel G, Kollen B, Twisk J. Impact of time on improvement of outcome after stroke. *Stroke* (2006) 37:2348–53. doi: 10.1161/01.STR.0000238594.91938.1e
51. van Duijnhoven HJ, Heeren A, Peters MA, Veerbeek JM, Kwakkel G, Geurts AC, et al. Effects of exercise therapy on balance capacity in chronic stroke: systematic review and meta-analysis. *Stroke* (2016) 47:2603–10. doi: 10.1161/STROKEAHA.116.013839
52. Inness EL, Mansfield A, Lakhani B, Bayley M, McIlroy WE. Impaired reactive stepping among patients ready for discharge from inpatient stroke rehabilitation. *Phys Ther.* (2014) 94:1755–64. doi: 10.2522/ptj.20130603
53. Godi M, Franchignoni F, Caligari M, Giordano A, Turcato AM, Nardone A. Comparison of reliability, validity, and responsiveness of the mini-BESTest and Berg Balance Scale in patients with balance disorders. *Phys Ther.* (2013) 93:158–67. doi: 10.2522/ptj.20120171

9

The Multidisciplinary Approach to Alzheimer's Disease and Dementia: A Narrative Review of Non-Pharmacological Treatment

Chiara Zucchella [1], Elena Sinforiani [2], Stefano Tamburin [1,3], Angela Federico [3], Elisa Mantovani [3], Sara Bernini [2], Roberto Casale [4] and Michelangelo Bartolo [4*]*

[1] Neurology Unit, University Hospital of Verona, Verona, Italy, [2] Alzheimer's Disease Assessment Unit, Laboratory of Neuropsychology, IRCCS Mondino Foundation, Pavia, Italy, [3] Department of Neurosciences, Biomedicine and Movement Sciences, University of Verona, Verona, Italy, [4] Neurorehabilitation Unit, Department of Rehabilitation, HABILITA, Bergamo, Italy

***Correspondence:**
Stefano Tamburin
stefano.tamburin@univr.it
Michelangelo Bartolo
bartolomichelangelo@gmail.com

Background: Alzheimer's disease (AD) and dementia are chronic diseases with progressive deterioration of cognition, function, and behavior leading to severe disability and death. The prevalence of AD and dementia is constantly increasing because of the progressive aging of the population. These conditions represent a considerable challenge to patients, their family and caregivers, and the health system, because of the considerable need for resources allocation. There is no disease modifying intervention for AD and dementia, and the symptomatic pharmacological treatments has limited efficacy and considerable side effects. Non-pharmacological treatment (NPT), which includes a wide range of approaches and techniques, may play a role in the treatment of AD and dementia.

Aim: To review, with a narrative approach, current evidence on main NPTs for AD and dementia.

Methods: PubMed and the Cochrane database of systematic reviews were searched for studies written in English and published from 2000 to 2018. The bibliography of the main articles was checked to detect other relevant papers.

Results: The role of NPT has been largely explored in AD and dementia. The main NPT types, which were reviewed here, include exercise and motor rehabilitation, cognitive rehabilitation, NPT for behavioral and psychological symptoms of dementia, occupational therapy, psychological therapy, complementary and alternative medicine, and new technologies, including information and communication technologies, assistive technology and domotics, virtual reality, gaming, and telemedicine. We also summarized the role of NPT to address caregivers' burden.

Conclusions: Although NPT is often applied in the multidisciplinary approach to AD and dementia, supporting evidence for their use is still preliminary. Some studies showed statistically significant effect of NPT on some outcomes, but their clinical significance is uncertain. Well-designed randomized controlled trials with innovative designs are needed to explore the efficacy of NPT in AD and dementia. Further studies are required to offer robust neurobiological grounds for the effect of NPT, and to examine its cost-efficacy profile in patients with dementia.

Keywords: Alzheimer's disease, dementia, non-pharmacological intervention, rehabilitation, caregiver, interprofessional team

INTRODUCTION

Dementia represents one of the major health problems in elderly individuals, with progressive deterioration of cognition, daily activity functioning and behavior that together lead to disability. Worldwide, approximately 40 million people over 65 years suffer from dementia, and 70% of them are affected by Alzheimer's disease (AD) that represents the most diffuse type of dementia. The incidence of dementia increases with age, which is the most important risk factor. Therefore, the prevalence of AD is expected to increase in the future, in parallel with the progressive aging of the population. In the European Union, the most reliable estimates forecast dementia cases to overcome 15 million in 2020 (1–3). Moreover, the improved life conditions in developing countries will lead to increased life expectancy, and therefore to higher incidence of dementia (4).

No disease-modifying treatment has been demonstrated to be effective in AD. Cholinesterase inhibitors and memantine, which are the only commercially available symptomatic drugs, may improve cognitive and behavioral outcomes, but their clinical impact remains modest and controversial (5–7). Despite research has been focused on the early [i.e., mild cognitive impairment (MCI) with biological evidence of AD] or preclinical stages of the disease, and new disease-modifying treatments have been tested to reduce the supposed pathophysiological changes of AD (i.e., amyloid deposition), no significant clinical effect has been achieved, to date (8).

Because of the limited efficacy of current pharmacological therapy and with the knowledge that caring for people with AD and dementia requires the involvement of a large number of professionals (e.g., psychologists, occupational therapists, etc.) and caregivers to offer a comprehensive and individualized management, research focused on non-pharmacological treatment (NPT). NPT may improve function, independence, and quality of life (QoL) in agreement with the International Classification of Functioning, Disability and Health (ICF) (9), is non-invasive, safe and has few side effects (10). NPT encompasses a wide range of interventions to improve patients' symptoms, reduce the stress of caregivers, and ameliorate the environment. NPT is based on different methodologies, ranging from simpler (e.g., environmental interventions) to complex approaches (e.g., virtual reality, home automation) (11). These interventions are not aimed to influence the underlying pathophysiological mechanisms but to maintain function and participation as long as possible, as the disease progresses, thus reducing disability and improving patient's and caregiver's QoL. However, a direct effect of NPT on cognition through neural plasticity/adaptation cannot be excluded in early disease stages.

The present narrative review summarized evidence on NPTs for AD and dementia. Because of the large bulk of data on this topic, we focused on the main NPT strategies. We did not report and discuss data on NPT in MCI, an intermediate state between intact cognition and dementia (12), because of the large number of studies that would have required a paper apart.

SEARCH STRATEGY

PubMed and the Cochrane database of systematic reviews were searched for studies published from 2000 to 2018 with a search string including the following terms: Alzheimer's disease, dementia, behavioral and psychological symptoms, non-pharmacological, intervention, therapy, exercise, motor, rehabilitation, neurorehabilitation, cognitive, training, stimulation, occupational, psychological, psychotherapy, multicomponent, multidimensional, complementary and alternative medicine, aromatherapy, music therapy, art therapy, massage and touch, technology, information and communication, assistive device, domotics, virtual reality, gaming, serious games, telemedicine, related terms, and MeSH. Only papers written in English were considered. The bibliography of the main articles (reviews, systematic reviews, meta-analyses) was also checked to detect other relevant papers.

In consideration of the great heterogeneity of interventions that are classified as NPT and of the variety of outcome measures reported in the different studies, this work was not conceived as a systematic review of the literature, but as a narrative one to provide a useful tool for clinicians on the state of the art of NPT in dementia.

EXERCISE AND MOTOR REHABILITATION

A growing amount of evidence suggests that a healthy lifestyle can reduce the risk of cardiovascular diseases (13, 14), osteoporosis, diabetes, and depression (15). A number of prospective cohort studies suggested that a regular physical activity may enhance cognitive function and reduce the risk of AD and other dementias and delay their onset or progression (16–24). A recent paper derived from the population-based Mayo Clinic study of aging on 280 MCI patients showed that moderate intensity midlife physical activity was significantly associated with a decreased risk of incident dementia (25). Regular physical exercise is recommended to all older adults, and indeed to those at increased risk of AD, as it may improve physical health, reduce frailty, lower the risk of depression, improve cognitive function in the short and long term (26–31).

Conversely, the evidence on the protecting role of short-term, single-component physical activity interventions seems to be largely insufficient (32).

Exercise has been documented to improve physical health and well-being (33), to reduce behavioral and psychological symptoms of dementia (BPSD) (34–36), and to enhance performance in the activities of daily living (ADL) (37, 38) in patients with AD or dementia.

A Cochrane review including 17 randomized controlled trials (RCTs) confirmed the positive effect of exercise programs in reducing the progression of dependence in ADL in people with dementia but showed limited evidence of benefit for the remaining outcomes (i.e., cognition, BPSD, QoL, depression, mortality, caregiver burden, and use of healthcare services) (39). This finding is of some relevance because preserving functional independence in ADL is critical for improving the QoL of people with dementia and their caregivers and delaying institutionalization.

The exercise interventions explored in dementia include a variety of training methods (e.g., aerobic exercise, resistance training or weightlifting, balance, and flexibility training), and the physical/motor outcome measures were quite different across studies (e.g., chair stand tests, timed up and go, timed walking tests). Comparative studies to explore the most effective exercise intervention, the amount of exercise, the most sensitive and significant outcome, and the role of physical activity in different patients' groups are needed.

According to animal models, a number of mechanisms may mediate the effects of exercise on brain and cognition (40). It has been suggested that exercise may improve vascular health by reducing blood pressure (41, 42), arterial stiffness (42), oxidative stress (43), systemic inflammation (44), and enhance endothelial dysfunction (45), all of which are associated with better cerebral perfusion (46, 47). Exercise may also preserve neurons and promote neurogenesis, synaptogenesis, (48–50), and neuronal plasticity (51–55).

Imaging studies in aging people confirmed the positive association between physical activity and gray matter volume. Both aerobic fitness and coordinative exercises was associated with reduced brain atrophy in the frontal and temporal regions and the hippocampus, all areas that are critical for higher cognitive function (56–58). A recent review on the association between fitness, physical activity and gray matter volume showed that both cross-sectional studies and randomized interventions consistently suggested a change in the size of prefrontal cortex and hippocampus after moderate intensity exercise in elderly people (59).

Neurotrophins, in particular the brain-derived neurotrophic factor, may be the common pathway of these mechanisms, may mediate the exercise-driven brain responses and can drive neuronal plasticity, improve cognition, and protect neurons against insult (60–63).

Future studies aimed to identify lifestyle, behavioral and/or biologic factors that may increase the likelihood of successful brain aging would help implementing preventive intervention to reduce age-related brain atrophy and consequently the risk for cognitive decline.

Conversely, the effect of physical exercise on other biological measures of AD pathology, such as cerebrospinal fluid biomarkers is still unclear (64, 65), and further studies are needed on this topic.

COGNITIVE INTERVENTION

Cognitive intervention is currently the NPT that has been better explored in dementia and represents the most robust alternative and/or complement to pharmacological treatment. Cognitive intervention is typically classified as cognitive stimulation (CS), cognitive training (CT), and cognitive rehabilitation (CR) (66). CS refers to a broad range of activities (i.e., reality orientation therapy, reminiscence therapy) aimed to enhance the general cognitive and social functioning of the individual (67). While CS consists in a global approach to arouse all cognitive domains, CT focuses on a particular cognitive function (e.g., attention, memory, executive functions, language) through a set of standard tasks to improve or maintain—as is the case for neurodegenerative diseases—its normal functioning as long as possible. CR refers to a tailor-made approach which sets realistic goals to help patients and their families in everyday life. To achieve these aims, the CR therapist may choose a restorative or a compensative approach (68).

Even though the distinction between CS, CT, and CR is clear, the literature on cognitive interventions is, to some extent, confused. These terms are often used interchangeably, even if they refer to distinct approaches with a different rationale. Moreover, CR has been rarely used in dementia, because it may be difficult to apply in this condition. For these reasons, our review will focus on studies exploring CS or CT for people with dementia.

CS is currently the intervention with the most robust evidence. Several studies reported an improvement of general cognitive functioning in patients with mild-to-moderate dementia after CS sessions of variable length (69–74). A recent meta-analysis showed that CS has a moderate effect size on the Mini Mental State Examination (75) and a small effect size on the Alzheimer's Disease Assessment Scale-cognitive subscale (76), which represent two commonly-used general cognitive functioning outcomes, in patients with dementia (73). There are still few data on the efficacy of CS on other outcomes, such as mood, behavioral symptoms, QoL, and well-being. However, preliminary results indicate that CS may improve QoL and well-being of caregivers of people with AD and dementia (69, 70, 74).

The evidence on CT for people with dementia is less robust. A recent systematic review indicated that CT may improve patient's performance in trained tasks and similar exercises but has no consistent effect on everyday functioning (77). Most RCTs showed no effect of CT on other outcomes, but their low quality impede any solid conclusion (70–72, 74, 77).

Some studies documented the association of CS and CT did not result in better outcomes than single interventions (73, 74).

The Cognitive Stimulation Therapy (CST) was proposed as a structured and methodologically sound CS protocol (78, 79). CST is currently considered the evidence-based NPT of choice for the cognitive symptoms of mild-to-moderate dementia of any etiology, including vascular one (80–83). Moreover, CST is at present, the only one for which international RCTs consistently demonstrated significant improvements to cognition and QoL, using the same CST program which has been culturally adapted using standardized guidelines. CST involves 14 or more sessions of themed activities, usually related to tasks including money use, word games, word association, object categorization, current affairs and famous faces, and is typically run twice weekly (78). Each CST session is aimed to stimulate cognitive abilities and social relationships with other members and operators (78, 79). Several studies suggested the area of major CST efficacy in people with mild-to-moderate dementia is general cognitive functioning, but some cognitive areas, namely memory, orientation and language comprehension seems to be those with larger improvement following CST in an open study (84).

Several issues (e.g., health or mobility problems, services not offering this treatment) could undermine the participation of patients with dementia to CST groups (85) and the interest for individualized CST (iCST) is increasingly growing (85, 86). However, a recent RCT showed that a home-based iCST program had neither effect on cognition and QoL of patients with mild-to-moderate dementia, nor on QoL of their caregivers (87). The reasons for this negative finding might include the lack of additional stimulation from participation in a group social context and the difficulty for the caregiver to administer the iCST program in the proper way, being not professional, and because of the difficult relationship with the person with dementia.

In conclusion, while the CST program—a precise technique with a specific manual and training—has a robust evidence-based body of data, the high heterogeneity in terms of duration of treatment, length, and number of single sessions and severity of dementia impede any definite conclusion on the efficacy of other CS and CT interventions (73).

NON-PHARMACOLOGICAL MANAGEMENT OF BEHAVIORAL AND PSYCHOLOGICAL SYMPTOMS OF DEMENTIA

Behavioral and psychological symptoms of dementia, i.e., the so-called BPSD, are characterized by alterations of perception (hallucinations, misidentification), thinking (delusions), mood (depression, anxiety, apathy), and behavior (aggression, agitation, disinhibition, wandering, socially or sexually inappropriate behavior) (88), being highly prevalent in all types of dementia, i.e., 50–80% in AD, >80% in fronto-temporal dementia, 50–70% in Lewy body dementia and vascular dementia (89, 90). BPSD may occur in all stages of AD, and even in people with MCI, but there is no agreement on the possible relationship with disease evolution. Indeed, although some studies showed that the prevalence and severity of BPSD increase with dementia severity, other reports suggest they are more frequent in the moderate AD stages, and diminish with disease progression (89, 90). Factors that may influence BPSD occurrence include premorbid personality, younger age, poor education, depression, high burden, concurrent medical conditions, and drugs. Environmental factors such as noise, overstimulation, isolation, inadequate temperature, change of routine, as well as inappropriate relationship between patient and caregiver (e.g., communication style, body language) or the inability of the patient to express his needs, may all trigger BPSD (91).

BPSD represent the most frequent cause of institutionalization and drug prescription, increase patient's disability, worsen patient's and caregiver's QoL, contribute to increase costs, but their influence on cognition is unclear (92).

According to consensus papers based on expert opinion and systematic revision of RCTs, the general principles for BPSD management include the following steps: symptoms evaluation (i.e., type, entity, frequency), recognition and treatment of possible organic causes or triggering factors, NPT, pharmacological therapy, educational, and psychological support for the caregiver (93–96).

Considering the limited evidence and concerns on the safety of drug treatment (94–99), all guidelines agree that individualized and person-centered NPT are the first-line treatment for BPDS and the use of a pharmacological strategy should be considered only later, using the least harmful drug for the shortest time.

Some theoretical models have been proposed to explain the role of non-pharmacological approaches to BPSD (100). The progressively lowered stress threshold (PLST) model suggests that, with disease progression, people with dementia experience increasing vulnerability to stress and external stimuli because of the environmental demand. According to the PLST model, minimizing environmental demands that exceed functional capacity, and regulating activity and stimulation levels throughout the day can reduce agitation. According to the competence-environmental press (CEP) model, the highest individual functioning results from optimal combinations of environmental conditions and personal competencies. The CEP model suggests that the right balance between individual ability and external environmental demands results in adaptive behaviors, while excessive or reduced environmental activities may result in BPSD. Both models suggest that BPSD can be reduced or managed by modifying environmental factors that place too much demand or pressure on the patient.

A different approach is provided by the need-driven, dementia-compromised behavior (NDB) that conceptualized BPSD as the result of the combination between the inability of the caregiver to understand patient's needs and the inability of the patient to express them. Therefore, BPSD may represent patient's attempts to express physical or emotional distress due to unmet needs. According to this model, NDB are induced by both background (i.e., cognitive, neurological, health, and psychosocial variables) and proximal factors (i.e., environmental and situational issues such as pain, fatigue, and noise); while background factors are quite stable, proximal ones are modifiable and represent the target for the interventions (101, 102).

The number of reports and reviews on the efficacy of NPT of BPSD has increased in recent years. Most studies have been performed in nursing homes on patients with advanced dementia. The interventions range from sensorial to psychological and behavioral approaches, and include environmental redesign, validation therapy, reminiscence therapy, light therapy, aromatherapy, massage and other sensory-based strategies, acupuncture, music therapy, pleasant events and activity engagement, behavioral management techniques, caregiver training (70, 99, 103–107). Potential benefits of these interventions have been documented, but the strength of evidence is overall low and the great heterogeneity in terms of type of intervention, follow-up duration, type of outcome measures hamper comparison across studies. In particular, there are no conclusive results for validation and reminiscence therapy, the effectiveness of light therapy is not clear, aromatherapy is better than no treatment. The small body of evidence for other sensory interventions, such as massage and touch therapy, suggests they could be viable treatment options, especially given the ease of implementation and minimal training involved. No effect has been documented for acupuncture and transcutaneous electrical nerve stimulation. Music therapy and behavioral management techniques seem to cause a short-term reduction of BPSD, but long-term efficacy is unclear.

In general, no conclusions can be drawn on the safety of these NPT, because this feature is largely unexplored (103). Some reports indicate the NPT to BPSD to be potentially cost-effective (70, 99, 106), but further research is needed on this point.

Factors that may predict a better response to these interventions include a higher level of cognitive functioning, fewer difficulties in ADL and communication, and relative preservation of speech, while staff barriers and pain are associated to worse outcome (108).

Independently from the results, all studies underline the relevance of a tailored individualized intervention and a careful and close monitoring of the outcomes to ameliorate and modulate the treatment (109, 110). Since pain and discomfort may cause difficulties in communication and self-management, and contribute to BPSD, these factors should be carefully searched and treated (111, 112).

In our opinion, the type of setting of interventions is an important point, as it may influence aims of the treatment and outcomes. The majority of studies on BPSD have been performed in nursing homes, where different health professionals (i.e., physicians, psychologists, nurses) are involved, and they may interact to offer a better outcome (111). In contrast, as caregiver is often the only figure that manage patients' BPSD at home, future studies should address the role of NPT for BPSD in non-institutionalized people with dementia (106).

OCCUPATIONAL THERAPY

Disease progression reduces the ability to participate in occupations—mainly ADL, IADL, leisure and social activities—in patients with dementia, leading to a negative impact on QoL and well-being of patients and caregivers (113–117). Therefore, improving and preserving ADLs is one of the most important patient-related outcome in dementia (118).

To increase functional abilities and enhance independence, occupational therapy (OT) uses a combined approach including activity simplification, environmental modification, adaptive aids, problem-solving strategies, skill training, and caregiver education (119, 120), according to the bio-psycho-social model of health proposed by the ICF (116). An RCT on patients with mild-to-moderate dementia living in the community showed that a multimodal OT approach, including cognitive and behavioral interventions to train patients to compensate for cognitive impairment and caregivers to cope with patients' abnormal behavior, was effective in improving ADL and in reducing caregiver's burden with effects lasting for up to 12 weeks (121). A review including seven RCTs showed that OT interventions may maintain physical function and ADL in community-dwelling persons with dementia (105, 122).

OT seems also effective in reducing BPSD, increasing patient's participation, improving physical performance, and QoL and reducing negative communication (123–129). These positive results have been confirmed in a recent review that showed OT interventions based on sensory stimulation, environmental modification and functionally oriented tasks, to be effective in improving BPSD and depression in dementia (130). Among environment-based interventions, ambient music, aromatherapy, and Snoezelen (i.e., a soothing and stimulating multisensory environment) were modestly effective in reducing agitation, but they did not have long-term effects, while the evidence to support bright light therapy for mood and sleep disorders was only preliminary (131).

An evidence-based review suggested that patient-centered leisure activities that involve social interaction may enhance caregiver satisfaction with visits for residential patients, while interventions focused on ADL and IADL may ameliorate patients' well-being and QoL. Social participation interventions, mainly involving people in the early or middle stage of the disease when verbal competence is still fairly spared, were shown to have at least short-term positive effect on patient's well-being (132).

Gitlin and collaborators proposed a 4-month structured home occupational therapy intervention, the Tailored Activity Program (TAP), that provided persons with dementia with activities tailored to their abilities, while caregivers were trained to effectively use these activities in daily life and to generalize them to different settings (133). Besides being effective in reducing caregiver burden, in that caregiver had significantly more free time, TAP was demonstrated to be highly cost-effective (123).

Some general considerations have been issued on OT: (a) programs should be tailored to elicit the patient's highest level of retained skill and interest; (b) cues for assisting people with AD to complete tasks should be short and provide clear direction; (c) compensatory strategies in the form of environmental modifications and simple adaptive equipment should be specifically tailored to the specific needs of single patients; (d) caregiver training and involvement are essential in implementing individualized programs (134).

OT is recommended by several guidelines for dementia management (135–137). The recently published clinical practice guidelines and principles of care for people with dementia in Australia reported important evidence-based recommendations for occupational therapists, based on the most updated high-quality evidence (138). However, well designed RCTs are lacking on this topic and often the studies use different approach, lacking specificity. Therefore, more research is needed to identify specific OT components and the optimal dosage of the intervention and to evaluate the long-term effects and the contraindications of OT in patients with dementia.

Subtle functional changes in highly cognitively demanding activities have been reported in individuals in the early stage of the disease, suggesting that, similarly to cognition, function declines along a continuum from healthy aging to dementia (139–141). Incorporating more challenging and high-level activities into the assessment of patients with early dementia may increase the sensitivity of functional measures, thus enabling early detection of impairment and expanding the window for timely OT interventions (142). These points may represent directions for future research on this topic.

PSYCHOLOGICAL THERAPY

In recent years, the growing awareness of the deep emotional impact of the diagnosis of dementia and of the need of a holistic and individualized approach to the disease, has led to a rising interest on the psychological care for persons with dementia (143).

Actually, experiencing depression and anxiety is very common in people with dementia, even if there is a lack of consensus on their prevalence rates as diagnostic criteria may vary among studies (144–147). All studies agree that depression and anxiety may have significant functional impact. Consistent evidence suggests that, in people with dementia, the severity of depression increases the severity of neurological impairment, institutionalization (148, 149), and caregiver burden (150), while anxiety is associated with decreased independence and increased risk of nursing home placement (151).

Although different from each other, depression often co-occurs with apathy. Apathy, which is defined as a loss or diminution of goal-directed behavior, cognition or emotion (152) is one the of the most common neuropsychiatric symptom in AD, with a prevalence ranging from 19 to 88% (153). Even if symptoms like social withdrawal or reduced initiation and motivation may occur both in apathy and depression, true apathy is usually not associated with depressive symptoms, such as sadness, guilt, or hopelessness (154). The presence of apathy seems to be related to greater caregiver burden, faster functional impairment, reduced QoL and increased morbidity, being a reliable longitudinal predictor of death in people with dementia (155–157).

Many recommendations underscored that the treatment of anxiety and depressive symptoms should be an essential part of the management of AD and other dementias (93, 152, 153) and suggested that psychological interventions could be effective for these patients (158). However, empirical evidence supporting the efficacy of psychological interventions is rather sparse (159), mainly because a broad group of interventions that are termed as psychological ones have been included in reviews (160, 161), but actually are not based on well-defined theory-driven psychological interventions.

According to the World Health Organization, cognitive behavioral therapy, psychodynamic therapy, interpersonal therapy, and supportive counseling (i.e., Rogersian person-centered therapy) are the main psychotherapeutic approaches with evidence of effectiveness in treating depression and anxiety in adults (162). Studies that have adopted one of these approaches have been included in a recent systematic review on psychological interventions for anxiety and depression in dementia or MCI (six RCTs, psychological treatment: $n = 216$ patients, usual care or placebo intervention: $n = 223$) (163). The Authors concluded that there is evidence that psychological interventions added to usual care can reduce symptoms of depression and clinician-rated anxiety in dementia and that psychological interventions have the potential to improve patient's well-being, while no effect was found on ADL, self- and caregiver-rated patient's QoL, BPSD, cognition, or caregivers' self-reported depressive symptoms (163).

A recent systematic review concluded that the strongest evidence supported the use of short-term group therapy soon after dementia diagnosis to reduce levels of depression and enhance QoL, while tailored and multi-component interventions seemed to reduce inappropriate behaviors in patients living in nursing homes with mild-to-moderate levels of impairment (164).

Systematic reviews indicated a variety of NPTs (e.g., one-to-one activities, activity programs tailored on patients' preferences, individualized cognitive rehabilitation, music therapy, art therapy) as potentially effective and safe in reducing apathy, although none of them is strictly a psychological intervention (165, 166).

Overall, the proposed psychological approaches were methodologically heterogeneous, some of them lacked specificity and conceptual clarity and often the description of the interventions was quite generic. Moreover, most studies included patients in the first stage of dementia, because cognitive decline prevents the understanding and feasibility of psychological therapy in advanced stages.

In conclusion, the current evidence for psychological support and psychotherapy in AD and dementia is limited and not conclusive. Therefore, further studies are needed to demonstrate which psychological interventions may lead to better outcome and to identify common factors across different approaches that may be effective in enhancing well-being of persons with dementia.

MULTICOMPONENT AND MULTIDIMENSIONAL STRATEGIES

The proposal of multidimensional protocols of treatment is based on the hypothesis that combining different approaches may be the most suitable intervention to improve different outcomes in AD. An Italian group developed the Multidimensional

Stimulation Therapy (MST), a multidimensional approach that combined cognitive stimulation, recreational activities, OT and physical exercises, and demonstrated that MST was more effective than a cognitive-specific intervention in improving both behavioral and functional outcomes in AD patients (167, 168). A recent fMRI study suggested restoration of neural functioning as the mechanism underlying the positive effects of MST (169).

Similarly, the Meeting Centers Support Program (MCSP), a supportive person-centered approach for mild-to-moderate dementia patients living in the community and their caregivers was implemented in the Netherlands. MCSP is based on the combination of recreational activities and psychomotor therapy for patients, psico-educational and support groups for caregivers, social activities for both, and regular center meetings (170). MCSP yielded promising results in terms of user satisfaction, reduction of patients' behavioral and emotional disturbances, decrease of caregivers' burden and delayed institutionalization (170–173). A study exploring the dissemination and implementation of MCSP to different European countries is currently ongoing (174).

Actually, some systematic reviews demonstrated that multicomponent interventions were more effective than single activities in improving general well-being of both persons with dementia and their caregivers (70, 175), and in hospitalized older adults with cognitive impairment (176, 177).

As dementia represents a complex disease with cognitive, psychological, functional and behavioral symptoms, the adoption of multicomponent approaches may represent a winning strategy, in agreement with the biopsychosocial model of care, upon which any rehabilitative intervention is founded. The encouraging results obtained so far suggest further studies in this area of research.

COMPLEMENTARY AND ALTERNATIVE MEDICINE

Complementary and alternative medicine (CAM) has become more commonly used over the last decade and has been applied to a wide range of health problems, including dementia. We will report evidence on the main CAM types, i.e., aromatherapy, music therapy, art therapy, massage, and touch. These NPTs are part of the main category of sensorial stimulation techniques, i.e., interventions aimed to promote the arousal of the patients' senses (178).

AROMATHERAPY

Among CAM, aromatherapy is probably the most familiar to consumers. Aromatherapy is part of phytotherapy and is based on the use of pure essential oils from fragrant plants to relieve health problems and improve QoL. The potential effects of essential oils are varied, including promotion of relaxation and sleep, relief of pain (179), reduction of depressive symptoms. Aromatherapy might be a useful intervention for people with cognitive disturbances, who are confused, or for whom verbal interaction is difficult and current conventional medicine provides only partial benefit (180). Indeed, aromatherapy has been used to address BPSD (181–186) and sleep disturbances (187–189) and to stimulate motivational behavior (190). A meta-analysis identified only seven RCTs and concluded that the benefits of aromatherapy for people with dementia are equivocal, mainly because of severe methodological problems (191). Therefore, the effects of aromatherapy in this condition should be better explored in high-quality RCTs.

MUSIC THERAPY

Music therapy (MT) can be defined as an NPT that uses music or sound as a non-verbal communication tool to induce educational, rehabilitative or therapeutic effects in several disease, including dementia. Music-based interventions can be conducted in single patients or in group, and they most consist of singing, listening, improvising or playing along on musical instruments (192). We can therefore classify MT in active and passive interventions. Since most studies on MT included both active and passive techniques, which type of intervention can be more effective in dementia is still unclear (193).

There is substantive literature reporting the importance and benefits of music and music therapy programs for older adults, and more specifically for those with dementia (194–199). Neurophysiologic and psychological data provide the theoretical basis for the use of music therapy. Studies showed that sound can exert a significant action on the brain (200–204) by activating a large number of cortical and subcortical areas, and, particularly, the limbic and paralimbic areas devoted to emotional processing (205). From a psychological point of view, music facilitates communicative and relational processes and emotional expression (206). Moreover, since music can stimulate both motor and cognitive functions, it can be an efficient tool for rehabilitation (207). A growing amount of evidence shows that patients with dementia can enjoy music, and their ability to respond to music is potentially preserved, even in the late to severe stages of disease when verbal communication may have ceased. Several studies reported the efficacy of music to treat BPSD (208–213), to enhance communications, relational processes and participation (199, 214–216), and to maintain or increase cognitive functions (217–222). However, reviews on this topic pointed out the methodological limitations and the scarce quality of previous studies and questioned the specificity of the effect of music that was found to be no more beneficial than other pleasant activities (223, 224).

A recent meta-analysis concluded that a music-based therapeutic intervention probably reduces depressive symptoms but has little or no effect on agitation or aggression, emotional well-being or QoL, overall behavioral problems and cognition in dementia, while effects on anxiety or social behavior, and long-term effects are unclear (192).

A recent RCT found that music therapy added to pharmacotherapy yielded no further benefits for language and verbal communication in comparison to pharmacotherapy alone, but this integrated approach could improve the psycho-behavioral profile (225).

In conclusion, the question whether music may have specific effects in patients with dementia is still open. Future studies should employ larger sample sizes, include all important outcomes, in particular positive ones, such as emotional and social well-being, and examine the duration of the effect in relation to the overall duration of the treatment and the number of sessions (192, 226).

ART THERAPY

The British Association of Art Therapists defines art therapy as "a form of psychotherapy that uses art media as its primary mode of communication" and underscored that (a) clients who are referred to an art therapist need not have experience or skill in art; (b) the art therapist is not primarily concerned with making an aesthetic or diagnostic assessment of the client's image; (c) the overall aim of its practitioners is to enable a client to change and grow on a personal level through the use of art materials in a safe and facilitating environment" (227).

Whether art therapy can be useful and may represent an effective rehabilitative strategy for people suffering from dementia is a debated issue (110, 228). It has been suggested that patients with dementia can produce and appreciate visual art and that aesthetic preference can remain stable, despite cognitive decline (229).

Case reports, observational studies, small trials and anecdotal evidence suggest that art therapy can engage attention, provide pleasure, and improve BPSD, social behavior, and self-esteem, contributing to the individual sense of well-being in dementia, and that these effects may be long-lasting (230–243). However, few high-quality studies have been performed so far on this topic, and there is too little empirical evidence to prove the effectiveness of this type of CAM. Therefore, RCTs with adequate methods and appropriate outcomes are needed to support the efficacy and define optimal conditions for the use of art therapy in dementia.

MASSAGE AND TOUCH

Massage and touch have been suggested as a CAM or supplement to other treatments to reduce a range of conditions associated with dementia. Evidence suggests that massage and touch may relax older people with dementia, reduce some BPSD, such as pacing, wandering and resisting care, improve appetite, sleep and communication problems, and, to some extent, counteract cognitive decline (244–250).

Massage seems to produce different physiological effects such as a decrease in pulse and respiration and an increase in body temperature (251). Physiological models suggest that the effects of massage may be mediated by the production of oxytocin that can reduce discomfort, agitation, blood pressure and heart rate, and improve mood. On the other hand, psychological models suggest that massage can help people with dementia to retain a sense of meaningful and reassuring communication even when words fail and may help to activate memories (252).

A recent meta-analysis of 11 RCTs showed that massage and touch interventions may have significant effect on physical non-aggressive, verbal aggressive and non-aggressive behavior, but the relatively small sample size and the low quality of the included studies do not allow to draw a firm conclusion on the effect on BPSD or any useful suggestion for clinical practice (253).

As for other CAM types, RCTs of better methodological quality are needed to provide evidence supporting the benefit of massage and touch in dementia.

NEW TECHNOLOGIES

The availability of new technologies, their diffusion and, for some of them, the relatively cheap price, resulted in a progressively larger number of studies exploring their role in dementia. We will briefly summarize evidence on the application of information and communication technologies (ICT), assistive devices, domotics, virtual reality, gaming and telemedicine to monitor, and treat people with dementia.

ICT, ASSISTIVE DEVICES AND DOMOTICS

Recent technological advances in ICT, including computational devices, robotics, machine learning algorithms, miniaturization of sensors and technologies, as well as the reduced costs of these devices increased the availability of intelligent devices and technology-embedded environments to support the daily life of persons with dementia and their caregivers, and to assess disease severity and progression (254–256). Nowadays, devices and sensors can be integrated into the patient's environment as part of a "smart" or automated home, or in the patient's clothes to offer healthcare professionals a much clearer view of the patient's condition and activity than that available from short periods of monitoring in a clinical setting (257). In particular, ICT allows continuous monitoring of patient's performance and actions in real time and real-life situations (258–260).

Moving freely outdoors is considered an important ADL outcome associated with the ability to maintain independence and participation. The development of technologies, which allow people with dementia to stay outdoors in a safe and secure way, is considered a priority research area. Therefore, tracking technologies that record the position of the patient based on global positioning system (GPS), and can localize him/her if lost is the most developed area of ICT research in dementia (261–265). Tracking technology devices can promote perceived safety and security among caregivers and relatives of people with dementia (266), in that they can locate the patient at any moment and represent a precious support in everyday life (263, 267). Many studies in this area focused on the perspective of relatives and/or healthcare staff, but only a limited number of them explored the experience of people when wearing a GPS tracking technology (259, 262, 268, 269).

Another application of ICT is represented by devices that can be used for surveillance and management of high-risk behaviors and may replace more severe forms of physical restraints (270–272). Acoustic sensors placed in the living room or bedroom can record noise, or patient's movement. Cameras or GPS devices can also be used to allow caregivers or staff to take actions when the patient is in a potentially dangerous condition, without restricting freedom of movement. Furthermore, patients can wear a chip in their clothes to give them access to certain parts of the building, while preventing them to move to other forbidden or dangerous areas (266).

However, the application of surveillance technologies to the care of people with dementia led to considerable ethical debate. Indeed, opponents of this approach claim that the continuous monitoring may represent a breach of patient's privacy and freedom and argue that tracking devices may diminish human contact between patients and the environment (273). A systematic review on the ethical and practical concerns of surveillance technologies in residential care for people with dementia concluded that there is no consensus and underlined the need for clearer policies on this topic (274). A recent descriptive review showed that a significant portion of current intelligent assistive technology is designed in the absence of explicit ethical considerations, and this may represent a structural limitation in the translation from designing labs to bedside (275). The Authors called for a coordinated effort to proactively incorporate ethical considerations early in the design and development of new ICT products (275).

ICT has also been applied to monitoring and prevention of falls in dementia. Body-worn gyroscopes measuring angular velocity, sensors to measure the acceleration of the trunk, and inertial sensors may detect when a fall occurs, along with the causes of the fall (276–279). Among non-wearable systems cameras, motion sensors, microphones and floor sensors have been applied to this aim (280, 281). Information obtained by accelerometers contained in a wristband may result in vibratory and visual feedback to increase the patient's awareness of their risk of falling (282). Similarly, a shoe insole that delivers vibration may prevent falls and improve gait and balance. Research projects are currently exploring how exoskeletons can correct and assist postural balance and improve overall function. Technology will hopefully provide many more options for assessment, prevention, and intervention in this area of health care (283).

Video and audio analysis techniques, computerized testing and actigraphy, besides being useful to promote patients' safety, may represent promising tools to improve functional and cognitive assessment of patients with AD (256). For instance, automatic speech analysis techniques through computerized speech recognition interfaces could represent a non-invasive and cheap method to collect information on verbal communication impairment in patients with cognitive disorders (284). Video processing technologies can be adopted to obtain pragmatic, ecological, and objective measures to improve assessment of ADL, and to provide additional information that cannot be gathered in a clinical setting (285).

ICT can be used for the assessment of agitation, one of the most challenging symptoms to manage for caregivers (286, 287). A core feature of agitation is excessive motor activity, and accelerometers can objectively measure abnormal motor activity, speech analyses may assess verbal aggression, and automated video analysis and activity recognition techniques can detect activities and movement sequences that underline physical aggression (288). Sensors measuring electrodermal activity could early detect agitation in persons with dementia. These devices could theoretically support nursing staff in recognizing early warning signs of BPSD, but further studies in a clinical setting are needed to confirm this hypothesis (289).

Overall, this is a challenging domain for clinicians, who should define the clinically relevant markers, and for ICT engineers, who should adapt the technical constraints to the clinical requirements.

Assistive technologies can support and facilitate disabled people in ADL (290). For instance, external cueing systems can assist people with cognitive disabilities by reminding them to perform a task at the appropriate time (e.g., take their pills), or by providing guidance through a task (291–293), and sensors recording a patient's position in space may help in navigation through environment (294). Moreover, assistive technologies may help to support decision-making in vocational and personal health domains (295), to read (296), or use the telephone (297).

Domotics is another important field of research, because nearly three quarters of older adults with dementia are cared for in their own homes (298), and there is a strong correlation between home environment and disability-related outcomes (299). Dementia-specific adapted home environment and related assistive devices may be helpful for both the patient and the caregiver (300–302). Changes to home environment may result in lack of familiarity for the patient, and earlier home modifications might enable individuals with dementia to adjust to their adapted environment (303).

Future smart homes will incorporate intelligent interfaces embedded in everyday objects, such as furniture, clothes, vehicles, and smart materials to observe the residents and provide proactive services (304). One of the key-supporting features of a smart home is the ability to monitor the ADL and safety of people, and to detect changes in their daily routines. With the availability of inexpensive low-power sensors, radios, and embedded processors, smart homes may be equipped with large amounts of networked sensors, which collaboratively process and make deductions from the acquired data on the state of the home, and the activity and behavior of its residents (305–310). Therefore, the smart home technology seems to be a promising and cost-effective way of improving home care for people with dementia in a non-obtrusive way, allowing greater independence, maintaining good health, preventing social isolation, and relieving the workload from family caregivers and health providers (311).

The data on domotics are encouraging but some factors, e.g., the accessibility and affordability of these devices and the limited caregiver's awareness of their availability and utility, may prevent a more widespread use of these technologies (312).

In conclusion, ICT applications are rapidly expanding to support assistive and clinical tasks in people with dementia, but structural limitations to successful adoption include partial lack of clinical validation and insufficient focus on patient's needs. Clinicians and stakeholders involved in the implementation and management of dementia care across ICT applications should collaborate to facilitate the translation of medical engineering research into clinical practice (313).

VIRTUAL REALITY AND GAMING

Virtual reality (VR) allows a user to navigate through, and interact with, a virtual environment that is a 3D digital space generated by computing technology and consisting of objects or entities seemingly "real" because they share at least one attribute of the real thing, without sharing all of its physical characteristics (e.g., volume, weight, surface friction) (314). The potential applications of VR systems to assess and train AD patients has been reported by several studies (315–320). Cognitively impaired patients can be exposed to computer-generated virtual environments, where they can safely perform quasi-naturalistic real-life activities and tasks to assess and/or treat cognitive and motor deficits under a range of conditions that are not easily controllable and quantifiable in the real world (321). The most specific domains for VR diagnostic and training purposes in AD patients include attention (322), executive functions (323–326), memory (327–333), orientation (322, 327, 334–336), and ADL (337, 338). Research is currently focusing on the design of VR based tests aimed to be more ecological and sensitive compared to common pen-and-paper tests. A recent study proposed a novel AD screening tests based on virtual environment and game principles to evaluate memory loss for common objects and recent events, and language changes (339).

The advantages of VR in comparison to traditional assessment and training tools are represented by the naturalistic situations, the safety from potential dangers that could occur in real-life situations and the enhancement of motivation because of its gaming, interactive, and immersive quality. For these reasons, computer-driven simulations of real-life environments can bridge the gap between traditional test outcomes and compensatory strategies that are transferable to daily life.

Since most of the evidence on the role of VR come from single case reports or to restricted samples, the debate on its role in patients with dementia is still open.

In this scenario, serious games (SG), i.e., interactive virtual simulations to represent real situations, otherwise hardly reproducible, allow the player to act in a real-life-like environment, or a fictitious scenario that serves as a gym for deliberately decontextualized learning. SG are widely recognized as promising non-pharmacological tools to assess patient's cognition and function (340, 341), and to treat, stimulate, and improve patient's well-being (342). Boosted by the publication of a Nature letter showing that video game training can enhance cognitive control in older adults (343), SG specifically adapted to people with AD have been developed and employed to train physical and cognitive abilities, showing preliminary but encouraging results (341, 344–348).

A recent literature review concluded that game-based interventions can positively affect both physical health by improving balance, gait and voluntary motor control and cognitive function by enhancing attention, memory, and visuo-spatial abilities in older adults and in patients with dementia (349). Both physical and cognitive games seem to have a positive impact on social and emotional function, improving mood and increasing positive affect and sociability (350).

Since the use of SG in neurodegenerative disorders is expanding, recent studies have provided recommendations in terms of ergonomic choices for their design, and to create customize SG specific to the target users (351). Considering that the actual recommendations are gathered from a relatively small group of experts working in the domain of SG for health, further work is needed to verify if they hold true for a wider expert population, and their applicability to patients.

On the basis of these preliminary data, clear evidence on the effectiveness of VR and SG for the assessment and training of people with AD requires further research that should adopt methodologies based upon best practices from clinical trials and incorporate behavioral and neurophysiological data.

TELEMEDICINE

Technology provides new opportunities for interventions to improve quality and access to health care. Since dementia is a chronic disease, with issues related to continuous long-term care and limited accessibility to medical service, telemedicine could be a valuable mean to provide assessment and care to dementia patients at home (352). Indeed, telemedicine can provide follow-up care to help people with dementia to maintain their independence and continue living in their own homes, improve their safety, (353, 354), ameliorate clinical outcomes, and reduce access to health services (355, 356). Moreover, likely because of the reduction of the discomfort due to travel, telemedicine was found to be an independent predictor for increased treatment duration (357). Telemedicine appears to be very promising and effective in the context of dementia assessment, especially in countries, such as the USA, where there are several rural retirement communities that are still medically underserved. A recent study conducted in a Southern California community showed not only that telemedicine was able to improve access and quality of dementia care, but also that most of the patients preferred the telemedicine consult compared to the traditional one (358).

Several studies confirmed the feasibility to perform cognitive assessment via telemedicine in elderly subjects with dementia and showed a good agreement with conventional face-to-face testing, and a high level of user satisfaction (359–362). However, since data are still preliminary, there is no consensus on the best practices for conducting neuropsychological assessment by telemedicine (362).

Besides the diagnostic evaluation and follow-up monitoring, telemedicine interventions for dementia include internet-based information and support groups, robotic companions, the use of smartphones to report symptoms (258, 363, 364), and cognitive rehabilitation training (365).

Telemedicine has been applied to support caregivers of people with dementia through in-home video monitoring and

TABLE 1 | Summary of the level of evidence, main positive outcomes, and limitations of the non-pharmacological treatment for Alzheimer's disease and dementia.

Treatment	Subtype	Evidence	Main positive outcomes	Limitations
Exercise and motor rehabilitation		Moderate	• Reduction of BPSD • Improvement of ADL	• Limited evidence for cognition, QoL, depression, mortality, caregiver burden • Few comparative studies exploring the most effective exercise intervention • Unclear duration and intensity of activity
Cognitive intervention	CS	Moderate	• Improvement of general cognitive function • Small effect on mood and QoL of patients and caregivers	• Unclear long-term effect on cognition • Heterogeneity of the outcomes
	CT	Small	• Enhancement of performance in trained and similar tasks	• No generalization effect to daily function • Low quality studies
	CS+CT	Small	• Improvement of general cognitive function	• Heterogeneity of treatment • Heterogeneity of dementia severity • Few high quality RCTs
	CST	Moderate	• Improvements of general cognitive function and specific cognitive domains • Small effect on QoL • Improvement of caregiving relationship • Small effect on depressive symptoms and QoL of caregivers	• Not all services offer this treatment • Unclear effect on BPSD and ADL
Occupational therapy		Small	• Improvement of ADL, social participation, QoL • Reduction of BPSD and depression • Reduction of caregiver burden	• Unclear optimal duration • Unclear long-term effect • Mixed approaches • Few high quality RCTs
Psychological therapy		Small	• Reduction of depression, anxiety, and apathy • Enhancement of patient's well-being	• No comparative studies between different psychological treatments • No long-term studies • Few high quality RCTs
Multicomponent/ multidimensional strategies		Small	• Reduction of BPSD • Improvement of some cognitive domains • Delayed institutionalization • Reduction of caregiver burden	• Persistence of effect • Generalization to everyday life • Limited implementation and dissemination • Few high quality RCTs
Aromatherapy		Very small	• Reduction of BPSD and sleep disturbances • Improvements in motivational behavior	• Severe methodological issues • Few high quality RCTs
Music therapy		Small	• Reduction of depression • Improvement in communication, social participation, relations and cognition	• Unclear long-term effect • Small sample size • Low-quality studies
Art therapy		Very small	• Reduction of BPSD • Improvement of attention • Improvement of social behavior and self-esteem	• Unclear long-term effect • No RCTs
Massage and touch		Very small	• Reduction of BPSD • Improvement of mood, sleep, appetite	• Small sample size • Low-quality studies

ADL, activities of daily living; BPSD, behavioral and psychological symptoms of dementia; CS, cognitive stimulation; CST, Cognitive Stimulation Therapy; QoL, quality of life; RCT, randomized controlled trial; CT, cognitive stimulation.

recording and feedback to help managing difficult situations (366). Telephone-based support groups is a promising way to provide support for caregivers, but research is only at the beginning (367). A systematic review on technology-driven telemedicine interventions, such as online training and support programs, for caregivers of persons with dementia concluded that included studies yielded positive findings in terms of mental health outcomes, but their marked heterogeneity impeded robust conclusions (368).

Overall, establishing systems for the care of dementia patients and their caregivers using telemedicine technologies seems to be feasible, but the evidence on clinical benefits is still scarce, cost-effectiveness data are lacking, and there is very little evidence of widespread practical applications (369).

LIMITATIONS OF THE STUDY

The main limitation of the present review is its narrative design, but a systematic one would have not been feasible because of the larger number of studies on NPT in AD and dementia. Another limitation is the use of two search engines, only (i.e., PubMed and the Cochrane database of systematic reviews). Searching in other databases (e.g., Embase, PsycINFO, Web of Science) would have yielded more pieces of literature, but it has been suggested that MEDLINE, which is completely covered by PubMed, may produce a sufficiently extensive coverage (370). A study comparing 15 databases for RCTs on CAM showed low overlap between databases and indicated that comprehensive CAM literature searches will require multiple databases (371) but this appear a minor problem in the present review because of the overall low quality of studies on CAM interventions.

CONCLUSIONS

Appropriate management of patients with AD and dementia is a significant public health concern, given the limited effectiveness of pharmacological therapies combined with their potentially life-threatening side effects. The development of effective NPT for these conditions is of paramount importance, and a large number of interventions has been proposed.

The interventions reviewed in this paper show different level of evidence of efficacy on different outcomes that are summarized in **Table 1**. Some of them share methodological problems that are common to all non-pharmacological studies, which are typically practice-oriented. They include small number of high-quality studies or double-blind RCTs, small sample sizes, heterogeneity in terms of study design, type of intervention and outcomes, uncertainty about the clinical significance of outcomes. The landscape of clinical trials has changed since the introduction of randomization 80 years ago, and new challenges in their design, conduction, and interpretation have emerged. Evidence-grading systems are biased toward RCTs, and they may lead to understatement of findings from non-RCT studies (372).The direct transposition of the traditional methods of drug RCTs to the rehabilitation and NPT scenarios raises some issues, and innovative trial designs would be helpful in these settings. Moreover, cost-effectiveness studies are needed to better address the role of NPT for dementia.

AUTHOR CONTRIBUTIONS

CZ, ES, and MB conceived and designed the study. All authors collected, analyzed, and interpreted the data. CZ, ES, AF, EM, SB, and MB drafted the manuscript. ST and RC revised critically the manuscript for important intellectual content. All authors approved the final version of the manuscript.

REFERENCES

1. World Alzheimer Report 2015. *The Global Impact of Dementia. An Analysis of Prevalence, Incidence, Cost and Trends*. Alzheimer Disease International, 2015.
2. Sosa-Ortiz AL, Acosta-Castillo I, Prince MJ. Epidemiology of dementias and Alzheimer's disease. *Arch Med Res.* (2012) 43:600–8. doi: 10.1016/j.arcmed.2012.11.003
3. Brodaty H, Breteler MM, Dekosky ST, Dorenlot P, Fratiglioni L, Hock C, et al. The world of dementia beyond 2020. *J Am Geriatr Soc.* (2011) 59:923–927. doi: 10.1111/j.1532-5415.2011.03365.x
4. Catindig JA, Venketasubramanian N, Ikram MK, Chen C. Epidemiology of dementia in Asia: insights on prevalence, trends and novel risk factors. *J Neurol Sci.* (2012) 321:11–6. doi: 10.1016/j.jns.2012.07.023
5. Birks J. Cholinesterase inhibitors for Alzheimer's disease. *Cochrane Database Syst Rev.* (2006) 1:CD005593. doi: 10.1002/14651858.CD005593
6. Birks JS, Grimley Evans J. Rivastigmine for Alzheimer's disease. *Cochrane Database Syst Rev.* (2015) 4:CD001191. doi: 10.1002/14651858.CD001191.pub3
7. Wong CW. Pharmacotherapy for dementia: a practical approach to the use of cholinesterase inhibitors and memantine. *Drugs Aging* (2016) 33:451–60. doi: 10.1007/s40266-016-0372-3
8. Scheltens P, Blennow K, Breteler MM, de Strooper B, Frisoni GB, Salloway S, et al. Alzheimer's disease. *Lancet* (2016) 388:505–17. doi: 10.1016/S0140-6736(15)01124-1
9. World Health Organization. *International Classification of Functioning, Disability and Health (ICF)*. Geneva: WHO (2001).
10. Poulos CJ, Bayer A, Beaupre L, Clare L, Poulos RG, Wang RH, et al. A comprehensive approach to reablement in dementia. *Alzheimers Dement.* (2017) 3:450–8. doi: 10.1016/j.trci.2017.06.005
11. McDermott O, Charlesworth G, Hogervorst E, Stoner C, Moniz-Cook E, Spector A, et al. Psychosocial interventions for people with dementia: a synthesis of systematic reviews. *Aging Ment Health* (2018) 17:1–11. doi: 10.1080/13607863.2017.1423031
12. Albert MS, DeKosky ST, Dickson D, Dubois B, Feldman HH, Fox NC, et al. The diagnosis of mild cognitive impairment due to Alzheimer's disease: recommendations from the National Institute on Aging-Alzheimer's Association workgroups on diagnostic guidelines for Alzheimer's disease. *Alzheimer Dement.* (2011) 7:270–9. doi: 10.1016/j.jalz.2011.03.008
13. NIH. Physical activity and cardiovascular health. NIH consensus development panel on physical activity and cardiovascular health. *JAMA* (1996) 276:241–6. doi: 10.1001/jama.1996.03540030075036
14. Thompson PD, Buchner D, Pina IL, Balady GJ, Williams MA, Marcus BH, et al. Exercise and physical activity in the prevention and treatment of atherosclerotic cardiovascular disease: a statement from the council on clinical cardiology (Subcommittee on exercise, rehabilitation, and prevention) and the council on nutrition, physical activity, and metabolism (subcommittee on physical activity). *Circulation* (2003) 107:3109–16. doi: 10.1161/01.CIR.0000075572.40158.77
15. World Health Organization. *Chronic Disease Information Sheets: Physical Activity*. Geneva: WHO (2006).
16. Lautenschlager NT, Cox K, Kurz AF. Physical activity and mild cognitive impairment and Alzheimer's disease. *Curr Neurol Neurosci Rep.* (2010) 10:352–8. doi: 10.1007/s11910-010-0121-7
17. Yaffe K, Barnes D, Nevitt M, Lui LY, Covinsky K. A prospective study of physical activity and cognitive decline in elderly women: women who walk. *Arch Intern Med.* (2001) 161:1703–8. doi: 10.1001/archinte.161.14.1703
18. Podewils LJ, Guallar E, Kuller LH, Fried LP, Lopez OL, Carlson M., et al. Physical activity, APOE genotype, and dementia risk: findings from the cardiovascular health cognition study. *Am J Epidemiol.* (2005) 161:639–51. doi: 10.1093/aje/kwi092
19. Barnes DE, Blackwell T, Stone KL, Goldman SE, Hillier T, Yaffe K, et al. Cognition in older women: the importance of daytime movement. *J Am Geriatr Soc.* (2008) 56:1658–64. doi: 10.1111/j.1532-5415.2008.01841.x
20. Middleton LE, Mitnitski A, Fallah N, Kirkland SA, Rockwood K. Changes in cognition and mortality in relation to exercise in late life: a population based study. *PLoS ONE* (2008) 3:e3124. doi: 10.1371/journal.pone.0003124
21. Brown BM, Pfeiffer JJ, Martins RN. Multiple effects of physical activity on molecular and cognitive signs of brain aging: can exercise slow neurodegeneration and delay Alzheimer's disease? *Mol Psychiatry* (2013) 18:864–74. doi: 10.1038/mp.2012.162
22. Hamer M, Muniz Terrera G, Demakakos P. Physical activity and trajectories in cognitive function: English longitudinal study of ageing. *J Epidemiol Community Health* (2018) 72:477–83. doi: 10.1136/jech-2017-210228
23. Loprinzi PD, Frith E, Edwards MK, Sng E, Ashpole N. The effects of exercise on memory function among young to middle-aged adults: systematic review and recommendations for future research. *Am J Health Promot.* (2018) 32:691–704. doi: 10.1177/0890117117737409
24. Song D, Yu DSF, Li PWC, Lei Y. The effectiveness of physical exercise on cognitive and psychological outcomes in individuals with mild cognitive impairment: A systematic review and meta-analysis. *Int J Nurs Stud.* (2018) 79:155–64. doi: 10.1016/j.ijnurstu.2018.01.002
25. Krell-Roesch J, Feder NT, Roberts RO, Mielke MM, Christianson TJ, Knopman DS, et al. Leisure-time physical activity and the risk of incident

dementia: the mayo clinic study of aging. *J Alzheimers Dis.* (2018) 63:149–55. doi: 10.3233/JAD-171141

26. Bray NW, Smart RR, Jakobi JM, Jones GR. Exercise prescription to reverse frailty. *Appl Physiol Nutr Metab.* (2016) 41:1112–6. doi: 10.1139/apnm-2016-0226
27. Santos-Lozano A, Pareja-Galeano H, Sanchis-Gomar F, Quindós-Rubial M, Fiuza-Luces C, Cristi-Montero C, et al. Physical activity and Alzheimer disease: a protective association. *Mayo Clin Proc.* (2016) 91:999–1020. doi: 10.1016/j.mayocp.2016.04.024
28. Schuch FB, Vancampfort D, Rosenbaum S, Richards J, Ward PB, Veronese N, et al. Exercise for depression in older adults: a metaanalysis of randomized controlled trials adjusting for publication bias. *Rev Bras Psiquiatr.* (2016) 38:247–54. doi: 10.1590/1516-4446-2016-1915
29. Law LL, Rol RN, Schultz SA, Dougherty RJ, Edwards DF, Koscik RL, et al. Moderate intensity physical activity associates with CSF biomarkers in a cohort at risk for Alzheimer's disease. *Alzheimers Dement.* (2018) 10:188–95. doi: 10.1016/j.dadm.2018.01.001
30. Martins RN, Villemagne V, Sohrabi HR, Chatterjee P, Shah TM, Verdile G, et al. Alzheimer's disease: a journey from amyloid peptides and oxidative stress, to biomarker technologies and disease prevention strategies-gains from AIBL and DIAN cohort studies. *J Alzheimers Dis.* (2018) 62:965–92. doi: 10.3233/JAD-171145
31. Northey JM, Cherbuin N, Pumpa KL, Smee DJ, Rattray B. Exercise interventions for cognitive function in adults older than 50: a systematic review with metaanalysis. *Br J Sports Med.* (2018) 52:154–60. doi: 10.1136/bjsports-2016-096587
32. Brasure M, Desai P, Davila H, Nelson VA, Calvert C, Jutkowitz E, et al. Physical activity interventions in preventing cognitive decline and alzheimer-type dementia: a systematic review. *Ann Intern Med.* (2018) 168:30–8. doi: 10.7326/M17-1528
33. Teri L, Logsdon RG, McCurry SM. Exercise interventions for dementia and cognitive impairment: the Seattle protocols. *J Nutr Health Aging* (2008) 12:391–4. doi: 10.1007/BF02982672
34. Scherder EJ, Bogen T, Eggermont LH, Hamers JP, Swaab DF. The more physical inactivity, the more agitation in dementia. *Int Psychogeriatr.* (2010) 22:1203–8. doi: 10.1017/S1041610210001493
35. Thune-Boyle IC, Iliffe S, Cerga-Pashoja A, Lowery D, Warner J. The effect of exercise on behavioural and psychological symptoms of dementia: towards a research agenda. *Int Psychogeriatr.* (2012) 24:1046–57. doi: 10.1017/S1041610211002365
36. Fleiner T, Dauth H, Gersie M, Zijlstra W, Haussermann P. Structured physical exercise improves neuropsychiatric symptoms in acute dementia care: a hospital-based RCT. *Alzheimers Res Ther.* (2017) 9:68. doi: 10.1186/s13195-017-0289-z
37. Kwak YS, Um SY, Son TG, Kim DJ. Effect of regular exercise on senile dementia patients. *Int J Sports Med.* (2008) 29:471–4. doi: 10.1055/s-2007-964853
38. Vidoni ED, Perales J, Alshehri M, Giles AM, Siengsukon CF, Burns JM. Aerobic exercise sustains performance of instrumental activities of daily living in early-stage Alzheimer disease. *J Geriatr Phys Ther.* 1. doi: 10.1519/JPT.0000000000000172
39. Forbes D, Forbes SC, Blake CM, Thiessen EJ, Forbes S. Exercise programs for people with dementia. *Cochrane Database Syst Rev.* (2015) 15:CD006489. doi: 10.1002/14651858.CD006489.pub3
40. Norman JE, Rutkowsky J, Bodine S, Rutledge JC. The potential mechanisms of exercise-induced cognitive protection: a literature review. *Curr Pharm Des.* (2018) 24:1827–31. doi: 10.2174/1381612824666180406105149
41. Colcombe SJ, Kramer AF, Erickson KI, Scalf P, McAuley E, Cohen NJ, et al. Cardiovascular fitness, cortical plasticity, and aging. *Proc Natl Acad Sci USA.* (2004) 101:3316–21. doi: 10.1073/pnas.0400266101
42. Fleg JL. Aerobic exercise in the elderly: a key to successful aging. *Discov Med.* (2012) 13: 223–8.
43. Covas MI, Elosua R, Fitó M, Alcántara M, Coca L, Marrugat J. Relationship between physical activity and oxidative stress biomarkers in women. *Med Sci Sports Exerc.* (2002) 34:814–9. doi: 10.1097/00005768-200205000-00014
44. Lavie CJ, Church TS, Milani RV, Earnest CP. Impact of physical activity, cardiorespiratory fitness, and exercise training on markers of inflammation. *J Cardiopulm Rehabil Prev.* (2011) 31:137–45. doi: 10.1097/HCR.0b013e3182122827
45. Ghisi GL, Durieux A, Pinho R, Benetti M. Physical exercise and endothelial dysfunction. *Arq Bras Cardiol.* (2010) 95:30–7. doi: 10.1016/B978-0-12-812348-5.00049-0
46. Churchill JD, Galvez R, Colcombe S, Swain RA, Kramer AF, Greenough WT. Exercise, experience and the aging brain. *Neurobiol Aging* (2002) 23:941–55. doi: 10.1016/S0197-4580(02)00028-3
47. Davenport MH, Hogan DB, Eskes GA, Longman RS, Poulin MJ. Cerebrovascular reserve: the link between fitness and cognitive function? *Exerc Sport Sci Rev.* (2012) 40:153–8. doi: 10.1097/JES.0b013e3182553430
48. Colcombe S, Kramer AF. Fitness effects on the cognitive function of older adults: a meta-analytic study. *Psychol Sci.* (2003) 14:125–30. doi: 10.1111/1467-9280.t01-1-01430
49. Kronenberg G, Bick-Sander A, Bunk E, Wolf C, Ehninger D, Kempermann G. Physical exercise prevents age-related decline in precursor cell activity in the mouse dentate gyrus. *Neurobiol Aging* (2006) 27:1505–13. doi: 10.1016/j.neurobiolaging.2005.09.016
50. Uda M, Ishido M, Kami K, Masuhara M. Effects of chronic treadmill running on neurogenesis in the dentate gyrus of the hippocampus of adult rat. *Brain Res.* (2006) 1104:64–72. doi: 10.1016/j.brainres.2006.05.066
51. Cotman CW, Berchtold NC. Exercise: a behavioural intervention toenhance brain health and plasticity. *Trends Neurosci.* (2002) 25:292–8. doi: 10.1016/S0166-2236(02)02143-4
52. Vaynman S, Gomez-Pinilla F. License to run: exercise impacts functional plasticity in the intact and injured central nervous system by using neurotrophins. *Neurorehabil Neural Repair* (2005) 19:283–95 doi: 10.1177/1545968305280753
53. Cotman CW, Berchtold NC. Physical activity and the maintenance of cognition: learning from animal models. *Alzheimers Dement* (2007) 3:S30–7. doi: 10.1016/j.jalz.2007.01.013
54. Voelcker-Rehage C, Niemann C. Structural and functional brain changes related to different types of physical activity across the life span. *Neurosci Biobehav Rev.* (2013) 37(9 Pt B):2268–95. doi: 10.1016/j.neubiorev.2013.01.028
55. Hamaide J, De Groof G, Van der Linden A. Neuroplasticity and MRI: a perfect match. *Neuroimage* (2016) 131:13–28. doi: 10.1016/j.neuroimage.2015.08.005
56. Weinstein AM, Voss MW, Prakash RS, Chaddock L, Szabo A,White SM, et al. The association between aerobic fitness and executive functions is mediated by prefrontal cortex volume. *Brain Behav Immun.* (2012) 26:811–9. doi: 10.1016/j.bbi.2011.11.008
57. Niemann C, Godde B, Voelcker-Rehage C. Not only cardiovascular, but also coordinative exercise increases hippocampal volume in older adults. *Front Aging Neurosci.* (2014) 6:170. doi: 10.3389/fnagi.2014.00170
58. Papenberg G, Ferencz B, Mangialasche F, Mecocci P, Cecchetti R, Kalpouzos G, et al. Physical activity and inflammation: effects on gray-matter volume and cognitive decline in aging. *Hum Brain Mapp.* (2016) 37:3462–73. doi: 10.1002/hbm.23252
59. Erickson KI, Leckie RL, Weinstein AM. Physical activity, fitness and gray matter volume. *Neurobiol Aging* (2014) 35(Suppl 2): S20–8. doi: 10.1016/j.neurobiolaging.2014.03.034
60. Cheng A, Wang S, Cai J, Rao MS, Mattson MP. Nitric oxide acts in a positive feedback loop with BDNF to regulate neural progenitor cell proliferation and differentiation in the mammalian brain. *Dev Biol.* (2003) 258:319–33. doi: 10.1016/S0012-1606(03)00120-9
61. Vaynman S, Ying Z, Gomez-Pinilla F. Hippocampal BDNF mediates the efficacy of exercise on synaptic plasticity and cognition. *Eur J Neurosci.* (2004) 20:2580–90. doi: 10.1111/j.1460-9568.2004.03720.x
62. Erickson KI, Weinstein AM, Lopez OL. Physical activity, brain plasticity, and Alzheimer's disease. *Arch Med Res.* (2012) 43:615–21. doi: 10.1016/j.arcmed.2012.09.008
63. Intlekofer KA, Cotman CW. Exercise counteracts declining hippocampal function in aging and Alzheimer's disease. *Neurobiol Dis.* (2013) 57:47–55. doi: 10.1016/j.nbd.2012.06.011
64. Jensen CS, Portelius E, Høgh P, Wermuth L, Blennow K, Zetterberg H, et al. Effect of physical exercise on markers of neuronal dysfunction in

cerebrospinal fluid in patients with Alzheimer's disease. *Alzheimers Dement.* (2017) 3:284–90. doi: 10.1016/j.trci.2017.03.007
65. Frederiksen KS, Gjerum L, Waldemar G, Hasselbalch SG. Effects of physical exercise on Alzheimer's disease biomarkers: a systematic review of intervention studies. *J Alzheimers Dis.* (2018) 61:359–72. doi: 10.3233/JAD-170567
66. Clare L, Woods RT. Cognitive training and cognitive rehabilitation for people with early-stage Alzheimer's disease: a review. *Neuropsychol Rehabil.* (2004) 14:385–401. doi: 10.1080/09602010443000074
67. D'Onofrio G, Sancarlo D, Seripa D, Ricciardi F, Giuliani F, Panza F, et al. Chapter 18: non-pharmacological approaches in the treatment of dementia. Update on dementia. In: D. Moretti, editor. *Update on Dementia.* Intech (2016). p. 477–491. Available online at: https://www.intechopen.com/books/update-on-dementia
68. Wilson BA. Towards a comprehensive model of cognitive rehabilitation. *Neuropsychol Rehabil.* (2002) 12:97–110. doi: 10.1080/09602010244000020
69. Woods B, Aguirre E, Spector AE, Orrell M. Cognitive stimulation to improve cognitive functioning in people with dementia. *Cochrane Database Syst Rev.* (2012) 15:CD005562. doi: 10.1002/14651858.CD005562.pub2
70. Olazarán J, Reisberg B, Clare L, Cruz I, Peña-Casanova J, Del Ser T, et al. Nonpharmacological therapies in Alzheimer's disease: a systematic review of efficacy. *Dement Geriatr Cogn Disord.* (2010) 30:161–78. doi: 10.1159/000316119
71. Kurz AF, Leucht S, Lautenschlager NT. The clinical significance of cognition-focused interventions for cognitively impaired older adults: a systematic review of randomized controlled trials. *Int Psychogeriatr.* (2011) 23:1364–75. doi: 10.1017/S1041610211001001
72. Bahar-Fuchs A, Clare L, Woods B. Cognitive training and cognitive rehabilitation for mild to moderate Alzheimer's disease and vascular dementia. *Cochrane Database Syst Rev.* (2013) 6:CD003260. doi: 10.1002/14651858.CD003260.pub2
73. Huntley JD, Gould RL, Liu K, Smith M, Howard RJ. Do cognitive interventions improve general cognition in dementia? A meta-analysis and meta-regression. *BMJ Open* (2015) 5:e005247. doi: 10.1136/bmjopen-2014-005247
74. Carrion C, Folkvord F, Anastasiadou D, Aymerich M. Cognitive Therapy for dementia patients: a systematic review. *Dement Geriatr Cogn Disord.* (2018) 46:1–26. doi: 10.1159/000490851
75. Folstein M, Folstein SE, McHugh PR. "Mini-mental state" a practical method for grading the cognitive state of patients for the clinician. *J Psychiatr Res.* (1975) 12:189–98.
76. Rosen WG, Mohs RC, Davis KL. A new rating scale for Alzheimer's disease. *Am J Psychiatry* (1984) 141:1356–64. doi: 10.1176/ajp.141.11.1356
77. Kallio EL, Öhman H, Kautiainen H, Hietanen M, Pitkälä K. Cognitive training interventions for patients with Alzheimer's disease: a systematic review. *J Alzheimers Dis.* (2017) 56:1349–72. doi: 10.3233/JAD-160810
78. Spector A, Orrell M, Davies S and Woods B. Can reality orientation be rehabilitated? Development and piloting of an evidence-based programme of cognition-based therapies for people with dementia. *Neuropsychol Rehabilitat.* (2001) 11:193–6. doi: 10.1080/09602010143000068
79. Spector A, Thorgrimsen L, Woods B, Royan L, Davies S, Butterworth M, et al. Efficacy of an evidence-based cognitive stimulation therapy programme for people with dementia: randomised controlled trial. *Br J Psychiatry* (2003) 183:248–54. doi: 10.1192/bjp.183.3.248
80. NICE-SCIE (2007). *Dementia: Supporting People With Dementia and Their Carers in Health and Social Care. NICE Clinical Guideline 42.* London: National Institute for Health and Clinical Excellence (Available online at: www.nice.org.uk)
81. Bacigalupo I, Mayer F, Lacorte E, Di Pucchio A, Marzolini F, Canevelli M, et al. *World Alzheimer Report: The Benefits of Early Diagnosis and Intervention.* Alzheimer's Disease International (ADI) (2011). Available online at: http://www.alz.co.uk/research/WorldAlzheimerReport2011.pdf
82. NHS Institute for Innovation and Improvement. *An Economic Evaluation of Alternatives to Antipsychotic Drugs for Individuals Living With Dementia.* Coventry: The NHS Institute for Innovation and Improvement (2011).
83. Piras F, Carbone E, Faggian S, Salvalaio E, Gardini S, Borella E. Efficacy of cognitive stimulation therapy for older adults with vascular dementia. *Dement Neuropsychol.* (2017) 11:434–41. doi: 10.1590/1980-57642016dn11-040014
84. Hall L, Orrell M, Stott J, Spector A. Cognitive Stimulation Therapy (CST): neurpsychological mechanisms of change. *Int Psychogeriatr.* (2013) 25:479–89. doi: 10.1017/S1041610212001822
85. Orrell M, Yates LA, Burns A, Russell I, Woods RT, Hoare Z, et al. Individual Cognitive Stimulation Therapy for dementia (iCST): study protocol for a randomized controlled trial. *Trials* (2012) 13:172. doi: 10.1186/1745-6215-13-172
86. Yates LA, Orgeta V, Leung P, Spector A, Orrell M. Field-testing phase of the development of individual cognitive stimulation therapy (iCST) for dementia. *BMC Health Services Res.* (2016) 16:233. doi: 10.1186/s12913-016-1499-y
87. Orrell M, Yates L, Leung P, Kang S, Hoare Z, Whitaker C, et al. The impact of individual Cognitive Stimulation Therapy (iCST) on cognition, quality of life, caregiver health, and family relationships in dementia: a randomised controlled trial. *PLoS Med.* (2017) 14:e1002269. doi: 10.1371/journal.pmed.1002269
88. Finkel SI, Costa e Silva J, Cohen G, Miller S, Sartorius N. Behavioural and psychological signs and symptoms of dementia: a consensus statement on current knowledge and implications for research and treatment. *Int Psychogeriatr.* (1996) 8(Suppl. 3):497–500. doi: 10.1017/S1041610297003943
89. Aalten P, Verhey FR, Boziki M, Brugnolo A, Bullock R, Byrne EJ, et al. Consistency of neuropsychiatric syndromes across dementias: results from the European Alzheimer disease consortium. Part II. *Dement Geriatr Cogn Disord.* (2008) 28:1–8. doi: 10.1159/000111082
90. Kazui H, Yoshiyama K, Kanemoto H, Suzuki Y, Sato S, Hashimoto M, et al. Differences of behavioural and psychological symptoms of dementia in disease severity in four major dementias. *PLoS ONE* (2016) 11:e0161092. doi: 10.1371/journal.pone.0161092
91. Gilhooly KJ, Gilhooly ML, Sullivan MP, McIntyre A, Wilson L, Harding E, et al. A meta-review of stress, coping and interventions in dementia and dementia caregiving. *BMC Geriatr.* (2016) 16:106–12. doi: 10.1186/s12877-016-0280-8
92. Herrmann N, Lanctôt KL, Sambrook R, Lesnikova N, Hébert R, McCracken P, et al. The contribution of neuropsychiatric symptoms to the cost of dementia care. *Int J Geriatr Psychiatry* (2006) 21:972–6. doi: 10.1002/gps.1594
93. Azermai M, Petrovic M, Elseviers MM, Bourgeois J, Van Bortel LM, Vander Stichele RH. Systematic appraisal of dementia guidelines for the management of behavioural and psychological symptoms. *Ageing Res Rev.* (2012) 11:78–86. doi: 10.1016/j.arr.2011.07.002
94. Sorbi S, Hort J, Erkinjuntti T, Fladby T, Gainotti G, Gurvit H, et al. EFNS-ENS guidelines on the diagnosis and management of disorders associated with dementia. *Eur J Neurol.* (2012) 19:1159–79. doi: 10.1111/j.1468-1331.2012.03784.x
95. Dyer SM, Harrison SL, Laver K, Whitehead C, Crotty M. An overview of systematic reviews of pharmacological and non-pharmacological interventions for the treatment of behavioural and psychological symptoms of dementia. *Int Psychogeriatr.* (2018) 30:295–309. doi: 10.1017/S1041610217002344
96. Gauthier S, Cummings J, Ballard C, Brodaty H, Grossberg G, Robert P, et al. Management of behavioral problems in Alzheimer's disease. *Int Psychogeriatr.* (2010) 22:346–72. doi: 10.1017/S1041610209991505
97. Seitz DP, Gill SS, Herrmann N, Brisbin S, Rapoport MJ, Rines J, et al. Pharmacological treatments for neuropsychiatric symptoms of dementia in long-term care: a systematic review. *Int Psychogeriatr.* (2013) 25:185–203. doi: 10.1017/S1041610212001627
98. Sultzer DL, Davis SM, Tariot PN, Dagerman KS, Lebowitz BD, Lyketsos CG, et al. Clinical symptom responses to atypical antipsychotic medications in Alzheimer's disease: phase 1 outcomes from the CATIE-AD effectiveness trial. *Am J Psychiatry* (2008) 165:844–54. doi: 10.1176/appi.ajp.2008.07111779
99. O'Connor DW, Ames D, Gardner B, King M. Psychosocial treatments of behaviour symptoms in dementia: a systematic review of reports

meeting quality standards. *Int Psychogeriatr.* (2009) 21:225–40. doi: 10.1017/S1041610208007588

100. Gitlin L, Earland TV. *Improving Quality of Life in Individuals With Dementia: The Role of Nonpharmacologic Approaches in Rehabilitation.* International Encycolpedia of Rehabilitation (2010) 2:22.
101. Norton MJ, Allen RS, Snow AL, Hardin JM, Burgio LD. Need-driven dementia-compromised behavior: an alternative view of disruptive behavior. *Am J Alzheimer's Dis Other Dem.* (1996) 11:10–9.
102. Kovach CR, Noonan PE, Schlidt AM, Wells T. A model of consequences of need-driven, dementia-compromised behavior. *J Nurs Scholarsh.* (2005) 37:134–40. doi: 10.1111/j.1547-5069.2005.00025_1.x
103. O'Neil ME, Freeman M, Christensen V, Telerant R, Addleman A, Kansagara D. *A Systematic Evidence Review of Non-pharmacological Interventions for Behavioural Symptoms of Dementia.* Washington DC, Department of Veterans Affairs (2011).
104. Brodaty H, Arasaratnam C. Meta-analysis of nonpharmacological interventions for neuropsychiatric symptoms of dementia. *Am J Psychiatry* (2012) 16:946–53. doi: 10.1176/appi.ajp.2012.11101529
105. McLaren AN, Lamantia MA, Callahan CM. Systematic review of non-pharmacologic interventions to delay functional decline in community-dwelling patients with dementia. *Aging Ment Health* (2013) 17:655–66. doi: 10.1080/13607863.2013.781121
106. Livingston G, Kelly L, Lewis-Holmes E, Baio G, Morris S, Patel N, et al. A systematic review of the clinical effectiveness and cost-effectiveness of sensory, psychological and behavioural interventions for managing agitation in older adults with dementia. *Health Technol Assess.* (2014) 18:1–226. doi: 10.3310/hta18610
107. Abraha I, Rimland JM, Trotta FM, Dell'Aquila G, Cruz-Jentoft A, Petrovic M, et al. Systematic review of systematic reviews of non-pharmacological interventions to treat behavioural disturbances in older patients with dementia. The SENATOR-On Top series. *BMJ Open* (2017) 7:e012759. doi: 10.1136/bmjopen-2016-012759
108. Cohen-Mansfield J, Thein K, Marx MS. Predictors of the impact of nonpharmacologic interventions for agitation in nursing home residents with advanced dementia. J Clin Psychiatry (2014) 75:666–71. doi: 10.4088/JCP.13m08649
109. Cohen-Mansfield J, Marx MS, Dakheel-Ali M, Thein K. The use and utility of specific nonpharmacological interventions for behavioural symptoms in dementia: an exploratory study. *Am J Geriatr Psychiatry* (2015) 23:160–70. doi: 10.1016/j.jagp.2014.06.006
110. Scales K, Zimmerman S, Miller SJ. Evidence-based nonpharmacological practices to address behavioural and psychological symptoms of dementia. *Gerontologist* (2018) 58(suppl_1):S88–102. doi: 10.1093/geront/gnx167
111. Cohen-Mansfield J, Jensen B, Resnick B, Norris M. Assessment and treatment of behaviour problems in dementia in nursing home residents: a comparison of the approaches of physicians, psychologists and nurse practitioners. *Int J Geriatr Psychiatry* (2012) 27:135–45. doi: 10.1002/gps.2699
112. Cohen-Mansfield J, Dakheel-Ali M, Marx MS, Thein K, Regier NG. Which unmet needs contribute to behaviour problems in persons with advanced dementia? *Psychiatry Res.* (2015) 30:59–64. doi: 10.1016/j.psychres.2015.03.043
113. Muò R, Schindler A, Vernero I, Schindler O, Ferrario E, Frisoni GB. Alzheimer's disease-associated disability: an ICF approach. *Disabil Rehabil.* (2005) 27:1405–13. doi: 10.1080/09638280500052542
114. Giebel CM, Sutcliffe C, Stolt M, Karlsson S, Renom-Guiteras A, Soto M, et al. Deterioration of basic activities of daily living and their impact on quality of life across different cognitive stages of dementia: a European study. *Int Psychogeriatr.* (2014) 26:1283–93. doi: 10.1017/S10416102140 00775
115. Prizer LP, Zimmerman S. Progressive support for activities of daily living for persons living with dementia. *Gerontologist* (2018) 58(suppl_1):S74–87. doi: 10.1093/geront/gnx103
116. Sun M, Mainland BJ, Ornstein TJ, Mallya S, Fiocco AJ, Sin GL, et al. The association between cognitive fluctuations and activities of daily living and quality of life among institutionalized patients with dementia. *Int J Geriatr Psychiatry* (2018) 33:e280–5. doi: 10.1002/gps.4788
117. Egan M, Hobson S, Fearing V. Dementia and occupation: a review of the literature. *Can J Occupat Ther.* (2006) 73:132–40. doi: 10.2182/cjot.05.0015
118. Georges J, Jansen S, Jackson J, Meyrieux A, Sadowska A, Selmes M. Alzheimer's disease in real life - the dementia carer's survey. *Int J Geriatr Psychiatry* (2008) 23:546–51. doi: 10.1002/gps.1984
119. Steultjens EM, Dekker J, Bouter LM, Leemrijse CJ, van den Ende CH. Evidence of the efficacy of occupational therapy in different conditions: an overview of systematic reviews. *Clin Rehabil.* (2005) 19:247–54. doi: 10.1191/0269215505cr870oa
120. Voigt-Radloff S, Graff M, Leonhart R, Schornstein K, Jessen F, Bohlken J, et al. A multicentre RCT on community occupational therapy in Alzheimer's disease: 10 sessions are not better than one consultation. *BMJ Open* (2011) 9:e000096. doi: 10.1136/bmjopen-2011-000096
121. Graff MJ, Vernooij-Dassen MJ, Thijssen M, Dekker J, Hoefnagels WH, Rikkert MG. Community based occupational therapy for patients with dementia and their caregivers: randomised controlled trial. *BMJ* (2006) 333:1196. doi: 10.1136/bmj.39001.688843.BE
122. Gitlin LN, Winter L, Corcoran M, Dennis MP, Schinfeld S, Hauck WW. Effects of the home environmental skill-building program on the caregiver-care recipient dyad: 6-month outcomes from the Philadelphia REACH Initiative. *Gerontologist* (2003) 43:532–46. doi: 10.1093/geront/43.4.532
123. Gitlin LN, Hodgson N, Jutkowitz E, Pizzi L. The cost-effectiveness of a nonpharmacologic intervention for individuals with dementia and family caregivers: the tailored activity program. *Am J Geriatr Psychiatry* (2010) 18:510–9. doi: 10.1097/JGP.0b013e3181c37d13
124. Kolanowski A, Litaker M, Buettner L, Moeller J, Costa PT Jr. A randomized clinical trial of theory-based activities for the behavioural symptoms of dementia in nursing home residents. *J Am Geriatr Soc.* (2001) 59:1032–41. doi: 10.1111/j.1532-5415.2011.03449.x
125. Rao AK, Chou A, Bursley B, Smulofsky J, Jezequel J. Systematic review of the effects of exercise on activities of daily living in people with Alzheimer's disease. *Am J Occup Ther.* (2014) 68:50–6. doi: 10.5014/ajot.2014.009035
126. Rao AK. Occupational therapy in chronic progressive disorders: enhancing function and modifying disease. *Am J Occup Ther.* (2014) 68:251–3. doi: 10.5014/ajot.2014.012120
127. Pimouguet C, Le Goff M, Wittwer J, Dartigues JF, Helmer C. Benefits of occupational therapy in dementia patients: findings from a real-world observational study. *J Alzheimers Dis.* (2017) 56:509–17. doi: 10.3233/JAD-160820
128. Gitlin LN, Winter L, Burke J, Chernett N, Dennis MP, Hauck WW. Tailored activities to manage neuropsychiatry behavior in persons with dementia and reduce caregiver burden. A randomized pilot study. *Am J Geriatr Psychiatry* (2008) 16:229–39. doi: 10.1097/01.JGP.0000300629.35408.94
129. Gitlin LN, Arthur P, Piersol C, Hessels V, Wu SS, Dai Y, et al. Targeting behavioral symptoms and functional decline in dementia: a randomized clinical trial. *J Am Geriatr Soc.* (2018) 66:339–45. doi: 10.1111/jgs.15194
130. Kim SY, Yoo EY, Jung MY, Park SH, Park JH. A systematic review of the effects of occupational therapy for persons with dementia: a meta-analysis of randomized controlled trials. *NeuroRehabilitation* (2012) 31:107–15.
131. Padilla R. Effectiveness of environment-based interventions for people with Alzheimer's disease and related dementias. *Am J Occup Ther.* (2011) 65:514–22. doi: 10.5014/ajot.2011.002600
132. Letts L, Edwards M, Berenyi J, Moros K, O'Neill C, O'Toole C, et al. Using occupations to improve quality of life, health and wellness, and client and caregiver satisfaction for people with Alzheimer's disease and related dementias. *Am J Occup Ther.* (2011) 65:497–504. doi: 10.5014/ajot.2011.002584
133. Gitlin LN, Winter L, Earland TV, Herge EA, Chernett NL, Piersol CV, et al. The Tailored Activity Program (TAP): a nonpharmacologic approach to improving quality of life at home for persons with dementia and their family caregivers. *Gerontol Practice Concepts* (2009) 49:428–39.
134. Padilla R. Effectiveness of interventions designed to modify the activity demands of the occupations of self-care and leisure for people with Alzheimer's disease and related dementias. *Am J Occup Ther.* (2011) 65:523–31. doi: 10.5014/ajot.2011.002618

135. National Collaborating Centre for Mental Health (commissioned by the Social Care Institute for Excellence and the National Institute for Health and Clinical Excellence). *Dementia. A NICE-SCIE Guideline on Supporting People with Dementia and their Carers in Health and Social Care. National Clinical Practice Guideline, Number 42*. London: The British Psychological Society and Gaskell (2007).
136. German Society for Psychiatry, Psychotherapy and Neurology and German Society for Neurology. *Consented Guideline 'Dementia'*. (2009). Available online at: https://www.dgn.org/leitlinien/3176-leitlinie-diagnose-und-therapie-von-demenzen-2016
137. Work Group on Alzheimer's Disease and other dementias. *Practice Guideline for the Treatment of Patients With Alzheimer's Disease and Other Dementias* (2007). Available online at: http://www.psychiatryonline.com/pracGuide/PracticePDFs/AlzPG101007.pdf
138. Laver K, Cumming R, Dyer S, Agar M, Anstey KJ, Beattie E, et al. Evidence-based occupational therapy for people with dementia and their families: What clinical practice guidelines tell us and implications for practice. *Aust Occup Ther J*. (2017) 64:3–10. doi: 10.1111/1440-1630.12309
139. Lindbergh CA, Dishman RK, Miller LS. Functional disability in mild cognitive impairment: a systematic review and meta-analysis. *Neuropsychol Rev*. (2016) 26:129–59. doi: 10.1007/s11065-016-9321-5
140. Kaur N, Belchior P, Gelinas I, Bier N. Critical appraisal of questionnaires to assess functional impairment in individuals with mild cognitive impairment. *Int Psychogeriatr*. (2016) 28:1425–39. doi: 10.1017/S104161021600017X
141. Reppermund S, Brodaty H, Crawford JD, Kochan NA, Draper B, Slavin MJ, et al. Impairment in instrumental activities of daily living with high cognitive demand is an early marker of mild cognitive impairment: the Sydney memory and ageing study. *Psychol Med*. (2013) 43:2437–45. doi: 10.1017/S003329171200308X
142. Fieo R, Zahodne L, Tang MX, Manly JJ, Cohen R, Stern Y. The historical progression from ADL scrutiny to IADL to advanced ADL: assessing functional status in the earliest stages of dementia. *J Gerontol A Biol Sci Med Sci*. (2017) 24:1035–1055. doi: 10.1093/gerona/glx235
143. Aminzadeh F, Byszewski A, Molnar FJ, Eisner M. Emotional impact of dementia diagnosis: exploring persons with dementia and caregivers' perspectives. *Aging Ment Health* (2007) 11:281–90. doi: 10.1080/13607860600963695
144. Enache D, Winblad B, Aarsland D. Depression in dementia: epidemiology, mechanisms, and treatment. *Curr Opin Psychiatry* (2011) 24:461–72. doi: 10.1097/YCO.0b013e32834bb9d4
145. Weiner MF, Doody RS, Sairam R, Foster B, Liao TY. Prevalence and incidence of major depressive disorder in Alzheimer's disease: findings from two databases. *Dement Geriatr Cog Disord*. (2002) 13:8–12. doi: 10.1159/000048627
146. Starkstein SE, Jorge R, Mizrahi R, Robinson RG. The construct of minor and major depression in Alzheimer's disease. *Am J Psychiatry* (2005) 162:2086–93. doi: 10.1176/appi.ajp.162.11.2086
147. Hwang TJ, Masterman DL, Ortiz F, Fairbanks LA, Cummings JL. Mild cognitive impairment is associated with characteristic neuropsychiatric symptoms. *Alzheimer Dis Assoc Disord*. (2004) 18:17–21.
148. Schultz SK, Hoth A, Buckwalter K. Anxiety and impaired social function in the elderly. *Ann Clin Psychiatry* (2004) 16:47–51. doi: 10.1080/10401230490281429
149. Gabryelewicz T, Styczynska M, Pfeffer A, Wasiak B, Barczak A, Luczywek E, et al. Prevalence of major and minor depression in elderly persons with mild cognitive impairment–MADRS factor analysis. *Int J Geriatr Psychiatry* (1998) 19:1168–72. doi: 10.1002/gps.1235
150. Lu PH, Edland SD, Teng E, Tingus K, Petersen RC, Cummings JL, et al. Donepezil delays progression to AD in MCI subjects with depressive symptoms. *Neurology* (2009) 72:2115–221. doi: 10.1212/WNL.0b013e3181aa52d3
151. Rozzini L, Chilovi BV, Peli M, Conti M, Rozzini R, Trabucchi M., et al. Anxiety symptoms in mild cognitive impairment. *Int J Geriatr Psychiatry* (2009) 24:300–5. doi: 10.1002/gps.2106
152. Alexopoulos GS, Jeste DV, Chung H, Carpenter D, Ross R, Docherty JP. The expert consensus guideline series. Treatment of dementia and its behavioural disturbances. Introduction: methods, commentary, and summary. *Postgrad Med Spec*. (2005) 6:22.
153. Salzman C, Jeste DV, Meyer RE, Cohen-Mansfield J, Cummings J, Grossberg GT, et al. Elderly patients with dementia-related symptoms of severe agitation and aggression: consensus statement on treatment options, clinical trials methodology, and policy. *J Clin Psychiatry* (2008) 69:889–98. doi: 10.4088/JCP.v69n0602
154. Starkstein SE, Ingram L, Garau ML, Mizrahi R. On the overlap between apathy and depression in dementia. *J Neurol Neurosurg Psychiatry* (2005) 76:1070–4. doi: 10.1136/jnnp.2004.052795
155. Spalletta G, Long JD, Robinson RG, Trequattrini A, Pizzoli S, Caltagirone C, et al. Longitudinal neuropsychiatric predictors of death in Alzheimer's disease. *J Alzheimers Dis*. (2015) 48:627–36. doi: 10.3233/JAD-150391
156. Dauphinot V, Delphin-Combe F, Mouchoux C, Dorey A, Bathsavanis A, Makaroff Z, et al. Risk factors of caregiver burden among patients with Alzheimer's disease or related disorders: a cross-sectional study. *J Alzheimers Dis*. (2015) 44:907–16. doi: 10.3233/JAD-142337
157. Hongisto K, Hallikainen I, Selander T, Törmälehto S, Väätäinen S, Martikainen J, et al. Quality of Life in relation to neuropsychiatric symptoms in Alzheimer's disease: 5-year prospective ALSOVA cohort study. *Int J Geriatr Psychiatry* (2018) 33:47–57. doi: 10.1002/gps.4666
158. Hogan DB, Bailey P, Black S, Carswell A, Chertkow H, Clarke B, et al. Diagnosis and treatment of dementia: non pharmacologic and pharmacologic therapy for mild to moderate dementia. *CMAJ* (2008) 179:1019–26. doi: 10.1503/cmaj.081103
159. Doody RS, Stevens JC, Beck C, Dubinsky RM, Kaye JA, Gwyther L, et al. Practice parameter: management of dementia (an evidence-based review). Report of the quality standards subcommittee of the American academy of neurology. *Neurology* (2001) 56:1154–66. doi: 10.1212/WNL.56.9.1154
160. Lyketsos CG, Olin J. Depression in Alzheimer's disease: overview and treatment. *Biol Psychiatry* (2002) 52:243–52. doi: 10.1016/S0006-3223(02)01348-3
161. Douglas S, James I, Ballard C. Non-pharmacological interventions in dementia. *Adv Psychiatr Treat*. (2004) 10:171–7. doi: 10.1192/apt.10.3.171
162. World Health Organization. *Evidence for Decision Makers*. World Health Organization, Regional Office for Europe, Health Evidence Network (2007). Available online at: http://www.euro.who.int/HEN/
163. Orgeta V, Qazi A, Spector AE, Orrell M. Psychological treatments for depression and anxiety in dementia and mild cognitive impairment. *Cochrane Database Syst Rev*. (2014) 22:CD009125. doi: 10.1002/14651858.CD009125.pub2
164. Cheston R, Ivanecka A.Individual and group psychotherapy with people diagnosed with dementia: a systematic review of the literature. *Int J Geriatr Psychiatry* (2017) 32:3–31. doi: 10.1002/gps.4529
165. Goris ED, Ansel KN, Schutte DL. Quantitative systematic review of the effects of non-pharmacological interventions on reducing apathy in persons with dementia. *J Adv Nurs*. (2016) 72:2612–28. doi: 10.1111/jan.13026
166. Theleritis C, Siarkos K, Politis AA, Katirtzoglou E, Politis A. A systematic review of non-pharmacological treatments for apathy in dementia. *Int J Geriatr Psychiatry* (2018) 33:e177–92. doi: 10.1002/gps.4783
167. Farina E, Mantovani F, Fioravanti R, Pignatti R, Chiavari L, Imbornone E, et al. Evaluating two group programmes of cognitive training in mild-to-moderate AD: is there any difference between a 'global' stimulation and a 'cognitive-specific' one? *Aging Ment Health* (2006) 10:211–8. doi: 10.1080/13607860500409492
168. Farina E, Mantovani F, Fioravanti R, Rotella G, Villanelli F, Imbornone E, et al. Efficacy of recreational and occupational activities associated to psychologic support in mild to moderate Alzheimer disease: a multicenter controlled study. *Alzheimer Dis Assoc Disord*. (2006) 20:275–82. doi: 10.1097/01.wad.0000213846.66742.90
169. Baglio F, Griffanti L, Saibene FL, Ricci C, Alberoni M, Critelli R, et al. Multistimulation group therapy in Alzheimer's disease promotes changes in brain functioning. *Neurorehabil Neural Repair* (2015) 29:13–24. doi: 10.1177/1545968314532833

170. Dröes RM, Breebaart E, Ettema TP, van Tilburg W, Mellenbergh GJ. The effect of integrated family support versus day care only on behavior and mood of patients with dementia. *Int Psychogeriatr.* (2000) 12:99–116. doi: 10.1017/S1041610200006232
171. Dröes RM, Breebaart E, Meiland FJM, Van Tilburg W, Mellenbergh GJ. Effect of Meeting Centres Support Programme on feeling of competence of family caregivers and delay of institutionalization of people with dementia. *Aging Ment Health* (2004) 8:201–11. doi: 10.1080/13607860410001669732
172. Dröes RM, Meiland FJM, Schmitz M, Van Tilburg W. Effect of combined support for people with dementia and carers versus regular day care on behaviour and mood of persons with dementia: results from a multi-centre implementation study. *Int J Geriatr Psychiatry* (2004) 19:1–12. doi: 10.1002/gps.1142
173. Dröes RM, Meiland FJM, Schmitz M, Van Tilburg W. An evaluation of the Meeting Centres Support Programme among persons with dementia and their carers. *Nonpharmacol Therapies Dementia* (2011) 2:19–39.
174. Dröes RM, Meiland FJ, Evans S, Brooker D, Farina E, Szcześniak D, et al. Comparison of the adaptive implementation and evaluation of the Meeting Centers Support Program for people with dementia and their family carers in Europe; study protocol of the MEETINGDEM project. *BMC Geriatr.* (2017) 17:79. doi: 10.1186/s12877-017-0472-x
175. Smits CH, de Lange J, Dröes RM, Meiland F, Vernooij-Dassen M, Pot AM. Effects of combined intervention programmes for people with dementia living at home and their caregivers: a systematic review. *Int J Geriatric Psychiatry* (2007) 22:1181–93. doi: 10.1002/gps.1805
176. Klapwijk MS, Caljouw MAA, Pieper MJC, Putter H, van der Steen JT, Achterberg WP. Change in quality of life after a multidisciplinary intervention for people with dementia: a cluster randomized controlled trial. *Int J Geriatr Psychiatry* (2018). 33:1213–19. doi: 10.1002/gps.4912
177. Sinvani L, Warner-Cohen J, Strunk A, Halbert T, Harisingani R, Mulvany C, et al. A multicomponent model to improve hospital care of older adults with cognitive impairment: a propensity score-matched analysis. *J Am Geriatr Soc.* (2018) 66:1700–7. doi: 10.1111/jgs.15452
178. Baker R, Bell S, Baker E, Gibson S, Holloway J, Pearce R, et al. A randomized controlled trial of the effects of multi-sensory stimulation (MSS) for people with dementia. *Br J Clin Psychol.* (2001) 40:81–96.
179. Scuteri D, Rombola L, Tridico L, Mizoguchi H, Watanabe C, Sakurada T, et al. Neuropharmacological properties of the essential oil of bergamot for the clinical management of pain-related BPSDs. *Curr Med Chem.* (2018) 25:1–10. doi: 10.2174/0929867325666180307115546
180. Forrester L, Maayan N, Orrell M, Spector AE, Buchan LD, Soares-Weiser K. Aromatherapy for dementia. *Cochr Datab Syst Rev.* (2014) 2:CD003150.
181. Brooker DJ, Snape M, Johnson E, Ward D, Payne M. Single case evaluation of the effects of aromatherapy and massage on disturbed behaviour in severe dementia. *Br J Clin Psychol.* (1997) 36:287–96. doi: 10.1111/j.2044-8260.1997.tb01415.x
182. Ballard CG, O'Brien JT, Reichelt K, Perry EK. Aromatherapy as a safe and effective treatment for the management of agitation in severe dementia: the results of a double-blind, placebo-controlled trial with Melissa. *J Clin Psychiatry* (2002) 63:553–58. doi: 10.4088/JCP.v63n0703
183. Lin PW, Chan WC, Ng BF, Lam LC. Efficacy of aromatherapy (Lavandula angustifolia) as an intervention for agitated behaviours in Chinese older persons with dementia: a cross-over randomized trial. *Int J Geriatr Psychiatry* (2007) 22:405–10. doi: 10.1002/gps.1688
184. Nguyen QA, Paton C. The use of aromatherapy to treat behavioural problems in dementia. *Int J Geriatr Psychiatry* (2008) 23:337–46. doi: 10.1002/gps.1886
185. Yang MH, Lin LC, Wu SC, Chiu JH, Wang PN, Lin JG. Comparison of the efficacy of aroma-acupressure and aromatherapy for the treatment of dementia-associated agitation. *BMC Complement Altern Med.* (2015) 29:93. doi: 10.1186/s12906-015-0612-9
186. VilelaI VC, PachecoI RL, Cruz LatorracaII CO, PachitoIII DV, Riera R. What do Cochrane systematic reviews say about non-pharmacological interventions for treating cognitive decline and dementia? *Sao Paulo Med J.* (2017) 135:309–20. doi: 10.1590/1516-3180.2017.0092060617
187. Wolfe, N, Herzberg J. Can aromatherapy oils promote sleep in severely demented patients? *Int J Geriatr Psychiatry* (1996) 11:926–7. doi: 10.1002/(SICI)1099-1166 (199610)11:10<926::AID-GPS473>3.0.CO;2-1
188. Johannessen B. Nurses experience of aromatherapy use with dementia patients experiencing disturbed sleep patterns. An action research project. *Complement Ther Clin Pract.* (2013) 19:209–13. doi: 10.1016/j.ctcp.2013.01.003
189. Takeda A, Watanuki E, Koyama S. Effects of inhalation aromatherapy on symptoms of sleep disturbance in the elderly with dementia. *Evid Based Complement Alternat Med.* (2017) 2017:1902807. doi: 10.1155/2017/19 02807
190. MacMahon S, Kermode S. A clinical trial of the effects of aromatherapy on motivational behaviour in a dementia care setting using a single subject design. *Aust J Holist Nurs.* (1998) 52:47–9.
191. Forrester LT, Maayan N, Orrell M, Spector AE, Buchan LD, Soares-Weiser K. Aromatherapy for dementia. *Cochrane Database Syst Rev.* (2014) 25:CD003150. doi: 10.1002/14651858.CD003150.pub2
192. van der Steen JT, van Soest-Poortvliet MC, van der Wouden JC, Bruinsma MS, Scholten RJ, Vink AC Music-based therapeutic interventions for people with dementia. *Cochrane Database Syst Rev.* (2017) 5:CD003477. doi: 10.1002/14651858.CD003477.pub3
193. Raglio A, Pavlic E, Bellandi D. Music listening for people living with dementia. *J Am Med Dir Assoc.* (2018) 19:722–3. doi: 10.1016/j.jamda.2018.05.027
194. Sherratt K, Thornton A, Hatton C. Music interventions for people with dementia: a review of the literature. *Aging Ment Health* (2004) 8:3–12. doi: 10.1080/13607860310001613275
195. Vink AC, Birks JS, Bruinsma MS, Scholten RJ. Music therapy for people with dementia. *Cochrane Database Syst Rev.* (2004) 3:CD003477. doi: 10.1002/14651858.CD003477.pub2
196. Raglio A, Bellelli G, Mazzola P, Bellandi D, Giovagnoli AR, Farina E, et al. Music, music therapy and dementia: a review of literature and the recommendations of the Italian psychogeriatric association. *Maturitas* (2012) 72:305–10. doi: 10.1016/j.maturitas.2012.05.016
197. McDermott O, Crellin N, Ridder HM, Orrell M. Music therapy in dementia: a narrative synthesis systematic review. *Int J Geriatr Psychiatry* (2013) 28:781–94. doi: 10.1002/gps.3895
198. Raglio A, Gianelli MV. Music and music therapy in the management of behavioral disorders in dementia. *Neurodegener Dis Manag.* (2013) 3:295–8. doi: 10.2217/nmt.13.27
199. Solé C, Mercadal-Brotons M, Galati A, De Castro M. Effects of group music therapy on quality of life, affect, and participation in people with varying levels of dementia. *J Music Ther.* (2014) 51:103–25. doi: 10.1093/jmt/thu003
200. Zatorre R. Music and the brain. *Ann N Y Acad Sci.* (2003) 999:4–14. doi: 10.1196/annals.1284.001
201. Zatorre R, McGill J. Music, the food of neuroscience? *Nature* (2005) 17:312–5. doi: 10.1038/434312a
202. Levitin DJ, Tirovolas AK. Current advances in the cognitive neuroscience of music. *Ann N Y Acad Sci.* (2009) 1156:211–31. doi: 10.1111/j.1749-6632.2009.04417.x
203. Koelsch S. A neuroscientific perspective on music therapy. *Ann N Y Acad Sci.* (2009) 1169:374–84. doi: 10.1111/j.1749-6632.2009.04592.x
204. Koelsch S. Towards a neural basis of music-evoked emotions. *Trends Cogn Sci.* (2010) 14:131–7. doi: 10.1016/j.tics.2010.01.002
205. Koelsch S. Brain correlates of music-evoked emotions. *Nat Rev Neurosci.* (2014) 15:170–80. doi: 10.1038/nrn3666
206. Gold C, Solli HP, Kruger V, Lie SA. Dose-response relationship in music therapy for people with serious mental disorders; systematic review and meta-analysis. *Clin Psychol Rev.* (2009) 29:193–207. doi: 10.1016/j.cpr.2009.01.001
207. Schlaug G. Part VI introduction: listening to and making music facilitates brain recovery processes. *Ann N Y Acad Sci.* (2009) 1169:372–3. doi: 10.1111/j.1749-6632.2009.04869.x
208. Raglio A, Bellelli G, Traficante D, Gianotti M, Ubezio MC, Gentile S, et al. Efficacy of music therapy treatment based on cycles of sessions: a randomized controlled trial. *Aging Ment Health* (2010) 14:900–4. doi: 10.1080/13607861003713158
209. Lin Y, Chu H, Yang CY, Chen CH, Chen SG, Chang HJ, et al. Effectiveness of group music intervention against agitated behavior in elderly persons with dementia. *Int J Geriatr Psychiatry* (2011) 26:670–8. doi: 10.1002/gps.2580
210. Sung HC, Lee WL, Li TL, Watson R. A group music intervention using percussion instruments with familiar music to reduce anxiety and agitation

of institutionalized older adults with dementia. *Int J Geriatr Psychiatry* (2012) 27:621–7. doi: 10.1002/gps.2761

211. Ridder HM, Stige B, Qvale LG, Gold C. Individual music therapy for agitation in dementia: an exploratory randomized controlled trial. *Aging Ment Health* (2013) 17:667–78. doi: 10.1080/13607863.2013.790926
212. Ueda T, Suzukamo Y, Sato M, Izumi S. Effects of music therapy on behavioral and psychological symptoms of dementia: a systematic review and meta-analysis. *Ageing Res Rev.* (2013) 12:628–41. doi: 10.1016/j.arr.2013.02.003
213. Craig J. Music therapy to reduce agitation in dementia. *Nurs Times* (2014) 110:12–5.
214. Raglio A, Bellelli G, Traficante D, Gianotti M, Ubezio MC, Villani D, et al. Efficacy of music therapy in the treatment of behavioral and psychiatric symptoms of dementia. *Alzheimer Dis Assoc Disord.* (2008) 22:158–62. doi: 10.1097/WAD.0b013e3181630b6f
215. Sakamoto M, Ando H, Tsutou A. Comparing the effects of different individualized music interventions for elderly individuals with severe dementia. *Int Psychogeriatr.* (2013) 25:775–84. doi: 10.1017/S1041610212002256
216. Jiménez-Palomares M, Rodríguez-Mansilla J, González-López-Arza MV, Rodríguez-Domínguez MT, Prieto-Tato M. Benefits of music therapy as therapy no pharmacology and rehabilitation moderate dementia. *Rev Esp Geriatr Gerontol.* (2013) 48:238–42. doi: 10.1016/j.regg.2013.01.008
217. Brotons M, Koger SM. The impact of music therapy on language functioning in dementia. *J Music Ther.* (2000) 37:183–95. doi: 10.1093/jmt/37.3.183
218. Cowles A, Beatty WW, Nixon SJ, Lutz LJ, Paulk J, Paulk K, et al. Musical skill in dementia: a violinist presumed to have Alzheimer's disease learns to play a new song. *Neurocase* (2003) 9:493–503. doi: 10.1076/neur.9.6.493.29378
219. Van de Winckel A, Feys H, De Weerdt W, Dom R. Cognitive and behavioral effects of music-based exercises in patients with dementia. *Clin Rehabil.* (2004) 18:253–60. doi: 10.1191/0269215504cr750oa
220. Cuddy LL, Duffin J. Music memory and Alzheimer's disease: is music recognition spared in dementia, and how can it be assessed? *Med Hypotheses* (2005) 64:229–35. doi: 10.1016/j.mehy.2004.09.005
221. Fornazzari L, Castle T, Nadkarni S, Ambrose M, Miranda D, Apanasiewicz N, et al. Preservation of episodic musical memory in a pianist with Alzheimer disease. *Neurology* (2006) 66:610–1. doi: 10.1212/01.WNL.0000198242.13411.FB
222. Ceccato E, Vigato G, Bonetto C, Bevilacqua A, Pizziolo P, Crociani S, et al. STAM protocol in dementia: a multicenter, single-blind, randomized, and controlled trial. *Am J Alzheimers Dis Other Demen.* (2012) 27:301–10. doi: 10.1177/1533317512452038
223. Baird A, Samson S. Music and dementia. *Prog Brain Res.* (2015) 217:207–35. doi: 10.1016/bs.pbr.2014.11.028
224. Samson S, Clément S, Narme P, Schiaratura L, Ehrlé N. Efficacy of musical interventions in dementia: methodological requirements of non-pharmacological trials. *Ann NY Acad Sci.* (2015) 1337:249–55. doi: 10.1111/nyas.12621
225. Giovagnoli AR, Manfredi V, Schifano L, Paterlini C, Parente A, Tagliavini F. Combining drug and music therapy in patients with moderate Alzheimer's disease: a randomized study. *Neurol Sci.* (2018) 39:1021–8. doi: 10.1007/s10072-018-3316-3
226. Fusar-Poli L, Bieleninik L, Brondino N, Xi-Jing C, Gold C. The effect of music therapy on cognitive functions in patients with dementia: a systematic review and meta-analysis. *Aging Ment Health* (2017) 10:1–10. doi: 10.1080/13607863.2017.1348474
227. British Association of Art Therapists website. Available online at: www.baat.org (Accessed on 25 September, 2018).
228. Chancellor B, Duncan A, Chatterjee A. Art therapy for Alzheimer's disease and other dementias. *J Alzheimers Dis.* (2014) 39:1–11. doi: 10.3233/JAD-131295
229. Silveri MC, Ferrante I, Brita AC, Rossi P, Liperoti R, Mammarella F, et al. The Memory of Beauty survives Alzheimer's disease (but cannot help memory). *J Alzheimers Dis.* (2015) 45:483–94. doi: 10.3233/JAD-141434
230. Sterritt PF, Pokorny ME. Art activities for patients with Alzheimer's and related disorders. *Geriatr Nurs.* (1994) 15:155–9. doi: 10.1016/S0197-4572(09)90043-X
231. Rentz CA. Memories in the making: outcome-based evaluation of an art program for individuals with dementing illnesses. *Am J Alzheimers Dis Other Demen.* (2002) 17:175–81. doi: 10.1177/153331750201700310
232. Bonner C. *Reducing Stress-Related Behaviours in People With Dementia-Care-Based Therapy.* London: Jessica Kingsley Publishers (2006).
233. Hannemann BT. Creativity with dementia patients. Can creativity and art stimulate dementia patients positively? *Gerontology* (2006) 52:59–65. doi: 10.1159/000089827
234. Rusted J. A multi-centre randomized control group trial on the use of art therapy for older people with dementia. *Group Analysis* (2006) 39:517–36. doi: 10.1177/0533316406071447
235. Flood M, Phillips KD. Creativity in older adults: a plethora of possibilities. *Issues Ment Health Nurs.* (2007) 28:389–411. doi: 10.1080/01612840701252956
236. Schmitt B, Frölich L. Creative therapy options for patients with dementia–a systematic review. *Fortschr Neurol Psychiatr.* (2007) 75:699–707. doi: 10.1055/s-2006-944298
237. Cummings JL, Miller BL, Christensen DD, Cherry D. Creativity and dementia: emerging diagnostic and treatment methods for Alzheimer's disease. *CNS Spectr.* (2008) 13(Suppl 2):1–20.
238. Stoukides J. Creative and sensory therapies enhance the lives of people with Alzheimers. *Med Health R I.* (2008) 91:154.
239. Peisah C, Lawrence G, Reutens S. Creative solutions for severe dementia with BPSD: a case of art therapy used in an inpatient and residential care setting. *Int Psychogeriatr.* (2001) 23:1011–3. doi: 10.1017/S1041610211000457
240. Safar LT. Use of art making in treating older patients with dementia. *Virtual Mentor.* (2014) 16:626–30. doi: 10.1001/virtualmentor.2014.16.08.stas1-1408
241. Seifert K, Spottke A, Fliessbach K. Effects of sculpture based art therapy in dementia patients—a pilot study. *Helyon* (2017) 3:1–13. doi: 10.1016/j.heliyon.2017.e00460
242. Pongan E, Tillmann B, Leveque Y, Trombert B, Getenet JC, Auguste N, et al. Can musical or painting interventions improve chronic pain, mood, quality of life, and cognition in patients with mild Alzheimer's disease? Evidence from a randomized controlled trial. *J Alzheimers Dis.* (2017) 60:663–77. doi: 10.3233/JAD-170410
243. Hsu TJ, Tsai HT, Hwang AC, Chen LY, Chen LK. Predictors of non-pharmacological intervention effect on cognitive function and behavioral and psychological symptoms of older people with dementia. *Geriatr Gerontol Int.* (2017) 17:28–35. doi: 10.1111/ggi.13037
244. Rowe M, Alfred D. The effectiveness of slow-stroke massage in diffusing agitated behaviours in individuals with Alzheimer's disease. *J Gerontol Nurs.* (1999) 25:22–34.
245. Remington R. Calming music and hand massage with agitated elderly. *Nurs Res.* (2002) 51:317–23. doi: 10.1097/00006199-200209000-00008
246. Nelson D. The power of human touch in Alzheimer's care. *Massage Ther J.* (2004) 43:82–92.
247. Moyle W, Johnston A, O'Dwyer S. Exploring the effect of foot massage on agitated behaviours in older people with dementia: a pilot study. *Aust J Ageing* (2011) 30:159–61. doi: 10.1111/j.1741-6612.2010.00504.x
248. Rodríguez-Mansilla J, González López-Arza MV, Varela-Donoso E, Montanero-Fernández J, González Sánchez B, Garrido-Ardila EM. The effects of ear acupressure, massage therapy and no therapy on symptoms of dementia: a randomized controlled trial. *Clin Rehabil.* (2015) 29:683–93. doi: 10.1177/0269215514554240
249. Moyle W, Cooke ML, Beattie E, Shum DH, O'Dwyer ST, Barrett S, et al. Foot massage and physiological stress in people with dementia: a randomized controlled trial. *J Altern Complement Med.* (2014) 20:305–11. doi: 10.1089/acm.2013.0177
250. Kapoor Y, Orr R. Effect of therapeutic massage on pain in patients with dementia. *Dementia* (2015) 1. doi: 10.1177/1471301215583391
251. Wang HL, Keck JF. Foot and hand massage as an intervention for postoperative pain. *Pain Manag Nurs.* (2004) 5:59–65. doi: 10.1016/j.pmn.2004.01.002
252. Bush E. The use of human touch to improve the well-being of older adults: a holistic nursing intervention. *J Holistic Nurs.* (2011) 19:256–70. doi: 10.1177/089801010101900306
253. Wu J, Wang Y, Wang Z. The effectiveness of massage and touch on behavioural and psychological symptoms of dementia: a quantitative

systematic review and meta-analysis. *J Adv Nurs.* (2017) 73:2283–95. doi: 10.1111/jan.13311
254. Culler D, Estrin D, Srivastava M. Guest editors' introduction: overview of sensor networks. *Computer* (2004) 37:41–9. doi: 10.1109/MC.2004.93
255. Cooper RA, Dicianno BE, Brewer B, LoPresti E, Ding D, Simpson R, et al. A perspective on intelligent devices and environments in medical rehabilitation. *Med Eng Phys.* (2008) 30:1387–98. doi: 10.1016/j.medengphy.2008.09.003
256. Robert PH, Konig A, Andrieu S, Bremond F, Chemin I, Chung PC, et al. Recommendations for ICT use in Alzheimer's disease assessment: Monaco CTAD expert meeting. *J Nutr Health Aging* (2013) 17:653–60. doi: 10.1007/s12603-013-0046-3
257. Rialle V, Duchene F, Noury N, Bajolle L, Demongeot J. Health "Smart" home: information technology for patients at home. *Telemed J E Health* (2002) 8:395–409. doi: 10.1089/15305620260507530
258. Powell J, Chiu T, Eysenbach G. A systematic review of networked technologies supporting carers of people with dementia. *J Telemed Telecare* (2008) 14:154–6. doi: 10.1258/jtt.2008.003018
259. Pilotto A, D'Onofrio G, Benelli E, Zanesco A, Cabello A, Margelí MC., et al. Information and communication technology systems to improve quality of life and safety of Alzheimer's disease patients: a multicenter international survey. *J Alzheimers Dis.* (2011) 23:131–41. doi: 10.3233/JAD-2010-101164
260. Romdhane R, Mulin E, Derreumeaux A, Zouba N, Piano J, Lee L, et al. Automatic video monitoring system for assessment of Alzheimer's disease symptoms. *J Nutr Health Aging* (2012) 16:213–8. doi: 10.1007/s12603-012-0039-7
261. Miskelly F. Electronic tracking of patients with dementia and wandering using mobile phone technology. *Age Ageing* (2005) 34:497–9. doi: 10.1093/ageing/afi145
262. Faucounau V, Riguet M, Orvoen G, Lacombe A, Rialle V, Extra J, et al. Electronic tracking system and wandering in Alzheimer's disease: a case study. *Ann Phys Rehabil Med.* (2009) 52:579–87. doi: 10.1016/j.rehab.2009.07.034
263. Bantry White E, Montgomery P, McShane R. Electronic tracking for people with dementia who get lost outside the home: a study of the experience of familial carers. *Br J Occup Ther.* (2010) 73:152–9. doi: 10.4276/030802210X12706313443901
264. Pot AM, Willemse BM, Horjus S. A pilot study on the use of tracking technology: feasibility, acceptability, and benefits for people in early stages of dementia and their informal caregivers. *Aging Ment Health* (2011) 16:127–34. doi: 10.1080/13607863.2011.596810
265. Teipel S, Babiloni C, Hoey J, Kaye J, Kirste T, Burmeister OK. Information and communication technology solutions for outdoor navigation in dementia. *Alzheimer Dement.* (2016) 12:695–707. doi: 10.1016/j.jalz.2015.11.003
266. Lauriks S, Reinersmann A, Van der Roest HG, Meiland FJ, Davies RJ, Moelaert F, et al. Review of ICT-based services for identified unmet needs in people with dementia. *Ageing Res Rev.* (2007) 6:223–46. doi: 10.1016/j.arr.2007.07.002
267. Olsson A, Engström M, Skovdahl K, Lampic C. My, your and our needs for safety and security: relatives' reflections on using information and communication technology in dementia care. *Scand J Caring Sci.* (2012) 26:104–12. doi: 10.1111/j.1471-6712.2011.00916.x
268. Robinson L, Hutchings D, Corner L, Finch T, Hughes J, Brittain K, et al. Balancing rights and risks: conflicting perspectives in the management of wandering in dementia. *Health Risk Soc.* (2007) 9:389–406. doi: 10.1080/13698570701612774
269. Landau R, Werner S, Auslander GK, Shoval N, Heinik J. Attitudes of family and professional care-givers towards the use of GPS for tracking patients with dementia: an exploratory study. *Br J Soc Work* (2009) 39:670–92. doi: 10.1093/bjsw/bcp037
270. Niemeijer AR, Frederiks BJ, Depla MF, Legemaate J, Eefsting JA, Hertogh CM. The ideal application of surveillance technology in residential care for people with dementia. *J Med Ethics* (2011) 37:303–10. doi: 10.1136/jme.2010.040774
271. Zwijsen SA, Depla MF, Niemeijer AR, Francke AL, Hertogh CM. Surveillance technology: an alternative to physical restraints? A qualitative study among professionals working in nursing homes for people with dementia. *Int J Nurs Stud.* (2012) 49:212–9. doi: 10.1016/j.ijnurstu.2011.09.002
272. Te Boekhorst S, Depla MF, Francke AL, Twisk JW, Zwijsen SA, Hertogh CM. Quality of life of nursing-home residents with dementia subject to surveillance technology versus physical restraints: an explorative study. *Int J Geriatr Psychiatry* (2013) 28:356–63. doi: 10.1002/gps.3831
273. Landau R, Werner S. Ethical aspects of using GPS for tracking people with dementia: recommendations for practice. *Int Psychogeriatr.* (2012) 24:358–66. doi: 10.1017/S1041610211001888
274. Niemeijer AR, Frederiks BJ, Riphagen II, Legemaate J, Eefsting JA, Hertogh CM. Ethical and practical concerns of surveillance technologies in residential care for people with dementia or intellectual disabilities: an overview of the literature. *Int Psychogeriatr.* (2010) 22:1129–42. doi: 10.1017/S1041610210000037
275. Ienca M, Wangmo T, Jotterand F, Kressig RW, Elger B. Ethical design of intelligent assistive technologies for dementia: a descriptive review. *Sci Eng Ethics* (2017) 73:1695–1700. doi: 10.1007/s11948-017-9976-1
276. Nelson A, Powell-Cope G, Gavin-Dreschnack D, Quigley P, Bulat T, Baptiste AS, et al. Technology to promote safe mobility in the elderly. *Nurs Clin North Am.* (2004) 39:649–71. doi: 10.1016/j.cnur.2004.05.001
277. Allum JH, Carpenter MG. A speedy solution for balance and gait analysis: angular velocity measured at the centre of body mass. *Curr Opin Neurol.* (2005) 18:15–21. doi: 10.1097/00019052-200502000-00005
278. Wu G, Xue S. Portable preimpact fall detector with inertial sensors. *IEEE Trans Neural Syst Rehabil Eng.* (2008) 16:178–83. doi: 10.1109/TNSRE.2007.916282
279. Schwickert L, Becker C, Lindemann U, Maréchal C, Bourke A, Chiari L, et al. Fall detection with body-worn sensors : a systematic review. *Z Gerontol Geriatr.* (2013) 46:706–19. doi: 10.1007/s00391-013-0559-8
280. Aud MA, Abbott CC, Tyrer HW, Neelgund RV, Shriniwar UG, Mohammed A, et al. Smart carpet: developing a sensor system to detect falls and summon assistance. *J Gerontol Nurs.* (2010) 36:8–12. doi: 10.3928/00989134-20100602-02
281. Chaudhuri S, Thompson H, Demiris G. Fall detection devices and their use with older adults: a systematic review. *J Geriatr Phys Ther.* (2014) 37:178–96. doi: 10.1519/JPT.0b013e3182abe779
282. Danielsen A, Olofsen H, Bremdal BA. Increasing fall risk awareness using wearables: a fall risk awareness protocol. *J Biomed Inf.* (2016) 63:184–94. doi: 10.1016/j.jbi.2016.08.016
283. Khanuja K, Joki J, Bachmann G, Cuccurullo S. Gait and balance in the aging population: Fall prevention using innovation and technology. *Maturitas* (2018) 110:51–6. doi: 10.1016/j.maturitas.2018.01.021
284. König A, Sacco G, Bensadoun G, Bremond F, David R, Verhey F, et al. The role of information and communication technologies in clinical trials with patients with Alzheimer's disease and related disorders. *Front Aging Neurosci.* (2015) 7:110. doi: 10.3389/fnagi.2015.00110
285. Sacco G, Joumier V, Darmon N, Dechamps A, Derreumaux A, Lee JH, et al. Detection of activities of daily living impairment in Alzheimer's disease and mild cognitive impairment using information and communication technology. *Clin Interv Aging* (2012) 7:539–49. doi: 10.2147/CIA.S36297
286. Okura T, Langa KM. Caregiver burden and neuropsychiatric symptoms in older adults with cognitive impairments: the aging, demographics, and memory study (ADAMS). *Alzheimer Dis Assoc Disord.* (2011) 25:116–21. doi: 10.1097/WAD.0b013e318203f208
287. Bankole A, Anderson M, Smith-Jackson T, Knight A, Oh K, Brantley J, et al. Validation of noninvasive body sensor network technology in the detection of agitation in dementia. *Am J Alzheimers Dis Other Demen.* (2012) 27:346–54. doi: 10.1177/1533317512452036
288. Cummings J, Mintzer J, Brodaty H, Sano M, Banerjee S, Devanand DP, et al. Agitation in cognitive disorders: international psychogeriatric association provisional consensus clinical and research definition. *Int Psychogeriatr.* (2015) 27:7–17. doi: 10.1017/S1041610214001963
289. Melander C, Martinsson J, Gustafsson S. Measuring electrodermal activity to improve the identification of agitation in individuals with dementia. *Dement Geriatr Cogn Disord Extra* (2017) 7:430–9. doi: 10.1159/000484890
290. Robinson L, Brittain K, Lindsay S, Jackson D, Olivier P. Keeping In Touch Everyday (KITE) project: developing assistive technologies with people with

dementia and their carers to promote independence. *Int Psychogeriatr.* (2009) 21:494–502. doi: 10.1017/S1041610209008448

291. Kime S, Lamb D, Wilson B. Use of a comprehensive program of external cueing to enhance procedural memory in a patient with dense amnesia. *Brain Inj.* (1996) 10:17–25. doi: 10.1080/026990596124683
292. Mihailidis A, Fernie GR, Barbenel JC. The use of artificial intelligence in the design of an intelligent cognitive orthosis for people with dementia. *Assist Technol.* (2001) 13:23–39. doi: 10.1080/10400435.2001.10132031
293. Hartin PJ, Nugent CD, McClean SI, Cleland I, Norton MC, Sanders C., et al. A smartphone application to evaluate technology adoption and usage in persons with dementia. *Conf Proc IEEE Eng Med Biol Soc.* (2014) 2014:5389–92. doi: 10.1109/EMBC.2014.6944844
294. Lancioni GE, Perilli V, O'Reilly MF, Singh NN, Sigafoos J, Bosco A, et al. Technology-based orientation programs to support indoor travel by persons with moderate Alzheimer's disease: impact assessment and social validation. *Res Dev Disabil.* (2013) 34:286–93. doi: 10.1016/j.ridd.2012.08.016
295. Stock SE, Davies DK, Secor RR, Wehmeyer ML. Self-directed career preference selection for individuals with intellectual disabilities: using computer technology to enhance self-determination. *J Vocat Rehabil.* (2003) 19:95–103.
296. Boman IL, Rosenberg L, Lundberg S, Nygard L. The first step in designing a videophone for people with dementia: identification of users' potentials and the requirements of communication technology. *Disabil Rehabil Assist Technol.* (2012) 7:256–363. doi: 10.3109/17483107.2011.635750
297. Perilli V, Lancioni GE, Singh NN, O'Reilly MF, Sigafoos J, Cassano G, et al. Persons with Alzheimer's disease make phone calls independently using a computer-aided telephone system. *Res Dev Disabil.* (2012) 33:1014–20. doi: 10.1016/j.ridd.2012.01.007
298. Wimo A, Winblad B, Jönsson L. An estimate of the total worldwide societal costs of dementia in 2005. *Alzheimers Dement.* (2007) 3:81–91. doi: 10.1016/j.jalz.2007.02.001
299. Wahl HW, Fänge A, Oswald F, Gitlin LN, Iwarsson S. The home environment and disability-related outcomes in aging individuals: what is the empirical evidence? *Gerontologist* (2009) 3:355–67. doi: 10.1093/geront/gnp056
300. Gitlin LN, Schinfeld S, Winter L, Corcoran M, Boyce AA, Hauck W. Evaluating home environments of persons with dementia: interrater reliability and validity of the Home Environmental Assessment Protocol (HEAP). *Disabil Rehabil.* (2002) 24:59–71. doi: 10.1080/09638280110066325
301. Marquardt G, Johnston D, Black BS, Morrison A, Rosenblatt A, Lyketsos CG, et al. A descriptive study of home modifications for people with dementia and barriers to implementation. *J Hous Elderly* (2011) 25:258–73. doi: 10.1080/02763893.2011.595612
302. Gitlin LN, Winter L, Dennis MP, Hodgson N, Hauck WW. Targeting and managing behavioral symptoms in individuals with dementia: a randomized trial of a nonpharmacological intervention. *J Am Geriatr Soc.* (2010) 58:1465–74. doi: 10.1111/j.1532-5415.2010.02971.x
303. Allen F, Cain R, Meyer C. How people with dementia and their carers adapt their homes. A qualitative study. *Dementia* (2017) 1:1471301217712294. doi: 10.1177/1471301217712294
304. Miori V, Russo D, Concordia C. Meeting people's needs in a fully interoperable domotic environment. *Sensors* (2012) 12:6802–24. doi: 10.3390/s120606802
305. Demiris G, Hensel BK. Technologies for an aging society: a systematic review of "smart home" applications. *Yearb Med Inform.* (2008) 2008:33–40.
306. Gentry T. Smart homes for people with neurological disability: state of the art. *NeuroRehabilitation* (2009) 25:209–17. doi: 10.3233/NRE-2009-0517
307. Aiello M, Aloise F, Baldoni R, Cincotti F, Guger C, Lazovik A, et al. Smart homes to improve the quality of life for all. *Conf Proc IEEE Eng Med Biol Soc.* (2011) 2011:1777–80. doi: 10.1109/IEMBS.2011.6090507
308. Ding D, Cooper RA, Pasquina PF, Fici-Pasquina L. Sensor technology for smart homes. *Maturitas* (2011) 69:131–6. doi: 10.1016/j.maturitas.2011.03.016
309. Frisardi V, Imbimbo BP. Gerontechnology for demented patients: smart homes for smart aging. *J Alzheimers Dis.* (2011) 23:143–6. doi: 10.3233/JAD-2010-101599
310. Blasco R, Marco Á, Casas R, Cirujano D, Picking R. A smart kitchen for ambient assisted living. *Sensors* (2014) 14:1629–53. doi: 10.3390/s140101629
311. Chan M, Campo E, Estève D, Fourniols JY. Smart homes - current features and future perspectives. *Maturitas* (2009) 64:90–7. doi: 10.1016/j.maturitas.2009.07.014
312. Bossen AL, Kim H, Williams KN, Steinhoff AE, Strieker M. Emerging roles for telemedicine and smart technologies in dementia care. *Smart Homecare Technol Telehealth.* (2015) 3:49–57. doi: 10.2147/SHTT.S59500
313. Ienca M, Fabrice J, Elger B, Caon M, Pappagallo AS, Kressig RW., et al. Intelligent assistive technology for Alzheimer's disease and other dementias: a systematic review. *J Alzheimers Dis.* (2017) 56:1301–40. doi: 10.3233/JAD-161037
314. Baus O, Bouchard S. Moving from virtual reality exposure-based therapy to augmented reality exposure-based therapy: a review. *Front Hum Neurosci.* (2014) 8:112. doi: 10.3389/fnhum.2014.00112
315. Gregg L, Tarrier N. Virtual reality in mental health: a review of the literature. *Soc Psychiatry Psychiatr Epidemiol.* (2007) 42:343–54. doi: 10.1007/s00127-007-0173-4
316. Cotelli M, Manenti R, Zanetti O, Miniussi C. Non-pharmacological intervention for memory decline. *Front Hum Neurosci.* (2012) 9:46. doi: 10.3389/fnhum.2012.00046
317. Déjos M, Sauzéon H, N'kaoua B. Virtual reality for clinical assessment of elderly people: early screening for Dementia. *Rev Neurol.* (2012) 168:404–14. doi: 10.1016/j.neurol.2011.09.005
318. Man DW, Chung JC, Lee GY. Evaluation of a virtual reality-based memory training programme for Hong Kong Chinese older adults with questionable dementia: a pilot study. *Int J Geriatr Psychiatry* (2012) 27:513–20. doi: 10.1002/gps.2746
319. García-Betances RI, Jiménez-Mixco V, Arredondo MT, Cabrera-Umpiérrez MF. Using virtual reality for cognitive training of the elderly. *Am J Alzheimers Dis Other Demen.* (2015) 30:49–54. doi: 10.1177/1533317514545866
320. Cogné M, Taillade M, N'Kaoua B, Tarruella A, Klinger E, Larrue F, et al. The contribution of virtual reality to the diagnosis of spatial navigation disorders and to the study of the role of navigational aids: a systematic literature review. *Ann Phys Rehab Med.* (2017) 60:164–76. doi: 10.1016/j.rehab.2015.12.004
321. Lange BS, Requejo P, Flynn SM, Rizzo AA, Valero-Cuevas FJ, Baker L, et al. The potential of virtual reality and gaming to assist successful aging with disability. *Phys Med Rehabil Clin N Am.* (2010) 21:339–56. doi: 10.1016/j.pmr.2009.12.007
322. Kalová E, Vlcek K, Jarolímová E, Bures J. Allothetic orientation and sequential ordering of places is impaired in early stages of Alzheimer's disease: corresponding results in real space tests and computer tests. *Behav Brain Res.* (2005) 159:175–86. doi: 10.1016/j.bbr.2004.10.016
323. Werner P, Rabinowitz S, Klinger E, Korczyn AD, Josman N. Use of the virtual action planning supermarket for the diagnosis of mild cognitive impairment: a preliminary study. *Dement Geriatr Cogn Disord.* (2009) 27:301–9. doi: 10.1159/000204915
324. Tarnanas I, Tsolaki M, Nef T, M Müri R, Mosimann UP. Can a novel computerized cognitive screening test provide additional information for early detection of Alzheimer's disease? *Alzheimers Dement.* (2014) 10:790–8. doi: 10.1016/j.jalz.2014.01.002
325. Zygouris S, Giakoumis D, Votis K, Doumpoulakis S, Ntovas K, Segkouli S, et al. Can a virtual reality cognitive training application fulfill a dual role? Using the virtual supermarket cognitive training application as a screening tool for mild cognitive impairment. *J Alzheimers Dis.* (2015) 44:1333–47. doi: 10.3233/JAD-141260
326. Sauzéon H, N'Kaoua B, Pala PA, Taillade M, Auriacombe S, Guitton P. Everyday-like memory for objects in ageing and Alzheimer's disease assessed in a visually complex environment: The role of executive functioning and episodic memory. *J Neuropsychol.* (2016) 10:33–58. doi: 10.1111/jnp.12055
327. Burgess N, Trinkler I, King J, Kennedy A, Cipolotti L. Impaired allocentric spatial memory underlying topographical disorientation. *Rev Neurosci.* (2006) 17:239–51. doi: 10.1515/REVNEURO.2006.17.1-2.239
328. Optale G, Urgesi C, Busato V, Marin S, Piron L, Priftis K., et al. Controlling memory impairment in elderly adults using virtual reality memory training: a randomized controlled pilot study. *Neurorehabil Neural Repair* (2010) 24:348–57. doi: 10.1177/1545968309353328
329. Weniger G, Ruhleder M, Lange C, Wolf S, Irle E. Egocentric and allocentric memory as assessed by virtual reality in individuals with

amnestic mild cognitive impairment. *Neuropsychologia* (2011) 49:518–27. doi: 10.1016/j.neuropsychologia.2010.12.031

330. Bellassen V, Iglói K, de Souza LC, Dubois B, Rondi-Reig L. Temporal order memory assessed during spatiotemporal navigation as a behavioral cognitive marker for differential Alzheimer's disease diagnosis. *J Neurosci.* (2012) 32:1942–52. doi: 10.1523/JNEUROSCI.4556-11.2012
331. Plancher G, Tirard A, Gyselinck V, Nicolas S, Piolino P. Using virtual reality to characterize episodic memory profiles in amnestic mild cognitive impairment and Alzheimer's disease: influence of active and passive encoding. *Neuropsychologia* (2012) 50:592–602. doi: 10.1016/j.neuropsychologia.2011.12.013
332. Jebara N, Orriols E, Zaoui M, Berthoz A, Piolino P. Effects of enactment in episodic memory: a pilot virtual reality study with young and elderly adults. *Front Aging Neurosci.* (2014) 6:338. doi: 10.3389/fnagi.2014.00338
333. Abichou K, La Corte V, Piolino P. Does virtual reality have a future for the study of episodic memory in aging? *Geriatr Psychol Neuropsychiatr Vieil.* (2017) 15:65–74. doi: 10.1684/pnv.2016.0648
334. Hort J, Laczó J, Vyhnálek M, Bojar M, Bures J, Vlcek K. Spatial navigation deficit in amnestic mild cognitive impairment. *Proc Natl Acad Sci USA.* (2007) 104:4042–47. doi: 10.1073/pnas.0611314104
335. Cushman LA, Stein K, Duffy CJ. Detecting navigational deficits in cognitive aging and Alzheimer disease using virtual reality. *Neurology* (2008) 71:888–95. doi: 10.1212/01.wnl.0000326262.67613.fe
336. Davis R, Ohman JM, Weisbeck C. Salient cues and wayfinding in Alzheimer's disease within a virtual senior residence. *Environm Behav.* (2017) 49:1038–65. doi: 10.1177/0013916516677341
337. Hofmann M, Rösler A, Schwarz W, Müller-Spahn F, Kräuchi K, Hock C, et al. Interactive computer-training as a therapeutic tool in Alzheimer's disease. *Compr Psychiatry* (2003) 44:213–9. doi: 10.1016/S0010-440X(03)00006-3
338. Allain P, Foloppe DA, Besnard J, Yamaguchi T, Etcharry-Bouyx F, Le Gall D, et al. Detecting everyday action deficits in Alzheimer's disease using a nonimmersive virtual reality kitchen. *J Int Neuropsychol Soc.* (2014) 20:468–77. doi: 10.1017/S1355617714000344
339. Fernandez Montenegro JM, Argyriou V. Cognitive evaluation for the diagnosis of Alzheimer's disease based on turing test and virtual environments. *Physiol Behav.* (2017) 173:42–51. doi: 10.1016/j.physbeh.2017.01.034
340. Zucchella C, Sinforiani E, Tassorelli C, Cavallini E, Tost-Pardell D, Grau S, et al. Serious games for screening pre-dementia conditions: from virtuality to reality? A pilot project. *Funct Neurol.* (2014) 29:153–8.
341. Manera V, Petit PD, Derreumaux A, Orvieto I, Romagnoli M, Lyttle G, et al. 'Kitchen and cooking,' a serious game for mild cognitive impairment and Alzheimer's disease: a pilot study. *Front Aging Neurosci.* (2015) 7:24. doi: 10.3389/fnagi.2015.00024
342. Robert PH, König A, Amieva H, Andrieu S, Bremond F, Bullock R, et al. Recommendations for the use of serious games in people with Alzheimer's Disease, related disorders and frailty. *Front Aging Neurosci.* (2014) 6:54. doi: 10.3389/fnagi.2014.00054
343. Anguera JA, Boccanfuso J, Rintoul JL, Al-Hashimi O, Faraji F, Janowich J, et al. Video game training enhances cognitive control in older adults. *Nature* (2013) 501:97–101. doi: 10.1038/nature12486
344. Nouchi R, Taki Y, Takeuchi H, Hashizume H, Akitsuki Y, Shigemune Y, et al. Brain training game improves executive functions and processing speed in the elderly: a randomized controlled trial. *PLoS ONE* (2012) 7:e29676. doi: 10.1371/journal.pone.0029676
345. Oei AC, Patterson MD. Enhancing cognition with video games: a multiple game training study. *PLoS ONE* (2013) 8:e58546. doi: 10.1371/journal.pone.0058546
346. Powers KL, Brooks PJ, Aldrich NJ, Palladino MA, Alfieri L. Effects of video-game play on information processing: a meta-analytic investigation. *Psychon Bull Rev.* (2013) 20:1055–79. doi: 10.3758/s13423-013-0418-z
347. Bisoglio J, Michaels TI, Mervis JE, Ashinoff BK. Cognitive enhancement through action video game training: great expectations require greater evidence. *Front Psychol.* (2014) 5:136. doi: 10.3389/fpsyg.2014.00136
348. Ben-Sadoun G, Sacco G, Manera V, Bourgeois J, König A, Foulon P, et al. Physical and cognitive stimulation using an exergame in subjects with normal aging, mild and moderate cognitive impairment. *J Alzheimers Dis.* (2016) 53:1299–314. doi: 10.3233/JAD-160268
349. McCallum S, Boletsis C. Dementia Games: a literature review of dementia-related Serious Games. In: Ma M, Oliveira MF, Petersen S, and Hauge JB, editors. *Serious Games Development and Applications-Lecture Notes in Computer Science.* Berlin, Heidelberg: Springer Publishing, 15–27. doi: 10.1007/978-3-642-40790-1_2
350. Narme P. Benefits of game-based leisure activities in normal aging and dementia. *Geriatr Psychol Neuropsychiatr Vieil.* (2016) 14:420–8. doi: 10.1684/pnv.2016.0632
351. Ben-Sadoun G, Manera V, Alvarez J, Sacco G, Robert P. Recommendations for the design of serious games in neurodegenerative diseases in neurodegenerative diseases. *Front Aging Neurosci.* (2018) 10:13. doi: 10.3389/fnagi.2018.00013
352. Lee JH, Kim JH, Jhoo JH, Lee KU, Kim KW, Lee DY, et al. A telemedicine system as a care modality for dementia patients in Korea. *Alzheimer Dis Assoc Disord.* 14:94–101. doi: 10.1097/00002093-200004000-00007
353. Barton C, Morris R, Rothlind J, Yaffe K. Video-telemedicine in a memory disorders clinic: evaluation and management of rural elders with cognitive impairment. *Telemed J E Health* (2011) 17:789–93. doi: 10.1089/tmj.2011.0083
354. Brims L, Oliver K. Effectiveness of assistive technology in improving the safety of people with dementia: a systematic review and meta-analysis. *Aging Ment Health* (2018) 10:1–10. doi: 10.1080/13607863.2018.1455805
355. Barlow J, Singh D, Bayer S, Curry R. A systematic review of the benefits of home telecare for frail elderly people and those with long-term conditions. *J Telemed Telecare* (2007) 13:172–9. doi: 10.1258/135763307780908058
356. Botsis T, Hartvigsen G. Current status and future perspectives in telecare for elderly people suffering from chronic diseases. *J Telemed Telecare* (2008) 14:195–203. doi: 10.1258/jtt.2008.070905
357. Cheong CK, Lim KH, Jang JW, Jhoo JH. The effect of telemedicine on the duration of treatment in dementia patients. *J Telemed Telecare* (2015) 21:214–8. doi: 10.1177/1357633X14566571
358. Tso JV, Farinpour R, Chui HC, Liu CY. A multidisciplinary model of dementia care in an underserved retirement community, made possible by telemedicine. *Front Neurol.* (2016) 7:225. doi: 10.3389/fneur.2016.00225
359. Mair F, Whitten P. Systematic review of studies of patient satisfaction with telemedicine. *BMJ* (2000) 320:1517–20. doi: 10.1136/bmj.320.7248.1517
360. Currell R, Urquhart C, Wainwright P, Lewis R. Telemedicine versus face to face patient care: effects on professional practice and health care outcomes. *Cochrane Database Syst Rev.* (2000) 2:CD002098. doi: 10.1002/14651858.CD002098
361. Asghar I, Cang S, Yu H. Usability evaluation of assistive technologies through qualitative research focusing on people with mild dementia. *Computers Human Behav.* (2018) 79:192–201. doi: 10.1016/j.chb.2017.08.034
362. Brearly TW, Shura RD, Martindale SL, Lazowski RA, Luxton DD, Shenal BV, et al. Neuropsychological test administration by videoconference: a systematic review and meta-analysis. *Neuropsychol Rev.* (2017) 27:174–86. doi: 10.1007/s11065-017-9349-1
363. Czaja SJ, Rubert MP. Telecommunications technology as an aid to family caregivers of persons with dementia. *Psychosom Med.* (2002) 64: 469–76. doi: 10.1097/00006842-200205000-00011
364. Klimova B. Mobile phone apps in the management and assessment of mild cognitive impairment and/or mild-to-moderate dementia: an opinion article on recent finding. *Front Human Neurosci.* (2017) 11:461. doi: 10.3389/fnhum.2017.00461
365. Jelcic N, Agostini M, Meneghello F, Bussè C, Parise S, Galano A, et al. Feasibility and efficacy of cognitive telerehabilitation in early Alzheimer's disease: a pilot study. *Clin Interv Aging* (2014) 24:1605–11. doi: 10.2147/CIA.S68145
366. Williams K, Arthur A, Niedens M, Moushey L, Hutfles L. In-home monitoring support for dementia caregivers: a feasibility study. *Clin Nurs Res.* (2013) 22:139–50. doi: 10.1177/1054773812460545
367. Berwig M, Dichter MN, Albers B, Wermke K, Trutschel D, Seismann-Petersen S, et al. Feasibility and effectiveness of a telephone - based social support intervention for informal caregivers of people with dementia: study protocol of the TALKING TIME project. *BMC Health Services Res.* (2017) 17:1–11. doi: 10.1186/s12913-017-2231-2

368. Egan KJ, Pinto-Bruno ÁC, Bighelli I, Berg-Weger M, van Straten A, Albanese E, et al. Online training and support programs designed to improve mental health and reduce burden among caregivers of people with dementia: a systematic review. *JAMDA* (2018) 19:200–6. doi: 10.1016/j.jamda.2017.10.023
369. Godwin KM, Mills WL, Anderson JA, Kunik ME. Technology-driven interventions for caregivers of persons with dementia: a systematic review. *Am J Alzheimers Dis Other Demen.* (2013) 28:216–22 doi: 10.1177/1533317513481091
370. Len Kelly, Natalie St Pierre-Hansen. So many databases, such little clarity: searching the literature for the topic aboriginal. *Can Fam Physician* (2008) 54:1572–3.e5.
371. Cogo E, Sampson M, Ajiferuke I, Manheimer E, Campbell K, Daniel R, Moher D. Searching for controlled trials of complementary and alternative medicine: a comparison of 15 databases. *Evid Based Complement Alternat Med.* (2011) 2011:858246. doi: 10.1093/ecam/nep038
372. Frieden TR. Evidence for health decision making - beyond randomized, controlled trials. *N Engl J Med.* (2017) 377:465–75. doi: 10.1056/NEJMra1614394

10

Prefrontal-Premotor Pathways and Motor Output in Well-Recovered Stroke Patients

Robert Schulz [1*†]***, Clemens G. Runge*** [1,2†]***, Marlene Bönstrup*** [1,3]***, Bastian Cheng*** [1]***, Christian Gerloff*** [1]***, Götz Thomalla*** [1] ***and Friedhelm C. Hummel*** [4,5,6*]

[1] Department of Neurology, University Medical Center Hamburg-Eppendorf, Hamburg, Germany, [2] Department of Neurology, University Medical Center Schleswig-Holstein, Lübeck, Germany, [3] Human Cortical Physiology and Neurorehabilitation Section, National Institute of Neurological Disorders and Stroke, National Institutes of Health, Bethesda, MD, United States, [4] Defitech Chair of Clinical Neuroengineering, Center for Neuroprosthetics and Brain Mind Institute, Swiss Federal Institute of Technology (EPFL), Geneva, Switzerland, [5] Defitech Chair of Clinical Neuroengineering, Clinique Romande de Réadaptation, Center for Neuroprosthetics and Brain Mind Institute, Swiss Federal Institute of Technology Valais (EPFL Valais), Sion, Switzerland, [6] Clinical Neuroscience, University of Geneva Medical School, Geneva, Switzerland

***Correspondence:**
Robert Schulz
rschulz@uke.de
Friedhelm C. Hummel
friedhelm.hummel@epfl.ch

† These authors have contributed equally to this work

Structural brain imaging has continuously furthered our knowledge how different pathways of the human motor system contribute to residual motor output in stroke patients. Tract-related microstructure of pathways between primary and premotor areas has been found to critically influence motor output. The motor network is not restricted in connectivity to motor and premotor areas but these brain regions are densely interconnected with prefrontal regions such as the dorsolateral (DLPFC) and ventrolateral (VLPFC) prefrontal cortex. So far, the available data about the topography of such direct pathways and their microstructural properties in humans are sparse. To what extent prefrontal-premotor connections might also relate to residual motor outcome after stroke is still an open question. The present study was designed to address this issue of structural connectivity of prefrontal-premotor pathways in 26 healthy, older participants (66 ± 10 years old, 15 male) and 30 well-recovered chronic stroke patients (64 ± 10 years old, 21 males). Probabilistic tractography was used to reconstruct direct fiber tracts between DLPFC and VLPFC and three premotor areas (dorsal and ventral premotor cortex and the supplementary motor area). Direct connections between DLPFC/VLPFC and the primary motor cortex were also tested. Tract-related microstructure was estimated for each specific tract by means of fractional anisotropy and alternative diffusion metrics. These measures were compared between the groups and related to residual motor outcome in the stroke patients. Direct prefrontal-premotor trajectories were successfully traceable in both groups. Similar in gross anatomic topography, stroke patients presented only marginal microstructural alterations of these tracts, predominantly of the affected hemisphere. However, there was no clear evidence for a significant association between tract-related microstructure of prefrontal-premotor connections and residual motor functions in the present group of well-recovered stroke patients. Direct prefrontal-motor connections between DLPFC/VLPFC and the primary motor cortex could not be reconstructed in the present healthy participants and stroke patients.

Keywords: diffusion, recovery, corticocortical, DLPFC, VLPFC, tractography

INTRODUCTION

Brain imaging has enhanced our understanding of plasticity-related functional reorganization after stroke. Within the motor domain, the focus of functional imaging based network analyses has been primarily the core motor network, comprising the primary motor cortices (M1) and secondary motor areas of the frontal lobe, such as the dorsal (PMd) and ventral (PMv) premotor cortex and the supplementary motor area (SMA). Such analyses could demonstrate that both active and passive network states and their temporal changes over time significantly relate to residual motor functioning and recovery processes (1). Diffusion-weighted imaging has shown that also the structural state of the underlying fiber tracts connecting these brain regions is associated with motor outcome. The body of literature of such structural connectivity analyses after stroke has been recently summarized (2).

Compared to the motor execution network showing prominent and clinically relevant changes in functioning and structure, much less is known about the prefrontal cortex (PFC) and its importance after ischemic stroke. Indeed, the PFC is a large brain area with multiple heterogeneous structurally and functionally defined brain regions. Studies in healthy participants have already evidenced its important role in the cognitive and higher-order motor domains including working memory (3–6). Herein, particularly the dorsolateral prefrontal cortex (DLPFC) activation has been reported in the cognitive control of task planning and learning of action sequences. Ventrolateral prefrontal cortices (VLPFC) have been found to influence emotional and visuomotor processing, action inhibition and updating of action plans, as well as object integration (3, 5). With regard to the underlying neuronal networks, animal tracing studies (7–11) and a study in healthy participants (12) have shown that DLPFC and VLPFC show various connections to other brain regions. Particularly with respect to the core motor network, both areas have been reported to show direct structural connections to multiple premotor areas; with DLPFC being primarily connected to PMd, and VLPFC to PMv. So far, neither the presence of such connections has been probed, nor have their topographical details been analyzed systematically in elderly healthy humans.

In patients after ischemic stroke, the present understanding of the contribution of PFC to motor functions is largely based on few functional imaging studies. These have reported, for instance, increased PFC activation after stroke for simple finger tapping (13), visuomotor grip tasks, particularly in more impaired patients (14), for timed hand movements (15) and during action-selection tasks (16). Motor imagery has been found to activate PFC in stroke patients (17) and to lead to enhanced excitatory coupling with PMd and SMA which might suggest a disease-specific role of cognitive related brain areas for movement preparation and planning to facilitate proper motor output (18). It has been argued that, in this way, PFC might contribute to the increasing neuronal output from the executive motor network to spinal cord motor neurons originating in premotor areas as well (14, 19). Moreover, the success of motor sequence learning after stroke has been related to PFC network activation (20, 21). This involvement in motor learning after stroke might render the PFC a potential substrate for continuous re-learning of lost motor functions during recovery (22).

Despite these data, most previous imaging studies, particularly those aiming at connectivity analyses like dynamic causal modeling (1), have largely neglected the PFC and its connections with premotor areas, often due to the lack of activation during simple motor tasks (1, 23). This is likely to continuously bias the present perception of the influence of the PFC after stroke in the motor domain besides its role in the cognitive domain (24). Similarly, a detailed analysis of the topography of prefrontal-premotor connections and their microstructural characteristics is still lacking, both in healthy participants and in stroke patients. Though, particularly such task-independent and tract-based structural analyses seem to be warranted and needed to extend our understanding of the importance of alternative brain networks (2) supporting motor outcome after stroke.

The present study was designed to address this topic of structural connectivity of prefrontal-premotor pathways. We aimed at reconstructing pathways between the DLPFC or the VLPFC and premotor areas such as PMd, PMv, and SMA, as well as the M1 by means of diffusion-based imaging and probabilistic tractography. On one hand, a group of older, healthy participants was examined to probe the presence and topography of these connections *in vivo*, and several diffusion metrics were used to quantify their microstructural properties. On the other hand, a group of well-recovered chronic stroke patients was analyzed. For this group, we hypothesized to find significant associations between the microstructural state of some of these fiber tracts and residual motor outcome. The presence or absence of such relationships might help to update priors for future studies aiming at analazing multiple motor networks simultaneously—both at the corticocortical and corticofugal level—to better understand the importance of various structural brain networks for motor recovery.

PARTICIPANTS AND METHODS

Subjects

Thirty well-recovered patients (64.2 $\pm$ 9.7 years old (SD), median 64, range 45-82, 21 male, 3 left-handed) were included 15.5 $\pm$ 7.7 months (range 6–44) after first-ever ischemic stroke with an upper extremity motor deficit. The lesions were mainly located in subcortical areas including the brainstem. **Figure 1** illustrates the distribution of stroke lesions. A subgroup of these patients ($n = 15$) has been already included in a previous study on parietofrontal structural connectivity (25).The patients were evaluated clinically by means of the Fugl-Meyer assessment of the upper extremity (UEFM) (26), a measure of motor function, that is active movement ranges and synergies of proximal and distal muscles, and grip and pinch force values (given as proportional values affected/unaffected hand, mean value over 3 consecutive measurements for each hand) (27), measures of force and residual motor output. In addition to these individual parameters, all three scores were also combined to one composite motor outcome score (MO) (27) using a factor analysis with principal component extraction (first eigenvariate accounting

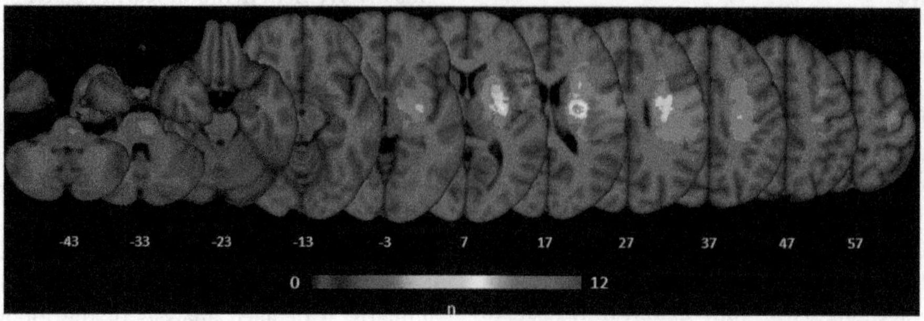

FIGURE 1 | Stroke lesions. All masks of stroke lesions were brought to the right side and overlaid on a T1 template in MNI standard space. The color bar indicates the number of subjects in which voxels lay within a stroke lesion.

for 67.6% of the variance in each variable). Demographic and clinical data are summarized in **Supplementary Table 1**. Twenty six healthy elderly participants of similar age and sex were also analyzed (66.4 ± 9.6 years old, median 69, range 48–79, 15 male, group comparison for age and sex, n.s.). The present study was approved by the local ethics committee (PV3777). All participants gave written informed consent according to the Declaration of Helsinki.

Brain Imaging

A 3T Siemens Skyra MRI scanner (Siemens, Erlangen, Germany) was used to acquire diffusion-weighted images as well as high-resolution T1-weighted images of the whole brain.

The diffusion-weighted images consisted of 75 axial slices with gradients (b = 1,500 s/mm^2) applied along 64 non-collinear directions. The sequence parameters were: repetition time (TR) = 10,000 ms, echo time (TE) = 82 ms, field of view (FOV) = 256 × 204, slice thickness (ST) = 2 mm, in-plane resolution (IPR) = 2 × 2 mm. A three-dimensional magnetization-prepared, rapid acquisition gradient-echo sequence (MPRAGE) was used for high-resolution T1-weighted images. The sequence parameters were: TR = 2,500 ms, TE = 2.12 ms, FOV = 256 × 208 mm, 256 axial slices, ST = 0.94 mm and IPR = 0.83 × 0.83 mm.

Pre-processing and Mask Creation

The FSL software package 5.1 (http://www.fmrib.ox.ac.uk/fsl) was used to analyze the diffusion-weighted and anatomical images. Prior to brain extraction, correction of eddy currents and head motion was conducted. The diffusion tensor model was fitted to each voxel and fractional anisotropy (FA) maps were calculated. FSL's *bedpostx* was used to estimate the distribution of diffusion parameters in each voxel, modeling crossing fibers using Markov Chain Monte Carlo sampling. A non-linear co-registration of the anatomical images to the individual FA maps was conducted. Both the FA maps as well as the anatomical images were then registered non-linearly to the Montreal Neurological Institute (MNI) standard space. Based on the tensor information, maps for alternative diffusion metrics that are mean diffusivity (MD), axial (AD), and radial diffusivity (RD) were also calculated. For T1 segmentation, cortical parcellation and the calculation of the cortical seed and target masks, that are SMA, PMv, PMd, M1, DLPFC, and VLPFC, we used FSL's *fast* and the Freesurfer software (http://surfer.nmr.mgh.harvard.edu/). An in-house Matlab script (Mathworks, Natick, MA, US) was used to bias the masks for SMA, PMv, PMd, and M1 toward hand representations. Details on the mask calculations are given in the **Supplementary Text 1** and also previous reports (25, 27).

Probabilistic Tractography

Structural connections were reconstructed from DLPFC and VLPFC to SMA, PMv, and PMd, respectively, applying probabilistic tractography via FSL's *probtrackx* in stroke patients and healthy participants. Also, we aimed to reconstruct probable trajectories between DLPFC and VLPFC and M1. First, 25,000 streamlines were sent from each voxel in the prefrontal seed masks VLPFC/DLPFC and also backward originating in the frontal motor masks. Both output distributions (backward/forward) (28) were then combined to estimate a tract-specific exclusion mask, in which a second tractography was conducted to control for erroneous trajectories. This procedure was already used in a previous study (25) and found to allow a reliable reconstruction of trajectories with, compared to others, small structural connectivity probabilities. The final probabilistic tractography distribution (28) was then analyzed applying four different thresholds from 1 to 10% (from more liberal to more restricted spatial extent). Tract-related mean FA, a widely used diffusion metric and surrogate parameter of white matter microstructure, was calculated for each tract and averaged across all four thresholds. Details on this procedure are given in **Supplementary Text 2**. Tract-related alternative diffusions metrics MD, AD, and RD values were also estimated to provide a more detailed picture about the microstructural characteristics of the prefrontal-premotor connections. Herein, as inverse measures of membrane density, MD and RD increases have been reported to parallel white matter demyelination, whereas AD decreases have been primarily correlated with axonal injury (29). Data of 26 healthy participants were also analyzed to allow for group comparisons. To account for the distribution of dominant and non-dominant hemispheres affected, the right and left hemispheres of the healthy participants were pseudo-randomly assigned to the "affected" (AH, right) and "unaffected" (UH, left) hemisphere, respectively. To assess the topographic distribution of each tract, we applied a center-of-gravity (COG) analysis along coronal slices in MNI space in steps of 2 mm from $y = -40$ to $y = 70$. Tract-related COG coordinate values were calculated for each participant, tract and threshold, and averaged across all thresholds in each slices. Only coordinates comprising values of at least two of the thresholds were considered.

As the corticospinal tract (CST) from M1 critically influences residual motor outcome after stroke (19), structure-function relationships for the corticocortical connections were analyzed by accounting for the integrity of the CST. Templates for this tract, originating from M1 hand area, derived from 26 healthy participants, were available for both sides from a previous study (27). Using these templates, tract-related FA values for the CST were calculated for the affected and unaffected hemispheres at the level from the mesencephalon to the cerebral peduncle (MNI: $z = -25$ to $z = -20$), given as proportional values affected/unaffected hemispheres.

Statistics

R (version 3.3.2) and RStudio (version 1.0.136) were used for the statistical analyses. R's *lmer* function for linear mixed-effects modeling with repeated measures was used to compare tract-related diffusion metrics (separate models for FA, MD, RD, AD values, each value as the dependent variable) for every tract of interest (effect TRACT) of both hemispheres (effect SIDE) between stroke patients and healthy participants (effect GROUP). Stepwise back elimination of relevant non-significant interactions (GROUP*TRACT*SIDE, GROUP*TRACT, GROUP*SIDE) and main effects was conducted for model simplification. The effects of age (AGE) and whether the dominant or non-dominant hemisphere was affected by the stroke (effect DOM) were included in the models as covariates. For group comparisons of COG coordinates of the tract locations, we used individual Student's *t*-tests (unpaired, 2-tailed). To explore structure-function relationships, we used R's *lm* function for multiple linear regression modeling. Separate models were fitted for each diffusion metric (FA, MD, RD, and AD) and with grip force, pinch force, UEFM, or MO, respectively, as the dependent variables. Here, AGE, DOM and also time after stroke (effect TAS) were included as covariates. Additionally, the level of damage to the CST was included in the models to account for its influence on motor outcome in chronic stroke patients (27). *Post-hoc*, we evaluated separate, additional models with lesion size (*log*-transformed) as another covariate to investigate its influence on structure-function relationships. Results are given as mean ± standard deviation (SD) or 95% confidence intervals (CI) as indicated. Statistical significance was assumed at $P < 0.05$ corrected by means of FDR correction (30), *P*-values were also reported as uncorrected values. The level of significance was indicated by asterisks, $^{*}P < 0.05$, $^{**}P < 0.01$, uncorrected.

RESULTS

Probabilistic Tractography of Prefrontal-Premotor Pathways

Probable trajectories connecting DLPFC and VLPFC with PMv, PMd, and SMA were reconstructed in the stroke patients and healthy participants. For PMv- and PMd-related connections we found similar spatial distributions across participants. As indicated by the center-of-gravity topographic analysis for DLPFC-derived tracts in **Figure 2** and VLPFC in **Figure 3** (see also **Table 1** and **Supplementary Figures 1, 2** for the results of the healthy participants), the majority of prefrontal-premotor pathways were located in the 2nd component of the superior longitudinal fascicle (SLF II). Trajectories connecting VLPFC and PMv appeared to be located rather in the 3rd than 2nd component (SLF III). With high spatial variability particularly in the stroke patients, SMA-related trajectories to DLPFC and VLPFC were partly located also in the 1st part of the superior longitudinal fascicle (SLF I) (25, 31, 32). Compared to the healthy participants, the patients showed a more laterocaudal mean distribution of DLPFC-SMA fibers in the unaffected hemisphere (**Table 1**). All other tracts did not show significant group differences in this coronal position. Overall, there was an anatomically plausible topographic distribution of prefrontal connections targeting SMA, PMv, and PMd with the connection of PMv to DLPFC/VLPFC being located in a ventrolateral position and DLPFC/VLPFC-PMd being located more medially. We also sought to reconstruct probable connections between DLPFC/VLPFC and M1. However, this did not result in successful tracking. In most cases the trajectories reconstructed by our approach included pathways through the primary sensory cortex (S1, postcentral gyrus). Hence, it was not possible to isolate direct connections from DLPFC/VLPFC to M1 from potential indirect connections via S1. Consequently, the connection between M1 and DLPFC/VLPFC was excluded from further analyses (data not shown).

Tract-Related White Matter Microstructure of Prefrontal-Premotor Connections

Linear mixed-effects models with repeated measures were estimated to compare tract-related microstructure between stroke patients and healthy participants. For tract-related FA, we did not find tract- and side-specific group differences (GROUP*TRACT*SIDE interaction: $F = 1.58$, $P = 0.17$). However, the simplified model showed a significant GROUP effect ($F = 5.54$, $P = 0.02$), indicating an unspecific, only marginal reduction of prefrontal-premotor FA in chronic stroke patients with estimated FA mean values [95% CI] of 0.33 [0.32–0.34] for patients and 0.34 [0.34–0.35] for healthy participants). **Table 2** summarizes tract-related mean FA values for both hemispheres and both groups. Triple interaction was similarly not significantly contributing to the models for the other diffusion metrics MD ($F = 1.75$, $P = 0.15$), RD ($F = 2.02$, $P = 0.10$), and AD ($F = 0.86$, $P = 0.51$). For MD however, there was a significant GROUP*SIDE interaction ($F = 13.80$, $P < 0.01$) with only marginally increased tract-related MD in the tracts on the affected hemisphere in stroke patients compared to the healthy participants. Likewise, also RD values (GROUP*SIDE, $F = 8.34$, $P < 0.01$) and AD values were slightly higher in the lesioned hemisphere of the patients (GROUP*SIDE interaction: $F = 20.50$, $P < 0.01$). MD, RD, and AD mean values are given in **Supplementary Table 3.**

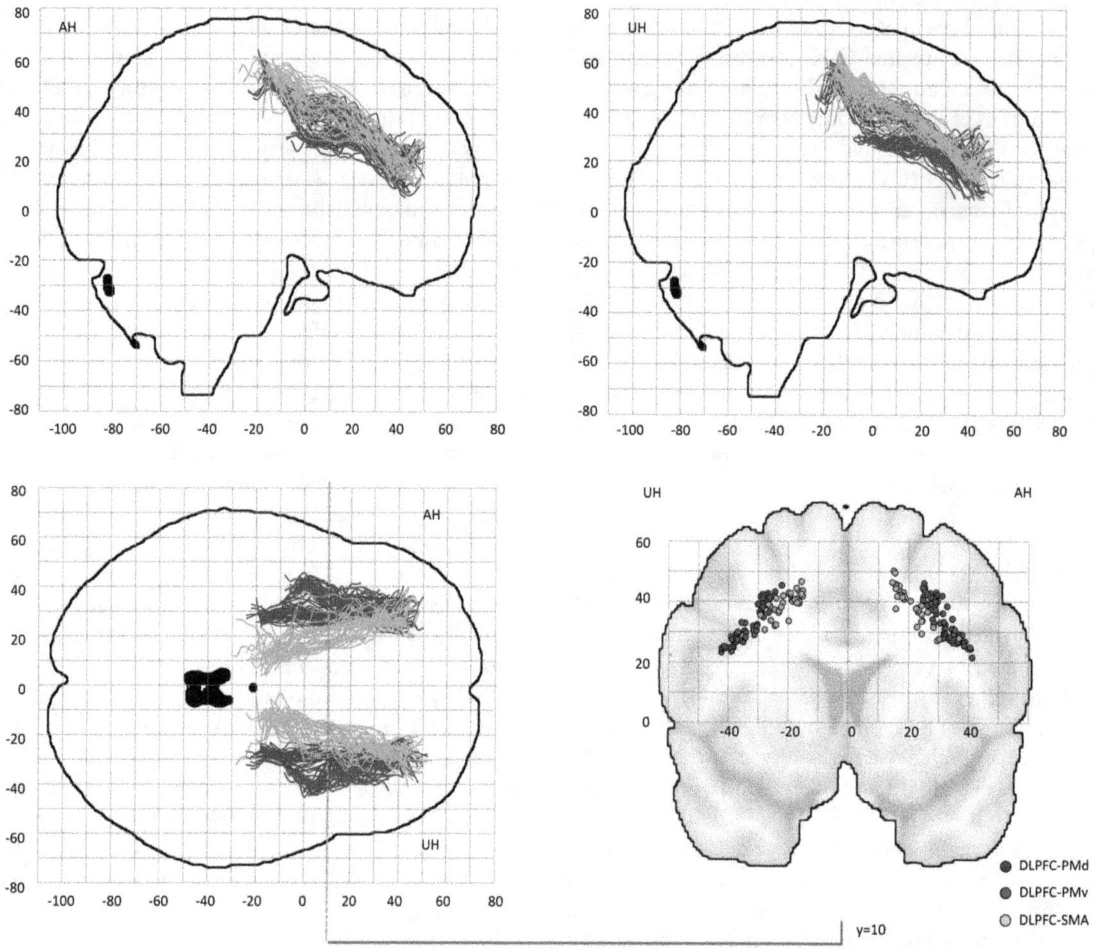

FIGURE 2 | Center-of-gravity analysis of prefrontal-premotor connections in chronic stroke patients (DLPFC). The mean center-of-gravity coordinate of all given tracts and patients was calculated from y = −40 to y = 70 (MNI standard space) in 2 mm steps. Notably, only those y-values were presented in which more than two thresholds contributed to the final coordinate. All individual tracts are shown on two sagital slices, one horizontal slice and one coronal slice at y = 10. **Table 1** provides statistics on the center-of-gravity analysis at the coronal level. DLPFC, dorsolateral prefrontal cortex; PMd, dorsal premotor cortex; PMv, ventral premotor cortex; SMA, supplementary motor area.

Tract-Related White Matter Microstructure and Residual Motor Outcome After Stroke

Individual multiple linear regression models were fitted for tract-related FA values for all prefrontal-premotor connections to estimate their influence on aspects of residual motor output in chronic stroke patients. **Table 3** summarizes the estimated coefficients for each tract with uncorrected *P*-values following the exploratory approach of the present study. Of note, after *post-hoc* false-discovery-rate (FDR) correction for 48 tests (30), there was no significant association for any of the tracts of interest, neither for residual motor output (grip, pinch forces), motor functions (UEFM) nor gross motor outcome (MO). Without correction though, we observed a significant positive influence of tract-related FA and pinch force ($P < 0.01$) for the connection DLPFC-PMv of the unaffected hemisphere. However, for whole-hand grip force and UEFM, the same tract did not show a similar structure-function association ($P = 0.46$ and $P = 0.47$, respectively). In order to explore the nature of this relationship in more detail, we also analyzed tract-related MD, RD and AD values. For DLPFC-PMv of the unaffected hemisphere, we found negative correlations with pinch force values for MD and RD values ($P < 0.01$), tract-related AD was not related to pinch forces. Similarly, all other behavioral measures were not related to MD, RD, or AD values of this specific tract. Finally, there was a negative correlation between UEFM and tract-related FA for DLPFC-PMv ($P = 0.045$) for the affected and a positive correlation between UEFM and tract-related AD for VLPFC-PMv ($P = 0.03$) of the unaffected hemisphere. All other models did not show significant results (see **Supplementary Tables 4–6** for estimated coefficients for tract-related MD, RD and AD values). *Post-hoc*, we explored whether lesion sizes (*log*-transformed) would influence these findings. However, including this additional covariate in the models did not change the present modeling results (see **Supplementary Tables 7–10**).

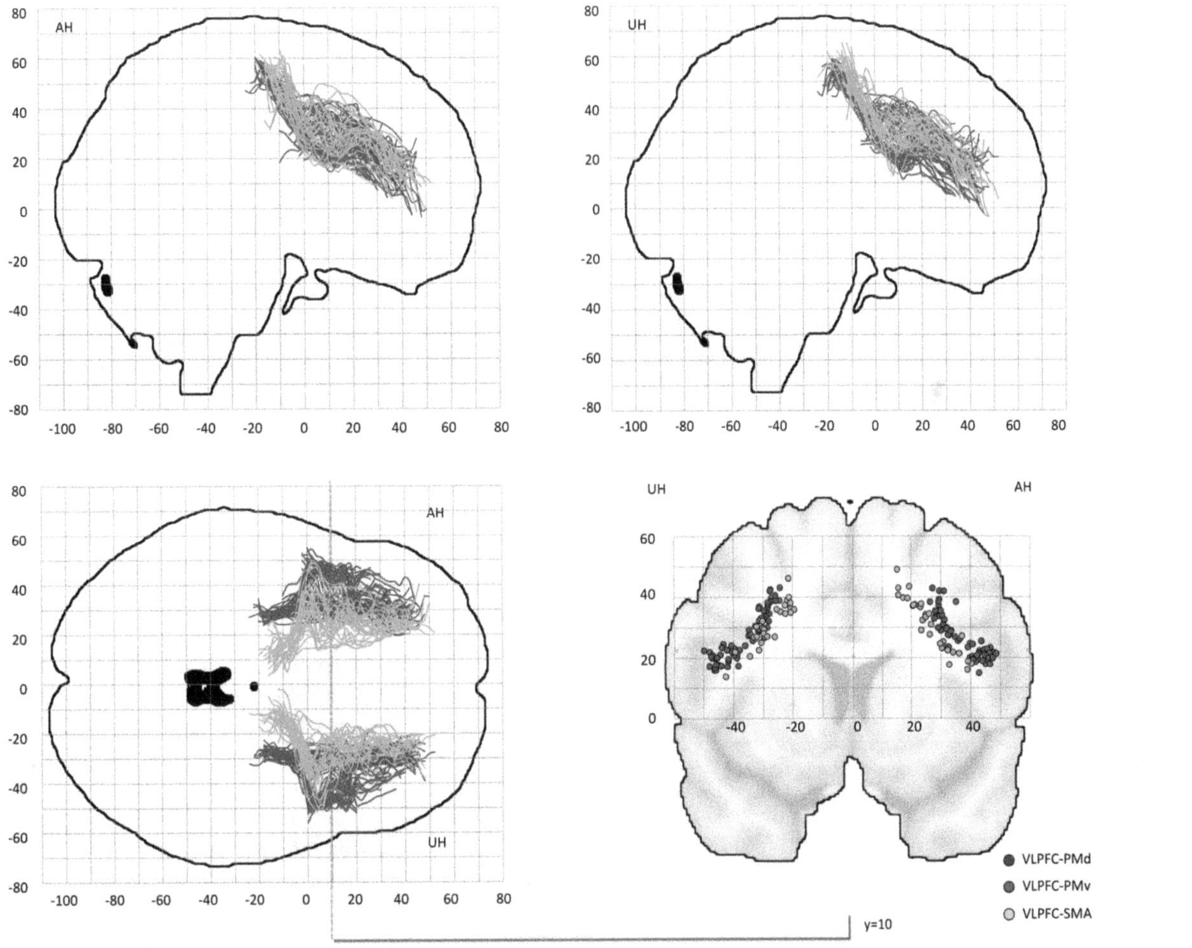

FIGURE 3 | Center-of-gravity analysis of prefrontal-premotor connections in chronic stroke patients (VLPFC). The mean center-of-gravity of all given tracts and patients was calculated from y = −40 to y = 70 (MNI standard space) in 2 mm steps. Notably, only those y-values were presented in which more than two thresholds contributed to the final coordinate. All individual tracts are shown on two sagital slices, one horizontal slice and one coronal slice at y = 10. **Table 1** provides statistics on the center-of-gravity analysis at the coronal level. VLPFC, ventrolateral prefrontal cortex; PMd, dorsal premotor cortex; PMv, ventral premotor cortex; SMA, supplementary motor area.

DISCUSSION

In the present study, we determined the topography and microstructural state of prefrontal-premotor connections of the human brain in a group of healthy aged participants and well-recovered chronic stroke patients. The data show that prefrontal-premotor trajectories are traceable in both groups. Similar in gross anatomic topography, stroke patients presented only marginal microstructural alterations of these tracts, predominantly of the affected hemisphere. However, there was no clear evidence for a significant association between tract-related microstructure of prefrontal-premotor connections and residual motor functions after stroke.

Using probabilistic tractography, we were able to reconstruct probable trajectories connecting DLPFC and VLPFC with PMd, PMv, and SMA in older healthy participants and chronic stroke patients. For DLPFC, this was in good agreement with tracing data in monkeys reporting strong connections between DLPFC and the whole extent of PMv equivalent areas. For SMA and PMd, DLPFC-premotor trajectories have been found to be restricted only to premotor regions, which are connected to M1, with higher connectivity for SMA than for PMd (7). Other tracing studies have reported variable connection strengths for DLPFC-PMd (8–10). Previous tractography data in humans have shown comparable connection strengths for DLPFC-PMv and DLPFC-PMd (12). For VLPFC, pathways have been traced in monkeys to PMv and, to a lesser extent, also to PMd equivalent brain regions (8, 10, 11). Similar findings have been reported for humans (12). Hence, the available data for direct DLPFC/VLPFC-SMA connections in monkeys seem to be rather inconclusive. Given increased spatial variability of these connections also in our sample, the allocation of prefrontal-SMA trajectories to SLF I remains relatively vague and should be interpreted with caution. As these trajectories were found to cross from the lateral to the medial surface of the frontal lobe, other crossing fibers of the SLF are likely to influence the present tract reconstructions.

TABLE 1 | Tract-related centers-of-gravity of DLPFC/VLPFC connections at y = 10 (MNI) for stroke patients and healthy participants.

	Group	DLPFC-PMd		DLPFC-PMv		DLPFC-SMA	
		AH	UH	AH	UH	AH	UH
X	Stroke	28.03 (±2.16)	−28.33 (±2.04)	35.22 (±3.12)	−37.18 (±3.40)	20.77 (±5.48)	−20.69** (±4.14)
	Control	27.43 (±1.68)	−27.64 (±2.91)	36.91 (±3.33)	−36.74 (±2.88)	18.99 (± 4.24)	−17.68 (±2.79)
Z	Stroke	39.73 (±3.58)	38.58 (±3.84)	28.60 (±3.53)	27.71 (±2.78)	39.46 (±6.13)	39.02** (±3.88)
	Control	40.29 (±2.38)	39.60 (±3.66)	27.89 (±2.68)	28.58 (±2.50)	41.63 (±3.70)	42.23 (±2.98)
	Group	**VLPFC-PMd**		**VLPFC-PMv**		**VLPFC-SMA**	
		AH	**UH**	**AH**	**UH**	**AH**	**UH**
x	Stroke	30.26 (±1.94)	−29.91 (±3.25)	42.86 (±3.55)	−43.45 (±3.50)	26.65 (±7.40)	−28.08 (±5.86)
	Control	29.92 (±1.82)	−30.79 (±3.12)	43.62 (±3.02)	−43.33 (±2.51)	29.22 (± 6.74)	−28.54 (±5.27)
z	Stroke	33.51 (±4.83)	34.20 (±5.74)	21.77 (±4.08)	20.36 (±2.50)	30.80 (±8.86)	30.49 (±6.85)
	Control	33.58 (±4.18)	32.31 (±6.79)	20.07 (±2.74)	20.65 (±2.18)	28.09 (±8.07)	28.59 (±6.33)

Centers-of-gravity of prefrontal-premotor connections at the mid-level of the connections (y = 10) for stroke patients and healthy participants. Individual x- and z-values are given as mean (±SD) for the affected (AH) and unaffected (UH) hemisphere for both groups. DLPFC, dorsolateral prefrontal cortex; VLPFC, ventrolateral prefrontal cortex; PMd, dorsal premotor cortex; PMv, ventral premotor cortex; SMA, supplementary motor area. Significant group differences are indicated by asterisks.

TABLE 2 | Tract-related white matter microstructure in stroke patients and healthy participants.

		DLPFC-PMd		DLPFC-PMv		DLPFC-SMA	
		AH	UH	AH	UH	AH	UH
FA	Stroke	0.34 (±0.03)	0.35 (±0.02)	0.31 (±0.03)	0.32 (±0.03)	0.36 (±0.03)	0.36 (±0.03)
	Control	0.35 (±0.03)	0.35 (±0.02)	0.32 (±0.03)	0.33 (±0.03)	0.37 (±0.03)	0.38 (±0.04)
		VLPFC-PMd		**VLPFC-PMv**		**VLPFC-SMA**	
		AH	**UH**	**AH**	**UH**	**AH**	**UH**
FA	Stroke	0.34 (±0.03)	0.35 (±0.02)	0.26 (±0.03)	0.26 (±0.02)	0.36 (±0.03)	0.37 (±0.03)
	Control	0.36 (±0.03)	0.36 (±0.02)	0.26 (±0.03)	0.26 (±0.03)	0.38 (±0.02)	0.38 (±0.03)

Overview of mean FA values presented as means (±SD) for the affected (AH) and unaffected (UH) hemisphere. FA, fractional anisotropy; DLPFC, dorsolateral prefrontal cortex; VLPFC, ventrolateral prefrontal cortex; PMd, dorsal premotor cortex; PMv, ventral premotor cortex; SMA, supplementary motor area.

More elaborated diffusion-based imaging techniques, e.g., based on constrained spherical deconvolution (33), might be helpful and needed to verify the present results. Nevertheless, the present study provides first topographic connectivity data for prefrontal-premotor pathways in healthy humans and also stroke patients *in vivo*. One study has already reported connection strengths for PMv and PMd in healthy participants, but has not investigated the topography of the underlying pathways (12). Here, PMv- and PMd-related connections of DLPFC and VLPFC could be largely allocated to SLF II and VLPFC-PMv trajectories to SLF III. In fact, these distributions are well in line with previous data in monkeys (34). Finally, for M1, our data corroborated previous monkey studies arguing against the existence of direct prefrontal-primary motor connection (7, 10, 35–37) indicating that prefrontal cortices are likely to influence the core motor network indirectly via premotor regions and not directly via M1.

We assessed tract-related microstructure by means of different diffusion metrics with a primary focus on tract-related mean FA as a surrogate parameter of white matter integrity, a complex, indirect measure influenced by axonal diameter and fiber density, coherence of fiber bundles and other biophysical properties (38). In order to draw a more complete picture, alternative diffusion metrics MD, RD and AD, were also assessed. We found an unspecific and only marginal reduction of tract-related FA of all tracts in the stroke patients with slightly increased tract-related MD, RD also AD values of the pathways of the affected hemisphere compared to that of the healthy participants. Previous whole brain analyses have revealed white matter changes in prefrontal-premotor brain regions in subacute (39) but not in chronic stroke patients (40, 41). The interpretation of these results (39) is neither simple nor straightforward due to technical limitations. The association fibers of the SLF investigated are crossed by corticofugal fibers, e.g., originating from the premotor areas. Thus, single voxels are likely to include multiple fiber populations with variable orientations. The validity of single-tensor derived measures is likely to be limited.

With regard to structure-function relationships, the present explorations of prefrontal-premotor and prefrontal-motor tracts did not reveal a relevant association between the microstructural properties of these tracts and residual motor outcome after stroke. There are some factors that might serve as potential explanations. First, the present sample included largely very well-recovered stroke patients in the chronic stage of recovery. In fact, previous task-related functional imaging studies have reported increased bilateral prefrontal brain activation for simple hand movements in severely impaired patients early after stroke (42) and in patients with variable deficits and intervals after stroke (41). Another study has found a negative correlation between bilateral DLPFC activation and CST integrity (14). In terms of network analyses, there is only very limited data on potential interactions of DLPFC with other brain regions and their relevance for motor output after stroke, both for task-dependent (18) and task-free resting-state analyses (43, 44). For instance, Park et al. have found in more impaired patients (mean UEFM at onset = 24) that early functional connectivity between ipsilesional M1 and contralesional DLPFC relates to motor output 6 months later (43). Hence, the present negative result overall might be explained by the high level of recovery and the time point after stroke and might change in more severely

TABLE 3 | Tract-related mean FA and residual motor output after stroke.

Parameter	Side	Tract	Estimated coefficient	Confidence interval		*T*-Value	*P*-Value
				Lower	Upper		
Grip	AH	DLPFC-PMd	0.35	−1.49	2.20	0.40	0.70
		DLPFC-PMv	−1.02	−2.92	0.89	−1.10	0.28
		DLPFC-SMA	0.07	−1.59	1.72	0.08	0.93
	UH	DLPFC-PMd	0.70	−1.71	3.10	0.60	0.56
		DLPFC-PMv	0.70	−1.22	2.63	0.76	0.46
		DLPFC-SMA	0.56	−1.46	2.57	0.57	0.57
	AH	VLPFC-PMd	0.05	−1.99	2.09	0.05	0.96
		VLPFC-PMv	0.03	−2.50	2.57	0.03	0.98
		VLPFC-SMA	−0.06	−1.83	1.72	−0.06	0.95
	UH	VLPFC-PMd	1.01	−1.46	3.49	0.85	0.41
		VLPFC-PMv	0.96	−2.56	4.47	0.56	0.58
		VLPFC-SMA	0.02	−1.97	2.01	0.02	0.99
Pinch	AH	DLPFC-PMd	1.72	−0.54	3.99	1.57	0.13
		DLPFC-PMv	0.66	−1.84	3.16	0.54	0.59
		DLPFC-SMA	0.56	−1.55	2.67	0.55	0.59
	UH	DLPFC-PMd	0.78	−2.32	3.88	0.52	0.61
		DLPFC-PMv	3.48	1.46	5.51	3.55	< 0.01**
		DLPFC-SMA	0.77	−1.82	3.35	0.61	0.55
	AH	VLPFC-PMd	2.29	−0.16	4.73	1.93	0.07
		VLPFC-PMv	0.53	−2.72	3.78	0.34	0.74
		VLPFC-SMA	0.89	−1.35	3.14	0.82	0.42
	UH	VLPFC-PMd	1.31	−1.87	4.48	0.85	0.41
		VLPFC-PMv	−0.77	−5.31	3.77	−0.35	0.73
		VLPFC-SMA	0.77	−1.76	3.31	0.63	0.53
UEFM	AH	DLPFC-PMd	−16.26	−63.79	31.26	−0.71	0.49
		DLPFC-PMv	−47.72	−94.34	−1.11	−2.11	0.045*
		DLPFC-SMA	−5.05	−47.95	37.84	−0.24	0.81
	UH	DLPFC-PMd	−11.05	−73.81	51.71	−0.36	0.72
		DLPFC-PMv	17.87	−32.09	67.82	0.74	0.47
		DLPFC-SMA	4.26	−48.41	56.92	0.17	0.87
	AH	VLPFC-PMd	−23.10	−75.24	29.04	−0.91	0.37
		VLPFC-PMv	−12.54	−78.19	53.11	−0.39	0.70
		VLPFC-SMA	−20.08	−65.27	25.10	−0.92	0.37
	UH	VLPFC-PMd	−12.48	−77.42	52.47	−0.40	0.70
		VLPFC-PMv	−10.95	−102.79	80.89	−0.25	0.81
		VLPFC-SMA	−9.52	−60.99	41.96	−0.38	0.71
MO	AH	DLPFC-PMd	4.37	−12.42	21.17	0.54	0.60
		DLPFC-PMv	−8.35	−25.86	9.16	−0.98	0.33
		DLPFC-SMA	1.29	−13.81	16.39	0.18	0.86
	UH	DLPFC-PMd	3.33	−18.77	25.42	0.31	0.76
		DLPFC-PMv	16.10	−0.32	32.53	2.02	0.05
		DLPFC-SMA	5.01	−13.41	23.43	0.56	0.58
	AH	VLPFC-PMd	4.11	−14.47	22.69	0.46	0.65
		VLPFC-PMv	0.00	−23.17	23.17	0.00	1.00
		VLPFC-SMA	−0.26	−16.43	15.92	−0.03	0.97
	UH	VLPFC–PMd	5.92	−16.87	28.70	0.54	0.60
		VLPFC-PMv	−0.65	−33.00	31.70	−0.04	0.97
		VLPFC-SMA	1.15	−17.01	19.31	0.13	0.90

Individual multiple linear regression models were estimated for each tract to test the relationship between tract-related mean FA values and the four behavioral parameter grip force (Grip), pinch force (Pinch) values, UEFM score, and the composite score MO. Estimated coefficients of the tract-related FA values were adjusted for age, lesioned hemisphere (dominant or non-dominant), time after stroke and CST integrity and are given with 95% confidence intervals. P-values are derived from each model separately and were not corrected for multiple testing. Note that after correction for 48 models (30), none of the tracts reached the level of significance. Estimated coefficients of the four covariates are not shown for the sake of clarity. AH, affected hemisphere, UH, unaffected hemisphere. Asterisks indicate significant tracts.

impaired patients in the acute or subacute phase after stroke. A future longitudinal study across various stages of recovery might add to a more detailed understanding of the importance of prefrontal-premotor connections for stroke recovery. Second, clinically relevant measures of residual motor output (grip and pinch forces) and motor function (UEFM) and their statistical combination via factor analysis were used to examine structure-behavior relationships in the stroke patients. Hence, the cognitive load of these tasks might have been too small for the present well-recovered stroke patients to uncover significant associations between prefrontal-premotor connections and motor function.

Some limitations of the present analysis are further worth to consider. First, patients with mainly subcortical lesions sparing prefrontal brain regions were included. To what extent our findings for prefrontal-premotor connections—remote from the lesion—can be generalized to patients with lesions directly affecting these connections remains a topic for future studies. Second, rather simple behavioral measures were used for structure-function analyses. To what extent structural properties of prefrontal-premotor connections might contribute to more complex functions (24), motor output and learning processes after stroke also remains to be investigated by future studies. For instance, cognitively more demanding tasks such as dual tasks might be able to uncover a functional importance of prefrontal-premotor structural connectivity in stroke patients. Third, based on clear a priori hypotheses, we focused on defined prefrontal-premotor connections at the cortical level. The present results are not exhaustive, and the state of other motor networks, such as prefrontal-subcortical (45) or prefrontal-cerebellar circuits, might also influence comparable analyses.

AUTHOR CONTRIBUTIONS

RS: study idea, study design, data acquisition, data analysis, interpretation, preparation of manuscript. CR: data analyses, interpretation, preparation of manuscript. MB and BC: data acquisition, revision of manuscript. GT and CG: providing data, interpretation, revision of manuscript. FH: study idea, study design, providing data, interpretation, and revision of manuscript.

REFERENCES

1. Rehme AK, Grefkes C. Cerebral network disorders after stroke: evidence from imaging-based connectivity analyses of active and resting brain states in humans. *J Physiol.* (2013) 591:17–31. doi: 10.1113/jphysiol.2012.243469
2. Koch P, Schulz R, Hummel FC. Structural connectivity analyses in motor recovery research after stroke. *Ann Clin Transl Neurol.* (2016) 3:233–44. doi: 10.1002/acn3.278
3. Miller EK, Freedman DJ, Wallis JD. The prefrontal cortex: categories, concepts and cognition. *Philos Trans R Soc Lond B Biol Sci.* (2002) 357:1123–36. doi: 10.1098/rstb.2002.1099
4. Funahashi S. Working memory in the prefrontal cortex. *Brain Sci.* (2017) 7:49. doi: 10.3390/brainsci7050049
5. Miller EK, Cohen JD. An integrative theory of prefrontal cortex function. *Annu Rev Neurosci.* (2001) 24:167–202. doi: 10.1146/annurev.neuro.24.1.167
6. Halsband U, Lange RK. Motor learning in man: a review of functional and clinical studies. *J Physiol Paris* (2006) 99:414–24. doi: 10.1016/j.jphysparis.2006.03.007
7. Lu M-T, Preston JB, Strick PL. Interconnections between the prefrontal cortex and the premotor areas in the frontal lobe. *J Comp Neurol.* (1994) 341:375–92. doi: 10.1002/cne.903410308
8. Saleem KS, Miller B, Price JL. Subdivisions and connectional networks of the lateral prefrontal cortex in the macaque monkey. *J Comp Neurol.* (2014) 522:1641–90. doi: 10.1002/cne.23498
9. Luppino G, Rozzi S, Calzavara R, Matelli M. Prefrontal and agranular cingulate projections to the dorsal premotor areas F2 and F7 in the macaque monkey. *Eur J Neurosci.* (2003) 17:559–78. doi: 10.1046/j.1460-9568.2003.02476.x
10. Dum RP, Strick PL. Frontal lobe inputs to the digit representations of the motor areas on the lateral surface of the hemisphere. *J Neurosci.* (2005) 25:1375–86. doi: 10.1523/JNEUROSCI.3902-04.2005
11. Gerbella M, Borra E, Tonelli S, Rozzi S, Luppino G. Connectional heterogeneity of the ventral part of the macaque area 46. *Cereb Cortex* (2013) 23:967–87. doi: 10.1093/cercor/bhs096
12. Tomassini V, Jbabdi S, Klein JC, Behrens TEJ, Pozzilli C, Matthews PM, et al. Diffusion-weighted imaging tractography-based parcellation of the human lateral premotor cortex identifies dorsal and ventral subregions with anatomical and functional specializations. *J Neurosci.* (2007) 27:10259–69. doi: 10.1523/JNEUROSCI.2144-07.2007
13. Wang LE, Fink GR, Diekhoff S, Rehme AK, Eickhoff SB, Grefkes C. Noradrenergic enhancement improves motor network connectivity in stroke patients. *Ann Neurol.* (2011) 69:375–88. doi: 10.1002/ana.22237
14. Ward NS. Motor system activation after subcortical stroke depends on corticospinal system integrity. *Brain* (2006) 129:809–19. doi: 10.1093/brain/awl002
15. Calautti C, Jones PS, Guincestre J-Y, Naccarato M, Sharma N, Day DJ, et al. The neural substrates of impaired finger tapping regularity after stroke. *Neuroimage* (2010) 50:1–6. doi: 10.1016/j.neuroimage.2009.12.012
16. Stewart JC, Dewanjee P, Shariff U, Cramer SC. Dorsal premotor activity and connectivity relate to action selection performance after stroke. *Hum Brain Mapp.* (2016) 37:1816–30. doi: 10.1002/hbm.23138
17. Dodakian L, Stewart J, Cramer S. Motor imagery during movement activates the brain more than movement alone after stroke: a pilot study. *J Rehabil Med.* (2014) 46:843–8. doi: 10.2340/16501977-1844
18. Sharma N, Baron J-C, Rowe JB. Motor imagery after stroke: relating outcome to motor network connectivity. *Ann Neurol.* (2009) 66:604–16. doi: 10.1002/ana.21810
19. Schulz R, Park C-H, Boudrias M-H, Gerloff C, Hummel FC, Ward NS. Assessing the integrity of corticospinal pathways from primary and secondary cortical motor areas after stroke. *Stroke* (2012) 43:2248–51. doi: 10.1161/STROKEAHA.112.662619
20. Meehan SK, Randhawa B, Wessel B, Boyd LA. Implicit sequence-specific motor learning after subcortical stroke is associated with increased prefrontal brain activations: an fMRI Study. *Hum Brain Mapp.* (2011) 32:290–303. doi: 10.1002/hbm.21019
21. Lefebvre S, Dricot L, Laloux P, Gradkowski W, Desfontaines P, Evrard F, et al. Neural substrates underlying motor skill learning in chronic hemiparetic stroke patients. *Front Hum Neurosci.* (2015) 9:320. doi: 10.3389/fnhum.2015.00320
22. Krakauer JW. Motor learning: its relevance to stroke recovery and neurorehabilitation. *Curr Opin Neurol.* (2006) 19:84–90. doi: 10.1097/01.wco.0000200544.29915.cc
23. Rehme AK, Eickhoff SB, Rottschy C, Fink GR, Grefkes C. Activation likelihood estimation meta-analysis of motor-related neural activity after stroke. *Neuroimage* (2012) 59:2771–82. doi: 10.1016/j.neuroimage.2011.10.023
24. Park J-Y, Kim Y-H, Chang WH, Park C, Shin Y-I, Kim ST, et al. Significance of longitudinal changes in the default-mode network for cognitive recovery after stroke. *Eur J Neurosci.* (2014) 40:2715–22. doi: 10.1111/ejn.12640
25. Schulz R, Koch P, Zimerman M, Wessel M, Bönstrup M, Thomalla G, et al. Parietofrontal motor pathways and their association with motor function after stroke. *Brain* (2015) 138:1949–60. doi: 10.1093/brain/awv100
26. Fugl-Meyer AR, Jääskö L, Leyman I, Olsson S, Steglind S. The post-stroke hemiplegic patient. 1. a method for evaluation of physical performance. *Scand J Rehabil Med.* (1975) 7:13–31.

27. Schulz R, Frey BM, Koch P, Zimerman M, Bönstrup M, Feldheim J, et al. Cortico-cerebellar structural connectivity is related to residual motor output in chronic stroke. *Cereb Cortex* (2017) 27:635–45. doi: 10.1093/cercor/bhv251
28. Hughes EJ, Bond J, Svrckova P, Makropoulos A, Ball G, Sharp DJ, et al. Regional changes in thalamic shape and volume with increasing age. *Neuroimage* (2012) 63:1134–42. doi: 10.1016/j.neuroimage.2012.07.043
29. Alexander AL, Hurley SA, Samsonov AA, Adluru N, Hosseinbor AP, Mossahebi P, et al. Characterization of cerebral white matter properties using quantitative magnetic resonance imaging stains. *Brain Connect.* (2011) 1:423–46. doi: 10.1089/brain.2011.0071
30. Benjamini Y, Yekutieli D. The control of the false discovery rate in multiple testing under dependency. *Ann Stat.* (2001) 29:1165–88. doi: 10.2307/2674075
31. Makris N, Kennedy DN, McInerney S, Sorensen AG, Wang R, Caviness VS, et al. Segmentation of subcomponents within the superior longitudinal fascicle in humans: a quantitative, *in vivo*, DT-MRI study. *Cereb Cortex* (2005) 15:854–69. doi: 10.1093/cercor/bhh186
32. Schmahmann JD, Pandya DN, Wang R, Dai G, D'Arceuil HE, de Crespigny AJ, et al. Association fibre pathways of the brain: parallel observations from diffusion spectrum imaging and autoradiography. *Brain* (2007) 130:630–53. doi: 10.1093/brain/awl359
33. Tournier JD, Calamante F, Connelly A. Robust determination of the fibre orientation distribution in diffusion MRI: non-negativity constrained super-resolved spherical deconvolution. *Neuroimage* (2007) 35:1459–72. doi: 10.1016/j.neuroimage.2007.02.016
34. Yeterian EH, Pandya DN, Tomaiuolo F, Petrides M. The cortical connectivity of the prefrontal cortex in the monkey brain. *Cortex* (2012) 48:58–81. doi: 10.1016/j.cortex.2011.03.004
35. Pandya DN, Dye P, Butters N. Efferent cortico-cortical projections of the prefrontal cortex in the rhesus monkey. *Brain Res.* (1971) 31:35–46. doi: 10.1016/0006-8993(71)90632-9
36. Pandya DN, Kuypers HGJM. Cortico-cortical connections in the rhesus monkey. *Brain Res.* (1969) 13:13–36. doi: 10.1016/0006-8993(69)90141-3
37. Jones EG, Powell TPS. An anatomical study of converging sensory pathways within the cerebral cortex of the monkey. *Brain* (1970) 93:793–820. doi: 10.1093/brain/93.4.793
38. Beaulieu C. The basis of anisotropic water diffusion in the nervous system - a technical review. *NMR Biomed.* (2002) 15:435–55. doi: 10.1002/nbm.782
39. Li Y, Wu P, Liang F, Huang W. The microstructural status of the corpus callosum is associated with the degree of motor function and neurological deficit in stroke patients. *PLoS ONE* (2015) 10:e0122615. doi: 10.1371/journal.pone.0122615
40. Schaechter JD, Fricker ZP, Perdue KL, Helmer KG, Vangel MG, Greve DN, et al. Microstructural status of ipsilesional and contralesional corticospinal tract correlates with motor skill in chronic stroke patients. *Hum Brain Mapp.* (2009) 30:3461–74. doi: 10.1002/hbm.20770
41. Wang LE, Tittgemeyer M, Imperati D, Diekhoff S, Ameli M, Fink GR, et al. Degeneration of corpus callosum and recovery of motor function after stroke: a multimodal magnetic resonance imaging study. *Hum Brain Mapp.* (2012) 33:2941–56. doi: 10.1002/hbm.21417
42. Rehme AK, Fink GR, Von Cramon DY, Grefkes C. The role of the contralesional motor cortex for motor recovery in the early days after stroke assessed with longitudinal fMRI. *Cereb Cortex* (2011) 21:756–68. doi: 10.1093/cercor/bhq140
43. Park C, Chang WH, Ohn SH, Kim ST, Bang OY, Pascual-Leone A, et al. Longitudinal changes of resting-state functional connectivity during motor recovery after stroke. *Stroke* (2011) 42:1357–62. doi: 10.1161/STROKEAHA.110.596155
44. Yin D, Song F, Xu D, Peterson BS, Sun L, Men W, et al. Patterns in cortical connectivity for determining outcomes in hand function after subcortical stroke. *PLoS ONE* (2012) 7:e52727. doi: 10.1371/journal.pone.0052727
45. Kalinosky BT, Berrios Barillas R, Schmit BD. Structurofunctional resting-state networks correlate with motor function in chronic stroke. *NeuroImage Clin.* (2017) 16:610–23. doi: 10.1016/j.nicl.2017.07.002

11

Assessment of the Efficacy of ReoGo-J Robotic Training Against Other Rehabilitation Therapies for Upper-Limb Hemiplegia after Stroke

Takashi Takebayashi[1], Kayoko Takahashi[2], Satoru Amano[3], Yuki Uchiyama[4], Masahiko Gosho[5], Kazuhisa Domen[6] and Kenji Hachisuka[7]*

[1] Department of Occupational Therapy, School of Health Science and Social Welfare, Kibi International University, Takahashi, Japan, [2] Department of Rehabilitation, School of Allied Health Science, Kitasato University, Sagamihara-shi, Japan, [3] Department of Rehabilitation, The Hospital of Hyogo College of Medicine, Nishinomiya-shi, Japan, [4] Department of Rehabilitation, Hyogo College of Medicine, Nishinomiya-shi, Japan, [5] Department of Biostatistics, Faculty of Medicine, University of Tsukuba, Tsukuba, Japan, [6] Department of Rehabilitation Medicine, Hyogo College of Medicine, Nishinomiya, Japan, [7] Kyushu Rosai Hospital, Moji Medical Center, Kita-kyushu-shi, Japan

***Correspondence:**
Takashi Takebayashi
takshi77@gmail.com;
takshi77@kiui.ac.jp

Background: Stroke patients experience chronic hemiparesis in their upper extremities leaving negative effects on quality of life. Robotic therapy is one method to recover arm function, but its research is still in its infancy. Research questions of this study is to investigate how to maximize the benefit of robotic therapy using ReoGo-J for arm hemiplegia in chronic stroke patients.

Methods: Design of this study is a multi-center parallel group trial following the prospective, randomized, open-label, blinded endpoint (PROBE) study model. Participants and setting will be 120 chronic stroke patients (over 6 months post-stroke) will be randomly allocated to three different rehabilitation protocols. In this study, the control group will receive 20 min of standard rehabilitation (conventional occupational therapy) and 40 min of self-training (i.e., sanding, placing and stretching). The robotic therapy group will receive 20 min of standard rehabilitation and 40 min of robotic therapy using ReoGo®-J device. The combined therapy group will receive 40 min of robotic therapy and 20 min of constraint-induced movement therapy (protocol to improve upper-limb use in ADL suggests). This study employs the Fugl-Meyer Assessment upper-limb score (primary outcome), other arm function measures and the Stroke Impact Scale score will be measured at baseline, 5 and 10 weeks of the treatment phase. In analysis of this study, we use the mixed effects model for repeated measures to compare changes in outcomes between groups at 5 and 10 Weeks. The registration number of this study is UMIN000022509.

Conclusions: This study is a feasible, multi-site randomized controlled trial to examine our hypothesis that combined training protocol could maximize the benefit of robotic therapy and best effective therapeutic strategy for patients with upper-limb hemiparesis.

Keywords: stroke, robotics, upper-extremity, paresis, constraint-induced movement therapy

INTRODUCTION

Severe, persistent paresis occurs in over 40% of stroke patients (1) and is reported to significantly decrease their quality of life (2). Thus, much research has been conducted to develop interventions, with many specifically targeting upper extremity hemiplegia. Among the many examples of neuroscience-based rehabilitation (neuro-rehabilitation) strategies, there is strong evidence supporting robotic therapy, constraint-induced movement therapy (CIMT), and task-oriented training (3, 4).

Robotic therapy is considered an effective intervention for mild to severe hemiplegic arm (5, 6), and is cost-effective for chronic stroke patients in terms of both manpower and medical costs (7, 8). However, its effects may be limited for some patients. Some researchers have found that robotic therapy effectively improves arm function as measured by the Fugl-Meyer Assessment (FMA) (9) and Action research arm test (ARAT) (10), but does not improve the use of the affected arm in activities of daily living (ADL) as measured by the Motor activity log (MAL)-14 (11) and by analysis of data from an accelerometer attached to the affected arm (6, 12–14).

On the contrary, CIMT is the most well-established intervention for improving the use of the affected arm in ADL (15). CIMT consists of three components: (1) a repeated task-oriented approach, (2) a behavioral approach to transfer the function gained during training to actual life (also called the "transfer package"), and (3) constraining use of the affected arm. Some researchers consider the transfer package the most important component of CIMT. In fact, research has shown that usage of the affected arm in daily life is significantly different between patients treated with and without the transfer package component (16, 17). However, many therapists question whether CIMT could benefit their patients because of the shortage of sites possessing the clinical resources to provide the intervention for the long duration required for effectiveness (18).

Therefore, there is an urgent need to establish an effective therapeutic approach, especially for upper-limb hemiplegia during the chronic stage of stroke recovery for which there are few clinical resources (In Japan, the insurance system only allows 260 min per month). Therefore, we will compare the efficacy of several therapy methods. As a control, we will monitor changes in arm function in patients undergoing a short, standard rehabilitation by a therapist and standard self-training (control group). This will be compared to similar self-training including robotic therapy with the ReoGo-J device as an adjuvant therapy (RT group). Finally, the robotic therapy will be compared to combined therapy including robotic therapy and CIMT (CT group). Through these comparisons, we will investigate the effect of robotic therapy, both alone and in combination with CIMT, which we hypothesize will complement each other in chronic stroke rehabilitation. Here, we report the structure and protocol of a multi-center, randomized controlled trial.

MATERIALS AND METHODS

Objective

This study is intended to verify the increased efficacy of self-training with robotic therapy compared with the commonly practiced traditional occupational therapy on upper-limb motor function and function in ADL in moderate to severe chronic post-stroke upper-limb hemiplegic patients. In addition, another objective of the study is to verify the degree of superiority of combination training including both robotic therapy and CIMT over training with robotic therapy alone in these patients. Therefore, in this study, primary objective is to compare the RT and control group, secondary objective is to compare the RT and the CT group. Additionally, to compare the CT and control group is auxiliary analysis. We hypothesize that robotic therapy will improve recovery over the usual care alone, and that combining robotic therapy with CIMT will further enhance its benefits.

Study Design

This study will be conducted as a multi-center, prospective, randomized, parallel group study. We aimed to enroll 120 chronic stroke patients from approval by the institutional review board until March 31, 2017. The chronic stroke patients enrolled will be randomized to three groups: a control group to receive conventional occupational therapy (usual care) and self-training that follows the concept of usual care; a group to receive usual care and self-training with robotic therapy; and a group to receive combination training that includes task-oriented training aimed at improving function in ADL and robotic therapy.

The principal investigator will register the study on the clinical trial registration system of the University Hospital Medical Information Network (UMIN000022509) after approval of this study by the clinical research institutional review board of the Hyogo College of Medicine (#2248) and before enrolling subjects.

Settings

The settings for this study include multiple hospitals and clinics throughout Japan. All sites provide outpatient rehabilitation for stroke patients at the chronic stage of recovery.

Recruitment

All patients will be screened for the inclusion and exclusion criteria described below. After the patient is determined to meet the criteria, the physician will obtain informed consent from the patient.

Inclusion and Exclusion Criteria

Patients will be considered eligible for this study if they are between 20 and 80 years of age, have chronic upper-limb hemiplegia from a supratentorial stroke that occurred at least 6 months before enrollment, are undergoing outpatient or ambulatory rehabilitation, and meet the following functional score requirements: FMA upper-limb scale (9) score of less than 44 points, Stroke Impairment Assessment Set (19) upper-limb distal function score of 1b or above, and modified Ashworth scale (MAS) (20) score of 2 or less.

Patients will be evaluated upon enrollment by their physician, and those with multiple strokes or a cerebellar/brain stem stroke, who have extreme upper-limb pain, or whose upper-limb function is deemed to be improving are not eligible for the study. To avoid complication with other medical conditions, patients with neuromuscular diseases, malignant tumors, balance or gait disturbance, or other serious uncontrolled diseases will be excluded. To ensure patients have the cognitive ability to participate in training and evaluation, patients will be excluded if they have serious aphasia or higher cortical dysfunction (a lack of lucid decision-making ability to participate this study, or a score of 24 points or less on the mini-mental state examination (21)). Possible confounding effects of other treatments will be avoided by excluding patients who have received intensive training with an upper-limb training robot or constraint-induced therapy for upper-limb hemiplegia at any time after their stroke, or a botulinum toxin injection within 16 weeks of enrollment. Additionally, before decision-making a participation of study, patients received the standard rehabilitation (physical and occupational therapy) who are not excluded in this study because (1) in study of rehabilitation area for chronic stroke patients, there are few studies that excluse patients receiving the standard rehabilitation before participation of the study from the participant (22–24); (2) in Japan which have health-insurance system that covers all of its citizens, there are few stroke patients in the chronic stroke phase who have not received physical therapy, if they are excluded, the feasibility of this study falls significantly. However, after decision-making a participation of this study, patients were forbidden to receive any other rehabilitation, out of study.

Withdrawal From Study

Patients will be withdrawn from the study if they undergo certain prohibited therapies after enrolling in the study. These include functional electrical stimulation, transcranial magnetic stimulation, and transcranial direct current stimulation. Training with any other upper-limb rehabilitation robot is also prohibited after informed consent. Patients must not receive botulinum toxin injections during the treatment period.

The investigator can decide to withdraw an enrolled and allocated patient from this study if they have difficulty beginning or continuing study participation, such as failure to attend study visits, withdrawal of informed consent, adverse events or complications, recovery of arm function so that no further rehabilitation is needed, or any other event judged by the investigator to warrant withdrawal. The investigators, after withdrawing a subject, shall perform the planned end-of-study examinations to the extent possible and record the observations, last date of training, and reasons for withdrawal on the case report form.

Enrollment And Randomization

Subjects who meet all of the inclusion criteria and none of the exclusion criteria, and have given informed consent, will be evaluated by the investigators for enrollment. At enrollment, information will be collected including demographic data, body measurements, stroke information, complications, lifestyle factors, and baseline function measures. The investigator will verify that the patient is eligible to participate and enter information into the electronic data capture and web allocation system as required.

Randomization will be done through the web allocation system. The patients will be randomized to one of the three treatment groups using dynamic allocation by the minimization method based on the baseline FMA upper-limb score, center, period after stroke, and age.

Blinding

This study integrates the prospective, randomized, open-label, blinded endpoint (PROBE) study model (25). Because the training methods differ between groups, it is not feasible to blind the subjects, therapists present at the training, and physicians to the treatment. Therefore, the individuals involved in endpoint evaluation, rather than those involved in the treatment, will be blinded. The primary endpoint (FMA) and one of the secondary endpoints (ARAT) will be assessed remotely through audio and visual evaluations of video footage that has undergone blinding. The remaining assessments involve each subject's subjective evaluation, and therefore cannot be blinded, and simple palpation, which will be performed by physicians or therapists who were not present at the training to ensure objectivity.

Interventions

All patients will receive training 3 times weekly for 10 weeks. During each training session, patients in the control arm of the study will receive 40 min of self-training (sanding, placing, stretching, and repetitive reaching/grasping/releasing practice) and 20 min of usual care (conventional occupational therapy including stretching, joint range-of-motion exercises, correct-movement exercises, and ADL exercises). The RT group intervention will consist of the same 20 min of usual care, and 40 min of self-training with the ReoGo®-J upper-limb rehabilitation device (certification No. 226AHBZX00029000). The CT group intervention will include 40 min of self-training with robotic therapy and 20 min of CIMT training (shaping, task-practice, and transfer package).

Outcomes

All outcomes will be measured at baseline, 5 and 10 weeks. The primary outcome examined will be changes in the FMA upper-limb score (9). This assessment examines motor and joint function, balance, and sensation in hemiplegic patients and results are represented as a numerical score with a maximum of 66 points.

Secondary outcomes include changes in: (1) the "amount of use" and "quality of movement" components of the MAL-14 scale (11), which assesses limb function in ADL; (2) the individual components of the FMA (9); (3) the ARAT score, another measure of upper-limb function (10); (4) the motricity index (26), an assessment of muscle strength in stroke patients; (5) the MAS score (20), which assesses muscle tone (i.e., spasticity); (6) the active range of motion of the shoulder, elbow, forearm, wrist, and fingers (27); and (7) the Stroke Impact Scale (28), a quality of life assessment scale for stroke patients.

Safety outcomes will include the occurrence of any adverse events. Adverse events will be assessed as either related or unrelated to the study treatment, and their severity graded using the CTCAE Ver 4.03 (29) as a reference. All adverse events will be recorded on the medical chart and case report form. In the case of serious adverse events, including those that are life-threatening or result in hospitalization, a "serious adverse event and malfunction report" will be prepared by the investigator and submitted to the hospital director promptly.

Data Monitoring and Management

The research director is responsible for monitoring the study, including ensuring that the data reported by the investigators are accurate, complete, and verifiable in comparison with the source documents and other records. An operating procedure for monitoring will be prepared by the principal investigator in advance, and the principal investigator shall appoint monitors to conduct this monitoring as appropriate. At each hospital, the investigator and the hospital director shall cooperate with all investigations by a monitor, the institutional review board, or a regulatory authority. The investigator and director must present all study-related records, such as source documents, when requested by the investigating body.

Because this study uses a medical device that has received marketing approval, together with the nature of the interventions and the sample size, specific quality assurance audits do not need to be planned. Rather, routine data monitoring as described above will ensure data quality.

The electronic case report form will be provided by the data center of the Tsukuba Clinical Research and Development Organization (T-CReDO). The data center will also perform quality control of the collected data, specifically by conducting logical checks. In cases where inconsistencies, missing values, or other issues are detected in the entered data, the investigator will be queried, and they will revise the electronic case report form if necessary. After completion of data quality control, a case review will be convened. The data center will create a dataset for analysis and transfer quality control records and datasets to the study statistician.

The investigator and director of each hospital are responsible for retaining all records, and the data center will retain the anonymized, transcribed case report form data. These data will be retained for 5 years after completion or termination of the study or 3 years after the last publication of results from the study, whichever is later, unless an individual study site has established a longer retention period.

Confidentiality

Data such as subject information and data collected from observations and examinations will be stored as an anonymized, linkable dataset using identification codes within the data center. Each participating study site shall manage the coding keys linking identification codes to respective subjects within its facility. All individuals involved in the study will take care to protect subjects' identifying information when handling documents, anonymizing case report forms, and incorporating data into publications.

Data Access and Dissemination

Subjects in this study may obtain or access the protocol and study-related documents by making a request to the treating physician, provided that doing so would not hinder the protection of personal information of other subjects or the assurance of originality of this study. After study completion, the principal investigator shall organize and publish the results promptly in an academic journal or academic conference, among other media. The ownership of any papers or presentations prepared using the data collected in this study shall be decided through consultations with the principal investigator. Any copyright will be shared by the lead author and coauthors.

Sample Size

The principal objective of the study is to verify the superiority of the RT group over the control group in the improvement of FMA upper-limb score. Using the minimal clinically important difference (MCID) as a reference, the mean difference between the patients in the RT and control groups with respect to the FMA upper-limb score is expected to be 4.25 points (30). Given that the subjects in this study will be chronic patients, the deviation is expected to be smaller than that in the pilot study conducted in recovering patients (standard deviation, 8.8) (6), and thus a standard deviation of 6 is expected. Based on a two-sided significance level of 0.05 and a power of 0.9 on Student's t-test, a sample size of 39 per group is needed. Considering some loss to follow-up, the sample size was increased from 39 to 40 per group. Additionally, in our similar previous study (6), we recruited 56 case in 6 facilities (about nine case per a facility). Therefore, considering difficulty to recruited case in chronic stage, we judged this study will be feasible to request more than 20 facilities to participate this study.

Statistical Analyses

Two analysis populations will be established: the safety analysis set and the efficacy analysis set. The safety analysis set will include all patients who were allocated, and the numbers and percentages of safety endpoints will be compared between groups by Fisher's exact test.

The subject characteristics collected upon enrollment will be analyzed by intergroup comparisons of continuous variables by analysis of variance and of categorical variables by Fisher's exact test.

The efficacy analysis set will include all patients for whom primary endpoint data are available based on intention-to-treat principle. Using the mixed effects model for repeated measures, we will perform intergroup comparisons of changes in the FMA upper-limb score at 5 and 10 Weeks of the treatment phase. This model will include the group, time point, group-by-time interaction term, baseline FMA upper-limb score, sex, and botulinum toxin injection. For multiplicity adjustment, Dunnett's test will be employed with the RT group used as a reference. The same analysis will be conducted for the secondary outcomes. The level of significance is set at 0.05.

DISCUSSION

Here, we describe an intervention protocol to improve upper-limb function in chronic stroke patients experiencing hemiplegia, which we are examining through a multi-center randomized clinical trial. This study is unique and innovative in the areas of neuro-rehabilitation, physical therapy, occupational therapy, and rehabilitation psychology. When establishing new interventions—whether they are drugs, medical techniques, neuro-rehabilitation techniques, or others—investigators must follow established scientific processes for building evidence. These processes begin with a discovery phase, followed by a pre-clinical trial, and finally several phases (I to IV) of clinical trials. The ReoGo-J study described here is a mid-sized phase IV randomized controlled clinical trial with two purposes: (1) to examine the efficacy of robotic therapy, and (2) to determine whether combined therapy consisting of CIMT and robotic therapy is an ideal rehabilitation protocol for chronic stroke patients. Furthermore, our study results could provide insight into whether the arm function gained by robotic therapy is generalizable to actual life.

Examining the efficacy of robotic therapy, there have been only a few studies conducted around the world to examine the efficacy of robotic therapy for patients in the chronic stage of stroke recovery (7, 16, 31–34). Hardly any of this research was conducted in East Asia, and thus our study would also be novel in this respect. The robot used in this study, ReoGo-J, is the successor of ReoGo, which was shown to be effective during stroke recovery (6). This study would be the first randomized controlled trial using this new robotic system.

Our combined therapy protocol could be an effective option for therapists in clinical settings. Our program is especially unique in that patients can gain the positive effects of both CIMT and robotic therapy, and favorable interaction effect: CIMT could complement the weakness of robotic therapy, which is the limited transfer of arm function gained to daily life, and robotic therapy could complement the weakness of CIMT, which needs large clinical resources. Therefore, by demonstrating the efficacy of our new program including training using ReoGo-J, we could establish a feasible robotic therapy protocol that could be easily carried out with limited clinical resources to treat chronic phase stroke patients.

For the each of the various measures we will use to assess rehabilitation, the MCID has been established. Of the measures that quantify general hemiplegic arm function, the MCID for FMA is 4.25–7.25 points (30), and that of the ARAT is 10% of the total score (10), or 5.7 points (35). The MCID of MAL, which measures the use of the affected arm in actual life, is 0.5 points for the amount of use scale (36) and 1.0–1.1 points for the quality of movement scale (37). Because clinical resources are limited, there are few interventions/approaches to achieve MCID in the measures of arm function and arm use. However, our pilot studies have shown that combined robot and CIMT therapy could improve arm function and use of the affected arm, and those increases were greater than MCID (38, 39). Those results suggest we will see a promising effect of CT in this ReoGo-J study, and that the combined therapy will overcome the weakness of robotic therapy and significantly increase the use of affected arm in real-life settings.

Currently in Japan, many elderly stroke patients receive one-on-one rehabilitation by physical or occupational therapist 20 min per day at an adult day-care center run by the long-term care insurance system. The protocol of the control group in this study is expected to represent the conventional rehabilitation usually done at such adult day-care center. Therefore, if this study proves RT or CT group exceeded control group, we could suggest a better protocol for rehabilitation for upper extremity hemiparesis for chronic stroke patients at adult day-care center. Furthermore, our suggestion may increase the recovery of upper extremity function and use of affected arm at the same resources and cost as conventional protocol.

However, there are some limitations in this study. For example, there are many factors affecting the prognosis of upper extremity hemiplegia caused by stroke: age, sex, baseline upper extremity motor function, time after stroke, degree of sensory deficit, patients' degree of motivation, family support, various approaches within robotic therapy and CIMT (i.e., types of movement, repetitions, clinical site). In this study, the allocation factor will be set based on previous studies to control for differences in the following characteristics between groups: (1) baseline FMA score (40), (2) time after stroke (41–43), (3) age (43, 44), and (4) clinical site. However, the other factors cannot be controlled by this method.

Another limitation is that we cannot blind the patient to their allocated intervention. To minimize the bias of placebo effect, we are modeling our study after the PROBE study design. However, in rehabilitation research, it is often impossible to blind patients to the intervention because we cannot provide sham intervention. Therefore, such studies cannot exclude bias caused by the placebo effect.

AUTHOR CONTRIBUTIONS

TT and KT contributed equally in the study design, writing and reviewing the manuscript. MG contributed in the analysis design. SA, YU, KD, and KH contributed to reviewing the manuscript.

ACKNOWLEDGMENTS

The authors thank associated facilities of this study for data acquisition, and Tsukuba Clinical Research and Development Organization, University of Tsukuba, for their support and assistance for the study initiation and implementation.

REFERENCES

1. Perker VM, Wade DT, Longton Hewer R. Loss of arm function after stroke: measurement, frequency, and recovery. *Int Rehabil Med.* (1986) 8:69–73. doi: 10.3109/03790798609166178
2. Nicholas-Larsen D, Clark PC, Zeringue A, Greenspan A, Blanton, S. Factors influencing stroke survivors' quality of life during subacute recovery. *Stroke* (2005) 36:1480–4. doi: 10.1161/01.STR.0000170706.13595.4f
3. Winstein CJ, Stein J, Arena R, Bates B, Cherney LR, Cramer SC, et al. Guidelines for adult stroke rehabilitation and recovery: A guideline for healthcare professionals form the American Heart Association/American Stroke Association. *Stroke* (2016) 47:e98–169. doi: 10.1161/STR.0000000000000098
4. Langhorne P, Bernhardt J, Kwakkel G. Stroke rehabilitation. *Lancet* (2011) 377:1693–702. doi: 10.1016/S0140-6736(11)60325-5
5. Hsieh YW, Wu CY, Lin KC, Yao G, Wu KY, Chang YJ. Dose-response relationship of robot-assisted stroke motor rehabilitation: the impact of initial motor status. *Stroke* (2012) 43:2729–34. doi: 10.1161/STROKEAHA.112.658807
6. Takahashi K, Domen K, Sakamoto T, Toshima M, Otaka Y, Seto M, et al. Efficacy of upper extremity robotic therapy in subacute poststroke hemiplegia: an exploratory randomized trial. *Stroke* (2016) 47:1385–8. doi: 10.1161/STROKEAHA.115.012520
7. Lo AC, Guarino PD, Richards LG, Haselkorn JK, Wittenberg GF, Federman DG, et al. Robotic-assisted therapy for long-term upper-limb impairment after stroke. *N Engl J Med.* (2010) 362:1772–83. doi: 10.1056/NEJMoa0911341
8. Bovolenta F, Goldoni M, Clerici P, Agosti M, Franceschini M. Robot therapy for functional recovery of the upper limbs: a pilot study on patients after stroke. *J Rehabil Med.* (2009) 41:971–5. doi: 10.2340/16501977-0402
9. Fugl-Meyer AR, Jääskö L, Leyman I, Olsson S, Steglind S. The post-stroke hemiplegic patient. 1. A method for evaluation of physical performance. *Scand J Rehabil Med.* (1975) 7:13–31.
10. Lyle, RC. A performance test for assessment of upper limb function in physical rehabilitation treatment and research. *Int J Rehabil Res.* (1981) 4:483–92. doi: 10.1097/00004356-198112000-00001
11. Uswatte G, Taub E, Morris D, Vignolo M, McCulloch K. Reliability and validity of the upper-extremity Motor Activity Log-14 for measuring real-world arm use. *Stroke* (2005) 36:2493–6. doi: 10.1161/01.STR.0000185928.90848.2e
12. Prange GB, Jannink MJ, Groothuis-Oudshoorn CG, Hermens HJ, Ijzerman MJ. Systematic review of the effect of robot-aided therapy on recovery of the hemiparetic arm after stroke. *J Rehabil Res Dev.* (2006) 43:171–84. doi: 10.1682/JRRD.2005.04.0076
13. Kwakkel G, Kokken BJ, Krebs HI. Effects of robot-assisted therapy on upper limb recovery after stroke: a systematic review. *Neurorehabil Neural Repair* (2008) 22:111–21. doi: 10.1177/1545968307305457
14. Mehrholz J, Platz T, Kugler J, Pohl M. Electromechanical and robot-assisted arm training for improving arm function and activities of daily living after stroke. *Cochrane Database Syst Rev.* (2008) 8:CD006876. doi: 10.1002/14651858.CD006876.pub2
15. Morris DM, Taub E, Mark VW. Constraint-induced movement therapy: characterizing the intervention protocol. *Eura Medicophys.* (2006) 42:257–68.
16. Taub E, Uswatte G, Mark VW, Morris DM, Barman J, Bowman MH, et al. Method for enhancing real-world use of a more affected arm in chronic stroke: the transfer package of constraint-induced movement therapy. *Stroke* (2013) 44:1383–8. doi: 10.1161/STROKEAHA.111.000559
17. Takebayashi T, Koyama T, Amano S, Hanada K, Tabusadani M, Hosomi M, et al. A 6-month follow-up after constraint-induced movement therapy with and without transfer package for patients with hemiparesis after stroke: a pilot quasi-randomized controlled trial. *Clin Rehabil.* (2013) 27:418–26. doi: 10.1177/0269215512460779
18. Page SJ, Levine P, Sisto S, Bond Q, Johnston MV. Stroke patients' and therapists' opinions of constraint-induced movement therapy. *Clin Rehabil.* (2002) 16:55–60. doi: 10.1191/0269215502cr473oa
19. Chino N, Sonoda S, Domen K, Saitoh E, Kimura A. Stroke Impairment assessment Set (SIAS). In: Chino N., Melvin J.L, editors. *Functional Evaluation of Stroke Patients.* Tokyo: Springer (1996) p. 19–31.
20. Bohannon RW, Smith MB. Interrater reliability of a modified Ashworth scale of muscle spasticity. *Phys Ther.* (1987) 67:206–07. doi: 10.1093/ptj/67.2.206
21. Folstein MF, Flostein SE, McHugh PR. "Mini-mental state". A practical method for grading the cognitive state of patients for the clinician. *J Psychiatr Res.* (1975) 12:189–98. doi: 10.1016/0022-3956(75)90026-6
22. Brazel A, Katels G, Tetzlaff B, Daubmann A, Wegsccheider K, van den Bussche H, et al. Home-besed constraint-induced movement therapy for patients with upper limb dysfunction after stroke (HomeCITE): a cluster-randomised, controlled trial. *Lancet Neurol.* (2015) 14:893–902. doi: 10.1016/S1474-4422(15)00147-7
23. Gauthier LV, Taub E, Perkins C, Ortmann M, Mark VW, Uswatte G. Remodeling the brain: plastic structural brain changes produced by different motor therapies after stroke. *Stroke* (2008) 39:1520–5. doi: 10.1161/STROKEAHA.107.502229
24. Taub E, Uswatte G, King DK, Morris D, Crago JE, Chatterjee A. A placebo-controlled trial of constraint-induced movement therapy for upper extremity after stroke. *Stroke* (2006) 37:1045–9. doi: 10.1161/01.STR.0000206463.66461.97
25. Hansson L, Hedner T, Dahlöf B. Prospective randomized open blinded end-point (PROBE) study. A novel design for intervention trials. Prospective randomized open blinded end-point. *Blood Press* (1992) 1:113–19. doi: 10.3109/08037059209077502
26. Demeurisse G, Demol O, Robaye E. Motor evaluation in vascular hemiplegia. *Eur Neurol.* (1980) 19:382–89. doi: 10.1159/0001151782
27. Hume MC, Gellman H, McKellop H, Brumfield RH. Functional range of motion of the joints of the hand. *J Hand Surg.* (1990) 15:240–43. doi: 10.1016/0363-5023(90)90102-W
28. Duncan PW, Bode RK, Lai SM, Perera S. Rasch analysis of a new stroke-specific outcome scale: the Stroke Impact Scale. *Arch Phys Med Rehabil.* (2003) 84:950–63. doi: 10.1016/S0003-9993(03)00035-2
29. Trotti A, Colevas AD, Setser A, Rusch V, Jaques D, Budach V, et al. National cancer institute cancer therapy evaluation program (CTEP). Common terminology criteria for adverse events (CTCAE), Version 4.03. *Semin Radiat Oncol.* (2010). 13:176–81. doi: 10.1016/S1053-4296(03)00031-6
30. Page SJ, Fulk GD, Boyne P. Clinically important differences for the upper-extremity Fugl-Meyer scale in people with minimal to moderate impairment due to chronic stroke. *Phys Ther.* (2012) 92:791–98. doi: 10.2522/ptj.20110009
31. Timmermans AA, Lemmens RJ, Monfrance M, Greers RP, Bakx W, Smeets RJ, et al. Effect of task-oriented robot training on arm function, activity, and quality of life in chronic stroke patients: a randomized controlled trial. *J Neuroeng Rehabil.* (2014) 11:45. doi: 10.1186/1743-0003-11-45
32. Housman SJ, Scott KM, Reinkensmeyer DJ. (2009). A randomized controlled trial of gravity-supported, computer-enhanced arm exercise for individuals with severe hemiparesis. *Neurorehabil Neural Repair.* (2009) 23:505–14. doi: 10.1177/1545968308331148
33. Kahn LE, Zygman ML, Rymer WZ, Reinkensmeyer DJ. Robot-assisted reaching exercise promotes arm movement recovery in chronic hemiparetic stroke: a randomized controlled pilot study. *J Neuroeng Rehabil.* (2006) 3:12. doi: 10.1186/1743-0003-3-12
34. Lemmens RJ, Timmermans AA, Janssen-potten YJ, Pulles SA, Geers RP, Bakx WG, et al. Accelerometry measuring the outcome of robot-supported upper limb training in chronic stroke: a randomized controlled trial. *PLoS ONE* (2013) 13:e96414. doi: 10.1371/journal.pone.0096414
35. van der Lee JH, De Groot V, Beckerman H, Wagenaar RC, Lankhorst GJ, Bouter LM, et al. The intra-and interrater reliability of the action research arm test: a practical test of upper extremity function in patients with stroke. *Arch Phys Med Rehabil.* (2001) 82:14–9. doi: 10.1053/apmr.2001.18668
36. van der Lee JH, Wagenaar RC, Lankhorst GJ, Vogelaar TW, Devillé WL, Bouter LM. Forced use of the upper extremity in chronic stroke patients: results from a single-blind randomized clinical trial *Stroke* (1999) 30:2369–75.
37. Lang CE, Edwards DF, Birkenmeier RL, Dromerick AW. Estimating minimal clinically important differences of upper-extremity measures early after stroke. *Arch Phys Med Rehabil.* (2008) 89:1693–1700 doi: 10.1016/j.apmr.2008.02.022
38. Takebayashi T, Amano S, Hanada K, Uchiyama Y, Domen K. Robotic therapy in multiple interventions for severe-to-moderate arm deficits in chronic stroke patients. *Jpn Occup Ther Res.* (2017) 36:148–58.
39. Takebayashi T, Amano S, Hanada K, Umeji A, Takahashi K, Koyama T, et al. Therapeutic synergism in the treatment of post-stroke arm paresis utilizing

botulinum toxin, robotic therapy, and constraint-induced movement therapy. *PMR* (2014) 6:1054–8. doi: 10.1016/j.pmrj.2014.04.014

40. Fritz SL, Light KE, Patterson TS, Behrman AL, Davis SB. Active finger extension predicts outcomes after constraint-induced movement therapy for individuals with hemiparesis after stroke. *Stroke* (2005) 36:1172–7. doi: 10.1161/01.STR.0000165922.96430.d0
41. Huang YH. Determinants of change in stroke-specific quality of life after distributed constraint-induced therapy. *Am J Occup Ther.* (2013) 67:54–63. doi: 10.5014/ajot.2013.004820
42. Jongbloed L. Prediction of function after stroke: a critical review. *Stroke* (1986) 17:765–76 doi: 10.1161/01.STR.17.4.765
43. Liou LM, Lin HF, Tsai CL, Lin RT, Lai CL. Timing of stroke onset determines discharge-functional status but not stroke severity: a hospital-based study. *Kaohsiung J Med Sci.* (2013) 29:32–3. doi: 10.1016/j.kjms.2012.08.005
44. Fritz SL, Light KE, Clifford SN, Patterson TS, Behrman AL, Davis SB. Descriptive characteristics as potential predictors of outcomes following constraint-induced movement therapy for people after stroke. *Phys Ther.* (2006) 86:825–32. doi: 10.1093/ptj/86.6.825

12

Oropharyngeal Muscle Exercise Therapy Improves Signs and Symptoms of Post-Stroke Moderate Obstructive Sleep Apnea Syndrome

Dongmei Ye[1*†], *Chen Chen*[2†], *Dongdong Song*[3], *Mei Shen*[4*], *Hongwei Liu*[1], *Surui Zhang*[1], *Hong Zhang*[1], *Jingya Li*[1], *Wenfei Yu*[1] *and Qiwen Wang*[1,4]

[1] Department of Rehabilitation, Affiliated Zhongshan Hospital of Dalian University, Dalian, China, [2] Department of Anatomy, Medical College of Dalian University, Dalian, China, [3] Department of Imaging, Affiliated Zhongshan Hospital of Dalian University, Dalian, China, [4] Department of Rehabilitation, People's Hospital of Longhua District of Shenzhen, Shenzhen, China

***Correspondence:**
Dongmei Ye
shuiyan_1980@163.com
Mei Shen
pyf0404@126.com

† These authors have contributed equally to this work

The primary aim of the current study was to assess the effects of oropharingeal muscle exercises in obstruction severity on stroke patients with OSAS. The secondary aims were to evaluate the effects of the exercises on rehabilitation of neurological function, sleeping, and morphology change of upper airway. An open-label, single-blind, parallel-group, randomized, controlled trial was designed. Fifty post-stroke patients with moderate OSAS were randomly assigned into 2 groups (25 in each group). For the therapy group, oropharyngeal muscle exercise was performed during the daytime for 20 min, twice a day, for 6 weeks. The control group was subjected to sham therapy of deep breathing. Primary outcomes were the obstruction severity by polysomnography. Secondary outcomes included recovery of motor and neurocognitive function, personal activities of daily living assessment (ADL), sleep quality and sleepiness scale. It also included upper airway magnetic resonance imaging (MRI) measurements. Assessments were made at baseline and after 6-week exercise. Finally, 49 patients completed the study. The apnea–hypopnea index, snore index, arousal index, and minimum oxygen saturation improved after exercise ($P < 0.05$). Oropharyngeal muscle exercises improved subjective measurements of sleep quality ($P = 0.017$), daily sleepiness ($P = 0.005$), and performance (both $P < 0.05$) except for neurocognition ($P = 0.741$). The changes in obstruction improvement, sleep characteristics and performance scale were also associated with training time, as detected by Pearson's correlation analysis. The anatomic structural remodeling of the pharyngeal airway was measured using MRI, including the lager retropalatal distance ($P = 0.018$) and shorter length of soft palate ($P = 0.044$) compared with the baseline. Hence, oropharyngeal muscle exercise is a promising alternative treatment strategy for stroke patients with moderate OSAS.

Clinical Trial Registration: http://www.chictr.org.cn. Unique identifier: ChiCTR-IPR-16009970

Keywords: MRI, obstructive sleep apnea syndrome, oropharyngeal muscles exercise, polysomnography, stroke

INTRODUCTION

Based on previous studies, 57% of stroke patients suffer from obstructive sleep apnea syndrome (OSAS) in rehabilitation units (1, 2). OSAS is associated with lower cognitive ability (3), motor ability (4), and daily activity (5) in patients admitted for stroke rehabilitation. Early use of continuous positive airway pressure (CPAP) appears to accelerate neurological recovery and delay cardiovascular events in patients with ischemic stroke (6). However, multiple randomized trials have demonstrated that the efficacy of CPAP has been limited due to poor clinical acceptance and adherence (7, 8). The poor treatment adherence, 12–15% as previously reported (9, 10), is a major limitation resulting in the overall poor efficacy for CPAP. Therefore, finding alternative therapies should help alleviate obstruction in the upper airway and improve compliance. Multiple imaging modalities have been used to study the airway passage and have demonstrated anatomical differences between patients with and without OSAS for physiologic dysfunction of muscles (10, 11). Electromyographic findings suggest reduced pharyngeal muscles and lingualis motility in patients with ischemic stroke (12, 13). Recent studies have demonstrated that training the upper airway muscles can ameliorate moderate OSAS (14, 15). The set of oropharyngeal exercises used in the present study was developed in 16 years and has previously been shown to be effective in patients with stroke-free OSAS in uncontrolled and controlled studies (14–16). However, its therapeutic effect on post-stroke OSAS has not been studied. The present study focused on patients with OSAS in stroke rehabilitation units. The primary aim of the study was to assess the effects of oropharingeal muscle exercises in obstruction severity. The secondary aims were to evaluate the effects of the exercises on recovery of neurological function, sleeping, and anatomic changing of upper airway. It was hypothesized that oropharyngeal muscle exercise could be beneficial for patients' recovery in the airway obstruction and in the motor, neurocognitive, and ADL performance after stroke.

METHODS

Trial Design and Oversight

The present study was an open-label, parallel-group, randomized, controlled trial (Clinical Trial Registration; http://www.chictr.org.cn. Unique identifier: ChiCTR-IPR-16009970). It was approved by the ethics committee of the affiliated Zhongshan Hospital of Dalian University in February 2016 (approval number 2016040). Patients were recruited from November 2016 to November 2017. All participants provided informed written consent.

Inclusion and Exclusion Criteria

Stroke patients visiting the rehabilitation center of the affiliated Zhongshan Hospital of Dalian University were recruited for the study from November 2016 to November 2017. Patients who experienced a first stroke that was either hemorrhagic or ischemic within 3 weeks were scheduled for stroke rehabilitation. The inclusion criteria included patients who snored, had the ability to participate in the sleep study, and complete the functional assessment. The patients' AHI should be >15 and <30 events/hour by polysomnography (PSG). Patients were excluded based on one or more of the following criteria: body mass index (BMI) 40 kg/m^2 or greater, craniofacial malformations, agomphosis, severe nasal disease, regular use of hypnotic medications, hypothyroidism, previous stroke, aphasia, neuromuscular disease, heart failure, or severe obstructive nasal disease. Sleep-disordered breathing was evaluated using a simple four-variable screening tool. The patients with screening scores below 10 were excluded (17, 18) (**Figure 1**).

Sleep Apnea Diagnosis

A respiratory sleep study was performed in the hospital ward within the first 48–72 h after transferring from the stroke unit to the rehabilitation unit. PSG was performed by trained staff at the patient's bedside before and after therapy. The PSG included electroencephalogram, respiratory inductive plethysmography, electrocardiogram, and oxygen saturation (SaO_2%). Portable unattended PSG (LifeShirt, Vivometrics, CA, USA) was used for the measurements (1). Apnea was defined as the reduction in peak signal excursion by ≥90% of the pre-event baseline that lasted for ≥10 s. Hypopnea was defined as a reduction in the peak signal excursion of ≥30% for ≥10 s with a corresponding oxygen desaturation event of ≥4%. The AHI was calculated using the total apneic and hypopneic events detected per hour of the recorded night data. Sleep apnea was diagnosed when the AHI ≥5 events/hour. Respiratory events in the presence of abdominal effort were scored as obstructive, and respiratory events in the absence of abdominal effort were scored as central events. A respiratory event was scored as a mixed apnea if it met the apnea criteria and was associated with the absence of inspiratory effort in the second portion of the event. For the purpose of distinguishing between obstructive and central sleep apnea, mixed apneas were classified as obstructive respiratory events (1).

Intervention

Oropharyngeal muscle exercises were derived from speech–language pathology and included soft palate, tongue, and facial muscle exercises. Patients were instructed by a single speech pathologist to perform the following tasks (14). The concrete proposal of the exercises see the **Table 1**. Patients would receive assistance from the therapist if they were unable to complete the motion or performed it inadequately. All the exercises were included in a 20-min training session and administered twice a day to the patients in the therapy group. The control group was subjected to 20-min deep breathing training twice a day.

Randomization

All the patients were randomized to receive either conventional treatment for stroke combined with oropharyngeal muscle exercise (therapy group) or deep breathing (control group) using a computer-generated random list (1:1 ratio) for 6 weeks. Patients' training time was recorded by the speech pathologist.

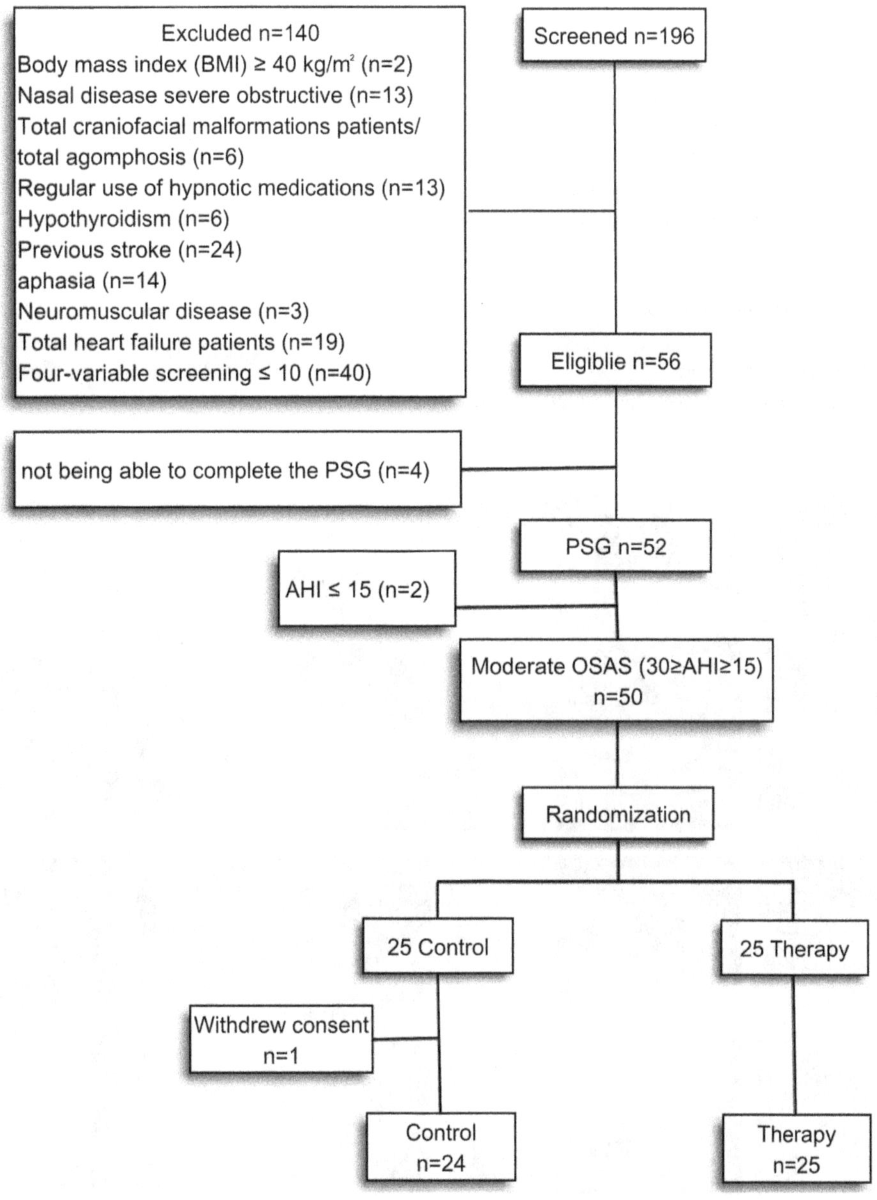

FIGURE 1 | Research design.

Outcomes

The primary outcomes were obstruction severity by PSG including apnea-hypopnea index (AHI), minimum SaO_2%, arousal index per sleep hour (AI), and snore index (SI). Several domains were evaluated as secondary outcomes. Motor recovery was evaluated using the Fugl–Meyer assessment (FMA), which included the upper or lower extremity motor performance (19). ADL was assessed by one occupational therapist using the basic Barthel Index (20). Cognition recovery was assessed using the Mini-Mental State Examination (MMSE) scale (21). Secondary outcomes also included sleep quality, sleepiness, and airway MRI measurements. The Stanford Sleepiness Scale (SSS) was administered to assess the level of sleepiness (22). The Pittsburgh Sleep Quality Index (PSQI) was used to determine the participants' sleep habits and quality (23). The participants with OSAS completed the functional, motor, and sleeping quality assessments between 9:00 and 11:00 a.m. administered by individuals who were blinded to subject randomization. Assessment scales were completed before and at the end of the intervention. Assessments were made at baseline and after 6-week exercise.

Airway MRI Measurements

The brain MRI examination was performed on 30 patients (15 from each group) at the beginning and end of the intervention. Images were obtained in the supine position with the head in

TABLE 1 | Oropharyngeal muscle exercises record.

Motion requirement	Times or duration	completion status
(1) pronouncing an oral vowel intermittently and continuously;	5 times	Yes/No
(2) brushing the superior and lateral surfaces of the teeth by tongue;	5 times	Yes/No
(3) placing the tip of the tongue against the front of the palate and sliding the tongue backward;	2 min	Yes/No
(4) forced tongue sucking upward against the palate, pressing the entire tongue against the palate;	2 min	Yes/No
(5) forcing the back of the tongue against the floor of the mouth while keeping the tip of the tongue in contact with the inferior incisive teeth;	2 min	Yes/No
(6) extended tongue;	200 times	Yes/No
(7) orbicularis oris muscle pressure with the mouth closed;	30 s × 4	Yes/No
(8) gargle without water;	200 times	Yes/No
(9) suction movements contracting only the buccinator;	5 s × 10	Yes/No
(10) ice stimulation on the soft palate, palatal arch, tongue root, and posterior wall of the pharynx.	5 s × 10	Yes/No

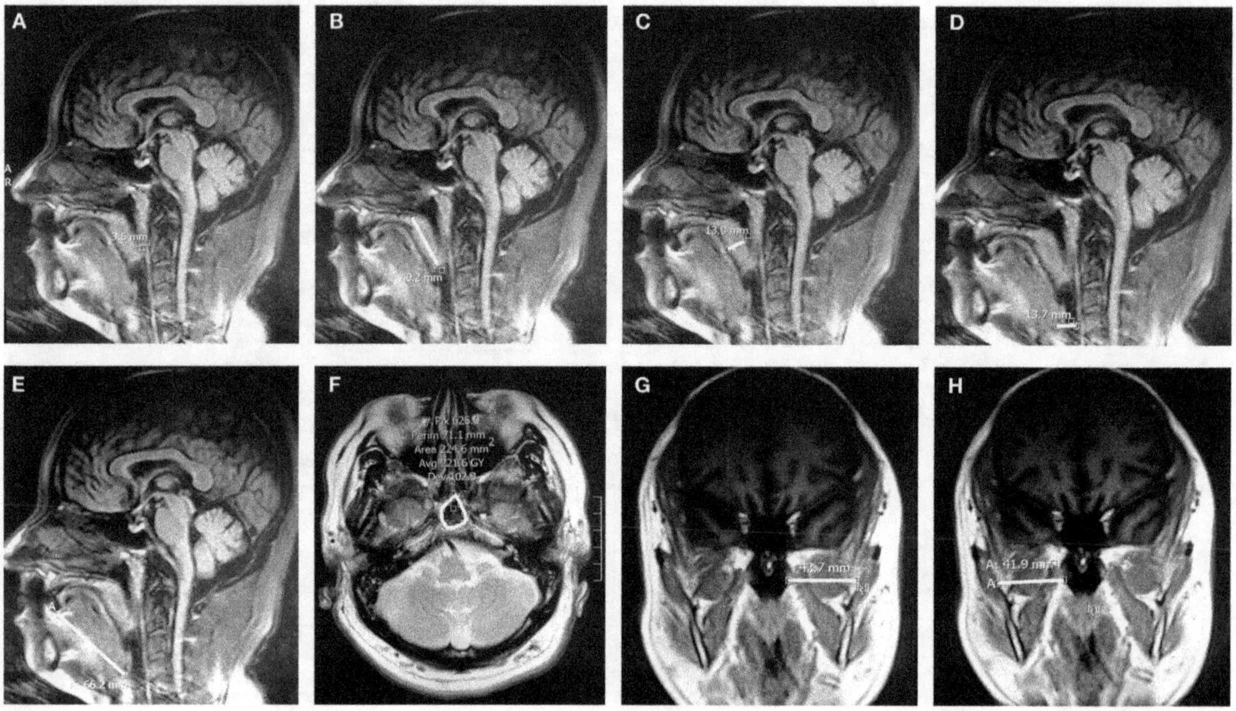

FIGURE 2 | MRI measurements. **(A)** Retropalatal distance on a sagittal T1-weighted image. **(B)** Palatal length on a sagittal T1-weighted image. **(C)** Palatal thickness on a sagittal T1-weighted image. **(D)** Retroglossal space on a sagittal T1-weighted image. **(E)** Tongue length on a sagittal T1-weighted image. **(F)** Cross-sectional area of the retropharyngeal region on an axial T2-weighted image. **(G,H)** Lateral pharyngeal wall thickness on a coronal T1-weighted image.

the neutral position. Brain MRI scans were retrieved from the hospital's PACS archives, and measurements were performed using the syngo.via image software (Siemens). Experienced neuroradiologists who were blinded to the interventions performed all the measurements. Measurements included the retropalatal distance (midsagittal T1), soft palatal length (midsagittal T1), soft palatal thickness (midsagittal T1), retroglossal space (midsagittal T1), tongue length (midsagittal T1), nasopharyngeal area (axial T2), and lateral pharyngeal wall thickness (coronal T1) (24) (**Figure 2**).

Statistical Analysis

At least 17 patients in each group were required to determine a 50% reduction in objective snoring in patients randomized to oropharyngeal exercises based on a previous study, using a two-sample design and the assumption of an α of 0.05 and 80% power (14). Data were expressed as mean [standard deviation (SD)] for normal distribution and as median (interquartile range 25–75%) for skewed variables. Data were analyzed using SPSS (version 22.0, IBM, NY, USA). The variables were tested for normal distribution using the Kolmogorov–Smirnov test. Variables not normally distributed were logarithmically transformed. Two-factor analysis of variance with adjustment for gender and calendar age was used to compare differences between groups for variables measured at baseline and after 6 weeks. Paired-samples t-tests were used to compare the difference in the value within a group between the baseline and after 6 weeks. Effect size values were calculated using Cohen's d. The effect size was computed by finding the difference between the control and treatment groups in the outcome measure after 6-week exercises and dividing this value by the pooled SD. As set forth by Cohen (1988), an effect size <0.2 was considered a small effect; 0.21–0.5 was a medium effect; and >0.8 was a large effect. The changes in PSG parameters, sleeping characteristics, performance scale, and MRI measurements were calculated using the difference in the values between 6 weeks and onset. The association between the changes and training time was assessed using the Pearson's correlation analysis. The correlation coefficient <0.2 was considered an extremely weak correlation or no correlation, 0.21–0.4 was considered a weak correlation, 0.41–0.6 was considered a moderate correlation, 0.61–0.8 was considered a strong correlation, and 0.41–0.6 was considered an extremely strong correlation (25). A $P < 0.05$ was considered significant.

TABLE 2 | Anthropometric data and baseline characteristics of the total sample.

Characteristic	Control (n = 24)	Therapy (n = 25)	P-value
Age	65.5 (10.4)	63.4 (9.9)	0.449[a]
Male, no.	17 (70.8)	19 (76.0)	0.399[b]
BMI, kg/m^2	27.8 (3.2)	26.7 (2.8)	0.182[a]
Neck circumference, cm	43.0 (42.0, 45.0)	43.0 (42.0, 44.5)	0.120[c]
NIHSS	8.4 (2.7)	7.7 (2.6)	0.370 [a]
MEDICAL HISTORY			
Snore history	18 (75.0)	16 (64.0)	0.404[b]
Hypertension	21 (87.5)	25 (100)	0.068[b]
Diabetes	14 (58.3)	13 (52.0)	0.656[b]
Hyperlipidemia	13 (54.2)	16 (64.0)	0.484[b]
Atrial fibrillation	7 (29.2)	11 (44.0)	0.282[b]
Current smoker	17 (70.8)	14 (56.0)	0.291[b]
Stroke type			0.102[b]
ischemia	21 (87.5)	17 (68.0)	
Hemorrhage	3 (12.5)	8 (32.0)	
PERFORMANCE SCALE			
MMSE	24.8 (2.4)	25.8 (2.5)	0.172[a]
FMA	33.3 (8.2)	30.5 (9.2)	0.266[a]
Barthel Index	30.0 (27.5, 37.5)	30.0 (26.6, 35.0)	0.837[c]
SLEEP CHARACTERISTICS			
SSS	6.0 (5.0, 6.0)	6.0 (5.0, 6.0)	0.675[c]
PSQI	8.0 (1.7)	7.6 (1.8)	0.750[a]
PSG RESULTS			
AHI	20.1 (3.0)	20.8 (4.0)	0.494[a]
Minimum SaO_2, %	81.2 (3.3)	80.8 (4.6)	0.724[a]
AI	17.3 (3.2)	18.2 (3.8)	0.411[a]
SI	19.4 (4.4)	18.4 (4.4)	0.472[a]
Central facial paralysis	12 (50.0)	18 (72.0)	0.114[b]
Days between onset to rehab unit	11.9 (2.6)	12.3 (3.5)	0.656 [a]
Training time, min	1482.7 (108.0)	1513.2 (102.7)	0.306[a]

BMI, body mass index; NIHSS, NIH Stroke Scale; MMSE, Mini-mental State Examination; FMA, Fugl-Meyer Assessment; SSS, Stanford sleepiness scale; PSQI, Pittsburg sleep quality index scale; PSG, polysomnogram; AHI, apnea-hypopnea index; AI, arousal index per sleep hour; SI, snore index. Values are presented as mean (standard deviation), n (%) or median (interquartile range). [a]Student t-test. [b]Fisher exact test, [c]Mann-Whitney U test.

RESULTS

A total of 196 stroke patients with snoring complaints were screened in this study. Fifty-six patients with screening scores above 10 were administered a polysomnography (PSG). Four patients who were unable to complete the PSG were excluded. Only two patients had an AHI $\leq$15. They were excluded for maintaining consistency of the moderate of apnea. Finally, 50 patients were selected for the study with $30 \geq \text{AHI} \geq 15$ events/hour. One patient in the control group withdrew due to recurrent strokes (**Figure 1**). The remaining patients achieved 81.5–100% of the expected training time. The demographic, sleep characteristics and training time, according to the group assigned, are presented in **Table 2**. Patients assigned to the control and therapy groups had similar baseline characteristics (**Table 2**). Obstructive sleep apnea was the predominant respiratory event, with central apneas being rare, while none of the patients had pure central sleep apnea.

Primary Outcomes

After 6 weeks of treatment, no significant changes were observed in the control group; however, significant changes were observed in the therapy group (**Table 3**). In contrast, patients who were randomized into the oropharyngeal muscle exercise group had a significant decrease in AHI ($P = 0.004$), AI ($P = 0.010$), and SI ($P = 0.006$), and an increase in minimum SaO_2% ($P = 0.039$) between the control and therapy groups with adjustment for gender and calendar age (**Table 3**). The values of effect size for AHI, AI, SI, and minimum SaO_2% were all > 0.8, indicating a large effect of exercises on the improvement in airway obstruction (**Table 4**). After the Pearson's correlation analysis, moderate correlations were found between the training time of oropharyngeal exercises and the changes in SI, AI, minimum SaO_2% (all $P < 0.05$), and a strong correlation between the training time and AHI change ($r = -0.833$, $P < 0.001$) (**Table 5**).

Secondary Outcomes

Patients assigned to the exercise group experienced a significant increase in motor function (FMA) ($P = 0.006$) and basic ADL score (Barthel Index) ($P < 0.001$) (**Table 3**), implying a large effect (**Table 4**). Despite an increase in cognitive function (MMSE), no significant difference between the two groups was observed. The results of Pearson's correlation analysis indicated that there were moderate correlations between the training time of oropharyngeal exercises and the changes in basic ADL scores ($r = 0.569$, $P = 0.003$), and a strong correlation between the training time and FMA change ($r = 0.627$, $P = 0.001$). However, no correlation was found between the training time and MMSE ($r = 0.358$, $P = 0.079$) (**Table 5**).

TABLE 3 | Polysomnographic, sleeping, and performance data.

	Control		Therapy		*P*-value
	Baseline	**6 weeks**	**Baseline**	**6 weeks**	
AHI	20.1 (3.0)	19.5 (3.5)	20.8 (4.0)	14.3 (4.1)†#	0.004
Minimum SaO_2, %	81.2 (3.3)	82.2 (4.2)	80.8 (4.6)	85.8 (4.2)†#	0.039
AI	17.3 (3.2)	16.9 (3.8)	18.2 (3.8)	13.0 (3.3)†#	0.010
SI	19.4 (4.4)	18.2 (4.5)	18.4 (4.4)	13.7 (5.6)†#	0.006
SSS	6.0 (5.0, 6.0)	5.5 (5.0, 6.0)	6.0 (5.0, 6.0)	4.0 (3.0, 4.5)†#	0.005
PSQI	8.0 (1.7)	7.6 (1.8)	7.6 (1.8)	5.7 (1.9)†#	0.017
MMSE	24.8 (2.5)	26.1 (1.9)†	25.8 (2.6)	26.9 (2.2)†	0.741
FMA	33.3 (8.2)	42.0 (10.3)†	30.5 (9.2)	57.5 (15.2)†#	0.006
Barthel Index	30.0 (27.5, 37.5)	45.0 (35.0, 55.0)†	30.0 (26.6, 35.0)	60.0 (51.3, 70.0)†#	<0.001

AHI, apnea-hypopnea index; SaO_2, oxygen saturation; AI, arousal index per sleep hour; SI, snore index; SSS, Stanford sleepiness scale; PSQI, Pittsburg sleep quality index scale; MMSE, Mini-mental State Examination; FMA, Fugl-Meyer Assessment. Values are presented as mean (standard deviation) or median (interquartile range). †*$P < 0.05$ baseline vs. 6 weeks.* #*$P < 0.05$ control (6 weeks) vs. therapy (6 weeks).*

TABLE 4 | The effect size measure for the difference between the groups after 6 weeks exercise.

	Control*	**Therapy***	***P*-value**	***t*-value**	**Cohen's *d* (95% confidence intervals)**
AHI	19.5 (3.5)	14.3 (4.1)	0.000	4.615	1.319 (0.693, 1.933)
Min SaO2, %	82.2 (4.2)	85.8 (4.2)	0.001	−3.520	1.006 (0.406, 1.597)
AI	16.9 (3.8)	13.0 (3.3)	0.003	3.146	0.899 (0.306, 1.483)
SI	18.2 (4.5)	13.7 (5.6)	0.000	4.366	1.248 (0.628, 1.856)
SSS	5.5 (5.0, 6.0)	4.0 (3.0, 4.5)	0.001	3.503	1.001 (0.401, 1.592)
PSQI	7.6 (1.8)	5.7 (1.9)	0.000	−1.216	1.187 (0.573, 1.791)
MMSE	26.1 (1.9)	26.9 (2.2)	0.230	−4.155	0.348 (−0.219, 0.910)
FMA	42.0 (10.3)	57.5 (15.2)	0.000	−4.941	1.415 (0.780, 2.037)
Barthel index	45.0 (35.0, 55.0)	60.0 (51.3, 70.0)	0.000	4.615	1.319 (0.692, 1.933)

*AHI, apnea-hypopnea index; SaO_2, oxygen saturation; AI, arousal index per sleep hour; SI, snore index; SSS, Stanford Sleepiness Scale; PSQI, Pittsburg sleep quality index scale; MMSE, Mini-mental State Examination; FMA, Fugl-Meyer Assessment, *Values are presented as mean (standard deviation) or median (interquartile range).*

The exercises significantly improved the scores for the sleep quality questionnaires ($P = 0.017$). The results of SSS decreased ($P = 0.005$), indicating that the excessive daytime sleepiness reduced (**Table 3**). The values of effect size for SSS and PSQI were >0.8, implying a large effect of exercises on the improvement in sleeping quality and daytime sleepiness (**Table 4**). Comparisons of MRI measurements between the therapy and control groups are shown in **Table 6**. After therapy, the retropalatal distance was significantly larger in the therapy group than in the control group ($P = 0.018$). The length of the soft palate was also found to be reduced significantly in the therapy group than in the control group ($P = 0.044$). Regarding the difference in the outcome measure after 6-week exercises between the control and treatment groups, the values of effect size showed that the exercises had a large effect on the retropalatal distance and soft palate length and small effects on other measurements (**Table 7**). The results of the Pearson's correlation analysis demonstrated the association between the MRI measurement changes and the training time of oropharyngeal exercises (**Table 8**). Larger retropalatal distance ($r = 0.800$, $P < 0.001$) and shorter soft palates ($r = -0.747$, $P = 0.001$) were strongly associated with longer training times.

DISCUSSION

The present study examined the effects of oropharyngeal exercise in stroke patients with moderate OSAS using objective polysomnography measurements and quantification of subjective symptoms, including snoring, daytime sleepiness, and sleep quality. Good compliance was observed in participation and time spent on the exercises. A satisfactory therapeutic effect of oropharyngeal exercise on OSAS was demonstrated by the decrease in AHI, AI, and SI and increase in minimum SaO_2%, suggesting the improvement in upper airway obstruction. According to the PSG results ($14 \geq$ AHI ≥ 5, $89 \geq SaO_2\% \geq 85$) (26), 52.0% (13 in 25) of subjects in treatment group was diagnosed with mild OSAS comparing with 4.1% (1 in 24) in control group after 6 weeks exercises. In cases of severe and moderate OSAS, treatment is necessary and CPAP is the first-line option (27). Significant increasing were observed on oxygen saturation CPAP titration (more than 15%), and also 90% decrease was recorded on AHI in patients with stroke-free OSAS (28). However, CPAP treats OSAS but is generally poorly tolerated by stroke patients. The result of previous study on nasal expiratory positive airway pressure (EPAP) for sleep apnea

TABLE 5 | Correlation of the training time and the change of PSG parameter, sleep characteristics, and performance in Pearson's correlation analysis.

	The length of training time	
	r	*P*-value
Δ AHI	−0.833	< 0.001
Δ Min SaO_2	0.487	0.014
Δ AI	−0.541	0.035
Δ SI	−0.605	0.001
Δ SSS	−0.450	0.024
Δ PSQI	−0.462	0.020
Δ MMSE	0.358	0.079
Δ FMA	0.627	0.001
Δ Barthel index	0.569	0.003

Δ, 6 weeks – baseline; AHI, apnea – hypopnea index; SaO_2, oxygen saturation; AI, arousal index per sleep hour; SI, snore index; SSS, Stanford sleepiness scale; PSQI, Pittsburg sleep quality index scale; MMSE, Mini-mental State Examination; FMA, Fugl-Meyer Assessment.

TABLE 6 | MRI measurement data (mm or mm^2).

	Control		Therapy		*P*-value
	Baseline	6 weeks	Baseline	6 weeks	
RPD	1.7 (0.1)	1.8 (0.2)	1.7 (0.1)	2.1 (0.2)†#	0.018
SPL	50.2 (3.1)	50.3 (4.8)	49.2 (2.7)	45.5 (1.9†#	0.044
MPT	9.9 (1.4)	10.0 (1.5)	9.6 (1.8)	10.0 (1.3)	0.656
RGS	9.1 (1.7)	10.0 (1.8)†	9.5 (2.2)	10.1 (1.8)†	0.747
TL	67.1 (8.7)	67.6 (6.8)	66.1 (8.4)	66.2 (9.4)	0.951
NPA	351.9 (24.5)	355.2 (22.6)	355.6 (28.2)	362.6 (32.5)	0.781
LPWT	79.4 (7.3)	78.9 (6.6)	79.2 (8.0)	80.3 (7.5)	0.659

RPD, Retropalatal distance; SPL, Soft palate length; MPT, Maximum palatal thickness; RGS, Retroglossal space; TL, Tongue length; NPA, Nasopharyngeal airway (mm^2); LPWT, lateral pharyngeal wall thickness. †$P < 0.05$ baseline vs. 6 weeks. #$P < 0.05$ control (6 weeks) vs. therapy (6 weeks).

TABLE 7 | The effect size measure for the difference between the groups after 6 weeks exercise.

	Control*	Therapy*	*P*-value	*t*-value	Cohen's *d* (95% confidence intervals)
DPR	1.8 (0.2)	2.1 (0.2)	0.000	4.02	1.468 (0.646, 2.269)
SPL	50.3 (4.8)	45.5 (1.9)	0.002	3.33	1.214 (0.423, 1.988)
MPT	10.0 (1.5)	10.0 (1.3)	0.886	−0.145	0.053 (−0.664, 0.769)
RGS	10.0 (1.8)	10.1 (1.8)	0.846	−0.195	0.071 (−0.645, 0.787)
TL	67.6 (6.8)	66.2 (9.4)	0.613	0.512	0.187 (−0.532, 0.903)
NPA	355.2 (22.6)	362.6 (32.5)	0.462	−0.745	0.272 (−0.450, 0.989)
LPWT	78.9 (6.6)	80.3 (7.5)	0.571	−0.573	0.209 (−0.510, 0.925)

*RPD, Retropalatal distance; SPL, Soft palate length; MPT, Maximum palatal thickness; RGS, Retroglossal space; TL, Tongue length; NPA, Nasopharyngeal airway (mm^2); LPWT, lateral pharyngeal wall thickness. *Values are presented as mean (standard deviation).*

TABLE 8 | Correlation of the training time and MRI measures change in Pearson's correlation analysis.

	The length of training time	
	r	*P*-value
Δ RPD	0.800	< 0.001
Δ SPL	−0.747	0.001
Δ MPT	0.200	0.474
Δ RGS	−0.043	0.879
Δ TL	−0.071	0.801
Δ NPA	0.067	0.814
Δ LPWT	0.333	0.225

Δ, 6 weeks-baseline; RPD, Retropalatal distance; SPL, Soft palate length; MPT, Maximum palatal thickness; RGS, Retroglossal space; TL, Tongue length; NPA, Nasopharyngeal airway (mm^2); TLPT, Total lateral pharyngeal soft tissue thickness.

after stroke shew a 33.5% decrease on AHI and a 11.4% increase on minimum SaO_2% (29). The results of the present research (a 25.5% decrease on AHI and a 6.19% increase on minimum SaO_2%) indicate that the effect of oropharyngeal exercise on improvement of airway obstruction seems to lower than CPAP and EPAP.

The genesis of post-stroke OSAS is multifactorial and includes anatomic and physiological factors. Upper airway dilator muscles are crucial for maintaining pharyngeal patency and may contribute to the genesis of OSAS (30). The influence of oropharyngeal exercise on the upper airway anatomy was explored in the present study. Retropalatal distance increased significantly after exercise. Additionally, the soft palate measurements showed that the obstruction in the pharyngeal morphology improved after exercise. The clinical significance of the change in upper airway anatomy was confirmed by effect size (Cohen's *d*). A previous study demonstrated that shorter retropalatal distances were associated with higher AHIs (24). Longer vertical soft palatal dimensions were observed in both non-stroke and stroke patients with OSAS (11, 24). The larger retropalatal distances and shorter soft palate length related to tonic activity were thought to enhance the stiffness in the rostral upper airway. Hence, it was believed that obstruction in the upper airway was alleviated by the exercises via the increase in muscular tension of the pharyngeal muscles. Epidemiological studies on stroke patients have shown that hypoactivation of the tongue is the major mechanism underlying narrowing and closing of the upper airway (14, 31). The neural modulation and motor output to the genioglossus muscle of the tongue are weak in wakefulness and natural sleep (32). Anatomically, movement of the tongue not only engages the lingualis but also the pharyngeal muscles around it. In the present study, 5 of the 10 movement exercises were related to the lingualis. Although the length of the tongue did not change significantly on MRI, the lingualis and pharyngeal muscles improved after exercise. A recent study indicated that single tongue treatment by intraoral electrical neurostimulation could reduce snoring but not AHI (33). In the present study, oropharyngeal and lingual muscle exercises reduced AHI. Hence, the muscle groups exercised for the upper airway benefited stroke patients with OSAS.

The training time of oropharyngeal muscle exercise was an important factor, as a kind of kinetotherapy. Both therapeutic effects and a good compliance need to be taken into account. Ieto et al. instructed patients to perform oropharyngeal exercises three times a day, including the six mastication patterns for approximately 8 min. Oropharyngeal exercises were effective in reducing objectively measured snoring (15). Guimarães's 30-min oropharyngeal exercises included six actions for linguales, five for facial muscles, and one for swallowing and chewing. It improved the snoring frequency, daytime sleepiness, and neck circumference (14). In Puhan's study on didgeridoo-playing treatment for OSAS, participants had to practice at home for at least 20 min on at least 5 days a week, which improved the daytime sleepiness and AHI (34). In the present study, the training time was 20 min twice a day. All the patients attainted 81.5–100% of training time. A positive correlation existed between the improvement in performance and training time. According to the results of Pearson's correlation analysis, reextension of time or frequency might lead to further improvement. However, the compliance likely declined because the exercise was a bit tedious in spots.

Previous studies demonstrated that OSAS was an independent predictor for worse functional outcome in post-stroke patients (35, 36). In a previous study, respiratory sleep disorders correlated with early neurological deterioration and less satisfactory functional outcomes as evaluated using the Barthel Index (37). Patients with recent stroke and sleep apnea were found to have a poorer functional outcome assessed using the Barthel Index at discharge from rehabilitation and 3 and 12 months after stroke onset (38). The present study focused on whether effective treatment of OSAS after stroke improved functional outcome. The results showed that recovery of motor function improved after oropharyngeal muscle exercise. The physical ADL estimated using the Barthel Index also improved significantly after the exercise intervention. Previous randomized studies on subacute stroke patients (in the range of 2–4 weeks) demonstrated the beneficial effects of CPAP on sleep architecture, motor function, and ADL (4, 7). The functional independence and motor improvements might have alleviated the adverse cerebrovascular effects of OSAS, possibly through enhanced neuroplasticity. A previous study found that unilateral nasal obstruction in rats during growth periods induced changes in arterial $SaO_2\%$ and altered the development of motor representation within the face primary cortex (39). The greater reduction in alveolar ventilation during REM sleep also resulted in transient declines in $SaO_2\%$ from a sustained level of hypoxia during NREM sleep for OSAS. Patients with OSAS demonstrated increased motor cortex inhibition by increasing GABAergic tone (40). The results of PSG in both previous studies and the present study indicated that the apnea–hypopnea events and minimum $SaO_2\%$ were ameliorated by both CPAP and oropharyngeal exercise. Therefore, the promotion of motor function and functional independence might enhance neuroplasticity by oropharyngeal muscle exercise, which may result from its positive cerebral $SaO_2\%$ effects. However, the difference in cognitive function after exercise between the two groups was not significant, which was also observed in studies using CPAP therapy for stroke patients with OSAS (7, 36, 41). The exact mechanism has yet to be deciphered and needs more investigation.

The present study had some limitations. First, patients enrolled in the study were required to complete the questionnaire evaluation and oropharyngeal muscle exercises. Patients with significant physical impairment or aphasia were excluded. Thus, the results of this study may not be applicable to patients with severe strokes. Second, based on the inclusion and exclusion criteria, most of the patients enrolled had moderate OSAS (AHI from 15 to 30). The therapeutic efficacy of exercise in mild and severe OSAS should be investigated further. Third, the sleep status of patients during MRI was not documented. Differences in MRI measurements on airway have been observed in awake patients with and without OSAS (24). Hence, it is believed that this method can be used to evaluate changes in the anatomic structures of the airway. Finally, CPAP is the clinically recommended treatment for stroke patients with OSAS. Unfortunately, the therapeutic efficacy of exercise and CPAP could not be compared due to limited resources. This is an important comparison and should be conducted in future studies.

CONCLUSIONS

In conclusion, oropharyngeal muscle exercises reduced OSAS severity and increased sleep quality in stroke patients with moderate OSAS. The oropharyngeal exercise also improved the rehabilitation of motor function and personal ADL. The anatomic structural remodeling of the upper airway (larger retropalatal distance and shorter soft palate) observed by MRI improved after exercise. The results suggested that the set of oropharyngeal muscle exercises used in the present study may serve as a promising alternative therapeutic strategy for stroke patients with moderate OSAS.

AUTHOR CONTRIBUTIONS

DY and MS conceived and designed the study. DS, SZ, HZ, JL, and WY performed the experiments. CC, HL, and QW analyzed the data. DY and CC wrote the manuscript.

ACKNOWLEDGMENTS

The authors wish to thank physiotherapists Yinliang Zhang and Yang Yang for their excellent work on performance assessment.

REFERENCES

1. Bravata DM, Concato J, Fried T, Ranjbar N, Sadarangani T, Mcclain V, et al. Continuous positive airway pressure: evaluation of a novel therapy for patients with acute ischemic stroke. *Sleep* (2011) 34:1271–7. doi: 10.5665/SLEEP.1254
2. Turkington PM, Bamford J, Wanklyn P, Elliott MW. Effect of upper airway obstruction on blood pressure variability after stroke. *Clin Sci.* (2004) 107:75–9. doi: 10.1042/CS20030404

3. Aaronson JA, van Bennekom CA, Hofman WF, van Bezeij T, van den Aardweg JG, Groet E, et al. Obstructive sleep apnea is related to impaired cognitive and functional status after stroke. *Sleep* (2015) 38:1431–7. doi: 10.5665/sleep.4984
4. Ryan CM, Bayley M, Green R, Murray BJ, Bradley TD. Influence of continuous positive airway pressure on outcomes of rehabilitation in stroke patients with obstructive sleep apnea. *Stroke* (2011) 42:1062–7. doi: 10.1161/STROKEAHA.110.597468
5. Benbir G, Karadeniz D. A pilot study of the effects of non-invasive mechanical ventilation on the prognosis of ischemic cerebrovascular events in patients with obstructive sleep apnea syndrome. *Neurol Sci.* (2012) 33:811–8. doi: 10.1007/s10072-011-0835-6
6. Parra O, Sanchez-Armengol A, Bonnin M, Arboix A, Campos-Rodriguez F, Perez-Ronchel J, et al. Early treatment of obstructive apnoea and stroke outcome: a randomised controlled trial. *Eur Respir J.* (2011) 37:1128–36. doi: 10.1183/09031936.00034410
7. Sandberg O, Franklin KA, Bucht G, Eriksson S, Gustafson Y. Nasal continuous positive airway pressure in stroke patients with sleep apnoea: a randomized treatment study. *Eur Respir J.* (2001) 18:630–4. doi: 10.1183/09031936.01.00070301
8. Brown DL, Chervin RD, Kalbfleisch JD, Zupancic MJ, Migda EM, Svatikova A, et al. Sleep apnea treatment after stroke (SATS) trial: is it feasible? *J Stroke Cerebrovasc Dis.* (2013) 22:1216–24. doi: 10.1016/j.jstrokecerebrovasdis.2011.06.010
9. Hui DS, Choy DK, Wong LK, Ko FW, Li TS, Woo J, et al. Prevalence of sleep-disordered breathing and continuous positive airway pressure compliance: results in chinese patients with first-ever ischemic stroke. *Chest* (2002) 122:852–60. doi: 10.1378/chest.122.3.852
10. Fusco G, Macina F, Macarini L, Garribba AP, Ettorre GC. Magnetic resonance imaging in simple snoring and obstructive sleep apnea-hypopnea syndrome. *Radiol Med.* (2004) 108:238–54.
11. Schwab RJ, Gupta KB, Gefter WB, Metzger LJ, Hoffman EA, Pack AI. Upper airway and soft tissue anatomy in normal subjects and patients with sleep-disordered breathing. Significance of the lateral pharyngeal walls. *Am J Respir Crit Care Med.* (1995) 152:1673–89. doi: 10.1164/ajrccm.152.5.7582313
12. Giannantoni NM, Minisci M, Brunetti V, Scarano E, Testani E, Vollono C, et al. Evaluation of pharyngeal muscle activity through nasopharyngeal surface electromyography in a cohort of dysphagic patients with acute ischaemic stroke. *Acta Otorhinolaryngol Ital.* (2016) 36:295–9. doi: 10.14639/0392-100X-1124
13. Brown DL, Chervin RD, Wolfe J, Hughes R, Concannon M, Lisabeth LD, et al. Hypoglossal nerve dysfunction and sleep-disordered breathing after stroke. *Neurology* (2014) 82:1149–52. doi: 10.1212/WNL.0000000000000263
14. Guimarães KC, Drager LF, Genta PR, Marcondes BF, Lorenzifilho G. Effects of oropharyngeal exercises on patients with moderate obstructive sleep apnea syndrome. *Am J Respir Critic Care Med.* (2009) 179:962–6. doi: 10.1164/rccm.200806-981OC
15. Ieto V, Kayamori F, Montes MI, Hirata RP, Gregório MG, Alencar AM, et al. Effects of oropharyngeal exercises on snoring : a randomized trial. *Chest* (2015) 148:683–91. doi: 10.1378/chest.14-2953
16. Kuna ST, Brennick MJ. Effects of pharyngeal muscle activation on airway pressure-area relationships. *Am J Respir Crit Care Med.* (2002) 166:972–7. doi: 10.1164/rccm.200203-214OC
17. Takegami M, Hayashino Y, Chin K, Sokejima S, Kadotani H, Akashiba T, et al. Simple four-variable screening tool for identification of patients with sleep-disordered breathing. *Sleep* (2009) 32:939–48.
18. Boulos MI, Wan A, Im J, Elias S, Frankul F, Atalla M, et al. Identifying obstructive sleep apnea after stroke/TIA: evaluating four simple screening tools. *Sleep Med.* (2016) 21:133–9. doi: 10.1016/j.sleep.2015.12.013
19. Gladstone DJ, Danells CJ, Black SE. The fugl-meyer assessment of motor recovery after stroke: a critical review of its measurement properties. *Neurorehabil Neural Repair* (2002) 16:232–40. doi: 10.1177/154596802401105171
20. Mahoney FI, Barthel DW. Functional evaluation: the barthel index. *Md State Med J.* (1965) 14:61–5.
21. Folstein MF, Folstein SE, Mchugh PR. Mini-mental state: a practical method for grading the state of patients for the clinician. *J Psychiatric Res.* (1975) 12:189–98. doi: 10.1016/0022-3956(75)90026-6
22. Hoddes E, Zarcone V, Smythe H, Phillips R, Dement WC. Quantification of sleepiness: a new approach. *Psychophysiology* (2010) 10:431–6. doi: 10.1111/j.1469-8986.1973.tb00801.x
23. Buysse D. The Pittsburgh sleep quality index (PSQI). An instrument for psychiatric practice and research. *Psychiatry Res.* (1988) 28:193–213.
24. Brown DL, Bapuraj JR, Mukherji SK, Chervin RD, Concannon M, Helman JI, et al. MRI of the pharynx in ischemic stroke patients with and without obstructive sleep apnea. *Sleep Med.* (2010) 11:540–4. doi: 10.1016/j.sleep.2010.01.008
25. Park SH, Kim SJ, Kim EK, Kim MJ, Son EJ, Kwak JY. Interobserver agreement in assessing the sonographic and elastographic features of malignant thyroid nodules. *AJR Am J Roentgenol.* (2009) 193:W416–23. doi: 10.2214/AJR.09.2541
26. Tingting X, Danming Y, Xin C. Non-surgical treatment of obstructive sleep apnea syndrome. *Eur Arch Otorhinolaryngol.* (2018) 275:335–46. doi: 10.1007/s00405-017-4818-y
27. Levy P, Kohler M, McNicholas WT, Barbe F, McEvoy RD, Somers VK, et al. Obstructive sleep apnoea syndrome. *Nat Rev Dis Primers* (2015) 1:15015. doi: 10.1038/nrdp.2015.15
28. Yetkin O, Aydogan D. Effect of CPAP on sleep spindles in patients with OSA. *Respir Physiol Neurobiol.* (2018) 247:71–3. doi: 10.1016/j.resp.2017.09.008
29. Wheeler NC, Wing JJ, O'Brien LM, Hughes R, Jacobs T, Claflin E, et al. Expiratory positive airway pressure for sleep apnea after stroke: a randomized, crossover trial. *J Clin Sleep Med.* (2016) 12:1233–8. doi: 10.5664/jcsm.6120
30. Schwartz AR, Patil SP, Laffan AM, Polotsky V, Schneider H, Smith PL. Obesity and obstructive sleep apnea: pathogenic mechanisms and therapeutic approaches. *Proc Am Thorac Soc.* (2008) 5:185–92. doi: 10.1513/pats.200708-137MG
31. Domzał T, Małowidzka-Serwinska M, Mróz K. Electrophysiological pattern of sleep after stroke. *Neurol Neurochir Pol.* (1994) 28:27–34.
32. Horner RL, Shea SA, Mcivor J, Guz A. Pharyngeal size and shape during wakefulness and sleep in patients with obstructive sleep apnoea. *Q J Med.* (1989) 72:719–35.
33. Randerath WJ, Galetke W, Domanski U, Weitkunat R, Ruhle KH. Tongue-muscle training by intraoral electrical neurostimulation in patients with obstructive sleep apnea. *Sleep* (2004) 27:254–9. doi: 10.1093/sleep/27.2.254
34. Punjabi NM. The epidemiology of adult obstructive sleep apnea. *Proc Am Thorac Soc.* (2008) 5:136. doi: 10.1513/pats.200709-155MG
35. Mansukhani MP, Bellolio MF, Kolla BP, Enduri S, Somers VK, Stead LG. Worse outcome after stroke in patients with obstructive sleep apnea: an observational cohort study. *J Stroke Cerebrovasc Dis.* (2011) 20:401–5. doi: 10.1016/j.jstrokecerebrovasdis.2010.02.011
36. Lefevre-Dognin C, Stana L, Jousse M, Lucas C, Sportouch P, Bradai N, et al. Lack of repercussions of sleep apnea syndrome on recovery and attention disorders at the subacute stage after stroke: a study of 45 patients. *Ann Phys Rehabil Med.* (2014) 57:618–28. doi: 10.1016/j.rehab.2014.09.008
37. Iranzo A, Santamaria J, Berenguer J, Sanchez M, Chamorro A. Prevalence and clinical importance of sleep apnea in the first night after cerebral infarction. *Neurology* (2002) 58:911–6. doi: 10.1212/WNL.58.6.911
38. Good DC, Henkle JQ, Gelber D, Welsh J, Verhulst S. Sleep-disordered breathing and poor functional outcome after stroke. *Stroke J Cereb Circu.* (1996) 27:252–9. doi: 10.1161/01.STR.27.2.252
39. Abe Y, Kato C, Uchima Koecklin KH, Okihara H, Ishida T, Fujita K, et al. Unilateral nasal obstruction affects motor representation development within the face primary motor cortex in growing rats. *J Appl Physiol.* (1985) (2017) 122:1494–503. doi: 10.1152/japplphysiol.01130.2016
40. Das A, Anupa AV, Radhakrishnan A. Reduced plastic brain responses to repetitive transcranial magnetic stimulation in severe obstructive sleep apnea syndrome. *Sleep Med.* (2013) 14:636–40. doi: 10.1016/j.sleep.2013.04.008

13

Unilateral Brachial Plexus Lesion Impairs Bilateral Touch Threshold

Bia Lima Ramalho [1,2*]***, Maria Luíza Rangel*** [1,2]***, Ana Carolina Schmaedeke*** [1,2]***, Fátima Smith Erthal*** [3] ***and Claudia D. Vargas*** [1,2]

[1] Laboratory of Neurobiology of Movement, Institute of Biophysics Carlos Chagas Filho, Federal University of Rio de Janeiro, Rio de Janeiro, Brazil, [2] Laboratory of Neuroscience and Rehabilitation, Institute of Neurology Deolindo Couto, Federal University of Rio de Janeiro, Rio de Janeiro, Brazil, [3] Laboratory of Neurobiology II, Institute of Biophysics Carlos Chagas Filho, Federal University of Rio de Janeiro, Rio de Janeiro, Brazil

****Correspondence:***
Bia Lima Ramalho
ramalhobsl@gmail.com

Unilateral brachial plexus injury (BPI) impairs sensory and motor functions of the upper limb. This study aimed to map in detail brachial plexus sensory impairment both in the injured and the uninjured upper limb. Touch sensation was measured through Semmes-Weinstein monofilaments at the autonomous regions of the brachial plexus nerves, hereafter called points of exclusive innervation (PEIs). Seventeen BPI patients (31.35 years $\pm$ 6.9 SD) and 14 age-matched healthy controls (27.57 years $\pm$ 5.8 SD) were tested bilaterally at six selected PEIs (axillary, musculocutaneous, median, radial, ulnar, and medial antebrachial cutaneous [MABC]). As expected, the comparison between the control group and the brachial plexus patients' injured limb showed a robust difference for all PEIs ($p \leq 0.001$). Moreover, the comparison between the control group and the brachial plexus uninjured limb revealed a difference for the median ($p = 0.0074$), radial ($p = 0.0185$), ulnar ($p = 0.0404$), and MABC ($p = 0.0328$) PEIs. After splitting the sample into two groups with respect to the dominance of the injured limb, higher threshold values were found for the uninjured side when it occurred in the right dominant limb compared to the control group at the median ($p = 0.0456$), radial ($p = 0.0096$), and MABC ($p = 0.0078$) PEIs. This effect was absent for the left, non-dominant arm. To assess the effect of the severity of sensory deficits observed in the injured limb upon the alterations of the uninjured limb, a K-means clustering algorithm ($k = 2$) was applied resulting in two groups with less or more severe sensory impairment. The less severely affected patients presented higher thresholds at the median ($p = 0.0189$), radial ($p = 0.0081$), ulnar ($p = 0.0253$), and MABC ($p = 0.0187$) PEIs in the uninjured limb in comparison with the control group, whereas higher thresholds at the uninjured limb were found only for the median PEI ($p = 0.0457$) in the more severely affected group. In conclusion, an expressive reduction in touch threshold was found for the injured limb allowing a precise mapping of the impairment caused by the BPI. Crucially, BPI also led to reduced tactile threshold in specific PEIs in the uninjured upper limb. These new findings suggest a superordinate model of representational plasticity occurring bilaterally in the brain after a unilateral peripheral injury.

Keywords: Semmens-Weinstein monofilaments, sensory threshold, brachial plexus neuropathy, impairment, light touch sensation, deafferentation, uninjured

INTRODUCTION

Brachial plexus injury (BPI) affects the sensory and motor functions of the upper limb to varying degrees resulting in complex patterns of sensorimotor dysfunction, often with very poor prognosis (1, 2). Affecting predominantly young male subjects [20–29 years, 89% male—(1)], BPI has major impacts on psychosocial well-being and quality of life (3, 4). A key aspect is that BPI often leads to loss of at least part of the upper limb movements (5) thus putatively compromising movements such as directional reaching, grasping and skilled manipulative movements with the upper limb. This is due not only to the loss of motor impairment, but also to the loss of sensation, known to be of particular importance in manipulative movements (6) [review in (7)]. Although most research in BPI has focused on motor impairment, relatively little has been done to further our understanding of its associated sensory dysfunction, despite its potential to inform both to clinicians and researchers about its severity and degree of impairment as well as to help improve strategies to increase the functionality of the upper limb.

Furthermore, current investigations of sensory dysfunction after a peripheral deafferentation consider the sensory deficit evaluation only in the injured limb and are often directed to a limited portion of the affected body surface (8–14). Given the heterogeneous nature of BPIs, it is important to make a complete investigation of all nerve territories of the BP, especially in its autonomous zones (2), corresponding to areas of skin in which each single nerve can be better assessed (15–17).

Although usually not evaluated after a peripheral nerve injury, changes in sensory function affecting the uninjured limb have been found in a variety of deafferentation models such as nerve block (18), nerve injury (19), amputation (20, 21), and in burned patients (22, 23). These changes have generally been interpreted as being the result of central nervous system adaptations occurring after the deafferentation.

Considering the lack of studies investigating the uninjured limb and possible sensory changes resulting from a BPI lesion, this study aimed to evaluate the sensory thresholds in BPI patients using Semmes-Weinstein monofilaments (SWM). We expected that a complete investigation of sensory thresholds in both upper limbs would allow not only the identification of the pattern of lesion-induced loss of sensation in the most affected limb but also reveal possible sensory deficits in the uninjured upper limb. This might expand the current knowledge on sensory changes after peripheral nerve lesions, providing novel approaches to clinical evaluation and also opening up new possibilities for the study of central reorganization after peripheral injury.

METHODS

Participants

Seventeen BPI patients (2 females) with a mean age of 31.35 years ± 6.9 SD (19–40), were recruited at the Institute of Neurology Deolindo Couto (INDC-UFRJ). Fifteen patients were right handed (1 left handed and 1 ambidextrous) (24). Inclusion criteria were age equal to or above 18 years, preserved ability to communicate and unilateral traumatic BPI (any level and severity, pre- or post- nerve surgery, see **Table 1**), diagnosed through clinical and complementary exams such as electromyography and magnetic resonance imaging. Exclusion criteria were a previous history of primary or secondary central and peripheral nervous system disease. Participants were consecutively recruited between the years 2014 and 2015.

Eighteen healthy right-handed participants were also evaluated, and from this sample fourteen age-matched healthy participants were included in the analysis (27.57 years ± 5.8 SD). The remaining four participants were excluded based on k-means clustering applied to homogenize the sample (see Statistics).

Before the evaluation, all participants were asked whether they felt comfortable enough to be evaluated. They were then informed about the experimental procedures and provided written informed consent to participate in the study, which was approved by the local ethics committee (Institute of Neurology Deolindo Couto—UFRJ, Brazil) and was in accordance with the declaration of Helsinki.

Semmes-Weinstein Monofilaments Assessment

In order to assess touch thresholds of the upper limb, a set of 20 Semmes-Weinstein Monofilaments (SWM, Bioseb, Vitrolles, France) were used. SWM are classified by the necessary force in grams to bend them against the skin, ranging from 0.007 to 160 g or, as expressed in log (10 × F; with F = force in milligrams), 1.84 to 6.20. The force values for each monofilament after the assessment using an analytical balance (Shimadzu Corp., Kyoto, Japan) were slightly different from the values specified by the manufacturer (see **Supplementary Material**). We decided to use the values we found rather than those of the manufacturer. Values for each monofilament are displayed in **Supplementary Table 1**.

Six stimulation points, called hereafter points of exclusive innervation (PEIs), were identified to perform the sensory test. The PEIs were within the five dermatomes (C5-T1) (25) of the BP and corresponded to the autonomous zones of six BP nerves: axillary, musculocutaneous, median, radial, ulnar and medial antebrachial cutaneous (MABC) (15) (**Figure 1A**).

During the assessment, participants sat in a chair in a quiet room together with the experimenters BR and AS. The upper limb to be tested rested on a pillow. Each limb was assessed separately. A black curtain blocked the volunteer's view of the assessed limb (**Figure 1B**). Both experimenters were trained to conduct the assessment the same way and while one experimenter was applying the filaments the other one was taking notes about the evoked sensations and the threshold values. The experimenters were not blind regarding the subject's condition since all the patients had the injured arm with some degree of paralysis and hypotrophy. The uninjured upper limb of the BPI patients was assessed first, or the right upper limb, in the case of healthy volunteers. The order of PEI stimulation was pseudo-randomized for each upper limb. For

Abbreviations: BPI, Brachial plexus injury; MABC, medial antebrachial cutaneous nerve; PEI, Point of exclusive innervation; SWM, Semmes-Weinstein monofilaments.

TABLE 1 | BPI patient characteristics and time between injury and surgery and time between injury and the assessment.

Id	Hand.	Lesion	Side	T1	Surgical procedures	T2
BPI01	R	S, M, I	R	x	x	5.3
BPI02	R	S, M, I	R	6.1	C5 graft and unsp. NT	15.2
BPI03	A	S, M, I	L	3.3/4.2	Int. to Musc. NT + Sup. NN	28.2
BPI04	L	S, M, I	L	3	Int. to Musc. NT + Acc. to Sup. NT	24
BPI05	R	S, M, I	L	12.2	C5, C6, and C7 NN	13.2
BPI06	R	S, M, I	L	8.4	Acc. to Sup. NT	36.1
BPI07	R	S	R	6.1	Ul. to Musc. NT + Acc. to Sup. NT + Rad. to Axi. NT	45.7
BPI08	R	S, M	R	4.9	Ul. to Musc. NT + Acc. to Sup. NT	7.7
BPI09	R	S, M	L	11.7	Ul. to Musc. NT	12.9
BPI10	R	I	R	x	x	3
BPI11	R	S, M	L	11.3	Ul. to Musc. NT	17.6
BPI12	R	S, M, I	L	5.6	Int. to Musc. NT + unsp. NN and neuroma dissection	7.5
BPI13	R	S, M	R	6/10.4	Ul. to Musc. NT + Acc. to Sup. NT	12.4
BPI14	R	S, M	L	4.6/10.7	Ul. to Musc. NT + unsp. NN	15
BPI15	R	S, M, I	L	x	x	14.1
BPI16	R	S, M, I	L	3	Int. to Musc. NT + Acc. to Sup. NT	5.5
BPI17	R	S, M, I	R	11.8/13.8	Int. to Musc. NT + Acc. to Sup. NT	18.4

Hand., handedness; R, right; L, left; A, ambidextrous; S, superior; M, middle; I, inferior; NT, nerve transfer; Int. to Musc, intercostal to musculocutaneous; Acc. to Sup., accessory to suprascapular; Ul. to Musc., ulnar to musculocutaneous; Rad. to Axil., radial to axillary; NN, nerve neurolysis; Sup., suprascapular nerve; unsp., unspecified procedures; T1, time between the injury and the surgery in months; T2, time between the injury and the sensory assessment in months.

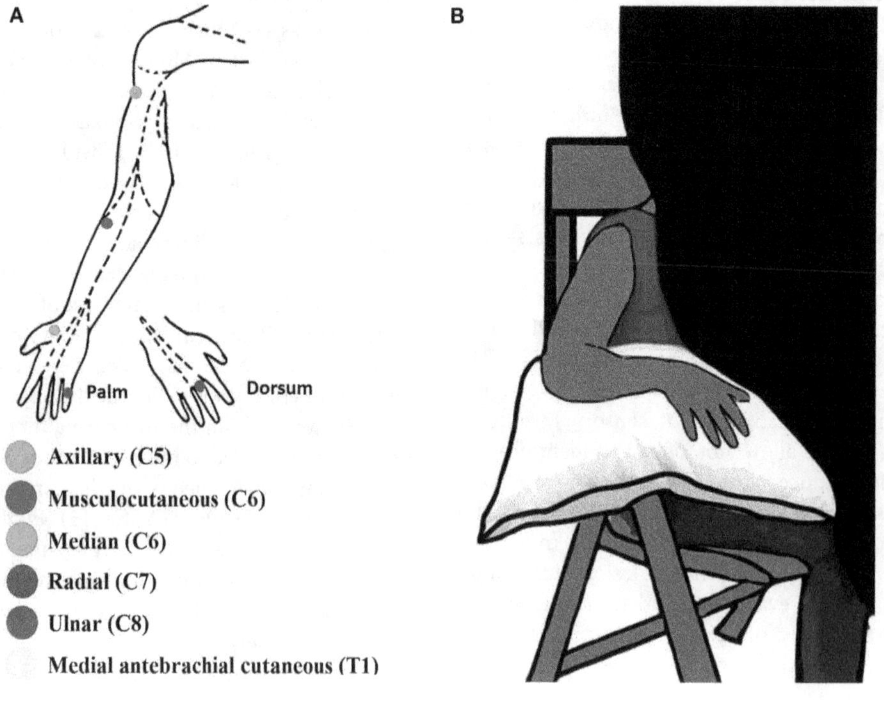

FIGURE 1 | (A) Illustration of the six Points of Exclusive Innervation (PEIs) in the upper limb. **(B)** Illustration of the experimental setup.

each PEI, monofilaments were applied in ascending order—from the thinnest to the thickest. The thinnest filament detected by the participant in 3 out of 5 applications was considered as the tactile threshold for that PEI (26). All the procedures were explained and demonstrated to the participants in advance. The intervals between each stimulation were arbitrary to avoid the learning of the stimulation sequence and, consequently, false positives. When the participant was not able to feel even the thickest filament (6.20, see **Supplementary Table 1**) his touch threshold was established at this filament (6.20).

Statistical Analysis

Threshold values for each participant were log transformed (10 × force in mg—see **Supplementary Table 1**). For each PEI, the threshold values were described as medians.

K-means Clustering

Both for the control and the patients' group we used k-means cluster analysis (27) to assign individuals to clusters based on their threshold values for the six PEIs. The k-means algorithm partitions the sample into k clusters based on variables of interest. The algorithm uses a heuristic to find centroid seeds for k-means clustering and then computes the squared Euclidean distance from each observation to each centroid, assigning each observation to its closest centroid. The goal of this procedure is to minimize the within-cluster variance and maximize the between-cluster variance.

The D'agostino-Pearson test was then used to assess normality of the groups. Since data from some PEIs did not respect Gaussian distribution, non-parametric tests were applied.

Control Group

For setting the control group, the K-means clustering algorithm was applied and resulted in a cluster comprising 14 participants (four participants were excluded from further analyses). The comparison between each PEI with its counterpart in the same control participant (right arm vs. left arm) was performed by means of the Wilcoxon signed-rank test. Since the comparison between right and left upper PEIs revealed no difference (axillary, $p = 0.5000$; musculocutaneous, $p = 0.7127$; median, $p = 0.3523$; radial, $p = 0.3493$; ulnar, $p = 1$; MABC, $p = 0.2123$), the mean between the corresponding right and left PEIs from both upper limbs was calculated. This procedure was performed to establish a single threshold value per PEI for each participant.

To investigate if the sensory threshold differed among the six PEIs of the control group, the Kruskal-Wallis test was applied, followed by Dunn's Multiple Comparison Test to compare the six PEIs with each other—alfa = 0.05.

Control vs. Patients

The Mann-Whitney test was applied to compare PEIs between control participants and BPI patients (control × injured; control × uninjured upper limbs). For each patient, threshold values for all PEIs of the uninjured limb were normalized to the median values of the control group and these normalized data were used to calculate Spearman correlation coefficients employing the patients' age and the time interval between the injury and the assessment (T2 from **Table 1**).

To investigate the effect of the side of the injury, patients were separated into two groups comprising BPI in the dominant right ($n = 7$) or non-dominant left limb ($n = 8$). BPI03 and BPI04 were excluded from the sample because they were ambidextrous and left handed, respectively (**Table 1**). The Mann-Whitney test was performed to compare the threshold values of the uninjured side of both patient groups (dominant and non-dominant injury) with those of the control group. In addition, a K-means clustering algorithm was applied to the BPI group to separate patients into two groups as a function of their sensory impairment ($k = 2$). Thus, based on their PEI threshold values on the injured side, patients were grouped into more or less severely affected. Sensory thresholds of the uninjured side of both patient groups were then compared with the control group using the Mann-Whitney test. This analysis aimed to investigate if different levels of sensory deficits in the injured side would result in different patterns of sensory changes in the uninjured side.

RESULTS

Control Values for Absolute Touch Threshold—"Typical" Index

A typical index per PEI was calculated for control subjects. The comparison among the six PEI threshold values in the control group revealed a significant difference ($p < 0.0001$). Dunn's Multiple Comparison Test (alfa = 0.05) revealed that the most proximal PEIs had lower threshold values than the most distal ones (**Figure 2**). Median (25th and 75th percentiles) PEI threshold values are presented in **Table 2.**

Control vs. Injured Side

The comparison between the control group and the BPI patients' injured side showed a clear difference for all evaluated PEIs (**Figure 3**). It confirms the important sensory deficit in the latter group. Touch thresholds on the injured side were highly variable among patients, ranging from 1.84 to 6.20 (**Table 2**). For several patients, even the thickest monofilament was not detectable in some PEIs.

Control vs. Uninjured Side

The comparison between the control group and the patients' uninjured side is shown in **Figure 4.** Statistical analysis showed differences for the median, radial, ulnar, and MABC PEIs, indicating that the uninjured side is also affected by the BPI. Moreover, sensory threshold values from the patients uninjured limb were globally considerably more variable than those of the control group, with several patient values lying above the control group range (**Table 2**).

Spearman correlation coefficients analysis showed no significant correlation between the normalized values of each uninjured PEI and patient age or for the time interval between the injury and the assessment ($p > 0.1$).

Side of Injury and Sensory Deficits in the Uninjured Side

After excluding the left handed and the ambidextrous patients we found that patients with BPI in the dominant right limb presented higher threshold values for the uninjured side compared to the control group at the median ($p = 0.0456$), radial ($p = 0.0096$) and MABC ($p = 0.0078$) PEIs (axillary: $p = 0.0732$; musculocutaneous: $p = 0.6531$; ulnar: $p = 0.0628$). Conversely, patients with BPI in the non-dominant left limb showed no PEI threshold difference from those of the control group (axillary: $p = 0.3762$; musculocutaneous: $p = 0.1157$; median: $p = 0.0568$; radial: $p = 0.2722$; ulnar: $p = 0.4035$; MABC: $p = 0.6539$). **Table 3** presents median threshold values of both groups. With respect to

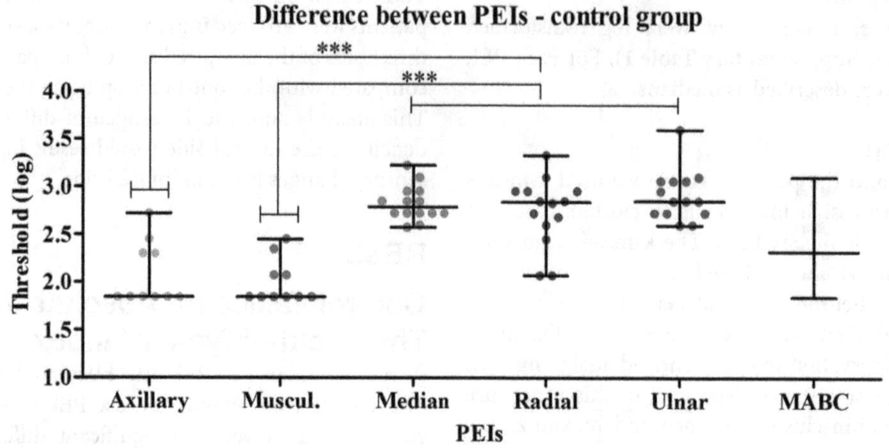

FIGURE 2 | Comparison between the six PEIs of the control group revealed a significant difference (Kruskal-Wallis test—$p < 0.0001$). Dunn's Multiple Comparison Test (alfa = 0.05) applied to compare all pairs of PEIs revealed that the most proximal PEIs (axillary and musculocutaneous) had lower thresholds than the distal PEIs (median, radial and ulnar). *** $p < 0.05$ at the Dunn's Multiple Comparison Test.

TABLE 2 | Median (Q1–Q3) threshold values for the control group and the injured and uninjured upper limbs of the BPI patients.

PEIs	Control ($n = 14$)	Injured ($n = 17$)	Uninjured ($n = 17$)
Axillary	1.84 (1.84–2.30)	6.02 (4.84–6.20)***	1.84 (1.84–2.30)
Musculoc.	1.84 (1.84–2.07)	6.20 (2.45–6.20)***	1.84 (1.84–1.84)
Median	2.79 (2.72–2.95)	4.65 (3.69–6.20)***	3.06 (2.95–3.60)*
Radial	2.84 (2.56–2.95)	4.65 (3.42–6.20)***	3.06 (2.85–3.69)*
Ulnar	2.85 (2.72–3.06)	4.11 (3.33–6.20)**	3.60 (2.85–3.69)*
MABC	2.32 (2.01–2.86)	4.11 (2.83–6.20)**	2.85 (2.45–3.60)*

*$p \leq 0.05$, **$p \leq 0.001$, ***$p \leq 0.0001$ compared to the control group ($n = 14$).

the ambidextrous and the left handed patients we cannot take any conclusion regarding the small sample size.

Severity of Injury and Sensory Deficits in the Uninjured Side

A K-means clustering algorithm applied to the BPI group (k = 2) resulted in the formation of two groups: one with less severe sensory impairment ($n = 10$: BPI01, BPI02, BPI03, BPI07, BPI08, BPI09, BPI10, BPI11, BPI13, and BPI14) and the other with more severe BPI impairment of sensory function ($n = 7$: BPI04, BPI05, BPI06, BPI12, BPI15, BPI16, and BPI17). For graphs depicting the patients' individual assessment of both limbs, see **Supplementary Figures 1, 2.**

The comparison between the control group and the uninjured side of the less severely affected patients ($n = 10$) revealed higher thresholds for patients at the median ($p = 0.0189$), radial ($p = 0.0081$), ulnar ($p = 0.0253$), and MABC ($p = 0.0187$) PEIs (axillary: $p = 0.6482$; musculocutaneous: $p = 0.3864$). Similar results were obtained after excluding the ambidextrous patient from the sample, with higher thresholds for the uninjured side in the less severely affected patients ($n = 9$) compared to the control group (axillary: $p = 0.5261$; musculocutaneous: $p = 0.4581$; median: $p = 0.0277$; radial: $p = 0.0161$; ulnar: $p = 0.0466$; and MABC: $p = 0.0367$).

From this sample of less severely affected patients, six have undergone ulnar to musculocutaneous nerve transfer. For these 6 patients the difference between the uninjured side and the control group was found only for the ulnar nerve ($p = 0.0332$) (axillary: $p = 0.5500$; musculocutaneous: $p = 0.1745$; median: $p = 0.0791$; radial: $p = 0.1582$; MABC: $p = 0.2452$).

The comparison between the uninjured side of the more severely affected patients and the control group showed statistical difference only for the median PEI ($p = 0.0457$) (axillary: $p = 0.3976$; musculocutaneous: $p = 0.3958$; radial: $p = 0.3109$; ulnar: $p = 0.3434$; MABC: $p = 0.3288$). This group comprised 6 right-handed and one left-handed patients. When the left handed patient was excluded from this group, no difference between the uninjured side and the control group was observed (axillary: $p = 0.7989$; musculocutaneous: $p = 0.1745$; median: $p = 0.1033$; radial: $p = 0.3002$; ulnar: $p = 0.6440$; MABC: $p = 0.4543$).

Taken together, these results suggest that more severe injuries are associated with minor sensory dysfunction in the uninjured upper limb. In contrast, for the less severe group, the unaffected upper limb presented a higher number of affected PEIs. **Table 4** presents median threshold values of both groups.

DISCUSSION

By applying Semmes-Weinstein monofilaments, we were able to characterize, for the first time, superficial sensibility deficits in points of exclusive innervation (PEI) both in the injured and the uninjured upper limbs in BPI patients as compared to an age-paired and sex-matched control group. The comparison between the control group and the BPI patients' injured side showed higher thresholds for all PEIs in the affected limb. Interestingly, the comparison between the sensory thresholds of the control group and those of the BPI patients' uninjured side also revealed higher thresholds for the median, radial, ulnar

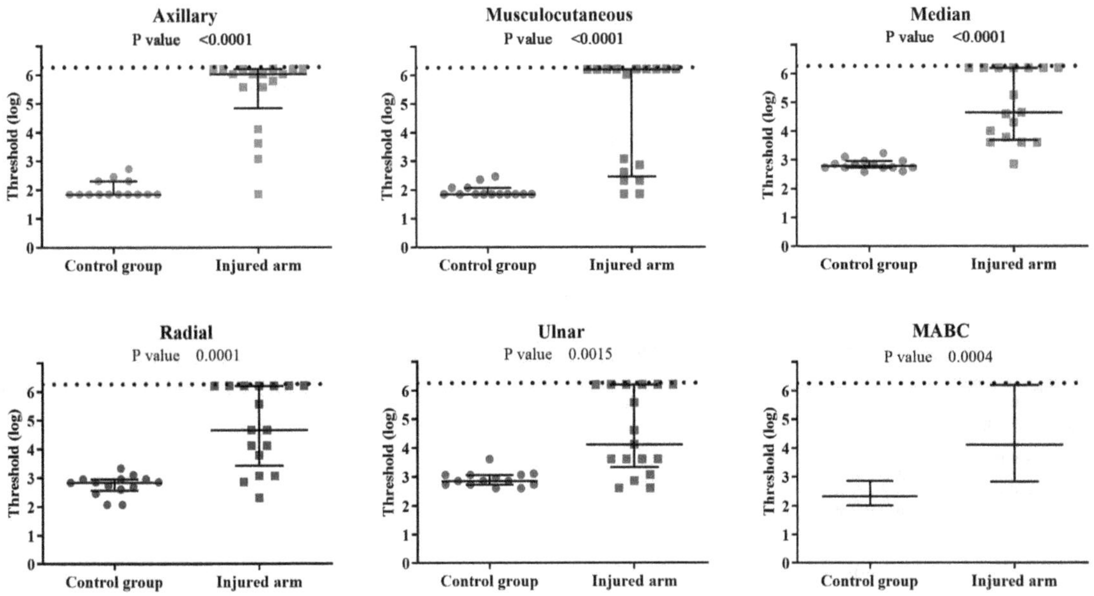

FIGURE 3 | Individual sensory threshold values in the 6 PEIs of the control group compared to the BPI patients' injured upper limb. Lines represent the median values of each group with the interquartile ranges. *P*-values of the statistical difference between groups (control × injured) are presented in each graph. The broken line represents the top limit of the set of monofilaments used (6.20). ● = control ($n = 14$) and ■ = BPI patients ($n = 17$).

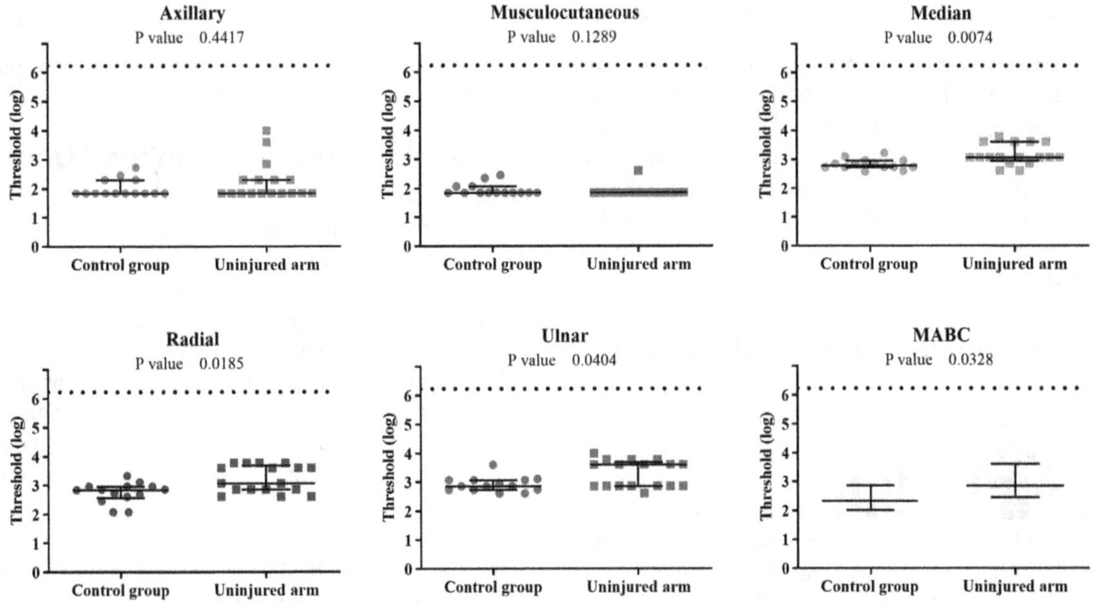

FIGURE 4 | Individual sensory threshold values of the 6 PEIs of the control group compared to the BPI patients' uninjured upper limb. Lines represent the median values and the interquartile ranges of each group. *P*-values of the difference between groups (control × uninjured) are presented in each graph. The broken line represents the top limit of the set of monofilaments used (6.20). ● = control ($n = 14$) and ■ = BPI patients ($n = 17$).

and MABC PEIs. After splitting the sample of right handed patients with respect to the dominance of the injured limb, we found higher threshold values for the uninjured side in the BPI patients in the right dominant limb compared to the control group at the median, radial and MABC PEIs. On the other hand, in patients with BPI in the left non-dominant arm, this effect was absent. Using the K-means clustering algorithm, the patient sample was then split into two groups based on the threshold values of the injured side. Thresholds of the uninjured side of the resulting two groups of patients were compared to those of the control group. Less severely affected BPI patients ($n = 10$) had higher thresholds for the median, radial, ulnar and MABC PEIs.

TABLE 3 | Median (Q1–Q3) threshold values for the injured and uninjured upper limbs after a BPI in the dominant and non-dominant limb.

	Dominant ($n = 7$)		Non-dominant ($n = 8$)	
PEIs	**Injured**	**Uninjured**	**Injured**	**Uninjured**
Axillary	6.02 (4.11–6.20)***	2.30 (1.84–3.60)	6.02 (5.62–6.20)**	1.84 (1.84–1.84)
Musculoc.	2.85 (1.84–6.20)*	1.84 (1.84–1.84)	6.20 (2.75–6.20)***	1.84 (1.84–1.84)
Median	3.78 (3.60–5.26)**	3.06 (2.85–3.60)*	6.20 (4.61–6.20)***	3.06 (2.90–3.06)
Radial	4.65 (2.85–5.57)*	3.60 (2.85–3.60)*	6.20 (3.863–6.20)**	2.95 (2.60–3.73)
Ulnar	3.60 (2.85–4.60)*	3.60 (2.85–3.60)*	5.88 (3.60–6.20)**	2.85 (2.85–3.73)
MABC	3.06 (2.30–4.90)*	3.06 (2.85–3.60)	6.11 (3.73–6.20)***	2.60 (1.95–2.60)

*$p \leq 0.05$, **$p \leq 0.001$, ***$p \leq 0.0001$ compared to the control group ($n = 14$).

TABLE 4 | Median (Q1–Q3) threshold values for the injured and uninjured upper limbs of the less and more severe BPI.

	Less severe ($n = 10$)		More severe ($n = 7$)	
PEIs	**Injured**	**Uninjured**	**Injured**	**Uninjured**
Axillary	5.67 (3.98–6.02)***	1.84 (1.84–2.30)	6.20 (6.02–6.20)**	1.84 (1.84–2.85)
Musculoc.	2.72 (2.18–6.06)*	1.84 (1.84–1.84)	6.20 (6.20–6.20)***	1.84 (1.84–1.84)
Median	3.89 (3.60–4.61)**	3.06 (3.01–3.19)*	6.20 (6.20–6.20)**	3.06 (2.85–3.60)*
Radial	3.94 (3.01–4.65)*	3.60 (2.85–3.78)*	6.20 (6.20–6.20)**	2.85 (2.60–3.60)
Ulnar	3.60 (2.79–3.73)	3.60 (2.85–3.64)*	6.20 (6.20–6.20)**	2.85 (2.85–3.78)
MABC	3.33 (2.30–3.73)*	3.06 (2.52–3.64)*	6.20 (6.02–6.20)**	2.60 (2.30–2.85)

*$p \leq 0.05$, **$p \leq 0.001$, ***$p \leq 0.0001$ compared to the control group ($n = 14$).

Conversely, more severe BPI patients showed higher thresholds only for the median PEI. These results suggest that both the laterality and the degree of sensory impairment of the injured arm associate to higher sensory thresholds in the uninjured side. These findings expand the current knowledge on sensory changes after peripheral nerve lesions, providing novel approaches to clinical evaluation and also opening up new possibilities for the study of central reorganization after peripheral injury.

"Typical" Threshold Values for the Upper Limb

In this study, it was possible to establish the control group's "typical" threshold for each PEI. The lack of difference between the sensory thresholds for the left and right upper limb in the control subjects corroborates previous findings (28). A "typical" threshold value has been previously described in healthy subjects (29). Many studies have employed this threshold value to evaluate all dermatomes of the upper limb (hand/arm/forearm) (11, 12, 14). Nevertheless, we found lower threshold values in proximal PEIs (axillary and musculocutaneous) than in distal PEIs (median, radial and ulnar). One possible explanation for this discrepancy may be related to the hairiness of the evaluated skin. Proximal PEIs are in hairy skin regions while the distal ones are in glabrous skin (30). The hair follicle shaft has collars of mechanoreceptor terminals, including at least three low threshold mechanoreceptor subtypes (31). Therefore, hair deflection might be associated with a lower threshold in the proximal PEIs. In this case, applying the normative threshold value of 2.85, which is higher than the "typical" threshold found for this population, to assess the entire upper limb could induce the detection of false negative sensory deficits.

Threshold Values in the Injured Upper Limb After a BPI

The assessment of the injured upper limb of the BPI patients at the six selected PEIs agreed with their clinical diagnoses. Indeed, in the majority of our sample BPI had been documented as affecting mainly the superior and middle trunk of the brachial plexus. Accordingly, axillary, musculocutaneous and the median PEIs presented the highest sensory thresholds when compared to the control group. The huge variability amongst threshold values found for most PEIs in the injured limb (**Figure 2**) can be attributed to the highly variable degree of severity that is commonly seen for BPI (1).

Unilateral BPI Induces Bilateral Touch Threshold Impairment

BPI led to increased tactile threshold in specific PEIs of the uninjured upper limb. These results are in agreement with a variety of deafferentation models that also found changes in sensory processing in the uninjured limb (18–23, 32). Both in burn patients (22, 23) and lower limb amputees (20), the assessment of cutaneous threshold presented higher values for the uninjured limb as compared to controls.

The sensory impairment in the uninjured limb found in BPI patients suggests that BPI leads to central modifications in the hemisphere contralateral to the uninjured limb, as shown in different models of deafferentation (33–41). As reviewed by Wall et al. (42), chronic nerve injuries (peripheral nerve injury, root injury, spinal injury, and amputation) in humans and primates promote not only cortical but also subcortical changes at all levels of the somatosensory system. In animal models, unilateral injuries also lead to bilateral changes in the somatosensory ascending pathway (43–46).

For contralateral alterations to be reflected in the ipsilateral hemibody there must be an interhemispheric transfer of information at some level in the brain. Sensory input is ordinarily processed in the contralateral primary somatosensory cortex but there is also to some extent an ipsilateral cortical response to peripheral stimulation (47, 48). As shown by Iwamura et al. (47), this ipsilateral response seems to depend on the opposite hemisphere via transcallosal connections between homotopic areas. In addition, as described by Preuss and Goldman-Rakic (49) in primates, the midline thalamic nuclei project bilaterally to the prefrontal cortex, an important path of top-down regulation of attention to a given stimulus (50). Thus, the altered ascending information coming from the injured limb could lead to reduced activity in the intralaminar nuclei and reduce the attentional network associated with the detection of ascending tactile stimuli, both for the injured and the uninjured limb.

BPIs of the Dominant Right Limb Are Linked to a Large Sensory Impairment in the Uninjured Side

When the injury occurred in the dominant right limb, higher sensory thresholds were observed in the non-dominant left uninjured limb. Thus, higher thresholds were found for the uninjured limb when the limb was the dominant one. With respect to the ambidextrous and the left handed patients we cannot take any conclusion due to the small sample size.

A behavioral study of tactile perception after bilateral hand transplant showed that the somatosensory perception of the right hand was largely reduced when the right side of the face was concurrently stimulated. The same was not true for the left side (51). After a bilateral hand allograft, Vargas et al. (52) showed that the motor cortical reorganization was faster and more extensive for the non-dominant hand than for the dominant hand. One possibility raised by these authors was that the hemisphere contralateral to the dominant hand is more "hardwired" (and thus less plastic) in the context of a bilateral hand allograft. Interestingly, the amputation of the dominant upper limb elicits more errors and slower responses in motor imagery and handedness judgment tasks (53).

Greater cortical functional reorganization is observed in patients with BPI when the dominant limb is affected as compared to the non-dominant limb (54). This suggests that a relatively more extensive adaptive process may occur following an injury to the dominant hand. The long-standing loss and/or disuse of the dominant limb may degrade the sensorimotor efficiency of both the dominant and the non-dominant upper limb. If this is correct, then it is possible that a dominant side BPI has a greater impact over sensorimotor representations, with reduced plasticity in the hemisphere contralateral to the dominant hand.

Reduced Sensory Impairments in the Injured Side Are Linked to Greater Sensory Impairment in the Uninjured Side

The group of patients with less severe sensory impairment presented a higher number of affected PEIs in their uninjured upper limb, while the more severe lesions were associated with lower sensory dysfunction in the uninjured upper limb. These results suggest that the severity of injury is inversely related to the impaired threshold detection observed in the uninjured upper limb. One possibility is that the less severe injury is associated with a higher sensorimotor disorganization in the hemisphere contralateral to the injured limb. This, in turn, would affect the representations of the uninjured limb to a greater extent. Indeed, Jain et al. (55) showed in owl monkeys that an incomplete unilateral cervical (C3–C4) dorsal column section leads to expanded cortical representations in the contralateral cortical somatosensory area 3b. Interestingly, the remaining parts of the hand in the deafferented cortical areas present larger receptive fields and abnormal response properties compared to complete lesions. It was also shown that the combination of median+radial nerve injury leads to far more silent regions in the primary somatosensory cortex (S1) than that of the median+ulnar lesion (56–58). These results suggest that both the type and extent of peripheral lesion matter when it comes to the cortical reorganization of S1 topographical maps. The manner by which these changes reflect modifications of the representation of the unaffected limb is unknown. The abnormal reorganization taking place in the less severe injuries can thus contribute to higher touch thresholds in the contralateral hemibody due to changes in interhemispheric communication of cortical maps (40, 41).

The group of patients classified as more severely impaired corresponded to those with extended lesions (superior, medium, and inferior trunks, SMI), most of them having undergone an intercostal to musculocutaneous nerve transfer. This surgery has already been proven to produce changes in the biceps cortical representation (59, 60). However, the small sample of patients with this type of surgery recruited in the present study precluded any further analysis on the effect of this nerve transfer upon sensory threshold impairment in the uninjured limb.

The group of less severely affected patients comprised those having undergone ulnar to musculocutaneous nerve transfer. Contrasting with the prevailing effect of higher threshold values found for the uninjured side, for these patients the difference between the uninjured side and the control group was found only for the ulnar nerve. As discussed above, a less severe injury would be associated with a higher sensorimotor disorganization in the hemisphere contralateral to the injured limb. This in turn would lead to a change in the cortical representation of the uninjured limb. In this context, the ulnar to musculocutaneous nerve transfer, already associated to functional improvement of the affected limb (61) and possibly of cortical representation restoration (62), could play a role by reducing the tactile threshold impairment of the uninjured limb through callosal modulatory effects (38).

CONCLUSION

This is the first report of superficial sensibility deficit in both injured and the uninjured upper limbs in BPI patients. Furthermore, the higher sensory deficits in the uninjured side were associated to BPI of the dominant limb and the lower severity of sensory deficits in the injured side. These findings corroborate previous results reported after other peripheral injuries such as in amputees and suggest a superordinate model of representational plasticity occurring bilaterally in the brain after unilateral peripheral deafferentation. Indeed, peripheral nerve lesion causes continuous, time-dependent adaptation in the cortical network (63, 64). Among the limitations of the current study we highlight the small sample size as well as its heterogeneity regarding the lesion extent, the occurrence and type of surgical intervention and the time elapsed from lesion. Expanding the knowledge on sensory changes after peripheral nerve lesions might provide novel approaches to understand and treat BPI.

The raw data supporting the conclusions of this manuscript will be made available by the authors, without undue reservation, to any qualified researcher.

AUTHOR CONTRIBUTIONS

BR: conception, data collection, analysis, and interpretation and drafting. MR: data collection, analysis, and interpretation and drafting. AS: conception and data collection. FE and CV: conception, data analysis, and interpretation and revision.

FUNDING

This work was funded by the Fundação de amparo à pesquisa do Estado de São Paulo (FAPESP) project NeuroMat (grant 2013/07699-0), Conselho Nacional de Pesquisa (CNPq) (grants 306817/2014-4 and 309560/2017-9), Fundação de Amparo à Pesquisa do Estado do Rio de Janeiro FAPERJ (grants E-26/111.655/ 2012 and E26/010.002902/2014), and Financiadora de Estudos e Projetos—FINEP (Pró-infra Hospitalar - 0.1.12.0308.00).

ACKNOWLEDGMENTS

The authors would like to thank José Fernando Guedes Correa, Paulo Leonardo Tavares, José Vicente Martins, and Michelle Miranda for their contribution to this work and Karen Reilly for her comments on a previous version of this manuscript.

SUPPLEMENTARY MATERIAL

Supplementary Figure 1 | Individual sensory threshold values in the 6 PEIs of each BPI patients' injured (dark gray) and uninjured (light gray) upper limbs of the more severe group. The black line represents the median values of the control group ($n = 14$). The top dashed line represents the higher threshold value possible to assess with our filaments set (6.20). ϕ = PEIs in which the subjects were unable to feel even the thickest filament assessed (6.20).

Supplementary Figure 2 | Individual sensory threshold values in the 6 PEIs of each BPI patients' injured (dark gray) and uninjured (light gray) upper limbs of the less severe group. The black line represents the median values of the control group ($n = 14$). The top dashed line represents the higher threshold value possible to assess with our filaments set (6.20). ϕ = PEIs in which the subjects were unable to feel even the thickest filament assessed (6.20).

Supplementary Table 1 | Calibration measures of the set of 20 SWM used. Forces in grams (g) and the log of the force (log) (10 × force in mg) needed to bend the filament (90° to the skin) in a "C" shape according to the manufacturer (Manufacturer's information) and after filaments calibration (Mean of the Calibrations).

REFERENCES

1. Midha R. Epidemiology of brachial plexus injuries in a multitrauma population. *Neurosurgery.* (1997) 40:1182–9. doi: 10.1097/00006123-199706000-00014
2. Moran SL, Steinmann SP, Shin AY. Adult brachial plexus injuries: mechanism, patterns of injury, and physical diagnosis. *Hand Clin.* (2005) 21:13–24. doi: 10.1016/j.hcl.2004.09.004
3. Mancuso CA, Lee SK, Dy CJ, Landers ZA, Model Z, Wolfe SW. Expectations and limitations due to brachial plexus injury: a qualitative study. *Hand.* (2015) 10:741–9. doi: 10.1007/s11552-015-9761-z
4. Franzblau L, Chung KC. Psychosocial outcomes and coping after complete avulsion traumatic brachial plexus injury. *Disabil Rehabil.* (2015) 37:135–43. doi: 10.3109/09638288.2014.911971
5. Thatte MR, Babhulkar S, Hiremath A. Brachial plexus injury in adults: diagnosis and surgical treatment strategies. *Ann Indian Acad Neurol.* (2013) 16:26–33. doi: 10.4103/0972-2327.107686
6. Johansson RS, Westling G. Roles of glabrous skin receptors and sensorimotor memory in automatic control of precision grip when lifting rougher or more slippery objects. *Exp Brain Res.* (1984) 56:550–64. doi: 10.1007/BF00237997
7. Johansson RS, Flanagan JR. Coding and use of tactile signals from the fingertips in object manipulation tasks. *Nat Rev Neurosci.* (2009) 10:345–59. doi: 10.1038/nrn2621
8. Novak CB. Evaluation of the nerve-injured patient. *Clin Physiol.* (2003) 30:127–38. doi: 10.1016/S0094-1298(02)00098-6
9. Bentolila V, Nizard R, Bizot P, Sedel L. Complete traumatic brachial plexus palsy. *J Bone Jt Surg.* (1999) 81A:20–8. doi: 10.2106/00004623-199901000-00004
10. Doi K, Muramatsu K, Hattori Y, Otsuka K, Tan S-H, Nanda V, et al. Restoration of prehension with the double free muscle technique following complete avulsion of the brachial plexus. *J Bone Jt Surg.* (2000) 82A:652–66. doi: 10.2106/00004623-200005000-00006
11. Htut M, Misra P, Anand P, Birch R, Carlstedt T. Pain phenomena and sensory recovery following brachial plexus avulsion injury and surgical repairs. *J Hand Surg Am.* (2006) 31B:596–605. doi: 10.1016/J.JHSB.2006.04.027
12. Bertelli JA, Ghizoni MF, Loureiro Chaves DP. Sensory disturbances and pain complaints after brachial plexus root injury: a prospective study involving 150 adult patients. *Microsurgery.* (2011) 31:93–7. doi: 10.1002/micr.20832
13. Bertelli JA, Ghizoni MF. Very distal sensory nerve transfers in high median nerve lesions. *J Hand Surg Am.* (2011) 36:387–93. doi: 10.1016/j.jhsa.2010.11.049
14. Bertelli JA. Distal sensory nerve transfers in lower-type injuries of the brachial plexus. *J Hand Surg Am.* (2012) 37A:1194–9. doi: 10.1016/j.jhsa.2012.02.047
15. Russel SM (ed). The diagnostic anatomy of the brachial plexus. In: *Examination of Peripheral Nerve Injuries: An Anatomical Approach.* New York, NY: Thieme Medical Publishers Inc. (2006). p. 66–89.
16. Highet WB. Procaine nerve block in the investigation of peripheral nerve injuries. *J Neurol Psychiatry.* (1942) 5:101–16. doi: 10.1136/jnnp.5.3-4.101
17. Haymaker W, Woodhall B. Causes and manifestations of peripheral nerve injuries. In: *Peripheral Nerve Injuries: Principles of Diagnosis.* Philadelphia, PA: WB Saunders (1953). p. 138–41.

18. Werhahn KJ, Mortensen J, Van Boven RW, Zeuner KE, Cohen LG. Enhanced tactile spatial acuity and cortical processing during acute hand deafferentation. *Nat Neurosci.* (2002) 5:936–8. doi: 10.1038/nn917
19. De La Llave-Rincón AI, Fernández-De-Las-Peñas C, Fernández-Carnero J, Padua L, Arendt-Nielsen L, Pareja JA. Bilateral hand/wrist heat and cold hyperalgesia, but not hypoesthesia, in unilateral carpal tunnel syndrome. *Exp Brain Res.* (2009) 198:455–63. doi: 10.1007/s00221-009-1941-z
20. Kavounoudias A, Tremblay C, Gravel D, Iancu A, Forget R. Bilateral changes in somatosensory sensibility after unilateral below-knee amputation. *Arch Phys Med Rehabil.* (2005) 86:633–640. doi: 10.1016/j.apmr.2004.10.030
21. Wahren LK. Changes in thermal and mechanical pain thresholds in hand amputeres. A clinical and physiological long term follow-up. *Pain.* (1990) 42:269–77. doi: 10.1016/0304-3959(90)91139-A
22. Malenfant A, Forget R, Amsel R, Papillon J, Frigon JY, Choinière M. Tactile, thermal and pain sensibility in burned patients with and without chronic pain and paresthesia problems. *Pain.* (1998) 77:241–51. doi: 10.1016/S0304-3959(98)00096-7
23. Hermanson A, Jonsson C-E, Lindblom U. Sensibility after burn injury. *Clin Physiol.* (1986) 6:507–21. doi: 10.1111/j.1475-097X.1986.tb00784.x
24. Oldfield RC. The assessment and analysis of handedness: the Edinburgh inventory. *Neuropsychologia.* (1971) 9:97–113. doi: 10.1016/0028-3932(71)90067-4
25. Gardner EP, Johnson KO. The somatosensory system: receptors and central pathways. In: Kandel ER, Schwartz JH, Jessell TM, Siegelbaum SA, Hudspeth AJ, editors. *Principles of Neural Science.* New York, NY: McGraw-Hill (2013). p. 475–97.
26. Gardner EP, Johnson KO. Sensory coding. In: Kandel ER, Schwartz JH, Jessell TM, Siegelbaum SA, Hudspeth AJ, editors. *Principles of Neural Science.* New York, NY: McGraw-Hill (2013). p. 449–74.
27. Hartigan JA, Wong MA. Algorithm AS 136 : a K-means clustering algorithm. *J R Stat Soc.* (1979) 28:100–8. doi: 10.2307/2346830
28. Jain S, Muzzafarullah S, Peri S, Ellanti R, Moorthy K, Nath I. Lower touch sensibility in the extremities of healthy Indians: further deterioration with age. *J Peripher Nerv Syst.* (2008) 13:47–53. doi: 10.1111/j.1529-8027.2008.00157.x
29. Bell-Krotoski JA, Fess EE, Figarola JH, Hiltz D. Threshold detection and Semmes-Weinstein monofilaments. *J Hand Ther.* (1995) 8:155–62. doi: 10.1016/S0894-1130(12)80314-0
30. Garn SM. Types and distribution of the hair in man. *Ann N Y Acad Sci.* (1951) 53:498–507. doi: 10.1111/j.1749-6632.1951.tb31952.x
31. Zimmerman A, Bai L, Ginty DD. The gentle touch receptors of mammalian skin. *Science.* (2014) 346:950–4. doi: 10.1126/science.1254229
32. Konopka KH, Harbers M, Houghton A, Kortekaas R, van Vliet A, Timmerman W, et al. Bilateral sensory abnormalities in patients with unilateral neuropathic pain; A quantitative sensory testing (QST) study. *PLoS ONE.* (2012) 7:e37524. doi: 10.1371/journal.pone.0037524
33. Capaday C, Richardson MP, Rothwell JC, Brooks DJ. Long-term changes of GABAergic function in the sensorimotor cortex of amputees. A combined magnetic stimulation and 11C-flumazenil PET study. *Exp Brain Res.* (2000) 133:552–6. doi: 10.1007/s002210000477
34. Werhahn KJ, Mortensen J, Kaelin-Lang A, Boroojerdi B, Cohen LG. Cortical excitability changes induced by deafferentation of the contralateral hemisphere. *Brain.* (2002) 125:1402–13. doi: 10.1093/brain/awf140
35. Fraiman D, Miranda MF, Erthal F, Buur PF, Elschot M, Souza L, et al. Reduced functional connectivity within the primary motor cortex of patients with brachial plexus injury. *NeuroImage Clin.* (2016) 12:277–84. doi: 10.1016/j.nicl.2016.07.008
36. Calford MB, Tweedale R. Interhemispheric transfer of plasticity in the cerebral cortex. *Science.* (1990) 249:805–7. doi: 10.1126/science.2389146
37. Elbert T, Sterr A, Flor H, Rockstroh B, Knecht S, Pantev C, et al. Input-increase and input-decrease types of cortical reorganization after upper extremity amputation in humans. *Exp Brain Res.* (1997) 117:161–4. doi: 10.1007/s002210050210
38. Simoes EL, Bramati I, Rodrigues E, Franzoi A, Moll J, Lent R, et al. Functional expansion of sensorimotor representation and structural reorganization of callosal connections in lower limb amputees. *J Neurosci.* (2012) 32:3211–20. doi: 10.1523/JNEUROSCI.4592-11.2012
39. Pawela CP, Biswal BB, Hudetz AG, Li R, Jones SR, Cho YR, et al. Interhemispheric neuroplasticity following limb deafferentation detected by resting-state functional connectivity magnetic resonance imaging (fcMRI) and functional magnetic resonance imaging (fMRI). *Neuroimage.* (2010) 49:1–25. doi: 10.1016/j.neuroimage.2009.09.054
40. Hsieh J-C, Cheng H, Hsieh H-M, Liao K-K, Wu Y-T, Yeh T-C, et al. Loss of interhemispheric inhibition on the ipsilateral primary sensorimotor cortex in patients with brachial plexus injury: fMRI study. *Ann Neurol.* (2002) 51:381–5. doi: 10.1002/ana.10149
41. Liu B, Li T, Tang WJ, Zhang JH, Sun HP, Xu WD, et al. Changes of inter-hemispheric functional connectivity between motor cortices after brachial plexuses injury: a resting-state fMRI study. *Neuroscience.* (2013) 243:33–9. doi: 10.1016/j.neuroscience.2013.03.048
42. Wall JT, Xu J, Wang X. Human brain plasticity: an emerging view of the multiple substrates and mechanisms that cause cortical changes and related sensory dysfunctions after injuries of sensory inputs from the body. *Brain Res Rev.* (2002) 39:181–215. doi: 10.1016/S0165-0173(02)00192-3
43. Behera D, Behera S, Jacobs KE, Biswal S. Bilateral peripheral neural activity observed *in vivo* following unilateral nerve injury. *Am J Nucl Med Mol Imaging.* (2013) 3:282–90.
44. Verge VM, Wiesenfeld-Hallin Z, Hökfelt T. Cholecystokinin in mammalian primary sensory neurons and spinal cord: *in situ* hybridization studies in rat and monkey. *Eur J Neurosci.* (1993) 5:240–50.
45. Chew DJ, Carlstedt T, Shortland PJ. A comparative histological analysis of two models of nerve root avulsion injury in the adult rat. *Neuropathol Appl Neurobiol.* (2011) 37:613–32. doi: 10.1111/j.1365-2990.2011.01176.x
46. Koltzenburg M, Wall PD, McMahon SB. Does the right hand know what the left hand is doing? *Trends Neurosci.* (1999) 22:122–7. doi: 10.1016/S0166-2236(98)01302-2
47. Iwamura Y, Taoka M, Iriki A. Bilateral activity and callosal connections in the somatosensory cortex. *Neuroscientist.* (2001) 7:419–29. doi: 10.1177/107385840100700511
48. Hansson T, Brismar T. Tactile stimulation of the hand causes bilateral cortical activation: a functional magnetic resonance study in humans. *Neurosci Lett.* (1999) 271:29–32. doi: 10.1016/S0304-3940(99)00508-X
49. Preuss TM, Goldman-Rakic PS. Crossed corticothalamic and thalamocortical connections of macaque prefrontal cortex. *J Comp Neurol.* (1987) 257:269–81. doi: 10.1002/cne.902570211
50. Hagen MC, Zald DH, Thornton TA, Pardo JV. Somatosensory processing in the human inferior prefrontal cortex. *J Neurophysiol.* (2002) 88:1400–6. doi: 10.1152/jn.2002.88.3.1400
51. Farnè A, Roy AC, Giraux P, Pawson T, Sirigu A. Face or hand, not both: perceptual correlates of reafferentation in a former amputee. *Curr Biol.* (2002) 12:1342–6. doi: 10.1016/S0960-9822(02)01018-7
52. Vargas CD, Aballéa A, Rodrigues EC, Reilly KT, Mercier C, Petruzzo P, et al. Re-emergence of hand-muscle representations in human motor cortex after hand allograft. *Proc Natl Acad Sci USA.* (2009) 106:7197–202. doi: 10.1073/pnas.0809614106
53. Nico D, Daprati E, Rigal F, Parsons L, Sirigu A. Left and right hand recognition in upper limb amputees. *Brain.* (2004) 127:120–32. doi: 10.1093/brain/awh006
54. Feng JT, Liu HQ, Xu JG, Gu YD, Shen YD. Differences in brain adaptive functional reorganization in right and left total brachial plexus injury patients. *World Neurosurg.* (2015) 84:702–8. doi: 10.1016/j.wneu.2015.04.046
55. Jain N, Catania KC, Kaas JH. Deactivation and reactivation of somatosensory cortex after dorsal spinal cord injury. *Nature.* (1997) 386:495–8. doi: 10.1038/386495a0
56. Merzenich MM, Kaas JH, Wall J, Nelson RJ, Sur M, Felleman D. Topographic reorganization of somatosensory cortical areas 3b and 1 in adult monkeys following restricted deafferentation. *Neuroscience.* (1983) 8:33–55. doi: 10.1016/0306-4522(83)90024-6
57. Garraghty PE, Kaas JH. Large-scale functional reorganization in adult monkey cortex after peripheral nerve injury. *Proc Natl Acad Sci USA.* (1991) 88:6976–80. doi: 10.1073/pnas.88.16.6976
58. Garraghty PE, Hanes DP, Florence SL, Kaas JH. Pattern of peripheral deafferentation predicts reorganizational limits in adult primate somatosensory cortex. *Somatosens Mot Res.* (1994) 11:109–17. doi: 10.3109/08990229409028864
59. Malessy MJ, van der Kamp W, Thomeer RT, van Dijk JG. Cortical excitability of the biceps muscle after intercostal-to-musculocutaneous nerve transfer. *Neurosurgery.* (1998) 42:787–94. doi: 10.1097/00006123-199804000-00062

60. Malessy MJ, Bakker D, Dekker AJ, Van Duk JG, Thomeer RT. Functional magnetic resonance imaging and control over the biceps muscle after intercostal-musculocutaneous nerve transfer. *Neurosurgery*. (2003) 98:261–8. doi: 10.3171/jns.2003.98.2.0261
61. Oberlin C, Beal D, Leechavengvongs S, Salon A, Dauge MC, Sarcy JJ. Nerve transfer to biceps muscle using part of ulnar nerve for C5-C6 avulsion of the brachial plexus: anatomical study and report of four cases. *J Hand Surg*. (1994) 19:232–7. doi: 10.1016/0363-5023(94)90011-6
62. de Sousa AC, Guedes-Corrêa JF. Post-Oberlin procedure cortical neuroplasticity in traumatic injury of the upper brachial plexus. *Radiol Bras*. (2016) 49:201–2. doi: 10.1590/0100-3984.2015.0082
63. Jiang S, Li Z-Y, Hua X-Y, Xu W-D, Xu J-G, Gu Y-D. Reorganization in motor cortex after brachial plexus avulsion injury and repair with the contralateral C7 root transfer in rats. *Microsurgery*. (2010) 30:314–20. doi: 10.1002/micr.20747
64. Qiu TM, Chen L, Mao Y, Wu JS, Tang WJ, Hu SN, et al. Sensorimotor cortical changes assessed with resting-state fMRI following total brachial plexus root avulsion. *J Neurol Neurosurg Psychiatry*. (2014) 85:99–105. doi: 10.1136/jnnp-2013-304956

14

What is the Role of the Placebo Effect for Pain Relief in Neurorehabilitation? Clinical Implications from the Italian Consensus Conference on Pain in Neurorehabilitation

Gianluca Castelnuovo[1,2], Emanuele Maria Giusti[1,2], Gian Mauro Manzoni[1,3], Donatella Saviola[4], Samantha Gabrielli[5], Marco Lacerenza[5], Giada Pietrabissa[1,2], Roberto Cattivelli[1,2], Chiara Anna Maria Spatola[1,2], Alessandro Rossi[1], Giorgia Varallo[1], Margherita Novelli[1], Valentina Villa[1], Francesca Luzzati[6], Andrea Cottini[6], Carlo Lai[7], Eleonora Volpato[2,8], Cesare Cavalera[2], Francesco Pagnini[2,9], Valentina Tesio[10], Lorys Castelli[10], Mario Tavola[11], Riccardo Torta[12], Marco Arreghini[13], Loredana Zanini[13], Amelia Brunani[13], Ionathan Seitanidis[13], Giuseppe Ventura[13], Paolo Capodaglio[13], Guido Edoardo D'Aniello[1,2], Federica Scarpina[1], Andrea Brioschi[14], Matteo Bigoni[14], Lorenzo Priano[12,14], Alessandro Mauro[12,14], Giuseppe Riva[1,2], Daniele Di Lernia[2], Claudia Repetto[2], Camillo Regalia[2], Enrico Molinari[1,2], Paolo Notaro[15], Stefano Paolucci[16], Giorgio Sandrini[17,18], Susan Simpson[19,20], Brenda Kay Wiederhold[21], Santino Gaudio[22], Jeffrey B. Jackson[23], Stefano Tamburin[24] and Fabrizio Benedetti[12] On Behalf of the Italian Consensus Conference on Pain in Neurorehabilitation*

[1] Istituto Auxologico Italiano IRCCS, Psychology Research Laboratory, San Giuseppe Hospital, Verbania, Italy, [2] Department of Psychology, Catholic University of Milan, Milan, Italy, [3] Faculty of Psychology, eCampus University, Novedrate, Italy, [4] Cardinal Ferrari Rehabilitation Center, Santo Stefano Rehabilitation Istitute, Fontanellato, Italy, [5] Pain Medicine Center, San Pio X Clinic, Humanitas, Milan, Italy, [6] IRCCS Galeazzi Orthopedic Institute, Milan, Italy, [7] Department of Dynamic and Clinical Psychology, Sapienza University of Rome, Rome, Italy, [8] HD Respiratory Rehabilitation Unit, IRCCS Fondazione Don Carlo Gnocchi, Milan, Italy, [9] Department of Psychology, Harvard University, Cambridge, MA, United States, [10] Department of Psychology, University of Turin, Turin, Italy, [11] Anesthesia and Intensive Care, ASST Lecco, Lecco, Italy, [12] Department of Neuroscience "Rita Levi Montalcini", University of Turin, Turin, Italy, [13] Istituto Auxologico Italiano IRCCS, Rehabilitation Unit, San Giuseppe Hospital, Verbania, Italy, [14] Istituto Auxologico Italiano IRCCS, Department of Neurology and Neurorehabilitation, San Giuseppe Hospital, Verbania, Italy, [15] Pain Medicine, Anesthesiology Department, A.O. Ospedale Niguarda ca Granda, Milan, Italy, [16] Fondazione Santa Lucia IRCCS, Rome, Italy, [17] C. Mondino National Neurological Institute, Pavia, Italy, [18] Department of Brain and Behavioral Sciences, University of Pavia, Pavia, Italy, [19] University of South Australia, Adelaide, SA, Australia, [20] Regional Eating Disorders Unit, NHS Lothian, Livingston, United Kingdom, [21] Virtual Reality Medical Institute, Brussels, Belgium, [22] Department of Neuroscience, Functional Pharmacology, Uppsala University, Uppsala, Sweden, [23] Virginia Tech, Falls Church, VA, United States, [24] Department of Neurosciences, Biomedicine and Movement Sciences, University of Verona, Verona, Italy

***Correspondence:**
Gianluca Castelnuovo
gianluca.castelnuovo@unicatt.it

Background: It is increasingly acknowledged that the outcomes of medical treatments are influenced by the context of the clinical encounter through the mechanisms of the placebo effect. The phenomenon of placebo analgesia might be exploited to maximize the efficacy of neurorehabilitation treatments. Since its intensity varies across neurological disorders, the Italian Consensus Conference on Pain in Neurorehabilitation (ICCP) summarized the studies on this field to provide guidance on its use.

Methods: A review of the existing reviews and meta-analyses was performed to assess the magnitude of the placebo effect in disorders that may undergo neurorehabilitation treatment. The search was performed on Pubmed using placebo, pain, and the names of neurological disorders as keywords. Methodological quality was assessed using a pre-existing checklist. Data about the magnitude of the placebo effect were extracted from the included reviews and were commented in a narrative form.

Results: 11 articles were included in this review. Placebo treatments showed weak effects in central neuropathic pain (pain reduction from 0.44 to 0.66 on a 0–10 scale) and moderate effects in postherpetic neuralgia (1.16), in diabetic peripheral neuropathy (1.45), and in pain associated to HIV (1.82). Moderate effects were also found on pain due to fibromyalgia and migraine; only weak short-term effects were found in complex regional pain syndrome. Confounding variables might have influenced these results.

Clinical implications: These estimates should be interpreted with caution, but underscore that the placebo effect can be exploited in neurorehabilitation programs. It is not necessary to conceal its use from the patient. Knowledge of placebo mechanisms can be used to shape the doctor–patient relationship, to reduce the use of analgesic drugs and to train the patient to become an active agent of the therapy.

Keywords: neurorehabilitation, placebo, pain, clinical psychology, health psychology, placebo effect, consensus conference

INTRODUCTION

The placebo effect can be defined as the improvement in the patient's symptoms after the administration of an inert substance in a context inducing positive expectations about its effects (1, 2). This phenomenon is raising a growing interest in the field of pain management in patients with neurological disorders. Neurorehabilitation treatments could be delayed or hampered by pain symptoms, whose management could be particularly difficult since the available treatments may provide only a moderate relief at the cost of various undesirable side effects (3–5). In this context, knowledge of the mechanisms of the placebo effect could be important. Rather than representing an alternative treatment modality, this phenomenon can be exploited to enhance the effectiveness of the care (6).

In the last decades, research has shifted its focus from the inert substance to the psychosocial context surrounding its administration. The placebo response can be considered as a form of *contextual healing*, since the beneficial outcome is due to the context of the clinical encounter, rather than to a specific efficacy of the actual treatment (7–9). This complex phenomenon can be described as the emerging effect of the doctor–patient relationship and of the psychosocial context in which it takes place (10). The patient's memory of previous treatments, personal characteristics, and expectations modulate and are modulated by the interaction with the doctor, whose characteristics and expectations, in turn, influence the context of the encounter. Therefore, the therapeutic ritual itself is the trigger of the placebo effect (11).

The placebo effect is grounded in physiological mechanisms. Different processes can be involved, depending both on the physical or psychological state of the patient and on the context. Various theoretical frameworks have been proposed to understand them, each focusing on a different set of variables, such as conditioning processes, patient expectations, individual attributions, and contextual factors (2, 12). Each of these processes was found to involve different neurobiological mechanisms, including opioid, endocannabinoid, or dopamine ones (13–20). The presence of various mechanisms seems to reflect the complexity of the phenomenon, as well as the variety of neurobiological, psychological, and psychosocial processes involved.

The placebo effect varies across individuals and disorders. Studies are increasingly shedding some light on the individual differences, focusing on the role of genetics (21–23), on differences in the activation of the reward system (16), on differences in expectancy mechanisms and in the emotional appraisal of situations (24), or on the role of psychological variables. Among them, preliminary data corroborate the role of dispositional optimism and state anxiety (25–27), various personality traits (28, 29), hypnotizability and suggestibility (30, 31), reappraisal ability (32), beliefs (33), learning mechanisms (34), and traits linked to dopaminergic mechanisms such as novelty seeking (35).

On the other hand, differences across disorders have received less attention, especially in the field of neurorehabilitation. To exploit the analgesic potential of placebo treatments in this field, knowledge about its differential effects is required. On behalf of The Italian Consensus Conference on Pain in Neurorehabilitation (ICCPN), a multidisciplinary board aimed at developing the national guidelines on the assessment and treatment of pain in neurorehabilitation, our working group was established to summarize the available studies on this topic.

METHODS

A review of the existing reviews and meta-analyses examining the role of the placebo effect in disorders that may undergo neurorehabilitation treatment was performed. This research design was chosen since (a) it allowed to summarize a high amount of studies on such a broad topic and (b) literature reviews focusing on each disorder were already present. Both systematic and non-systematic reviews were considered for inclusion since it was hypothesized that the quality of the existing literature about each disorder would be heterogeneous. Studies were, therefore, included if they reported reviews, with or without meta-analysis, presenting data about the effects of a placebo treatment on pain intensity in disorders that may undergo neurorehabilitation treatment. Only articles written in English language were considered. Studies were excluded if they did not report summary data about the effects of placebo treatments.

An initial search was performed on July 2014, imposing no restraints on the articles' publication date. Subsequently, a research update took place on March 2017, restraining the search to articles published from 2014 to 2017. Both the searches were performed on PubMed using the following keywords: "placebo" (research restricted to the title) "nervous system disease" (as a MeSH word), the names of the primary neurological disorders and "pain." The inclusion and exclusion criteria were used by one of the authors to judge the eligibility of the studies based on the articles' titles, abstracts and, finally, full texts. The bibliographies of the selected articles were analyzed to identify other potentially relevant reviews. The methodological quality of included studies was then assessed using the Critical Appraisal Checklist for Systematic Reviews (**Table 1**) (36). When assessing the methodological quality of non-systematic reviews, items from 5 to 8 of this checklist were not considered.

The following data were extracted from the included reviews: study design of the review, disorder addressed by the review, participants' details, study design of the included studies, number of electronic databases accessed during the search, date range of the search, number of studies included, number of subjects included in placebo arms, total number of subjects, instruments used by the studies to assess pain intensity, and quantitative results. Since the aim of the present review was not to assess if placebo treatments are evidence-based interventions, the quality of evidence was not graded and no recommendations were made. Instead, the results of the reviews were synthesized in a narrative form. Results from excluded reviews or from primary studies that were found during the search that were considered relevant to give insight to areas not explored by the included reviews were also commented.

TABLE 1 | Critical Appraisal Checklist for Systematic Reviews.

1	Is the review question clearly and explicitly stated?
2	Were the inclusion criteria appropriate for the review question?
3	Was the search strategy appropriate?
4	Were the sources and resources used to search for studies adequate?
5	Were the criteria for appraising studies appropriate?
6	Was critical appraisal conducted by two or more reviewers independently?
7	Were the methods used to combine studies appropriate?
8	Was the likelihood of publication bias assessed?
9	Were recommendations for policy and/or practice supported by the reported data?
10	Were the specific directives for new research appropriate?

RESULTS

Overall, the searches yielded 872 records. From this sample, 11 reviews were included in the present review. The flowchart of the study search and selection is reported in **Figure 1**.

Among the included reviews, 10 out of 11 were systematic and 9 included a meta-analysis. Five of these reviews focused on peripheral and/or central neuropathic pain disorders, three on migraine and the remaining on chronic regional pain syndrome, fibromyalgia, or mixed chronic pain conditions. The characteristics of the studies are reported in **Table 2**.

The methodological quality of the included reviews was variable (**Table 3**). Among the systematic reviews, three studies did not meet at least six items of the critical appraisal checklist (39, 40, 44), but none of them showed substantial biases that may hinder the interpretation of their results.

PLACEBO EFFECT IN PAIN CONDITIONS IN NEUROREHABILITATION

The main quantitative results of the included reviews generally show that the placebo effect has a low to moderate effect on pain across the various disorders (**Table 4**). However, differences are visible, especially when neuropathic and non-neuropathic pain disorders are contrasted.

Various reviews and meta-analyses addressed the role of placebo in neuropathic pain disorders and found a noticeable heterogeneity between peripheral and central ones (43–46). In general, the placebo effect was found to be more intense in the former than in the latter. A meta-analytic study estimated the intensity of the placebo effect in various neuropathic pain disorders, and explored both the average pain reduction and the percentage of patients who positively responded to the placebo treatment (44). On a 0–10 scale, the average decrease in pain severity was 1.82 in pain associated with HIV (percentage of positive responders: 48.2%), 1.45 in painful diabetic peripheral neuropathy (percentage of positive responders: 20%), 1.16 in postherpetic neuralgia (percentage of positive responders: 11.5%), and between 0.44 and 0.64 in central neuropathic pain (percentage of positive responders: 7.2%) (42, 44). Other studies confirmed that, among the disorders associated with peripheral neuropathic pain, the placebo effect was higher in painful diabetic peripheral neuropathy than in postherpetic neuralgia (43). In contrast, the placebo effect in complex regional pain syndrome, a disorder with some neuropathic characteristics (48), seems to be nearly absent, with only weak short-term effects (37). In neuropathic pain disorders, the intensity of the placebo effect is modulated by the duration of treatment, with longer treatments associated with increased effects, and by the duration and intensity of initial pain, with longer duration of and higher intensity associated with a reduced placebo response (42, 43, 45).

The intensity of the placebo effect is generally higher in non-neuropathic pain disorders. A meta-analysis by Madsen et al. (47) compared the effects of acupuncture, placebo acupuncture, and a no-treatment condition on pain from various disorders, including headache (tension type, migraine), nociceptive pain (osteoarthritis, low back pain), iatrogenic pain (postoperative,

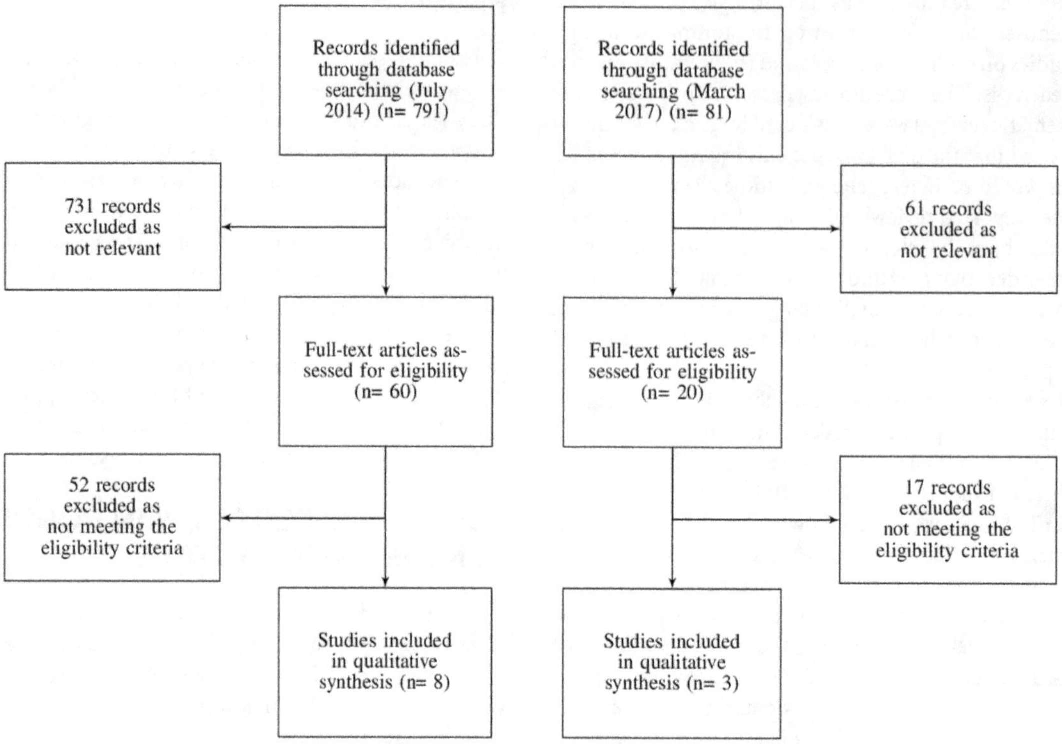

FIGURE 1 | Flowchart of the records search and selection.

procedural pain during colonoscopy, abdominal scar pain), and fibromyalgia. In this study, acupuncture was found to have slightly stronger effects (i.e., 0.4 points on a 0–10 scale) than placebo acupuncture, whereas a moderate difference (i.e., 1.0 points) was found between placebo acupuncture and no acupuncture conditions.

Hauser et al. (38) studied both the placebo and the nocebo effect in the management of fibromyalgia, and estimated that the percentage of patients experiencing a 50% pain reduction after a placebo treatment was 18.6% and that the dropout rate due to adverse events was 10.9%. In contrast, groups receiving a true drug showed a higher rate of responders (31.6%) and a higher dropout rate due to adverse events (20.4%). This study did not compare the improvement in the placebo group with that in the untreated groups.

Despite the variability of their effects, placebo treatments were found to be associated with both short- and long-term improvements in migraine sufferers (39, 41). Placebo groups showed an improvement of pain symptoms in 26% of cases, and 21% of patients taking placebo for migraine prophylaxis improved. For both outcomes, the efficacy of the placebo treatment was estimated to be half of that of active drugs. The placebo treatment type influenced its efficacy, with sham acupuncture and sham surgery being more effective than oral placebos (41). These effects were accompanied by a high rate of adverse events (39–41). The presence of adverse events in case of placebo administration is in line with the nature of placebo, since their characteristics are generally similar to the characteristics of the active drugs against which placebo is compared (49).

The size of the placebo effect and its variability across disorders and type of placebo treatment is apparent also when non-neurological disorders are considered. It was estimated that placebo treatments for osteoarthritis resulted in an overall moderate effect (effect size = 0.51) and that topical and intra-articular placebos are more effective than oral ones (effect size differences of 0.20 and 0.29, respectively) (50, 51). Other estimates show that the size of the placebo effect is equivalent to 72% of that of the drug treatment in burning mouth syndrome (52) and that it leads to pain remission rates of 19.9% in chronic pancreatitis (53).

IMPLICATIONS FOR CLINICAL PRACTICE

The effectiveness of placebo treatments should not be overestimated. Most of the studies on this topic showed high heterogeneity and did not take into account confounding variables, such as spontaneous remission of symptoms or regression toward the mean, thus potentially overestimating the intensity of the placebo response. In addition, various authors underlined that (a) placebo effect is higher when subjective rather than objective outcome measures are explored (54); (b) bias may be present in patients' responses (54); (c) each individual responds differently to placebos (55, 56), and (d) outcomes vary consistently across studies and methodological design (57). These limitations are prominent in studies on placebo treatments, and may impede

TABLE 2 | Description of the included reviews.

Reference	Type of review	Disorder	Participants details	Study design of the included studies	Number of databases searched	Date range of the database search	Number of trials included	Number of subjects in placebo arms	Total number of subjects
Mbizvo et al. (37)	Meta-analysis	Complex regional pain Syndrome	Patients with complex regional pain syndrome I and II	RCT and controlled studies	5 (+ other sources)	1966–2013	20 (18 included in the meta-analysis)	340	Not reported
Hauser et al. (38)	Meta-analysis	Fibromyalgia	Patients with fibromyalgia, both males and females	Double-blind RCT	3	up to 2012	18	3,546	6,589
Loder et al. (39)	Meta-analysis	Migraine	Acute migraine sufferers	RCT and controlled trials	1	1991–2002	31	Not reported	Not reported
Macedo et al. (40)	Meta-analysis	Migraine	Migraine sufferers	Double-blind RCT	1	1998–2004	32 (22 included in the meta-analysis)	1,416	4,519
Meissner et al. (41)	Meta-analysis	Migraine	Migraine sufferers	RCT	4	up to 2012	102 (79 included in the meta-analysis)	Not reported	9,287
Cragg et al. (42)	Meta-analysis	Neuropathic pain (central)	Patients with spinal cord injury, stroke or multiple sclerosis	Placebo-controlled trials	1	up to 2015	39	1,153	Not reported
Arakawa et al. (43)	Meta-analysis	Neuropathic pain	Patients with peripheral or central neuropathic pain	Placebo-controlled trials	3	1995–2014	71	Not reported	6,126
Cepeda et al. (44)	Meta-analysis	Neuropathic pain	Diabetic neuropathy, postherpetic neuralgia, central neuropathic pain, HIV-associated neuropathic pain	RCT	1 (+ other sources)	1995–2009	141	Not reported	6,239
Quessy and Rowbotham (45)	Topical review	Neuropathic pain	Patients with painful diabetic neuropathy or postherpetic neuralgia	RCT	Not reported	Not reported	35	3,355	Not reported
Tuttle et al. (46)	Systematic review	Neuropathic pain	Patients with various types of neuropathic pain	Double-blind RCT	3	1980–2013	84	Not reported	Not reported
Madsen et al. (47)	Meta-analysis	Chronic pain	Patients with headache, migraine, osteoarthritis, low back pain, postoperative pain, colonoscopy, fibromyalgia or scar pain	3-armed RCT	5	up to 2008	13	943	3,025

RCT, randomized controlled trials.

TABLE 3 | Quality assessment of the included reviews.

Reference	Item 1	Item2	Item 3	Item 4	Item 5	Item 6	Item 7	Item 8	Item 9	Item 10
Mbizvo et al. (37)	✓	✓	✓	✓	✓	✓	✓	✓	✓	✓
Hauser et al. (38)	✓	✓	✓	✓	×	×	✓	×	✓	✓
Loder et al. (39)	✓	×	×	×	✓	×	✓	×	✓	×
Macedo et al. (40)	✓	✓	✓	×	×	×	✓	×	×	×
Meissner et al. (41)	✓	✓	✓	✓	✓	✓	✓	×	✓	✓
Cragg et al. (42)	✓	✓	✓	×	×	×	✓	✓	✓	✓
Arakawa et al. (43)	✓	✓	✓	✓	×	×	✓	×	✓	✓
Cepeda et al. (44)	✓	✓	✓	×	×	×	✓	×	✓	×
Quessy and Rowbotham (45)	×	✓	×	×	n\a	n\a	n\a	n\a	✓	×
Tuttle et al. (46)	✓	✓	✓	✓	×	×	✓	✓	✓	✓
Madsen et al. (47)	✓	✓	✓	✓	✓	✓	✓	×	✓	✓

TABLE 4 | Quantitative findings of the included reviews.

Reference	Disorder	Instruments or outcome data	Results	Comments
Mbizvo et al. (37)	Complex Regional Pain Syndrome	VAS, NRS (if other scales were used, scores were converted)	Mean change in 0–100 VAS or NRS at 15–30 min posttreatment: 18,423, 95% CI [−33.15, −3.65] Mean change in 0–100 VAS or NRS at 1 week posttreatment: −6,772, 95% CI [−14.92, 1.38] Mean change in 0–100 VAS or NRS at 3–4 weeks posttreatment: 0.326, 95% CI [−2.329, 2.981] Mean change in 0–100 VAS or NRS at 6 weeks posttreatment: −3.87, 95% CI [−9.48, 1.71]	Only mean change at 15–30 min posttreatment was significant. Study design and invasiveness of the placebo treatment affected placebo response
Hauser et al. (38)	Fibromyalgia	0–10 or 0–100 VAS or NRS	Percentage of patients with a 50% reduction of pain intensity in placebo arms: 18.6%, 95% CI [17.4–19.9] vs 31.6%, 95% CI [30.5, 32.7] of patients in active drugs arms	Nocebo effect: dropout due to adverse events: 10.9%, 95% CI [9.9–11.9]. Confounders: percentage of women or Caucasians included and study duration are positively correlated with placebo effect, number of continents is negatively associated with placebo effect
Loder et al. (39)	Migraine	Percentage of pain-free patients, response rate, adverse events rate	Percentage of pain-free patients at two hours: 6.08% (±4.83) Response rate at 2 h: 28.90% (±8.55) Adverse events rate at 2 h: 23.4% (±14.05)	Migraine prophylaxis: percentage of pain-free patients: 6.02%; response rate: 25.52%; adverse events rate: 19.56%
Macedo et al. (40)	Migraine	Percentage of improved patients, attacks per month reduction, adverse events rate	Migraine prophylaxis: percentage of improved patients: 21%, 95% CI [13%, 28%] Attacks per month reduction: −0.8, 95% CI [0.4, 1.1] Adverse events rate: 30%, 95% CI [17%, 43%]	Significant confounders: study design and country
Meissner et al. (41)	Migraine	Proportion of responders (directly extracted or calculated from: number of days with migraine, number of days with headache, or 50% decrease in headache scales scores)	Proportion of placebo responders at 3–4 months: 0.26, 95% CI [0.22, 0.30] vs responders to active treatments: 0.42, 95% CI [0.38, 0.45] Difference between placebo treatments: sham surgery: 0.58, 95% CI [0.37, 0.77]; sham acupuncture: 0.38, 95% CI [0.30, 0.47]; oral placebo: 0.22, 95% CI [0.17, 0.28]	Subgroup analysis: when all confounders are considered, blinding of subjects and type of placebo treatment is positively correlated with placebo magnitude
Cragg et al. (42)	Neuropathic pain (central)	VAS, NRS	Overall mean change in pain rating (0–10): −0.64 95% CI [−0.83, −0.45]	Meta-regression: weaker placebo effect associated with higher chronic pain duration, baseline pain variability, cross-over study design. High heterogeneity
Arakawa et al. (43)	Neuropathic pain	VAS, NRS	Neuropathic pain (both central and peripheral): percentage of patients with 50% pain intensity reduction: 23%, 95% CI [20%, 25%], percentage of patients with 30% pain intensity reduction: 37%, 95% CI [34%, 41%] Peripheral neuropathic pain: percentage of patients with 50% pain intensity reduction: 23%, 95% CI [21, 26], percentage of patients with 30% pain intensity reduction: 39%, 95% CI [34%, 42%]	Among the results of the multivariable analysis, baseline pain intensity was found to be negatively correlated with placebo response in postherpetic neuralgia and in painful diabetic peripheral neuropathy

(Continued)

TABLE 4 | Continued

Reference	Disorder	Instruments or outcome data	Results	Comments
			Central neuropathic pain: percentage of patients with 50% pain intensity reduction: 14%, 95% CI [10, 19], percentage of patients with 30% pain intensity reduction: 26%, 95% CI [19%, 33%]	
Cepeda et al. (44)	Neuropathic pain	Mean decrease in 0–10 pain intensity, responder rate (percentage of patients with 50% pain intensity reduction)	Overall: 1.2 (±1.0) mean reduction in pain intensity, RR 17% (range: 0–43%) Diabetic neuropathy: 1.45, 95% CI [1.35–1.55] mean reduction in pain intensity, RR of 20.2%, 95% CI [14.6–25.8] Postherpetic neuralgia: 1.16, 95% CI [1.03–1.29] mean reduction in pain intensity, RR of 11.5%, 95% CI [8.4–14.5] Central neuropathic pain 0.53, 95% CI [0.19–0.86] mean reduction in pain intensity, RR of 7.2%, 95% CI [2.1–12.3] HIV-associated neuropathic pain: 1.82, 95% CI [1.51–2.12], RR of 42.8%, 95% CI [34.9–50.7]	Trials evaluating NMDA blockers showed weaker placebo response, age was positively correlated with placebo response
Quessy and Rowbotham (45)	Neuropathic pain	VAS, NRS	Median change in pain intensity in PDN: 26% (range 11–35%); in PHN 15–16 (range 4–44%)	The placebo response was found to vary throughout the time course of trials and to be influenced by trial duration
Tuttle et al. (46)	Neuropathic pain	VAS, NRS	Mean change in pain intensity: 18.3%, 95% CI [15.2%, 21.4%]	Multivariable analysis: placebo magnitude is positively correlated with sample size; in studies performed in the US the placebo magnitude is positively correlated with study duration
Madsen et al. (47)	Various types of pain	SMD based on WOMAC, VAS or Likert-type rating scales	Acupuncture vs placebo SMD: −0.17, 95% CI [−0.26, −0.08]; placebo vs nontreated controls SMD: −0.42, 95% CI [−0.60, −0.23]	High heterogeneity

VAS, Visual Analogue Scale; NRS, Numeric Rating Scale; MPQ, McGill Pain Questionnaire; WOMAC, Western Ontario and McMaster Universities Osteoarthritis Index Pain Score; CI, Confidence Interval; SMD, standardized mean difference; RR, responders rate.

to predict their effects in routine clinical practice. It is recommended to take these treatments into consideration in neurorehabilitation settings only after traditional ones have failed or are contraindicated (58–64).

Rather than simply representing an alternative type of treatment, the placebo effect is a phenomenon that can increase the effectiveness of the care, since it constitutes the process through which the doctor–patient relationship becomes therapeutic. The knowledge of relevance of the placebo effect for each specific pain disorder is recommended to exploit its potential. For example, placebo response is generally small in central neuropathic pain, where pharmacological and non-pharmacological treatments have also limited efficacy, while it appears to represent half of the effect of active treatments in the prophylaxis of primary headaches. This information is central to shape the communication with the patient, allowing to provide a trustworthy explanation of the positive effects of the therapeutic context.

It is increasingly acknowledged that concealment is not necessary for the placebo effect to take place. Research on open-label placebos treatments, i.e., non-deceptive treatments in which the participants are alerted that the therapeutic mean is inert, but are informed about the effects of the administration of placebos, corroborates this claim. Further studies are needed, but open-label placebo treatments seem to have a similar or even higher efficacy than deceptive ones and are associated with marked improvement of symptoms of a variety of conditions (65–70). These treatments are more easily accepted by patients (71) and overcome the ethical and legal implications of the deceitful prescription of placebos, which violates the principle of the informed consent and may affect the trust that shape the doctor–patient relationship (72, 73).

Various techniques can be used to improve the patient's symptoms through placebo mechanisms. A possible strategy is to maximize the patient's expectations regarding the treatment. This can be done by informing the patient on the nature and effects of placebo analgesia, by assessing the appropriateness of the patient's beliefs about his disorder and its treatment and providing information in case they are excessively positive or negative. In this case, it would be important to balance the information regarding the positive and negative effects of the treatment, underlying the role of the positive ones despite its undesired effects, and by cognitively reinforcing the impact of the positive outcomes as they appear (74–76). Furthermore, it is possible to exploit conditioning mechanisms to support the pharmacological therapy. Once the person associates the characteristics of the analgesic agent, such as appearance and taste, to the reduction of pain, it could be possible to employ inert substitutes with the same characteristics to obtain similar results (6). Using similar methods, it would be possible, after an adequate initial conditioning, to progressively reduce the administration of medication by alternatively switching to a placebo with similar characteristics (74, 77). Finally, the patient can also be trained to create those conditions that maximize the placebo effect, for example by focusing on the characteristics of the analgesic agent or by increasing his own expectations through appropriate information (75).

It should be underscored that all these techniques need to take place within the context of a doctor–patient relationship. The relational aspect of the placebo effect resides in the person's feeling of being taken care for and in the process by which he himself becomes an active agent of the therapy (78). Having an empathic attitude, reassuring the patient, helping him to self-manage his symptoms, emphasizing the role of interpersonal resources and creating therapeutic rituals during therapy represent key aspects of the relationship.

In conclusion, the neurorehabilitation team needs to address a variety of disorders, each of which responds differently to the placebo effect. It is, therefore, necessary to personalize all these features depending on the disorder and on the patient's characteristics. Studies are beginning to clarify the genetic, biological, psychological, and contextual factors that may enable to identify subjects with high or low likelihood of experiencing a placebo response (22, 28). To exploit the placebo effect, the doctor should collect information regarding not only about the patient's disorder, but also about his personal characteristics and his context (74). The context of the doctor–patient relationship should be shaped so that the doctor does not focus only on the treatment of pain as a symptom of the neurological disorder, but is able to take care of the person as a whole.

THE ITALIAN CONSENSUS CONFERENCE ON PAIN IN NEUROREHABILITATION

The following Authors, who are listed in alphabetical order, contributed to the work of the Italian Consensus Conference on Pain in Neurorehabilitation: **Michela Agostini**, Neurorehabilitation Department, Foundation IRCCS San Camillo Hospital, Venice, Italy; **Enrico Alfonsi**, C. Mondino National Institute of Neurology Foundation, IRCCS, Pavia, Italy; **Anna Maria Aloisi**, Department of Medicine, Surgery and Neuroscience, University of Siena, Siena, Italy; **Elena Alvisi**, Department of Brain and Behavioural Sciences, University of Pavia, Pavia, Italy; **Irene Aprile**, Don Gnocchi Foundation, Milan, Italy; **Michela Armando**, Department of Neuroscience and Neurorehabilitation, Bambin Gesù Children's Hospital, IRCCS, Rome, Italy; **Micol Avenali**, C. Mondino National Institute of Neurology Foundation, IRCCS, Pavia, Italy, Department of Brain and Behavioural Sciences, University of Pavia, Pavia, Italy; **Eva Azicnuda**, IRCCS Santa Lucia Foundation, Rome, Italy; **Francesco Barale**, Department of Brain and Behavioural Sciences, University of Pavia, Pavia, Italy; **Michelangelo Bartolo**, Neurorehabilitation Unit, IRCCS INM Neuromed, Pozzilli, Italy; **Roberto Bergamaschi**, C. Mondino National Institute of Neurology Foundation, IRCCS, Pavia, Italy; **Mariangela Berlangieri**, Department of Brain and Behavioural Sciences, University of Pavia, Pavia, Italy; **Vanna Berlincioni**, Department of Brain and Behavioural Sciences, University of Pavia, Pavia, Italy; **Laura Berliocchi**, Department of Health Sciences, University Magna Graecia of Catanzaro, Catanzaro, Italy; **Eliana Berra**, C. Mondino National Institute of Neurology Foundation, IRCCS, Pavia, Italy; **Giulia Berto**, Department of Neurological and Movement Sciences, University of Verona, Verona, Italy; **Silvia Bonadiman**, Department of Neurological and Movement Sciences, University of Verona, Verona, Italy; **Sara Bonazza**, Department of Surgery, University of Verona, Verona, Italy; **Federica Bressi**, Campus Biomedico University, Rome, Italy; **Annalisa Brugnera**, Department of Neurological and Movement Sciences, University of Verona, Verona, Italy; **Stefano Brunelli**, IRCCS Santa Lucia Foundation, Rome, Italy; **Maria Gabriella Buzzi**, IRCCS Santa Lucia Foundation, Rome, Italy; **Carlo Cacciatori**, Department of Neurological and Movement Sciences, University of Verona, Verona, Italy; **Andrea Calvo**, Rita Levi Montalcini Department of Neuroscience, University of Turin, Turin, Italy; **Cristina Cantarella**, Physical and Rehabilitation Medicine Unit, Tor Vergata University, Rome, Italy; **Augusto Caraceni**, Palliative Care, Pain Therapy and Rehabilitation, Fondazione IRCCS Istituto Nazionale dei Tumori di Milano, Milan, Italy; **Roberto Carone**, Neuro- Urology Department, City Hospital Health and Science of the City of Turin, Turin, Italy; **Elena Carraro**, Neuropediatric Rehabilitation Unit, E. Medea Scientific Institute, Conegliano, Italy; **Roberto Casale**, Department of Clinical Neurophysiology and Pain Rehabilitation Unit, Foundation Salvatore Maugeri IRCCS, Montescano, Italy; **Paola Castellazzi**, Department of Neurological and Movement Sciences, University of Verona, Verona, Italy; **Gianluca Castelnuovo**, Psychology Research Laboratory, Istituto Auxologico Italiano IRCCS, Ospedale San Giuseppe, Verbania, Italy, Department of Psychology, Catholic University of Milan, Italy; **Adele Castino**, ASL of the Province of Lodi, Lodi, Italy; **Rosanna Cerbo**, Hub Terapia del Dolore Regione Lazio, Policlinico Umberto I, Sapienza University, Rome Italy; **Adriano Chiò**, Rita Levi Montalcini Department of Neuroscience, University of Turin, Turin, Italy; **Cristina Ciotti**, Physical and Rehabilitation Medicine Unit, Tor Vergata University, Rome, Italy; **Carlo Cisari**, Department of Health Sciences, Università del Piemonte Orientale, Novara, Italy; **Daniele Coraci**, Department of Orthopaedic Science, Sapienza University, Rome, Italy; **Elena Dalla Toffola**, Department of Clinical, Surgical, Diagnostic and Pediatric Sciences, University of Pavia, Pavia, Italy, IRCCS Policlinico San Matteo Foundation, Pavia; **Giovanni Defazio**, Department of Basic Medical Sciences, Neuroscience and Sensory Organs, Aldo Moro University of Bari, Bari, Italy; **Roberto De Icco**, C. Mondino National Institute of Neurology Foundation, IRCCS, Pavia, Italy, Department of Brain and Behavioural Sciences, University of Pavia, Pavia, Italy; **Ubaldo Del Carro**, Section of Clinical Neurophysiology and Neurorehabilitation, San Raffaele Hospital, Milan, Italy; **Andrea Dell'Isola**, Department of Health Sciences, Università del Piemonte Orientale, Novara, Italy; **Antonio De Tanti**, Cardinal Ferrari Rehabilitation Center, Santo Stefano Rehabilitation Institute, Fontanellato, Italy; **Mariagrazia D'Ippolito**, IRCCS Santa Lucia Foundation, Rome, Italy; **Elisa Fazzi**, Childhood and Adolescence Neurology and Psychiatry Unit, City Hospital,

Brescia, Italy, Department of Clinical and Experimental Sciences, University of Brescia, Brescia, Italy; **Adriano Ferrari**, Children Rehabilitation Unit, IRCCS Arcispedale S.Maria Nuova, Reggio Emilia, Italy; **Sergio Ferrari**, Department of Neurological and Movement Sciences, University of Verona, Verona, Italy; **Francesco Ferraro**, Section of Neuromotor Rehabilitation, Department of Neuroscience, Azienda Ospedaliera Carlo Poma, Mantova, Italy; **Fabio Formaglio**, Palliative Care, Pain Therapy and Rehabilitation, Fondazione IRCCS Istituto Nazionale dei Tumori di Milano, Milan, Italy; **Rita Formisano**, IRCCS Santa Lucia Foundation, Rome, Italy; **Simone Franzoni**, Poliambulanza Foundation Istituto Ospedaliero, Geriatric Research Group, Brescia, Italy; **Francesca Gajofatto**, Department of Neurological and Movement Sciences, University of Verona, Verona, Italy; **Marialuisa Gandolfi**, Department of Neurological and Movement Sciences, University of Verona, Verona, Italy; **Barbara Gardella**, IRCCS Policlinico San Matteo Foundation, Pavia; **Pierangelo Geppetti**, Department of Health Sciences, Section of Clinical Pharmacology and Oncology, University of Florence, Florence, Italy; **Alessandro Giammò**, Neuro-Urology Department, City Hospital Health and Science of the City of Turin, Turin, Italy; **Raffaele Gimigliano**, Department of Physical and Mental Health, Second University of Naples, Naples, Italy; **Emanuele Maria Giusti**, Department of Psychology, Catholic University of Milan, Italy; **Elena Greco**, Department of Neurological and Movement Sciences, University of Verona, Verona, Italy; **Valentina Ieraci**, Department of Oncology and Neuroscience, University of Turin, City Hospital Health and Science of the City of Turin, Turin, Turin, Italy; **Marco Invernizzi**, Department of Health Sciences, Università del Piemonte Orientale, Novara, Italy; **Marco Jacopetti**, University of Parma, Parma, Italy; **Marco Lacerenza**, Casa di Cura San Pio X S.r.l., HUMANITAS, Milan, Italy; **Silvia La Cesa**, Department of Neurology and Psychiatry, University Sapienza, Rome, Italy; **Davide Lobba**, Department of Neurological and Movement Sciences, University of Verona, Verona, Italy; **Gian Mauro Manzoni**, Psychology Research Laboratory, Istituto Auxologico Italiano IRCCS, Ospedale San Giuseppe, Verbania, Italy, Department of Psychology, Catholic University of Milan, Italy; **Francesca Magrinelli**, Department of Neurological and Movement Sciences, University of Verona, Verona, Italy; **Silvia Mandrini**, Department of Clinical, Surgical, Diagnostic and Pediatric Sciences, University of Pavia, Pavia, Italy; **Umberto Manera**, Rita Levi Montalcini Department of Neuroscience, University of Turin, Turin, Italy; **Paolo Marchettini**, Pain Medicine Center, Hospital San Raffaele, Milan, Italy; **Enrico Marchioni**, C. Mondino National Institute of Neurology Foundation, IRCCS, Pavia, Italy; **Sara Mariotto**, Department of Neurological and Movement Sciences, University of Verona, Verona, Italy; **Andrea Martinuzzi**, Neuropediatric Rehabilitation Unit, E. Medea Scientific Institute, Conegliano, Italy; **Marella Masciullo**, IRCCS Santa Lucia Foundation, Rome, Italy; **Susanna Mezzarobba**, Department of Medicine, Surgery and Health Sciences, University of Trieste, Trieste, Italy; **Danilo Miotti**, Palliative Care and Pain Therapy Unit, Fondazione Salvatore Maugeri IRCCS, Scientific Institute of Pavia, Pavia, Italy; **Angela Modenese**, Department of Neurological and Movement Sciences, University of Verona, Verona, Italy; **Marco Molinari**, IRCCS Santa Lucia Foundation, Rome, Italy; **Salvatore Monaco**, Department of Neurological and Movement Sciences, University of Verona, Verona, Italy; **Giovanni Morone**, IRCCS Santa Lucia Foundation, Rome, Italy; **Rossella Nappi**, Department of Clinical, Surgical, Diagnostic and Pediatric Sciences, University of Pavia, Pavia, Italy, IRCCS Policlinico San Matteo Foundation, Pavia; **Stefano Negrini**, Don Gnocchi Foundation, Milan, Italy, Department of Clinical and Experimental Sciences, University of Brescia, Brescia, Italy; **Andrea Pace**, Neuro-Oncology Unit, Regina Elena National Cancer Institute of Rome, Rome, Italy; **Luca Padua**, Don Gnocchi Foundation, Milan, Italy, Institute of Neurology, Catholic University, Rome, Italy; **Emanuela Pagliano**, Developmental Neurology Unit, C. Besta Neurological Institute Foundation, Milan, Italy; **Valerio Palmerini**, Hub Terapia del Dolore Regione Lazio, Policlinico Umberto I, Sapienza University, Rome Italy; **Stefano Paolucci**, IRCCS Santa Lucia Foundation, Rome, Italy; **Costanza Pazzaglia**, Don Gnocchi Foundation, Milan, Italy; **Cristiano Pecchioli**, Don Gnocchi Foundation, Milan, Italy; **Alessandro Picelli**, Department of Neurological and Movement Sciences, University of Verona, Verona, Italy; **Carlo Adolfo Porro**, Department of Biomedical, Metabolic and Neural Sciences, University of Modena and Reggio Emilia, Modena, Italy; **Daniele Porru**, IRCCS Policlinico San Matteo Foundation, Pavia; **Marcello Romano**, Neurology Unit, Azienda Ospedaliera Ospedali Riuniti Villa Sofia Cervello, Palermo, Italy; **Laura Roncari**, Department of Neurological and Movement Sciences, University of Verona, Verona, Italy; **Riccardo Rosa**, Hub Terapia del Dolore Regione Lazio, Policlinico Umberto I, Sapienza University, Rome Italy; **Marsilio Saccavini**, ASL 2 Bassa Friulana-Isontina, Italy; **Paola Sacerdote**, Department of Pharmacological and Biomolecular Sciences, University of Milano, Milano, Italy; **Giorgio Sandrini**, C. Mondino National Institute of Neurology Foundation, IRCCS, Pavia, Italy, Department of Brain and Behavioural Sciences, University of Pavia, Pavia, Italy; **Donatella Saviola**, Cardinal Ferrari Rehabilitation Center, Santo Stefano Rehabilitation Institute, Fontanellato, Italy; **Angelo Schenone**, Department of Neuroscience, Rehabilitation, Ophthalmology, Genetics, Maternal and Child Health (DiNOGMI), University of Genoa, Genoa, Italy; **Vittorio Schweiger**, Department of Surgery, University of Verona, Verona, Italy; **Giorgio Scivoletto**, IRCCS Santa Lucia Foundation, Rome, Italy; **Nicola Smania**, Department of Neurological and Movement Sciences, University of Verona, Verona, Italy; **Claudio Solaro**, Neurology Unit, ASL3, Genoa, Italy; **Vincenza Spallone**, Department of Systems Medicine, University Tor Vergata, Rome, Italy; **Isabella Springhetti**, Functional Recovery and Rehabilitation Unit, IRCCS Fondazione S. Maugeri, Pavia, Italy; **Stefano Tamburin**, Department of Neurological and Movement Sciences, University of Verona, Verona, Italy; **Cristina Tassorelli**, C. Mondino National Institute of Neurology Foundation, IRCCS, Pavia, Italy, Department of Brain and Behavioural Sciences, University of Pavia, Pavia, Italy; **Michele Tinazzi**, Department of Neurological and Movement Sciences, University of Verona, Verona, Italy; **Rossella Togni**, Department of Clinical, Surgical, Diagnostic and Pediatric Sciences, University of Pavia, Pavia, Italy; **Monica Torre**, IRCCS Santa Lucia Foundation, Rome, Italy; **Riccardo Torta**, Department of Oncology and Neuroscience, University of Turin, City Hospital

Health and Science of the City of Turin, Turin, Turin, Italy; **Marco Traballesi**, IRCCS Santa Lucia Foundation, Rome, Italy; **Marco Tramontano**, IRCCS Santa Lucia Foundation, Rome, Italy; **Andrea Truini**, Department of Neurology and Psychiatry, University Sapienza, Rome, Italy; **Valeria Tugnoli**, Neurological Unit, University Hospital of Ferrara, Ferrara, Italy; **Andrea Turolla**, Neurorehabilitation Department, Foundation IRCCS San Camillo Hospital, Venice, Italy; **Gabriella Vallies**, Department of Neurological and Movement Sciences, University of Verona, Verona, Italy; **Elisabetta Verzini**, Department of Neurological and Movement Sciences, University of Verona, Verona, Italy; **Mario Vottero**, Neuro-Urology Department, City Hospital Health and Science of the City of Turin, Turin, Italy; **Paolo Zerbinati**, Neuro- orthopaedic Program, Hand Surgery Department, Santa Maria Hospital MultiMedica, Castellanza, Italy.

AUTHOR'S NOTE

This paper has been written and shared in the Consensus Conference modality.

AUTHOR CONTRIBUTIONS

All authors listed have made a substantial, direct and intellectual contribution to the work, and approved it for publication.

REFERENCES

1. Benedetti F, Frisaldi E, Carlino E, Giudetti L, Pampallona A, Zibetti M, et al. Teaching neurons to respond to placebos. *J Physiol* (2016) 594:5647–60. doi:10.1113/JP271322
2. Dodd S, Dean OM, Vian J, Berk M. A review of the theoretical and biological understanding of the nocebo and placebo phenomena. *Clin Ther* (2017) 39:469–76. doi:10.1016/j.clinthera.2017.01.010
3. Benrud-Larson LM, Wegener ST. Chronic pain in neurorehabilitation populations: prevalence, severity and impact. *NeuroRehabilitation* (2000) 14:127–37.
4. Magrinelli F, Zanette G, Tamburin S. Neuropathic pain: diagnosis and treatment. *Pract Neurol* (2013) 13:292–307. doi:10.1136/practneurol-2013-000536
5. Tamburin S, Paolucci S, Magrinelli F, Musicco M, Sandrini G. The Italian Consensus Conference on Pain in Neurorehabilitation: rationale and methodology. *J Pain Res* (2016) 9:311–8. doi:10.2147/JPR.S84646
6. Klinger R, Flor H. Clinical and ethical implications of placebo effects: enhancing patients' benefits from pain treatment. *Handb Exp Pharmacol* (2014) 225:217–35. doi:10.1007/978-3-662-44519-8_13
7. Miller FG, Kaptchuk TJ. The power of context: reconceptualizing the placebo effect. *J R Soc Med* (2008) 101:222–5. doi:10.1258/jrsm.2008.070466
8. Price DD, Finniss DG, Benedetti F. A comprehensive review of the placebo effect: recent advances and current thought. *Annu Rev Psychol* (2008) 59:565–90. doi:10.1146/annurev.psych.59.113006.095941
9. Crane GS. Harnessing the placebo effect: a new model for mind-body healing mechanisms. *Int J Trans Stud* (2016) 35:39–51. doi:10.24972/ijts.2016.35.1.39
10. Benedetti F. Placebo and the new physiology of the doctor-patient relationship. *Physiol Rev* (2013) 93:1207–46. doi:10.1152/physrev.00043.2012
11. Benedetti F. Placebo-induced improvements: how therapeutic rituals affect the patient's brain. *J Acupunct Meridian Stud* (2012) 5:97–103. doi:10.1016/j.jams.2012.03.001
12. Colagiuri B, Schenk LA, Kessler MD, Dorsey SG, Colloca L. The placebo effect: from concepts to genes. *Neuroscience* (2015) 307:171–90. doi:10.1016/j.neuroscience.2015.08.017
13. Levine JD, Gordon NC, Fields HL. The mechanism of placebo analgesia. *Lancet* (1978) 2:654–7. doi:10.1016/S0140-6736(78)92762-9
14. Benedetti F, Amanzio M, Casadio C, Oliaro A, Maggi G. Blockade of nocebo hyperalgesia by the cholecystokinin antagonist proglumide. *Pain* (1997) 71:135–40. doi:10.1016/S0304-3959(97)03346-0
15. Amanzio M, Benedetti F. Neuropharmacological dissection of placebo analgesia: expectation-activated opioid systems versus conditioning-activated specific subsystems. *J Neurosci* (1999) 19:484–94. doi:10.1523/JNEUROSCI.19-01-00484.1999
16. Scott DJ, Stohler CS, Egnatuk CM, Wang H, Koeppe RA, Zubieta JK. Individual differences in reward responding explain placebo-induced expectations and effects. *Neuron* (2007) 55:325–36. doi:10.1016/j.neuron.2007.06.028
17. Scott DJ, Stohler CS, Egnatuk CM, Wang H, Koeppe RA, Zubieta JK. Placebo and nocebo effects are defined by opposite opioid and dopaminergic responses. *Arch Gen Psychiatry* (2008) 65:220–31. doi:10.1001/archgenpsychiatry.2007.34
18. Eippert F, Bingel U, Schoell ED, Yacubian J, Klinger R, Lorenz J, et al. Activation of the opioidergic descending pain control system underlies placebo analgesia. *Neuron* (2009) 63:533–43. doi:10.1016/j.neuron.2009.07.014
19. Zubieta J-K, Stohler CS. Neurobiological mechanisms of placebo responses. *Ann N Y Acad Sci* (2009) 1156:198–210. doi:10.1111/j.1749-6632.2009.04424.x
20. Benedetti F, Amanzio M, Rosato R, Blanchard C. Nonopioid placebo analgesia is mediated by CB1 cannabinoid receptors. *Nat Med* (2011) 17:1228–30. doi:10.1038/nm.2435
21. Carlino E, Piedimonte A, Benedetti F. Nature of the placebo and nocebo effect in relation to functional neurologic disorders. *Handb Clin Neurol* (2017) 139:597–606. doi:10.1016/B978-0-12-801772-2.00048-5
22. Wang RS, Hall KT, Giulianini F, Passow D, Kaptchuk TJ, Loscalzo J. Network analysis of the genomic basis of the placebo effect. *JCI Insight* (2017) 2:93911. doi:10.1172/jci.insight.93911
23. Hall KT, Loscalzo J, Kaptchuk T. Pharmacogenomics and the placebo response. *ACS Chem Neurosci* (2018) 9(4):633–5. doi:10.1021/acschemneuro.8b00078
24. Wager TD, Atlas LY, Leotti LA, Rilling JK. Predicting individual differences in placebo analgesia: contributions of brain activity during anticipation and pain experience. *J Neurosci* (2011) 31:439–52. doi:10.1523/JNEUROSCI.3420-10.2011
25. Geers AL, Helfer SG, Kosbab K, Weiland PE, Landry SJ. Reconsidering the role of personality in placebo effects: dispositional optimism, situational expectations, and the placebo response. *J Psychosom Res* (2005) 58:121–7. doi:10.1016/j.jpsychores.2004.08.011
26. Morton DL, Watson A, El-Deredy W, Jones AK. Reproducibility of placebo analgesia: effect of dispositional optimism. *Pain* (2009) 146:194–8. doi:10.1016/j.pain.2009.07.026
27. Geers AL, Wellman JA, Fowler SL, Helfer SG, France CR. Dispositional optimism predicts placebo analgesia. *J Pain* (2010) 11:1165–71. doi:10.1016/j.jpain.2010.02.014
28. Pecina M, Azhar H, Love TM, Lu T, Fredrickson BL, Stohler CS, et al. Personality trait predictors of placebo analgesia and neurobiological correlates. *Neuropsychopharmacology* (2013) 38:639–46. doi:10.1038/npp.2012.227
29. Darragh M, Booth RJ, Consedine NS. Who responds to placebos? Considering the "placebo personality" via a transactional model. *Psychol Health Med* (2015) 20:287–95. doi:10.1080/13548506.2014.936885
30. De Pascalis V, Chiaradia C, Carotenuto E. The contribution of suggestibility and expectation to placebo analgesia phenomenon in an experimental setting. *Pain* (2002) 96:393–402. doi:10.1016/S0304-3959(01)00485-7
31. Raz A. Genetics and neuroimaging of attention and hypnotizability may elucidate placebo. *Int J Clin Exp Hypn* (2008) 56:99–116. doi:10.1080/00207140701506482
32. Van Der Meulen M, Kamping S, Anton F. The role of cognitive reappraisal in placebo analgesia: an fMRI study. *Soc Cogn Affect Neurosci* (2017) 12(7):1128–37. doi:10.1093/scan/nsx033
33. Watkinson A, Chapman SC, Horne R. Beliefs about pharmaceutical medicines and natural remedies explain individual variation in placebo analgesia. *J Pain* (2017) 18(8):908–22. doi:10.1016/j.jpain.2017.02.435
34. Colloca L, Benedetti F. How prior experience shapes placebo analgesia. *Pain* (2006) 124:126–33. doi:10.1016/j.pain.2006.04.005
35. Schweinhardt P, Seminowicz DA, Jaeger E, Duncan GH, Bushnell MC. The anatomy of the mesolimbic reward system: a link between personality and

the placebo analgesic response. *J Neurosci* (2009) 29:4882–7. doi:10.1523/JNEUROSCI.5634-08.2009

36. Aromataris E, Fernandez R, Godfrey CM, Holly C, Khalil H, Tungpunkom P. Summarizing systematic reviews: methodological development, conduct and reporting of an umbrella review approach. *Int J Evid Based Healthc* (2015) 13:132–40. doi:10.1097/XEB.0000000000000055
37. Mbizvo GK, Nolan SJ, Nurmikko TJ, Goebel A. Placebo responses in long-standing complex regional pain syndrome: a systematic review and meta-analysis. *J Pain* (2015) 16:99–115. doi:10.1016/j.jpain.2014.11.008
38. Hauser W, Sarzi-Puttini P, Tolle TR, Wolfe F. Placebo and nocebo responses in randomised controlled trials of drugs applying for approval for fibromyalgia syndrome treatment: systematic review and meta-analysis. *Clin Exp Rheumatol* (2012) 30:78–87.
39. Loder E, Goldstein R, Biondi D. Placebo effects in oral triptan trials: the scientific and ethical rationale for continued use of placebo controls. *Cephalalgia* (2005) 25:124–31. doi:10.1111/j.1468-2982.2004.00817.x
40. Macedo A, Banos JE, Farre M. Placebo response in the prophylaxis of migraine: a meta-analysis. *Eur J Pain* (2008) 12:68–75. doi:10.1016/j.ejpain.2007.03.002
41. Meissner K, Fassler M, Rucker G, Kleijnen J, Hrobjartsson A, Schneider A, et al. Differential effectiveness of placebo treatments: a systematic review of migraine prophylaxis. *JAMA Intern Med* (2013) 173:1941–51. doi:10.1001/jamainternmed.2013.10391
42. Cragg JJ, Warner FM, Finnerup NB, Jensen MP, Mercier C, Richards JS, et al. Meta-analysis of placebo responses in central neuropathic pain: impact of subject, study, and pain characteristics. *Pain* (2016) 157:530–40. doi:10.1097/j.pain.0000000000000431
43. Arakawa A, Kaneko M, Narukawa M. An investigation of factors contributing to higher levels of placebo response in clinical trials in neuropathic pain: a systematic review and meta-analysis. *Clin Drug Investig* (2015) 35:67–81. doi:10.1007/s40261-014-0259-1
44. Cepeda MS, Berlin JA, Gao CY, Wiegand F, Wada DR. Placebo response changes depending on the neuropathic pain syndrome: results of a systematic review and meta-analysis. *Pain Med* (2012) 13:575–95. doi:10.1111/j.1526-4637.2012.01340.x
45. Quessy SN, Rowbotham MC. Placebo response in neuropathic pain trials. *Pain* (2008) 138:479–83. doi:10.1016/j.pain.2008.06.024
46. Tuttle AH, Tohyama S, Ramsay T, Kimmelman J, Schweinhardt P, Bennett GJ, et al. Increasing placebo responses over time in U.S. clinical trials of neuropathic pain. *Pain* (2015) 156:2616–26. doi:10.1097/j.pain.0000000000000333
47. Madsen MV, Gotzsche PC, Hrobjartsson A. Acupuncture treatment for pain: systematic review of randomised clinical trials with acupuncture, placebo acupuncture, and no acupuncture groups. *BMJ* (2009) 338:a3115. doi:10.1136/bmj.a3115
48. Naleschinski D, Baron R. Complex regional pain syndrome type I: neuropathic or not? *Curr Pain Headache Rep* (2010) 14:196–202. doi:10.1007/s11916-010-0115-9
49. Amanzio M, Corazzini LL, Vase L, Benedetti F. A systematic review of adverse events in placebo groups of anti-migraine clinical trials. *Pain* (2009) 146:261–9. doi:10.1016/j.pain.2009.07.010
50. Zhang W, Robertson J, Jones AC, Dieppe PA, Doherty M. The placebo effect and its determinants in osteoarthritis: meta-analysis of randomised controlled trials. *Ann Rheum Dis* (2008) 67:1716–23. doi:10.1136/ard.2008.092015
51. Bannuru RR, Mcalindon TE, Sullivan MC, Wong JB, Kent DM, Schmid CH. Effectiveness and implications of alternative placebo treatments: a systematic review and network meta-analysis of osteoarthritis trials. *Ann Intern Med* (2015) 163:365–72. doi:10.7326/M15-0623
52. Kuten-Shorrer M, Kelley JM, Sonis ST, Treister NS. Placebo effect in burning mouth syndrome: a systematic review. *Oral Dis* (2014) 20:e1–6. doi:10.1111/odi.12192
53. Capurso G, Cocomello L, Benedetto U, Camma C, Delle Fave G. Meta-analysis: the placebo rate of abdominal pain remission in clinical trials of chronic pancreatitis. *Pancreas* (2012) 41:1125–31. doi:10.1097/MPA.0b013e318249ce93
54. Hrobjartsson A, Gotzsche PC. Is the placebo powerless? Update of a systematic review with 52 new randomized trials comparing placebo with no treatment. *J Intern Med* (2004) 256:91–100. doi:10.1111/j.1365-2796.2004.01355.x
55. Wager TD, Fields HL. Placebo analgesia. 6th ed. In: Mcmahon SB, Koltzenburg M, Tracey I, Turk D, editors. *Wall and Melzack's Textbook of Pain*. Philadelhia, PA: Elsevier Saunders (2013). p. 362–73.
56. Vase L, Skyt I, Hall KT. Placebo, nocebo, and neuropathic pain. *Pain* (2016) 157(Suppl 1):S98–105. doi:10.1097/j.pain.0000000000000445
57. Vase L, Petersen GL, Riley JL III, Price DD. Factors contributing to large analgesic effects in placebo mechanism studies conducted between 2002 and 2007. *Pain* (2009) 145:36–44. doi:10.1016/j.pain.2009.04.008
58. Bartolo M, Chio A, Ferrari S, Tassorelli C, Tamburin S, Avenali M, et al. Assessing and treating pain in movement disorders, amyotrophic lateral sclerosis, severe acquired brain injury, disorders of consciousness, dementia, oncology and neuroinfectivology. Evidence and recommendations from the Italian Consensus Conference on Pain in Neurorehabilitation. *Eur J Phys Rehabil Med* (2016) 52:841–54.
59. Castelnuovo G, Giusti EM, Manzoni GM, Saviola D, Gatti A, Gabrielli S, et al. Psychological considerations in the assessment and treatment of pain in neurorehabilitation and psychological factors predictive of therapeutic response: evidence and recommendations from the Italian consensus conference on pain in neurorehabilitation. *Front Psychol* (2016) 7:468. doi:10.3389/fpsyg.2016.00468
60. Castelnuovo G, Giusti EM, Manzoni GM, Saviola D, Gatti A, Gabrielli S, et al. Psychological treatments and psychotherapies in the neurorehabilitation of pain: evidences and recommendations from the Italian consensus conference on pain in neurorehabilitation. *Front Psychol* (2016) 7:115. doi:10.3389/fpsyg.2016.00115
61. Ferraro F, Jacopetti M, Spallone V, Padua L, Traballesi M, Brunelli S, et al. Diagnosis and treatment of pain in plexopathy, radiculopathy, peripheral neuropathy and phantom limb pain. Evidence and recommendations from the Italian Consensus Conference on Pain on Neurorehabilitation. *Eur J Phys Rehabil Med* (2016) 52:855–66.
62. Paolucci S, Martinuzzi A, Scivoletto G, Smania N, Solaro C, Aprile I, et al. Assessing and treating pain associated with stroke, multiple sclerosis, cerebral palsy, spinal cord injury and spasticity. Evidence and recommendations from the Italian Consensus Conference on Pain in Neurorehabilitation. *Eur J Phys Rehabil Med* (2016) 52:827–40.
63. Picelli A, Buzzi MG, Cisari C, Gandolfi M, Porru D, Bonadiman S, et al. Headache, low back pain, other nociceptive and mixed pain conditions in neurorehabilitation. Evidence and recommendations from the Italian Consensus Conference on Pain in Neurorehabilitation. *Eur J Phys Rehabil Med* (2016) 52:867–80.
64. Tamburin S, Lacerenza MR, Castelnuovo G, Agostini M, Paolucci S, Bartolo M, et al. Pharmacological and non-pharmacological strategies in the integrated treatment of pain in neurorehabilitation. Evidence and recommendations from the Italian Consensus Conference on Pain in Neurorehabilitation. *Eur J Phys Rehabil Med* (2016) 52:741–52.
65. Kaptchuk TJ, Friedlander E, Kelley JM, Sanchez MN, Kokkotou E, Singer JP, et al. Placebos without deception: a randomized controlled trial in irritable bowel syndrome. *PLoS One* (2010) 5:e15591. doi:10.1371/journal.pone.0015591
66. Kam-Hansen S, Jakubowski M, Kelley JM, Kirsch I, Hoaglin DC, Kaptchuk TJ, et al. Altered placebo and drug labeling changes the outcome of episodic migraine attacks. *Sci Transl Med* (2014) 6:218ra215. doi:10.1126/scitranslmed.3006175
67. Carvalho C, Caetano JM, Cunha L, Rebouta P, Kaptchuk TJ, Kirsch I. Open-label placebo treatment in chronic low back pain: a randomized controlled trial. *Pain* (2016) 157:2766–72. doi:10.1097/j.pain.0000000000000700
68. Charlesworth JEG, Petkovic G, Kelley JM, Hunter M, Onakpoya I, Roberts N, et al. Effects of placebos without deception compared with no treatment: a systematic review and meta-analysis. *J Evid Based Med* (2017) 10:97–107. doi:10.1111/jebm.12251
69. Locher C, Frey Nascimento A, Kirsch I, Kossowsky J, Meyer A, Gaab J. Is the rationale more important than deception? A randomized controlled trial of open-label placebo analgesia. *Pain* (2017) 158(12):2320–8. doi:10.1097/j.pain.0000000000001012
70. Mundt JM, Roditi D, Robinson ME. A comparison of deceptive and non-deceptive placebo analgesia: efficacy and ethical consequences. *Ann Behav Med* (2017) 51:307–15. doi:10.1007/s12160-016-9854-0
71. Martin AL, Katz J. Inclusion of authorized deception in the informed consent process does not affect the magnitude of the placebo effect for experimentally induced pain. *Pain* (2010) 149:208–15. doi:10.1016/j.pain.2009.12.004
72. Brody H. The lie that heals: the ethics of giving placebos. *Ann Intern Med* (1982) 97:112–8. doi:10.7326/0003-4819-97-1-112

73. Finniss DG, Kaptchuk TJ, Miller F, Benedetti F. Placebo effects: biological, clinical and ethical advances. *Lancet* (2010) 375:686–95. doi:10.1016/S0140-6736(09)61706-2
74. Enck P, Bingel U, Schedlowski M, Rief W. The placebo response in medicine: minimize, maximize or personalize? *Nat Rev Drug Discov* (2013) 12:191–204. doi:10.1038/nrd3923
75. Klinger R, Colloca L, Bingel U, Flor H. Placebo analgesia: clinical applications. *Pain* (2014) 155:1055–8. doi:10.1016/j.pain.2013.12.007
76. Bystad M, Bystad C, Wynn R. How can placebo effects best be applied in clinical practice? A narrative review. *Psychol Res Behav Manage* (2015) 8:41–5. doi:10.2147/PRBM.S75670
77. Doering BK, Rief W. Utilizing placebo mechanisms for dose reduction in pharmacotherapy. *Trends Pharmacol Sci* (2012) 33:165–72. doi:10.1016/j.tips.2011.12.001
78. Barrett B, Muller D, Rakel D, Rabago D, Marchand L, Scheder JC. Placebo, meaning, and health. *Perspect Biol Med* (2006) 49:178–98. doi:10.1353/pbm.2006.0019

15

Tablet App Based Dexterity Training in Multiple Sclerosis (TAD-MS)

Judith J. W. van Beek [1,2]*, *Erwin E. H. van Wegen* [3], *Cleo D. Bol* [1], *Marc B. Rietberg* [3], *Christian P. Kamm* [1,4] *and Tim Vanbellingen* [1,2]*

[1] Neurocenter, Lucerne Cantonal Hospital, Lucerne, Switzerland, [2] Gerontechnology and Rehabilitation Group, University of Bern, Bern, Switzerland, [3] Department of Rehabilitation Medicine, Amsterdam Movement Sciences, MS Center Amsterdam, Amsterdam University Medical Center VUmc, Amsterdam, Netherlands, [4] Department of Neurology, Inselspital University Hospital Bern, University of Bern, Bern, Switzerland

***Correspondence:**
Judith J. W. van Beek
judith.vanbeek@luks.ch
Tim Vanbellingen
tim.vanbellingen@luks.ch;
tim.vanbellingen@artorg.unibe.ch

Introduction: Patients with Multiple Sclerosis exhibit disturbed dexterity, leading to difficulties in fine motor skills such as buttoning a T-shirt or hand-writing. Consequently, activities of daily living and quality of life are affected. The aim of the present study is to investigate the effectiveness of a tablet app-based home-based training intervention to improve dexterity in patients with Multiple Sclerosis.

Methods: An observer-blinded randomized controlled trial will be performed. Seventy patients with Multiple Sclerosis with self-reported difficulties in dexterity while executing activities of daily living will be recruited. After baseline assessment, participants are randomized to either an intervention group (n = 35) or control group (n = 35) by a computerized procedure. Blinded assessments will be done at baseline, post-intervention (after 4 weeks) and 12 weeks follow-up. The home-based intervention consists of a 4-week tablet app-based dexterity program. The app contains six dexterity games in which finger coordination, tapping, pinch grip is required. The control group will receive a Thera-band training program focused on strengthening the upper limb. The primary outcome is the Arm function of Multiple Sclerosis Questionnaire, a measure of patient-reported activities of daily living related dexterity. Secondary outcomes are dexterous function, hand strength, and quality of life.

Discussion: This study will evaluate the effects of tablet app-based training for dexterity in patients with Multiple Sclerosis. We hypothesize that a challenging app-based dexterity program will improve dexterity both in the short term and the long-term. The improved finger and hand functions are expected to generalize to improved activities of daily living and quality of life.

Keywords: randomized controlled trial, app-based training, dexterity, multiple sclerosis, arm function in multiple sclerosis questionnaire

BACKGROUND

Multiple sclerosis (MS) is a chronic inflammatory disease of the central nervous system and the most common cause of non-traumatic disability in young adults (1–3). It is a heterogeneous disease, which is associated with long-term disability, leading to reduced Health related Quality of Life (HrQoL). While disease-modifying pharmacological therapies can decrease disease activity and progression, and symptomatic pharmacological treatments reduce complaints to a certain extent (3), patients with MS (PwMS) often still suffer from various neurological deficits during the course of their disease (1). Consequently, specific non-pharmacological rehabilitation is needed in order to further reduce disability and improve HrQoL (2, 4, 5). Evidence is accumulating that targeted rehabilitation drives neuroplasticity in MS (6).

Impaired dexterity is a frequently observed impairment, affecting up to 76% of PwMS (7). The different neurological deficits caused by MS, such as ataxia, spasticity, sensory-motor deficits, and apraxia may by themselves or in combination, impair dexterity (8, 9). Anatomically, it has been shown by Bonzano et al. (10) that reduced microstructural integrity of the corpus callosum, caused by the MS pathology, is associated with deficits in bimanual finger movements, therefore possibly explaining impaired dexterity (10). Consequently, PwMS report impairments in the performance of several activities of daily living (ADL), such as grooming, cooking, which may have a huge impact on the self-reported general health perception (11). Sometimes these problems are even associated with loss of work, and lack of social integration (12). Two systematic reviews by Lamers et al. highlighted the importance of a thorough standardized assessment and treatment of upper limb dysfunction in MS, more specifically impaired dexterity (4, 13). In a previous randomized controlled trial (RCT) we showed that a home-based unsupervised dexterity program can improve dexterity in MS (14). The program however did not allow for online monitoring of the patient's performance, meaning that no direct feedback could be given by the therapist, possibly explaining the lack of long term efficacy.

To obtain an optimal training effect, work load must be "shaped" (adjusting the task difficulty to the subjects' performance), and the intensiveness of training should be progressive and challenging. Based on these motor learning principles, Bonzano et al. (15) found in a small pilot RCT that task-oriented upper limb rehabilitation in PwMS had a positive impact on white matter architecture. They demonstrated that connection fibers in the corpus callosum and corticospinal fibers bundles, which are in general affected by the disease, were preserved through active motor training (15). This suggests that upper limb rehabilitation may promote neuroplasticity in MS. Furthermore, the involved tasks should also stimulate subjects' motivation, should be fun, and sustain arousal (16).

With recent technological innovations, such as the development of applications (apps) for mobile phones and/or tablets there are new possible treatment options. The advantages of such apps, certainly build on the premise that these are often mentally stimulating, are game-based, attractive, fun, all aspects which are fundamental to possibly stimulate neuroplasticity in MS. Training with mobile apps may also allow flexible training at home, so PwMS can exercise whenever they want at a convenient time of the day. Recently such an app, called COGNI-TRAck, was developed to train cognition in MS, which was found to be feasible, highly motivating and well-accepted among PwMS (17). A follow-up pilot RCT evaluated the effectiveness of the COGNI-TRAck and demonstrated improved cognitive function, more specifically working memory (18). With respect to dexterity, a first new app has been developed called "Finger Zirkus©," by a team of experts including an occupational therapist (AO, see for acknowledgments), graphic designer, and IT expert. The app is already available to be downloaded from Google Play store or Apple Store (see for more details: www.fingers-in-motion.de). The app specifically contains six dexterous exercises, which are explained more in the methods. The exercises are goal oriented, repetitive, give direct feedback and most importantly are fun to to. To ensure constant improvement, the speed and difficulty of the exercises are progressively adapted to the individuals' performance limit. To our knowledge the efficacy of this tablet app-based training has not been investigated in MS.

The aim of the present study will therefore be to investigate the effectiveness of a tablet app-based dexterity home-based intervention in MS (TAD-MS). The short and long-term benefits of this training program will be compared with a Thera-band® training program. For these purposes, an observer-blinded proof-of-concept RCT will be performed. We hypothesize that TAD-MS will improve dexterity, leading to improved ADL, and HrQoL in PwMS.

METHODS AND DESIGN

Trial Design

An observer-blinded RCT will be performed with random allocation of intervention, with pre- (baseline) and post-intervention measurements, at 4 weeks immediately after intervention and a follow-up 12 weeks later, after finishing the training. The study flow chart is shown in see **Figure 1**. Ethical approval has been given by the Ethics committee of the State of Luzern (EKNZ/2017-00768), Switzerland. Trial registration is Clinicaltrials.gov NCT03369470 and SNCTP clinical trials registry SNCTP000002451. The study will be performed according to the CONSORT (Consolidated Standards of Reporting Trials) statement, http://www.consort-statement.org/.

Participants

We aim to recruit 70 PwMS. The inclusion criteria are as follows: males and females, age 18–75, diagnosis of MS (primary or secondary progressive, relapsing-remitting) following the

Abbreviations: Abbreviations: MS, Multiple Sclerosis; ADL, Activities of daily living; RCT, Randomized controlled trial; AMSQ, Arm Function in Multiple Sclerosis Questionnaire; MSIS-29, Multiple Sclerosis Impact Scale 29; 9-HPT, Nine-hole peg test; CR, Coin rotation; PT, Physical therapy; HrQoL, Health related Quality of life; CI, confidence interval; ITT, Intention to treat CRF, Case Report Form; PwMS, Patients with Multiple Sclerosis.

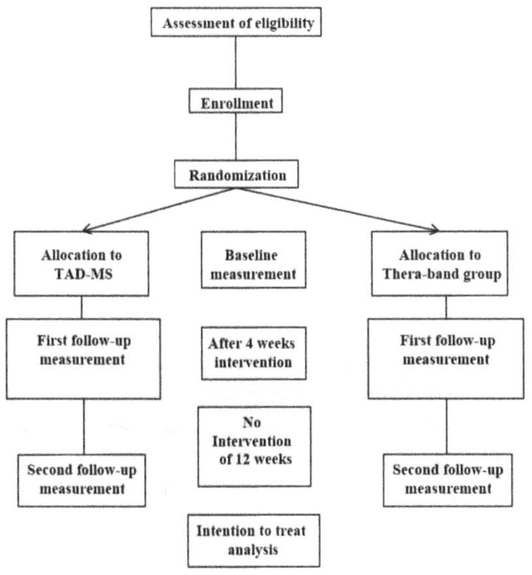

FIGURE 1 | Study flow chart.

revised McDonald criteria (19). In addition, patients must report difficulties in dexterity that impact ADL and/or have a pathological Nine Hole Peg Test (9HPT) according to cut-off values (20). The exclusion criteria will be other conditions that may limit hand function training or, impaired cognitive functioning (Mini Mental Status Examination score <24).

Sample Size Calculation

The significance level alpha is defined two-tailed at *p*-value of 0.05 for detecting 20% difference between groups on the Arm Function in Multiple Sclerosis Questionnaire (AMSQ) in favor of the App-based dexterity group. Based on mean expected baseline values of 50.2 ±14.0 (pooled mean and standard deviations values) of the whole group, a 20% difference would reflect a 10-point improvement. Following Cohen's guidelines (21), the probability to prevent type II error is set at 0.20 assuming a 1-beta value of 0.80. The power analysis (clinical superiority trial), with the above-mentioned parameters, resulted in a total sample size of 62 persons, i.e., 31 people per group. Considering a maximal drop-out rate of 10% we aim to recruit 70 patients in total.

Recruitment

Potential participants will be recruited from the MS center, Luzerner Kantonsspital, Luzern. In addition, Swiss Multiple Sclerosis Society, which is a non-profit patient organization, will be contacted and asked to inform their members about the ongoing study. Prior to study participation, written informed consent will be obtained from all patients according to the latest Declaration of Helsinki.

Randomization and Blinding

An independent biostatistician (DC, see acknowledgments) will execute a balanced (1:1 ratio) group allocation using a computerized randomization protocol. Two clinicians (JvB, CB), with experience in the field of MS rehabilitation, will be responsible for the assessments and instruction of both interventions. All outcome measures (baseline, post-intervention and follow-up measures) will be videotaped and rated by an independent rater blinded to randomization procedure and group allocation.

Treatment Interventions

Two home-based treatment conditions are investigated in this study: the experimental condition (TAD-MS) and the control condition (Thera-band®). Patients will receive instructions for their home-based training programs by a trained clinician (JvB, CB). Both groups will train 5 days per week (approximately 30 min per day) for 4 weeks. All exercises will be performed with both hands. Besides therapist instructions, for each exercise the app contains a demonstration video and a text explaining how to perform the exercises. The app is linked with a website in which a clinician can log in and track the patient's performance, so compliance to the protocol can be monitored. Patients exercising with Thera-band® receive a booklet explaining all exercises with pictures and text instructions. This booklet also contains a diary to document if an exercise is performed and, if applicable, the time needed to accomplish the exercise.

Tablet App-Based Dexterity Intervention (TAD-MS)

PwMS allocated to the TAD-MS will receive a tablet with the app on it. The app contains six different exercises. During a first training session PwMS receive instructions about the log-in procedure and functionality of the web-interface and exercise app. The therapist can pre-select the exercises for the patient. For more information about TAD-MS a step by step manual is presented in **Supplementary File 1**.

Control Intervention

PwMS allocated to the control group will receive Thera-band-exercises on paper [see (14)]. PwMS will perform seven upper extremity strength-training exercises using a Thera-band®, which are illustrated in detail in **Supplementary File 2**. As TAD-MS, both arms will be trained equally long.

Outcome Measures

Primary End Point

The AMSQ measures manual dexterity in MS patients and shows good validity, test-retest reliability and inter-observer reliability (22). Recently, a German version of the AMSQ was validated (23). It contains 31 questions on a unidimensional scale that are formulated as "during the past 2 weeks, to what extent has MS limited your ability to ...?." Response categories are "not at all," "a little," "moderately," "quite a lot," "extremely," and "no longer able to." One final sum score is obtained ranging from 0 to 100 with higher scores indicating more dexterous difficulties.

Secondary End Points

The 9HPT is a reliable, valid and sensitive test to quantify impaired dexterity, and has been validated in patients with MS (13). While seated at a table, patients have to put nine pegs out of a shallow container into nine holes one at a time and then remove them again one at a time back into the shallow container. The time to perform the task is measured. Age and gender-dependent normal values are available (20).

The Coin rotation Task (CRT) is a sensitive measure to quantify fine coordinated finger movements in MS (9). Participants have to rotate a 20 swiss rappen coin (corresponding to a dime), as quickly as possible between their thumb, index and middle finger. The time to perform 20 half turns is measured twice on both hands and mean values are taken for each hand. We found values of 18.75 s for the dominant and 19.25 s for the non-dominant hand to be optimal cut-offs that are highly sensitive and specific for detecting impaired dexterity (9).

The hand-held JAMAR dynamometer (Sammons Preston Rolyan, 1000 Remington Blvd, Bolingbrook, IL, 60440) is a reliable and valid test to measure isometric grip strength in healthy subjects and PwMS (13, 24). Testing will be performed in a seated position with 90° flexion of the elbow next to the body. Mean values (kilograms force) of three maximum voluntary grip strength movements are taken for each hand.

The Multiple Sclerosis Impact Scale 29 (MSIS-29) is a HrQoL questionnaire assessing the impact of MS on physical and psychological functions (25, 26). It is formed by 29 items: 20 about physical activity and ADL and 9 on psychological status of the person. Each item can be scored with a value from 0 to 5; total score is given by the sum of all the items and is then transformed to a range from 0 to 100. A higher value corresponds to a worse perception of subject's HrQoL.

Statistical Analysis

Descriptive statistics will be used to present baseline characteristics and results of outcome measurements. The main analysis will be an analysis of covariance (ANCOVA) with between-group factor Intervention (2 levels) and within group factor Time (3 levels). Baseline scores will be used as covariates. Two-sided 95% confidence intervals (CI) will also be calculated, as well as effect size (Cohen's d). *Post-hoc* Tukey test will be used to test for pairwise comparisons. The Benjamini–Hochberg procedure will be applied to control the false discovery rate (27). According to the Intention to treat (ITT) principle every randomized PwMS, including the drop-outs, will be included for final evaluation. Multiple imputation methods will be used to handle missing data, caused by random drop outs. For all analyses the level of significance will be set at $p < 0.05$. Statistical analyses will be performed using PASW for Windows (version 23.0; SPSS, Inc. Chicago, IL).

Availability of Data and Materials

In accordance with Good Clinical Practice Guidelines members of the ethics committees will be granted access to the original clinical data (coded) for audits or inspections, via the principal investigator. Throughout the entire study, strict confidentiality is ensured. All data will be coded and archived at the Luzerner Kantonsspital throughout the whole study period and archived for 15 years. All measurements (AMSQ, 9HPT, CRT, Jamar, MSIS-29), which are specifically related to the study design, will be entered directly into electronic Case Report Forms (eCRF).

DISCUSSION

Impaired dexterity is a frequently reported problem in MS, leading to reduced HrQoL (2, 4, 7). However, evidence-based upper limb therapies are still scarce mainly due to lack of methodologically well-conducted trials in this neglected field (4). New technology such as tablet app-based training, has been shown to improve working memory in MS (18).

The aim of the present proof-of-concept RCT is to investigate the effectiveness of a tablet app-based dexterity training at home, compared with a non-dexterity focused Thera-band program. The exercises within the TAD-MS intervention focus on different components of dexterity such as pinch grip, coordinated finger movements, consequently being highly specific to improve dexterity. In addition, all exercises are game-based and designed to be challenging and to trigger motivation. During the performance of the dexterity exercises the app provides direct feedback of performance which can lead to immediate perception of error and correction of movement, increasing the effectiveness of progressive motor learning training (28, 29). Instead, the Thera-band® program includes non-specific upper limb and hand strength exercises.

The total dosage of the TAD-MS intervention is 600 min of dexterity training (30 min five times a week, 4 weeks), representing a trade-off between feasibility and adequate dosage. Although no studies have investigated tablet-app based dexterity training in MS, a previous home-based sensory re-education training (3 weeks, five times a week 15 min, 300 min total training) induced significant in manual dexterity (30), with stronger effect size when compared with another dexterity interventions (4) Additionally, another home-based dexterity program achieved adequate effect sizes with a 4-week program and 600 min of dexterity training (14). Therefore, the choice of the dosage of our TAD-MS seems appropriate to significantly improve dexterity. The TAD-MS has the potential to be easily implemented in the daily routine of PwMS, since no extensive instruction is needed and the program is not time consuming. Furthermore, TAD-MS is efficient in terms of staff resources as patients can train independently at home without continuous guidance from a therapist. Such cost-effectiveness should be investigated in future studies.

In sum, we expect that the presented tablet app-based program, TAD-MS, through provision of challenging, stimulating dexterity training in the patients' home-environment will be effective in PwMS.

DISSEMINATION

When protocol amendments are needed (e.g., to include another participating center), ethical approval will be obtained first. After having obtained this approval, relevant adaptations will be made in the relevant clinical trial registry databases.

After completing recruitment, according to the inclusion and exclusion criteria, statistical analyses are planned. When completed, submission to a peer-reviewed journal is planned. In addition, results will be published in patient and healthcare professional magazines and will be presented at national and international congresses.

AUTHOR CONTRIBUTIONS

JvB physical therapist, junior researcher and movement scientist, responsible for patient recruitment, provides data collection, manuscript writing. EvW senior researcher and movement scientist, gave critical review of concept and design of the study, and critically revised the manuscript. CB research assistant, responsible for patient recruitment, provides data collection, she critically revised the manuscript. MR senior researcher and movement scientist, gave critical review of concept and design of the study, and critically revised the manuscript. CK neurologist, provided concept and design of the study and critically revised the manuscript. TV is a senior researcher and principal investigator, obtained funding, conceived the idea for the present study, overall project coordination, manuscript writing. All authors contributed to the design of the interventions and outcome measures. All authors assisted in editing and reviewing the submitted manuscript. They all read and approved the final form.

REFERENCES

1. Kamm CP, Uitdehaag BM, Polman CH. multiple sclerosis: current knowledge and future outlook. *Eur Neurol.* (2014) 72:132–41. doi: 10.1159/000360528
2. Vanbellingen T, Kamm CP. Neurorehabilitation topics in patients with multiple sclerosis: from outcome measurements to rehabilitation interventions. *Semin Neurol.* (2016) 36:196–202. doi: 10.1055/s-0036-1579694
3. Thompson AJ, Baranzini SE, Geurts J, Hemmer B, Ciccarelli O. Multiple sclerosis *Lancet* (2018) 21:1622–36. doi: 10.1016/S0140-6736(18)30481-1
4. Lamers I, Maris A, Severijns D, Dielkens W, Geurts S, Van Wijmeersch B, et al. Limb rehabilitation in people with multiple sclerosis: a systematic review. *Neurorehabil Neural Repair.* (2016) 30:773–93. doi: 10.1177/1545968315624785
5. Boesen F, Nørgaard M, Trénel P, Rasmussen PV, Petersen T, Løvendahl B, et al. Longer term effectiveness of inpatient multidisciplinary rehabilitation on health-related quality of life in MS patients: a pragmatic randomized controlled trial - The Danish MS hospitals rehabilitation study. *Mult Scler.* (2018) 24:340–9. doi: 10.1177/1352458517735188
6. Straudi S, Basaglia N. Neuroplasticity-based technologies and interventions for restoring motor functions in multiple sclerosis. *Adv Exp Med Biol.* (2017) 958:171–85. doi: 10.1007/978-3-319-47861-6_11
7. Johansson S, Ytterberg C, Claesson IM, Lindberg J, Hillert J, Andersson M, et al. High concurrent presence of disability in multiple sclerosis. Associations with perceived health. *J Neurol.* (2007) 254:767–73. doi: 10.1007/s00415-006-0431-5
8. Kamm CP, Heldner MR, Vanbellingen T, Mattle HP, Müri R, Bohlhalter S. Limb apraxia in multiple sclerosis: Prevalence and impact on manual dexterity and activities of daily living. *Arch Phys Med Rehab.* (2012) 93:1081–5. doi: 10.1016/j.apmr.2012.01.008
9. Heldner MR, Vanbellingen T, Bohlhalter S, Mattle HP, Müri RM, Kamm CP. The coin rotation task: a valid test for manual dexterity in multiple sclerosis. *Phys Ther.* (2014) 94:1644–51. doi: 10.2522/ptj.20130252
10. Bonzano L, Tacchino A, Roccatagliata L, Abbruzzese G, Mancardi GL, Bove M. Callosal contributions to simultaneous bimanual finger movements. *J Neurosci.* (2008) 28:3227–33. doi: 10.1523/JNEUROSCI.4076-07.2008
11. Mansson E, Lexell J. Performance of activities of daily living in multiple sclerosis. *Disabil Rehabil.* (2004) 26:576–85. doi: 10.1080/09638280410001684587
12. Chruzander C, Johansson S, Gottberg K, Einarsson U, Fredrikson S, Holmqvist LW, et al. A 10-year follow-up of a population-based study of people with multiple sclerosis in Stockholm, Sweden: Changes in disability and the value of different factors in predicting disability and mortality *J Neurol Sci.* (2013) 332:121–7. doi: 10.1016/j.jns.2013.07.003
13. Lamers I, Kelchtermans S, Baert I, Feys P. Upper limb assessment in multiple sclerosis: a systematic review of outcome measures and their psychometric properties. *Arch Phys Med Rehabil.* (2014) 95:1184–200. doi: 10.1016/j.apmr.2014.02.023
14. Kamm CP, Mattle HP, Müri RM, Heldner MR, Blatter V, Bartlome S, et al. Home-based training to improve manual dexterity in patients with multiple sclerosis: a randomized controlled trial. *Mult Scler.* (2015) 21:1546–56. doi: 10.1177/1352458514565959

13. Lamers I, Kelchtermans S, Baert I, Feys P. Upper limb assessment in multiple sclerosis: a systematic review of outcome measures and their psychometric properties. *Arch Phys Med Rehabil.* (2014) 95:1184–200. doi: 10.1016/j.apmr.2014.02.023
14. Kamm CP, Mattle HP, Müri RM, Heldner MR, Blatter V, Bartlome S, et al. Home-based training to improve manual dexterity in patients with multiple sclerosis: a randomized controlled trial. *Mult Scler.* (2015) 21:1546–56. doi: 10.1177/1352458514565959

15. Bonzano L, Tacchino A, Brichetto G, Roccatagliata L, Dessypris A, Dessypris A, et al. Upper limb motor rehabilitation impacts white matter microstructure in multiple sclerosis. *Neuroimage* (2014) 90:107–16. doi: 10.1016/j.neuroimage.2013.12.025
16. Fasczewski KS, Gill DL. A model of motivation for physical activity in individuals diagnosed with multiple sclerosis. *Disabil Rehabil.* (2018) 10:1–8. doi: 10.1080/09638288.2018.1459883
17. Tacchino A, Pedullà L, Bonzano L, Vassallo C, Battaglia MA, Mancardi G, et al. A new app for At-home cognitive training: description and pilot testing on patients with multiple sclerosis. *JMIR Mhealth Uhealth.* (2015) 31:e85. doi: 10.2196/mhealth.4269
18. Pedullà L, Brichetto G, Tacchino A, Vassallo C, Zaratin P, Battaglia MA, et al. Adaptive vs. non-adaptive cognitive training by means of a personalized App: a randomized trial in people with multiple sclerosis. *J Neuroeng Rehabil.* (2016) 13:88. doi: 10.1186/s12984-016-0193-y
19. Thompson AJ, Banwell BL, Barkhof F, Carroll WM, Coetzee T, Comi G, et al. Diagnosis of multiple sclerosis: 2017 revisions of the McDonald criteria. *Lancet Neurol.* (2018) 17:162–73. doi: 10.1016/S1474-4422(17)30470-2
20. Mathiowetz V, Weber K, Kashman N, Volland G. Adult norms for the nine-hole peg test of finger dexterity. *Occ Ther J Res.* (1985) 5:24–38. doi: 10.1177/153944928500500102
21. Cohen J. A power primer. *Psychol Bull.* (1992) 112:155–9. doi: 10.1037/0033-2909.112.1.155
22. Mokkink LB, Knol DL, Van der Linden FH, Sonder JM, D'hooghe M, Uitdehaag BM. The Arm Function in Multiple Sclerosis Questionnaire (AMSQ): development and validation of a new tool using IRT methods. *Disabil Rehabil.* (2015) 26:1–7. doi: 10.3109/09638288.2015.10 27005
23. Steinheimer S, Wendel M, Vanbellingen T, Westers LT, Hodak J, Blatter V, et al. The Arm Function in Multiple Sclerosis Questionnaire was successfully translated to German. *J Hand Ther.* (2018) 31:137–40.e1. doi: 10.1016/j.jht.2017.09.010
24. Paltamaa J, West H, Sarasoja T, Wikström J, Mälkiä E. Reliability of physical functioning measures in ambulatory subjects with MS. *Physiother Res Int.* (2005) 10:93–109. doi: 10.1002/pri.30
25. Hobart JC, Riazi A, Lamping DL, Fitzpatrick R, Thompson AJ. How responsive is the multiple sclerosis impact scale (MSIS-29)? A comparison with some other self report scales. *J Neurol Neurosurg Psychiatry* (2005) 76:1539–43. doi: 10.1136/jnnp.2005.064584
26. Hobart J, Lamping D, Fitzpatrick R, Riazi A, Thompson A. The multiple sclerosis impact scale (MSIS-29): a new patient-based outcome measure. *Brain* (2001). 124(Pt 5):962–73. doi: 10.1093/brain/124.5.962
27. Benjamini Y, Hochberg Y. Controlling the false discovery rate: a practical and powerful approach to multiple testing. *J R Stat Soc.* (1995) 57: 289–300.

16

Diffusion Tensor Tractography Studies on Injured Anterior Cingulum Recovery Mechanisms

*Sung Ho Jang and Jeong Pyo Seo**

Department of Physical Medicine and Rehabilitation, College of Medicine, Yeungnam University, Daegu, South Korea

***Correspondence:**
Jeong Pyo Seo
raphael0905@hanmail.net

The cingulum, a major structure in the limbic system, contains the medial cholinergic pathway, which originates from the basalis nucleus of Meynert (Ch 4) in the basal forebrain. The cingulum is involved in various cognitive functions, including memory, attention, learning, motivation, emotion, and pain perception. In this mini-review, 10 studies reporting on recovery mechanisms of injured cinguli in patients with brain injury were reviewed. The recovery mechanisms of the injured anterior cinguli reported in those 10 studies are classified as follows: Mechanism 1, recovery via the normal pathway of the cingulum between the injured cingulum and Ch 4; mechanism 2, recovery through the neural tract between the injured cingulum and the brainstem cholinergic nuclei; mechanism 3, recovery via the lateral cholinergic pathway between the injured cingulum and the white matter of the temporo-occipital lobes; mechanism 4, recovery through the neural tract between the contralesional basal forebrain and the ipsilesional basal forebrain via the genu of the corpus callosum; and mechanism 5, recovery through the neural tract between the injured cingulum and Ch 4 via an aberrant pathway. Elucidation of the recovery mechanisms of injured anterior cinguli might be useful for neurorehabilitation of patients with anterior cingulum injuries. Diffusion tensor tractography appears to be useful in the detection of recovery mechanisms of injured anterior cinguli in patients with brain injury. However, studies on cingulum injury recovery mechanisms are still in the early stages because most of the above studies are case reports confined to a few brain pathologies. Therefore, further studies involving large numbers of subjects with various brain pathologies should be encouraged. In addition, studies on the influencing factors and clinical outcomes associated with each recovery mechanism are warranted.

Keywords: diffusion tensor imaging, diffusion tensor tractography, cingulum, recovery mechanism, brain injury

INTRODUCTION

There are several cholinergic nuclei in the human brain (1–4). Four cholinergic nuclei are located in the basal forebrain and septal region (the medial septal nucleus [Ch 1], the vertical nucleus of the diagonal band [Ch 2], the horizontal limb of the diagonal band [Ch 3], and the nucleus basalis of Meynert [Ch 4]), three in the brainstem (the pedunculopontine nucleus [Ch 5], the laterodorsal tegmental nucleus [Ch 6], and the parabigeminal nucleus [Ch 8]), and one in the thalamus (the medial habenular nucleus [Ch 7]) (2, 3). Ch 4 provides the major cholinergic projections to the cerebral cortex and hippocampus, and the pontine cholinergic system acts mainly through thalamic intralaminar nuclei and provides only minor innervation of the cortex (5, 6). In addition, cholinergic neurons (Ch 1 and Ch 2) in the medial septum innervate mostly the hippocampus, while those of the vertical diagonal band (Ch 3) project to the anterior cingulate cortex (5, 6). As a result, the brain cholinergic system has roles in cortical activity, the sleep-wake cycle, modulating cognitive function, and cortical plasticity, and pathology of the brain cholinergic system can lead to cognitive impairment, age-related cognitive decline, and Alzheimer's disease (4, 7–9). Thus, the cholinergic system of the human brain is important in cognition, especially memory (10).

The cholinergic system of the cerebral cortex is innervated by the medial and lateral cholinergic pathways which mainly originate from Ch 4 (1). After originating from Ch 4, the medial cholinergic pathway joins the white matter of the gyrus rectus and then curves around the rostrum of the corpus callosum to enter the cingulum (1). It supplies cholinergic innervation to the parolfactory, cingulate, paracingulate, and retrosplenial cortices. The lateral cholinergic pathway innervates the remaining portion of the fronto-parieto-temporal cortex (1). As a result, the cingulum is involved in various cognitive functions, especially memory, and an injury of the cingulum could interfere with the corticopetal flow of cholinergic pathways to the above cortical areas (1, 11, 12).

Elucidation of recovery mechanisms following brain injury is important in neurorehabilitation because such information provides a scientific basis for developing neurorehabilitation strategies and predicting prognosis. The recovery mechanisms of the injured brain are based on the following classical concepts for brain plasticity: (1) unmasking of reserve axons and synapses for particular functions following injury of the ordinarily dominant system, and (2) collateral sprouting from an intact neuron to a denervated region (13–15). Recently, the recovery mechanisms of an injured neural tract have been elucidated in more detail; for example, the recovery mechanisms of the corticospinal tract, which have been actively researched, include recoveries through restoration of a normal pathway, perilesional reorganization, and recovery via a collateral pathway or transcallosal or transpontine pathways (16–19). However, relatively little has been reported about the recovery mechanisms of other neural tracts.

Research on the recovery mechanisms of injured cinguli has been limited because identification of the cingulum by using conventional brain magnetic resonance imaging has been impossible because it cannot discern the cingulum from other adjacent structures (20). However, the recently introduced diffusion tensor tractography (DTT) method, which is a derivation of diffusion tensor imaging (DTI), has enabled three-dimensional reconstruction and estimation of the cingulum (21). Several studies have used DTT to describe the recovery mechanisms of injured anterior cinguli in patients with brain injury (20, 22–30).

In this mini-review, DTT studies reporting on injured cingulum recovery mechanisms in patients with brain injury are reviewed. Relevant studies in the period 1990 to 2018 were identified by searching within the PubMed, Google Scholar, and MEDLINE electronic databases. The following keywords/abbreviations were used: DTI, DTT, cingulum, anterior cingulum, memory, traumatic brain injury (TBI), stroke, intracerebral hemorrhage (ICH), cerebral infarct, hypoxic-ischemic brain injury (HI-BI), brain tumor, brain injury, brain plasticity, and recovery mechanism. This review was limited to studies of humans with brain injury. We selected the relevant studies according to the flow diagram presented in **Figure 1**. As a result, ten studies were selected and reviewed (20, 22–30).

RECOVERY MECHANISMS OF AN INJURED ANTERIOR CINGULUM

The recovery mechanisms of the injured anterior cinguli reported in the ten reviewed studies are classified as follows: Mechanism 1, recovery via the normal pathway of the cingulum between an injured cingulum and Ch 4; mechanism 2, recovery through the neural tract between the injured cingulum and the brainstem cholinergic nuclei; mechanism 3, recovery through the lateral cholinergic pathway between the injured cingulum and the white matter of the temporo-occipital lobes; mechanism 4, recovery through the neural tract between the contralesional basal forebrain and the ipsilesional basal forebrain via the genu of the corpus callosum; and mechanism 5, recovery through the neural tract between the injured cingulum and Ch 4 via an aberrant pathway (**Figure 2**, **Table 1**) (20, 22–30).

Mechanism 1: Recovery via the Normal Pathway of the Cingulum

In 2013, Jang and Seo reported on neural recovery of an injured cingulum in a patient who had HI-BI and a subarachnoid hemorrhage (SAH) that was observed on follow-up DTT (20). The patient showed severe cognitive impairment; therefore, the authors were unable to perform an evaluation using

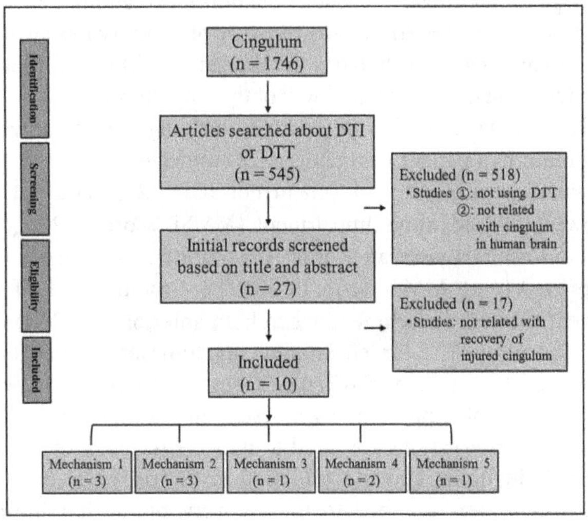

FIGURE 1 | Flow diagram of the approach used to select the studies to be reviewed.

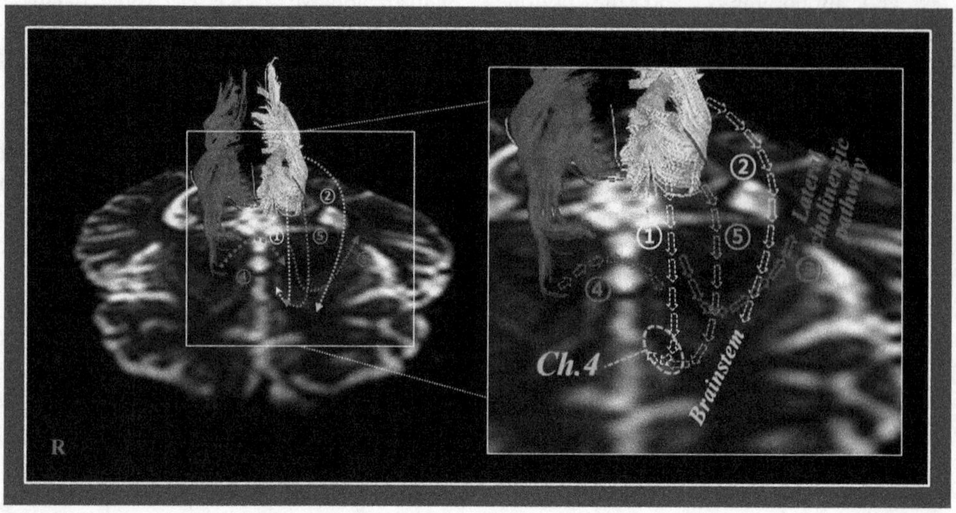

FIGURE 2 | Previously reported recovery mechanisms associated with injured anterior cinguli. ① Mechanism 1: recovery via the normal pathway of the cingulum between an injured cingulum and the basalis nucleus of Meynert (Ch 4). ② Mechanism 2: recovery through a neural tract between an injured cingulum and brainstem cholinergic nuclei. ③ Mechanism 3: recovery through a lateral cholinergic pathway between an injured cingulum and the white matter of the temporo-occipital lobes. ④ Mechanism 4: recovery through a neural tract between the contralesional basal forebrain and the ipsilesional basal forebrain via the genu of the corpus callosum. ⑤ Mechanism 5: recovery through a neural tract between an injured cingulum and Ch 4 via an aberrant pathway.

the Mini-Mental State Examination (MMSE: full score=30) or other cognitive function tests (31). At 14 months after onset, the patient's cognition had improved and she scored 24 on the MMSE. Other cognitive function test results were as follows: Total intelligence quotient (IQ) on the Wechsler adult intelligence scale (WAIS: 81); Memory assessment scale (MAS) scores: short-term memory, 88 (21%ile); verbal memory, 62 (1%ile); visual memory, 68 (2%ile); and global memory, 56 (<1%ile) (32, 33). On DTT at 7 days after brain injury, discontinuations of both cinguli anterior to the genu of the corpus callosum were observed. However, on 14-month follow-up DTT, the right cingulum was observed to have elongated to the right basal forebrain through the normal cingulum pathway. The authors suggested that the recovery of memory impairment in this patient was attributed to the elongation of the right injured cingulum via the normal pathway of the cingulum (20).

In 2016, Jang and Kwon reported on changes to the anterior cingulum in a patient who underwent craniectomy and removal of meningioma and had concurrent ICH (27). The patient showed mild cognitive impairment (MMSE score = 22) (31). By contrast, at 4 years after onset, his cognitive impairment had improved to an MMSE score of 28. The 4-month DTT of the patient showed discontinuations in both anterior cinguli. On 4-year follow-up DTT, the left anterior cingulum was shown to have elongated to the basal forebrain through the normal pathway of the anterior cingulum. As a result, the authors concluded that their observations appeared to indicate recovery of the left injured cingulum, and the reduction in the patient's cognitive impairment was ascribed to the recovery of the left injured cingulum (27).

In 2018, Jang et al. reported on a patient with mild TBI who, on follow-up DTT, showed recovery of an injured cingulum concurrent with improvement of short-term memory (29). The patient showed mild memory impairment at 3 months after onset: MAS scores: global memory, 95 (37%ile); short-term memory, 75 (5%ile); verbal memory, 80 (9%ile); and visual memory, 112 (79%ile) (33). By contrast, 2 years after onset, his mild memory impairment had reduced and his memory scores indicated a normal state: MAS scores: global memory, 104 (61%ile); short-term memory, 95 (37%ile); verbal memory, 101 (53%ile); and visual memory, 106 (66%ile) (33). On 3-month DTT, discontinuation of the right anterior cingulum over the genu of the corpus callosum was observed; however, on 2-year DTT, the discontinued right anterior cingulum was observed to have elongated to the right basal forebrain. As a result, the authors concluded that elongation to the right basal forebrain of the discontinued anterior cingulum appeared to be the recovery mechanism associated with the injured cingulum following a mild TBI (29).

Mechanism 2: Recovery Through the Neural Tract Between an Injured Cingulum and the Brainstem Cholinergic Nuclei

In 2012, Yeo et al. presented a case report on a patient who had experienced a traffic accident and underwent conservative management for SAH in the right frontal and left Sylvian fissure (22). The patient revealed severe cognitive impairment (MMSE score = 15) (31). In contrast, at a 6-month post-onset cognitive evaluation, there was a reduction in cognitive impairment (MMSE score = 24 and WAIS score = 83) (31, 32). Moreover, on 6-month DTT of the patient, they observed discontinuations of both cinguli above the genu of the corpus callosum; in contrast, the left cingulum was observed to be connected to the left Ch 5 in the brainstem via a neural tract that passed through the anterior

TABLE 1 | Previous diffusion tensor imaging studies on the recovery mechanisms of injured cinguli.

Authors	Publication year	Number of patients	Clinical evaluation method	Duration to DTI	Pathology of brain injury	Recovery mechanism
Yeo et al. (22)	2012	1	MMSE WAIS	6 months	TBI	2
Seo and Jang (20)	2013	1	MMSE WAIS MAS	7 days 14 months	Hypoxic-ischemic brain injury	1
Seo and Jang (23)	2014	1	WAIS MAS	1 month 7 months	SAH	2
Yoo et al. (24)	2014	20	WAIS MAS	Average 6.98 months	TBI	2
Jang et al (25)	2015	1	WAIS MAS	2 weeks 6 months	TBI	4
Jang et al. (26)	2016	1	MMSE WAIS	4 weeks 9 months	TBI	3
Jang and Kwon (27)	2016	1	MMSE	4 months 4 years	Brain tumor, ICH	1
Jang and Seo (28)	2016	1	MMSE WAIS	6 weeks 6 months 10 months	TBI	5
Jang et al. (29)	2018	1	MAS	3 months 2 years	TBI	1
Jang et al. (30)	2018	1	MMSE	3 weeks	ICH IVH SAH	4

DTI, Diffusion Tensor Imaging; TBI, Traumatic Brain Injury; MMSE, Mini-Mental State Examination; WAIS, Wechsler Adult Intelligence Scale; MAS, Memory Assessment Scale.

corona radiata and the thalamus. As a result, the authors assumed that the cognitive improvement in this patient was related to the recovery of the neural connection between the injured cingulum and Ch 5 in the brainstem (22).

In 2014, Seo and Jang reported on a patient who showed unusual neural connections between the anterior portions of injured cinguli and the brainstem cholinergic nuclei following SAH (23). The patient showed memory impairment at 5 weeks after onset but his memory function showed improvement to within the normal range at 7 months after onset: His total IQ on WAIS increased from 104 to 125; moreover, there were widespread improvements in MAS scores: global memory, from 79 (8%ile) to 104 (61%ile); short-term memory, from 111 (77%ile) to 114 (83%ile); verbal memory, from 94 (35%ile) to 111 (77%ile); and visual memory, from 71 (3%ile) to 97 (42%ile) (32, 33). On both 1- and 7-month DTT of the patient, discontinuations of both cinguli above the genu of the corpus callosum were observed. On the 1-month DTT, both cinguli were connected to their respective bilateral Ch 5 via neural tracts that passed through the thalamus; in contrast, on the 7-month DTT, the left neural tract was not visible, and the right neural tract was connected to the right Ch 6. The authors suggested that this unusual neural connection between the anterior portions of injured cinguli and the brainstem cholinergic nuclei was the recovery mechanism associated with cholinergic innervation of the injured cinguli (23).

During the same year (2014), Yoo et al. investigated the relationship between cognition and the neural connections from injured cinguli to brainstem cholinergic nuclei in patients with TBI (24). Twenty chronic TBI patients who showed discontinuation between both anterior cinguli and the basal forebrain on DTT were recruited for the study. Eight patients who had neural connections between their injured cinguli and various brainstem cholinergic nuclei (Ch 5, Ch 6, and Ch 8) had better MAS short-term memory scores than 12 patients who did not have such connections. The authors concluded that the observed neural connections between the injured cinguli and the brainstem cholinergic nuclei appeared to be a recovery mechanism of injured cinguli (24).

Mechanism 3: Recovery Through the Lateral Cholinergic Pathway Between an Injured Cingulum and the White Matter of the Temporo-Occipital Lobes

In 2016, Jang et al. reported on a patient with TBI who showed recovery of an injured cingulum that progressed via the lateral cholinergic pathway (26). At 4 weeks after TBI onset, the patient exhibited mild cognitive impairment; however, cognition had improved at the 9-month evaluation (MMSE from 21 to 29; total IQ from 85 to 96; verbal IQ from 86 to 96; performance IQ from 84 to 97; verbal immediate recall from 26.76 to 56.75%ile; visual immediate recall from 29.81 to 89.49%ile; verbal delayed recall from 24.51 to 78.23%ile; visual delayed recall from 11.70 to 89.07%ile; verbal recognition from 43.25 to 85.31%ile; and visual recognition from 0.94 to 93.06%ile) (31–33). On 4-week DTT, discontinuations in both cinguli were observed superior to the genu of the corpus callosum. However, on 9-month DTT, the discontinued anterior part of the right cingulum was observed to have elongated inferoposteriorly via an unusual neural tract that passed through the external capsule and the white matter of the temporo-occipital lobes. The authors concluded that recovery of an injured cingulum via a lateral cholinergic pathway is a recovery mechanism of an injured cingulum (26).

Mechanism 4: Recovery Through a Neural Tract Between the Contralesional Basal Forebrain and the Ipsilesional Basal Forebrain via the Genu of the Corpus Callosum

In 2015, Jang et al. reported on changes in DTT results for the cingulum that coincided with changes in cognitive impairment in a patient with TBI (25). Upon evaluation of cognitive function performed 2 weeks after onset, the patient revealed severe cognitive impairment; however, cognition was improved at the 6-month evaluation. Improvements include total IQ from 65 to 82; MAS global memory from 61 (1%ile) to 102 (55%ile); and MAS immediate memory from 83 (13%ile) to 107 (68%ile) (32, 33). On DTT 2 weeks after onset, the authors observed discontinuations in both cinguli anterior to the genu of the corpus callosum. However, on a 6-month follow-up DTT, the left cingulum had elongated to the left basal forebrain and the right cingulum was connected to left basal forebrain by a new tract that passed anterior to the genu of the corpus callosum. That new tract was not observed on the DTT results obtained at 2 weeks after onset (25).

Recently, Jang et al. reported on a patient who had developed new neural tracts between the injured anterior cinguli and the basal forebrain following ICH, intraventricular hemorrhage, and SAH after the rupture of an aneurysm in the left middle cerebral artery (30). When beginning rehabilitation at 3 weeks after onset, the patient showed severe cognitive impairment (MMSE: uncheckable) (31). At that time, DTT revealed the discontinued right anterior cingulum was connected to the left basal forebrain via the genu of the corpus callosum. In addition, the discontinued left anterior cingulum was shown to be connected via an unusual neural tract from the right anterior cingulum to the left basal forebrain. The authors suggested that development of this unusual neural tract between the basal forebrain and the injured cinguli via the genu of the corpus callosum, after interruption of cholinergic innervation from the basal forebrain by complete injury of the anterior cingulum, might have been the result of reorganization of cholinergic innervations following the stroke (30).

Mechanism 5: Recovery Through a Neural Tract Between an Injured Cingulum and the Basalis Nucleus of Meynert via an Aberrant Pathway

In 2016, Jang et al. reported on a patient who, following TBI, appeared to show recovery of an injured anterior cingulum via an aberrant neural tract between an injured cingulum and Ch 4 (28). The patient showed improvement of cognitive function on the MMSE with scores of 10 at 2 months, 13 at 6 months, and 26 at 10 months after onset (31). Total IQ was 90 on the WAIS at 10 months after onset (32). DTT at 6 weeks after onset showed discontinuation superior to the genu of the corpus callosum in both cinguli. However, on a 6-month DTT, the discontinued anterior part of the right cingulum was shown to have elongated anteriorly through the anterolateral subcortical white matter of the cingulum. On 10-month DTT, this elongated neural tract of the right cingulum was connected to the right Ch 4 in the basal forebrain. The authors concluded that the aberrant neural tract between the injured anterior cingulum and Ch 4 appeared to be a recovery mechanism of an injured cingulum (28).

CONCLUSIONS

In this mini-review article, 10 studies (six TBI studies; three stroke studies; and one HI-BI study) reporting recovery mechanisms of injured cinguli in patients with brain injuries were reviewed (20, 22–30). The frequencies of occurrence of the five different recovery mechanisms of injured cinguli are: Mechanism 1, 3 papers; mechanism 2, 3 papers; mechanism 4, 2 papers; mechanism 3, 1 paper; and mechanism 5, 1 paper. Based on the presence of multiple reports describing mechanisms 1 and 2, recovery mechanisms through the normal pathway of the anterior cingulum and the neural tract between an injured cingulum and the brainstem cholinergic nuclei appeared to be reliable. However, the other recovery mechanisms are less assured because of the shortage of published reports on those mechanisms.

Based on the observations in the reviewed papers, it appears that injured cingulum recovery mechanisms are based on reorganization of the cholinergic innervation between the injured cingulum and the cholinergic nuclei as a means to obtain cholinergic innervation after the loss of cholinergic innervation between the basal forebrain and the anterior cingulum (1, 34–36). Studies of injured anterior cinguli that describe recovery mechanisms might be useful in the neurorehabilitation of patients with anterior cingulum injury; for example, neuromodulation such as that provided by repetitive transcranial magnetic stimulation or transcranial direct current stimulation, which have been popularly applied in neurorehabilitation in recent years, can be applied to facilitate or induce a possible recovery mechanism of injured cinguli in patients with brain injuries (37–40). In addition, the information provided in those papers suggests that DTT appears to be useful in the detection of the particular recovery mechanism associated with injured anterior cinguli in a patient with brain injury. However, studies on this topic are uncommon, and research into such recovery mechanisms is still in the early, descriptive stage because most of the reviewed studies were case reports and were confined to a few brain pathologies including TBI, stroke, and HI-BI. Therefore, further studies involving large numbers of subjects and a wider variety of brain pathologies should be encouraged. In addition, studies into the influencing factors and clinical outcomes associated with each recovery mechanism are warranted. Despite the advantages of DTT, the limitations of DTT also need to be considered because three-dimensional reconstruction of brain regions that involve fiber complexity and fiber crossing can prevent DTT from fully reflecting the underlying fiber architecture, resulting in a possible underestimation of the status of the neural tract of interest (41–43).

AUTHOR CONTRIBUTIONS

SHJ: study concept and design, manuscript development, and writing. JPS: study concept and design, acquisition and analysis of data, and manuscript authorization.

ACKNOWLEDGMENTS

This research was supported by Basic Science Research Program through the National Research Foundation of Korea (NRF) funded by the Ministry of Education (NRF-2016R1A6A3A11933121).

REFERENCES

1. Selden NR, Gitelman DR, Salamon-Murayama N, Parrish TB, Mesulam MM. Trajectories of cholinergic pathways within the cerebral hemispheres of the human brain. *Brain* (1998) 121(Pt. 12):2249–57. doi: 10.1093/brain/121.12.2249
2. Nieuwenhuys R, Voogd J, Huijzen CV. *The Human Central Nervous System*. New York, NY: Springer (2008). doi: 10.1007/978-3-540-34686-9
3. Naidich TP, Duvernoy HM. *Duvernoy's Atlas of the Human Brain Stem and Cerebellum: High-Field MRI: Surface Anatomy, Internal Structure, Vascularization and 3d Sectional Anatomy*. Wien; New York, NY: Springer (2009).
4. Mesulam MM. Human brain cholinergic pathways. *Prog Brain Res.* (1990) 84:231–41. doi: 10.1016/S0079-6123(08)60908-5
5. Schliebs R, Arendt T. The significance of the cholinergic system in the brain during aging and in alzheimer's disease. *J Neural Transm.* (2006) 113:1625–44. doi: 10.1007/s00702-006-0579-2
6. Bigl V, Arendt T, Biesold D. The nucleus basalis of Meynert during aging and in dementing neuropsychiatric disorders. In: Steriade M, Biesold D, IBR Organization, editors. *Brain Cholinergic Systems*. Oxford: Oxford University Press (1990). p. 364–86.
7. Detari L, Rasmusson DD, Semba K. The role of basal forebrain neurons in tonic and phasic activation of the cerebral cortex. *Prog Neurobiol.* (1999) 58:249–77. doi: 10.1016/S0301-0082(98)00084-7
8. Lee MG, Hassani OK, Alonso A, Jones BE. Cholinergic basal forebrain neurons burst with theta during waking and paradoxical sleep. *J Neurosci.* (2005) 25:4365–9. doi: 10.1523/JNEUROSCI.0178-05.2005
9. Arendt T, Bigl V. Alzheimer plaques and cortical cholinergic innervation. *Neuroscience* (1986) 17:277–9. doi: 10.1016/0306-4522(86)90243-5
10. Hampel H, Mesulam MM, Cuello AC, Farlow MR, Giacobini E, Grossberg GT, et al. The cholinergic system in the pathophysiology and treatment of Alzheimer's disease. *Brain* (2018) 141:1917–33. doi: 10.1093/brain/awy132
11. Vogt BA, Finch DM, Olson CR. Functional heterogeneity in cingulate cortex: the anterior executive and posterior evaluative regions. *Cereb Cortex* (1992) 2:435–43. doi: 10.1093/cercor/2.6.435-a
12. Bush G, Luu P, Posner MI. Cognitive and emotional influences in anterior cingulate cortex. *Trends Cogn Sci.* (2000) 4:215–22. doi: 10.1016/S1364-6613(00)01483-2
13. Bach-y-Rita P. Brain plasticity as a basis of the development of rehabilitation procedures for hemiplegia. *Scand J Rehabil Med.* (1981) 13:73–83.
14. Bach y Rita P. Central nervous system lesions: sprouting and unmasking in rehabilitation. *Arch Phys Med Rehabil.* (1981) 62:413–7.
15. Jang SH, Kwon HG. Perspectives on the neural connectivity of the fornix in the human brain. *Neural Regen Res.* (2014) 9:1434–6. doi: 10.4103/1673-5374.139459
16. Lindenberg R, Renga V, Zhu LL, Betzler F, Alsop D, Schlaug G. Structural integrity of corticospinal motor fibers predicts motor impairment in chronic stroke. *Neurology* (2010) 74:280–7. doi: 10.1212/WNL.0b013e3181ccc6d9
17. Pannek K, Chalk JB, Finnigan S, Rose SE. Dynamic corticospinal white matter connectivity changes during stroke recovery: a diffusion tensor probabilistic tractography study. *J Magn Reson Imag.* (2009) 29:529–36. doi: 10.1002/jmri.21627
18. Schaechter JD, Fricker ZP, Perdue KL, Helmer KG, Vangel MG, Greve DN, et al. Microstructural status of ipsilesional and contralesional corticospinal tract correlates with motor skill in chronic stroke patients. *Hum Brain Mapp.* (2009) 30:3461–74. doi: 10.1002/hbm.20770
19. Jang SH. A review of diffusion tensor imaging studies on motor recovery mechanisms in stroke patients. *NeuroRehabilitation* (2011) 28:345–52. doi: 10.3233/NRE-2011-0662
20. Seo JP, Jang SH. Recovery of injured cingulum in a patient with brain injury: diffusion tensor tractography study. *NeuroRehabilitation* (2013) 33:257–61. doi: 10.3233/NRE-130953
21. Concha L, Gross DW, Beaulieu C. Diffusion tensor tractography of the limbic system. *AJNR Am J Neuroradiol.* (2005) 26:2267–74.
22. Yeo SS, Chang MC, Kim SH, Son SM, Jang SH. Neural connection between injured cingulum and pedunculopontine nucleus in a patient with traumatic brain injury. *NeuroRehabilitation* (2012) 31:143–6. doi: 10.3233/NRE-2012-0783
23. Seo JP, Jang SH. Unusual neural connection between injured cingulum and brainstem in a patient with subarachnoid hemorrhage. *Neural Regen Res.* (2014) 9:498–9. doi: 10.4103/1673-5374.130068
24. Yoo JS, Kim OL, Kim SH, Kim MS, Jang SH. Relation between cognition and neural connection from injured cingulum to brainstem cholinergic nuclei in chronic patients with traumatic brain injury. *Brain Inj.* (2014) 28:1257–61. doi: 10.3109/02699052.2014.901557
25. Jang SH, Kim SH, Kwon HG. Recovery of injured cingulum in a patient with traumatic brain injury. *Neural Regen Res.* (2015) 10:323–4. doi: 10.4103/1673-5374.170321
26. Jang SH, Kim SH, Kwon HG. Recovery of an injured cingulum via the lateral cholinergic pathway in a patient with traumatic brain injury. *Am J Phys Med Rehabil.* (2016) 95:e18–21. doi: 10.1097/PHM.0000000000000439
27. Jang SH, Kwon HG. Recovery of an injured anterior cingulum to the basal forebrain in a patient with brain injury: a 4-year follow-up study of cognitive function. *Neural Regen Res.* (2016) 11:1695–6. doi: 10.4103/1673-5374.193252
28. Jang SH, Seo JP. Recovery of an injured cingulum via an aberrant neural tract in a patient with traumatic brain injury: a case report. *Medicine* (2016) 95:e4686. doi: 10.1097/MD.0000000000004686
29. Jang SH, Kim SH, Seo JP. Recovery of an injured cingulum concurrent with improvement of short-term memory in a patient with mild traumatic brain injury. *Brain Inj.* (2018) 32:144–6. doi: 10.1080/02699052.2017.1367960
30. Jang SH, Chang CH, Lee HD. Reorganization of injured anterior cingulums in a stroke patient. *Neural Regen Res.* (2018) 13:1486–7. doi: 10.4103/1673-5374.235308
31. Folstein MF, Folstein SE, McHugh PR. "Mini-mental state." a practical method for grading the cognitive state of patients for the clinician. *J Psychiatr Res.* (1975) 12:189–98.
32. Wechsler D. *Wais-r Manual: Wechsler Adult Intelligence Scale-Revised*. San Antonio, TX: Psychological Corporation (1981).
33. Williams JM. *Mas: Memory Assessment Scales: Professional Manual*. Odessa, FL: Psychological Assessment Resources (1991).
34. Lucas-Meunier E, Fossier P, Baux G, Amar M. Cholinergic modulation of the cortical neuronal network. *Pflugers Arch.* (2003) 446:17–29. doi: 10.1007/s00424-002-0999-2

35. Mesulam MM. The cholinergic innervation of the human cerebral cortex. *Prog Brain Res.* (2004) 145:67–78. doi: 10.1016/S0079-6123(03)45004-8
36. Hong JH, Jang SH. Neural pathway from nucleus basalis of Meynert passing through the cingulum in the human brain. *Brain Res.* (2010) 1346:190–4. doi: 10.1016/j.brainres.2010.05.088
37. Henrich-Noack P, Sergeeva EG, Sabel BA. Non-invasive electrical brain stimulation: from acute to late-stage treatment of central nervous system damage. *Neural Regen Res.* (2017) 12:1590–4. doi: 10.4103/1673-5374.217322
38. Dionisio A, Duarte IC, Patricio M, Castelo-Branco M. The use of repetitive transcranial magnetic stimulation for stroke rehabilitation: a systematic review. *J Stroke Cerebrovasc Dis.* (2018) 27:1–31. doi: 10.1016/j.jstrokecerebrovasdis.2017.09.008
39. Hanlon CA, Dowdle LT, Henderson JS. Modulating neural circuits with transcranial magnetic stimulation: implications for addiction treatment development. *Pharmacol Rev.* (2018) 70:661–83. doi: 10.1124/pr.116.013649
40. Nasios G, Messinis L, Dardiotis E, Papathanasopoulos P. Repetitive transcranial magnetic stimulation, cognition, and multiple sclerosis: an overview. *Behav Neurol.* (2018) 2018:8584653. doi: 10.1155/2018/8584653
41. Parker GJ, Alexander DC. Probabilistic anatomical connectivity derived from the microscopic persistent angular structure of cerebral tissue. *Philos Trans R Soc Lond B Biol Sci.* (2005) 360:893–902. doi: 10.1098/rstb.2005.1639
42. Wedeen VJ, Wang RP, Schmahmann JD, Benner T, Tseng WY, Dai G, et al. Diffusion spectrum magnetic resonance imaging (dsi) tractography of crossing fibers. *Neuroimage* (2008) 41:1267–77. doi: 10.1016/j.neuroimage.2008.03.036
43. Yamada K, Sakai K, Akazawa K, Yuen S, Nishimura T. Mr tractography: a review of its clinical applications. *Magn Reson Med Sci.* (2009) 8:165–74. doi: 10.2463/mrms.8.165

17

Effects of High-Intensity Robot-Assisted Hand Training on Upper Limb Recovery and Muscle Activity in Individuals with Multiple Sclerosis

Marialuisa Gandolfi[1], Nicola Valè[1], Eleonora Kirilova Dimitrova[1], Stefano Mazzoleni[2], Elena Battini[2], Maria Donata Benedetti[1], Alberto Gajofatto[1], Francesco Ferraro[3], Matteo Castelli[4], Maruo Camin[4], Mirko Filippetti[1], Carola De Paoli[1], Elena Chemello[1], Alessandro Picelli[1,5], Jessica Corradi[1], Andreas Waldner[6], Leopold Saltuari[7,8] and Nicola Smania[1,5]*

[1]Department of Neurosciences, Biomedicine and Movement Sciences, University of Verona, Verona, Italy, [2] The BioRobotics Institute, Scuola Superiore Sant' Anna, Polo Sant' Anna Valdera, Pontedera, Italy, [3] Section of Neuromotor Rehabilitation, Department of Neuroscience, ASST Carlo Poma, Mantova, Italy, [4] Centro di riabilitazione Franca Martini—ATSM ONLUS, Trento, Italy, [5] UOC Neurorehabilitation, AOUI Verona, Verona, Italy, [6] Department of Neurological Rehabilitation, Private Hospital Villa Melitta, Bolzano, Italy, [7] Research Department for Neurorehabilitation South Tyrol, Bolzano, Italy, [8] Department of Neurology, Hochzirl Hospital, Zirl, Austria

***Correspondence:**
Marialuisa Gandolfi
marialuisa.gandolfi@univr.it

Background : Integration of robotics and upper limb rehabilitation in people with multiple sclerosis (PwMS) has rarely been investigated.

Objective: To compare the effects of robot-assisted hand training against non-robotic hand training on upper limb activity in PwMS. To compare the training effects on hand dexterity, muscle activity, and upper limb dysfunction as measured with the International Classification of Functioning.

Methods: This single-blind, randomized, controlled trial involved 44 PwMS (Expanded Disability Status Scale:1.5–8) and hand dexterity deficits. The experimental group (n = 23) received robot-assisted hand training; the control group (n = 21) received non-robotic hand training. Training protocols lasted for 5 weeks (50 min/session, 2 sessions/week). Before (T0), after (T1), and at 1 month follow-up (T2), a blinded rater evaluated patients using a comprehensive test battery. Primary outcome: Action Research Arm Test. Secondary outcomes: Nine Holes Peg Test; Fugl-Meyer Assessment Scale–upper extremity section; Motricity Index; Motor Activity Log; Multiple Sclerosis (MS) Quality of Life—54; Life Habits assessment—general short form and surface electromyography.

Results: There were no significant between-group differences in primary and secondary outcomes. Electromyography showed relevant changes providing evidence increased activity in the extensor carpi at T1 and T2.

Conclusion: The training effects on upper limb activity and function were comparable between the two groups. However, robot-assisted training demonstrated remarkable effects on upper limb use and muscle activity. https://clinicaltrials.gov NCT03561155.

Keywords: upper limb abnormalities, quality of life, rehabilitation, robotics, electromyography, learning

INTRODUCTION

Multiple sclerosis (MS) is the most common non-traumatic cause of neurologic disability in young adults worldwide (1). The major causes of disability are inflammatory demyelination and axonal loss[2], which result in the hallmark motor, sensory, cognitive, and autonomic dysfunctions found in people with MS (2, 3). In the first year of disease onset up to 66% of patients will develop upper limb impairment that will continue to worsen over the following three decades (3–5) and diminish participation and quality of life (5, 6) Temporal fluctuations and fatigue render clinical management extraordinarily complex (3).

In the last decade, integration of robot-assisted devices in upper limb training programs has gained increasing interest for their capability to provide early, intensive, task-specific and multisensory stimulation especially in stroke patients (7). There is consensus on the effectiveness of upper limb rehabilitation also in people with MS (8). In their review, Lamers et al. emphasized the importance of multidisciplinary rehabilitation to improve upper limb capacity, along with body function and they suggested that upper limb capacity could be enhanced by robot-assisted training (8). Despite differences in sample characteristics and methodologies, the literature generally supports the benefits of upper limb robot-assisted training in people with MS. However, studies differ considerably in primary outcomes (activity vs. function), study design [uncontrolled vs. randomized controlled trial [RCT]], and therapy content and dosage. Only two controlled trials on upper limb robot-assisted training in people with MS have used devices designed for rehabilitating the proximal upper limb (shoulder and elbow) (9, 10). No studies to date have been performed using a robot-assisted device specifically designed for the hand in people with MS.

The Amadeo® (Tyromotion-Austria) is a modern, mechatronic end-effector robotic device. Its most distinctive feature is that it simulates natural grasping motion and executes automated movement sequences. Results from its application in stroke rehabilitation suggest that robot-assisted hand rehabilitation reduces motor impairment and increases use of the affected hand, with possible generalization to the entire upper limb (11, 12). It is not clear, however, whether these improvements can translate to increased upper limb use in everyday activities (11).

The primary aim of this study was to compare the effects of robot-assisted hand training and robot-unassisted rehabilitation on upper limb activity. The secondary aim was to compare the training effects on hand dexterity and upper limb function, disability, and quality of life. We hypothesized that, because it boosts greater use of the hand, upper limb activity would improve more after robot-assisted hand training than after non-robotic training. To explore the potential mechanisms involved in such improvements the electromyographic activity of 6 upper limb muscles was investigated. Given the multiplicity of symptoms that often need to be addressed in MS, the integration of robotics and rehabilitation holds promise for developing high-intensity, repetitive, task-specific, interactive treatment of upper limb impairment.

MATERIALS AND METHODS

Trial Design

This single-blind RCT compared the effects of robot-assisted [experimental group (EG)] vs. non-robotic [control group (CG)] training. The examiner was blinded to group assignment (**Figure 3**).

Participants

From March 2014 to March 2017, consecutive outpatients with MS and hand dexterity deficits referred to our Neurorehabilitation Unit (AOUI Verona) were assessed. Inclusion criteria were: confirmed MS diagnosis (13), age between 18 and 65 years, Expanded Disability Status Scale (EDSS) score $1.5 \leq x \leq 8$ (13), Mini-Mental State Evaluation (MMSE) score $\geq$24/30 (14), Modified Ashworth Scale (MAS) score <2 evaluated at the elbow, wrist, and fingers (15), Nine Hole Peg Test (NHPT) score between 30 and 300 s (9). Exclusion criteria were: relapse or relapse-related treatments in the 3 months before entering the study, musculoskeletal impairments or visual analog scale (VAS) for pain score > 7/10 in any joint that could interfere with the training program, severe visual dysfunction, any type of rehabilitation in the month prior to recruitment, other concomitant neurological or orthopedic diseases involving the upper limb and interfering with their function. Patients gave their written, informed consent after being informed about the experimental nature of the study. The study was carried out in accordance with the Helsinki Declaration, approved by the local Ethics Committee (prog n.230CESC), and registered at clinical trial (NCT03561155).

Interventions

One experienced physical therapist per treatment group supervised the training sessions. Patients received individualized treatment for 50 min/day, 2 days/week for 5 weeks at the physical therapy facility of the Neurorehabilitation Unit (AOUI Verona). At the end of each session, upper limb passive mobilization was performed in supine position for 10 min. Based on baseline assessment, the weaker upper limb was selected for evaluation and treatment. When both upper limbs were equally impaired, the participant's preference was taken into account.

Experimental Group

Patients underwent robot-assisted hand training on an Amadeo® (Tyromotion, Austria). This modern, mechatronic end-effector computer-assisted robotic device is specifically designed to improve sensorimotor functions in patients with restricted hand function (**Figure 1**). Therapy sessions were conducted by a physical therapist experienced in use of the device. The patient was seated in a comfortable position and the arm strapped into an adjustable stabilizing splint attached to the robotic device, with the wrist in neutral position and the forearm pronated. The wrist was stabilized to the body of the device by means of a spring-loaded hinge, which allowed for some degree of passive flexion and extension during use. The height of the device was adjusted to an angle of about 30° of elbow flexion. Each finger was attached to the robotically driven slide with magnets taped to the distal phalanx of each finger. Three different training modes were performed: (1) continuous passive motion (CPM) during which the hand is passively stimulated in finger flexion and extension (10 min); (2) assistive therapy in which the hand is functional but is actively trained at the patient's limit of performance (10 min); (3) interactive therapy via active training with specifically developed virtual therapy games (10 min) in which the patient exerts isometric force in flexion or extension to avoid obstacles or to reach a target (fire) shown on the video. The isometric force produces proportional movement of a virtual figure. The physiotherapist sets task difficulty from among 30 pre-selected levels graded by duration, force, and accuracy in completing the task. Each exercise was repeated several times according to the patient's ability and task complexity was increased as performance improved. The physiotherapist recorded on the patient's chart the exercises (i.e., type of exercise, number of repetitions) and any adverse events that occurred during the study.

Control Group

The protocol for upper limb rehabilitation was designed according to the neurodevelopmental technique and consisted of upper limb mobilization (shoulder girdle, elbow, wrist, and finger joints), facilitation of movements, and active tasks chosen out of 15 that are challenging for patients (16, 17). The exercises were focused on improving muscle strength in flexion and extension, dexterity, and motor control. At the end of each treatment session, the patient received feedback about her/his performance in terms of the number of errors and comments on execution of movement.

Outcomes

Demographic and clinical data (EDSS score, disease duration, and Tremor Severity Scale score) were collected at baseline (18). A comprehensive test battery was administered before (T0), after (T1), and again at 1 month of follow-up (T2).

The primary outcome was the change in upper limb activity as measured with the Action Research Arm Test (ARAT) at T1 compared to T0 (19). Secondary outcomes: upper limb activity measured using the Nine Holes Peg Test (NHPT) (20–22); manual dexterity speed calculated as the number of pegs placed

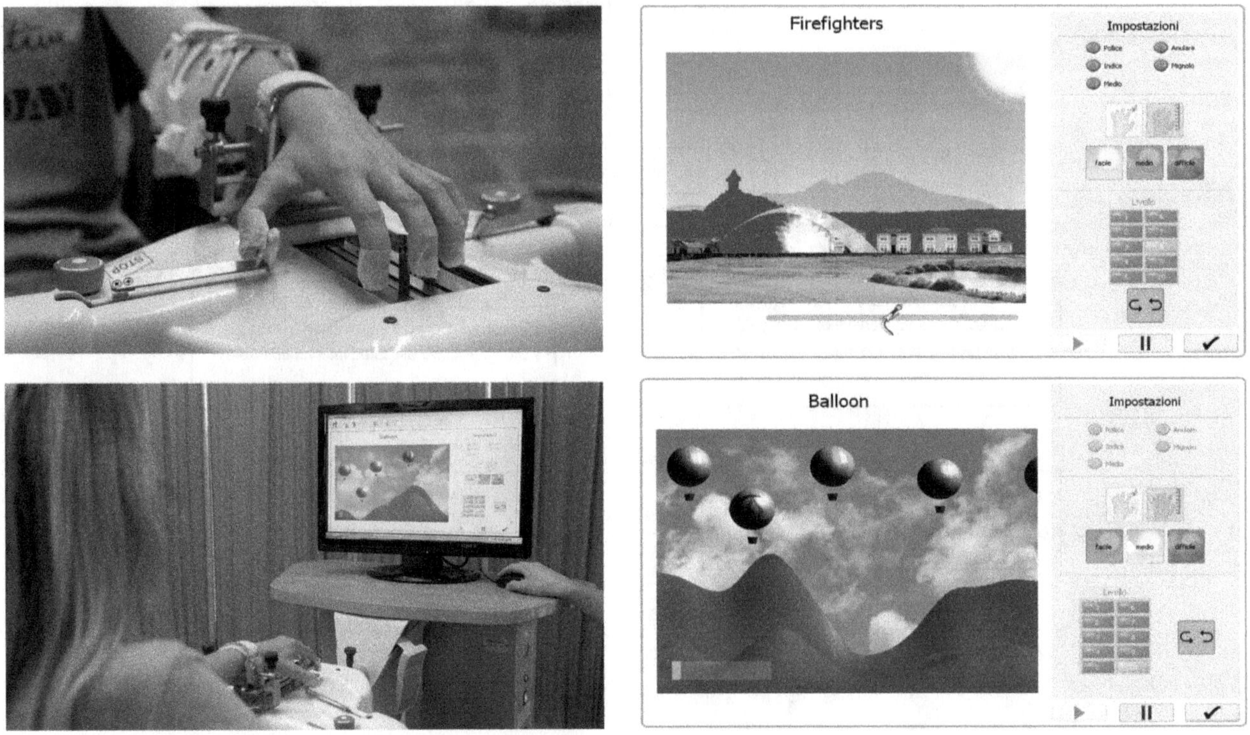

FIGURE 1 | Hardware set-up of the Amadeo System, finger slings, and visual display.

per second. Trials in which patients were unable to place any peg within the time limit of 300 s were scored as 0 peg per second (6). Upper limb function was measured by means of the Fugl-Meyer Assessment Scale–upper extremity section (FMA) (range, 0–66 where higher scores indicate better performance) (23) and the Motricity Index (MI) (range, 0–100 where higher scores indicate better performance) (24). The Motor Activity Log (MAL) was used to assess changes in the amount and quality of arm use in accomplishing 30 daily activities (range, 0–168 where higher scores indicate better performance) (25). The MS Quality

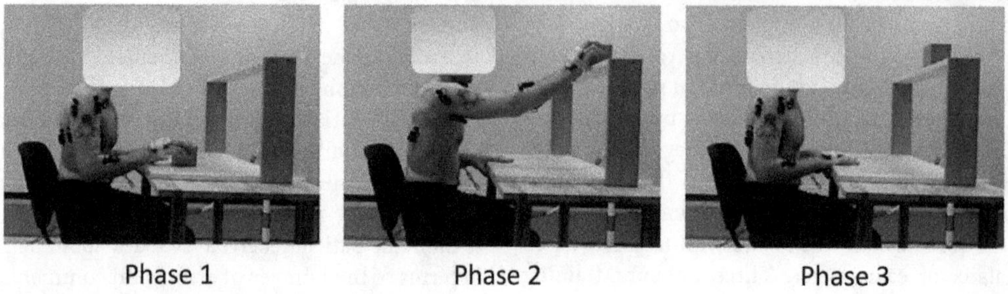

FIGURE 2 | Experimental set-up with the surface EMG electrodes placement.

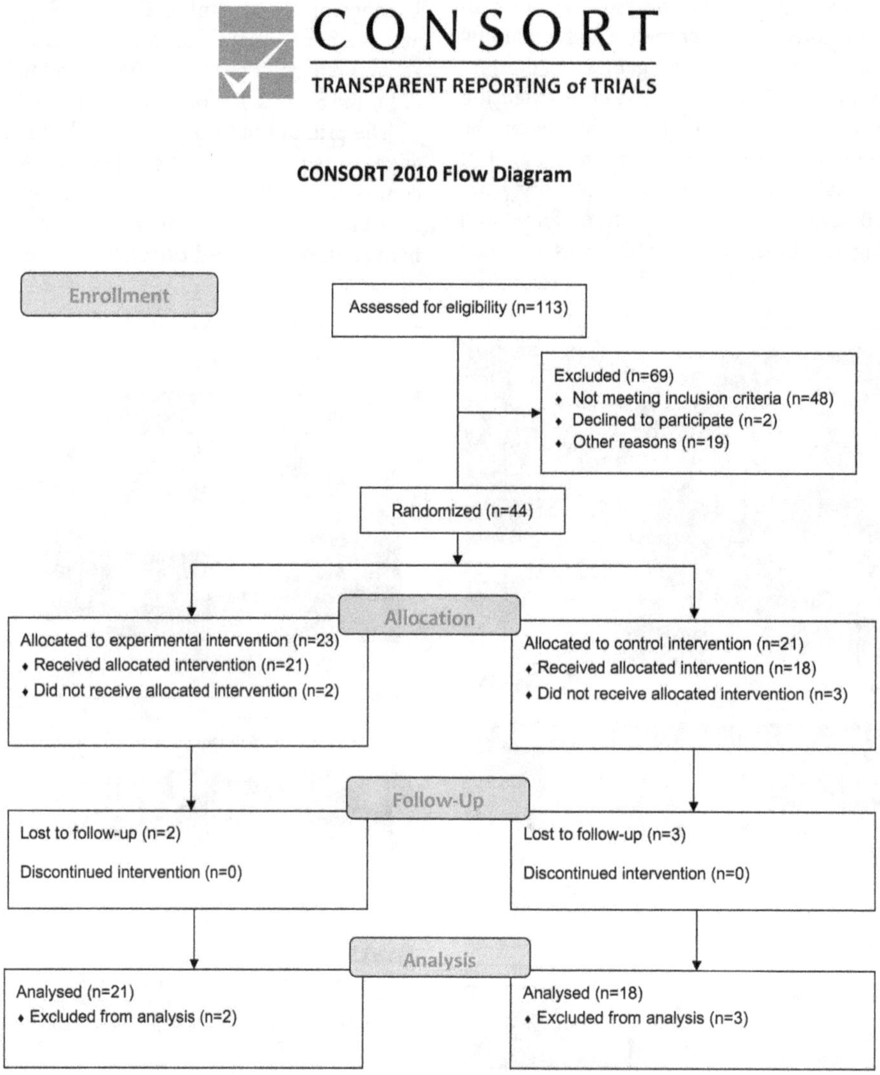

FIGURE 3 | CONSORT flowchart.

of Life−54 (MSQoL-54), with the physical health (PHC) and mental health (MHC) domains, were used to investigate generic and MS-specific domains of health-related QoL (range, 0–100 where higher scores indicate better performance) (26). Patient satisfaction with daily activities or social roles was assessed using the Life Habits assessment—general short form (LifeH) (27).

Electromyography (EMG)

The EMG activity of 6 upper limb muscles of the more affected side (deltoid scapular, deltoid clavicular, triceps brachii, biceps brachii, flexor carpi radialis, and extensor carpi radialis) was measured using pairs of self-adhesive surface electrodes. Disposable Ag-AgCl electrodes were placed according to SENIAM guidelines with an inter-electrode spacing of 0.02 m. Before electrode placement, the skin was shaved with a disposable, single-use razor and cleaned with alcohol (28). Raw EMG signals were collected using BTS FREEEMG 300 wireless surface EMG sensors (BTS spa, Milan, Italy) at a sampling rate of 1000 Hz. Raw EMG signals were processed with a customized routine developed in MATLAB environment (MathWorks, USA). The raw EMG signal was bandpass filtered at 20–450 Hz and then smoothed using a 20 ms root mean square (RMS) algorithm to obtain the envelope. Signals were recorded in three conditions: 30 s during resting position (basal), 5 s of maximal voluntary isometric contraction (MVIC), and during a reach-to-grasp task (ARAT subscale). Patients were asked to grasp and place a 7.5 cm wooden-cube on a shelf of standardized height. The movement was divided in three phases by identifying 4 temporal events (start, grasping the cube, placing the cube on the shelf, returning to base position). The task was repeated 3 times and the signals were time-normalized. Normative data were collected from 14 healthy age-matched controls undergoing one surface EMG acquisition. The EMG tasks are illustrated in **Figure 2**.

Sample Size

A sample size of 36 patients (18 per group) was estimated to have 80% power to detect a mean difference of 3 on the primary outcome measure (ARAT) and an alpha (probability of type 1 error) of 5% (10). Assuming a 10% drop-out rate, 40 patients were necessary to perform the study.

Randomization

Eligible patients were assigned to either the EG or the CG by a simple randomization scheme using an automated randomization system (www.randomization.com). Group allocation was kept concealed. The randomization list was locked in a desk drawer accessible only to the principal investigator.

Blinding

Primary and secondary outcomes were measured by the same blinded examiner at each session.

Statistical Analysis

A per-protocol analysis was used. Descriptive statistics included means and standard deviation. The X^2 test was utilized for categorical variables. Since the data were normally distributed (Shapiro-Wilk Test), parametric tests were used for inferential statistics. Two-way mixed ANOVA was applied using "Time" as the within-group factor and "Group" as the between-group factor. Two-tailed Student's t-test for unpaired data was used

TABLE 1 | Demographic and clinical characteristics of treated subjects.

	Experimental Group (*n* = 23)	Control Group (*n* = 21)	Between-group analysis
Age (years) [mean (SD)]	51.96 (10.87)	50.67 (10.80)	n.s.
Gender (Male/Female)	10/13	41487	n.s.
Disease onset age (years) [mean(SD)]	37.57 (11.91)	36.57 (8.82)	n.s.
Disease duration since diagnosis (years) [mean(SD)]	13.48 (7.82)	14.19 (9.78)	n.s.
Type of MS (RR/PP/SP, respectively)	16/01/06	10/02/09	n.s.
EDSS score [median (Q1–Q3)]	6.00 [5.00–6.60]	6.00 [4.00–7.25]	n.s.
Cerebellar Functions	1 [0–1]	1 [0–3]	n.s.
Dominant hand (R/L)	19/4	20/1	n.s.
Trained hand (DH/NDH)	11/12	9/11	n.s.
MAS [median (Q1–Q3)]			
Elbow	0 [0–1]	0 [0–1]	n.s.
Wrist	0 [0–0]	0 [0–0.5]	n.s.
Fingers	0 [0–1]	0 [0–1]	n.s.
TSS Score [median (Q1–Q3)]			
Rest tremor	0 [0–0]	0 [0–0]	n.s.
Postural tremor	0 [0–1]	0 [0–1]	n.s.
Kinetic tremor	0 [0–1]	0 [0–1]	n.s.

RR, Relapsing Remitting; PP, Primarly Progressive; SP, Secondary Progressive; EDSS, Expanded Disability Status Scale; DH, Dominant Hand; NDH, Non Dominant Hand; MAS, Modified Ashworth Scale; TSS, Tremor Severity Scale; MI, Motricity Index.

for between-group comparisons. The level of significance was set at $p < 0.05$. Bonferroni's correction was applied for multiple comparisons ($p < 0.025$). Statistical analysis was performed with SPSS 20.0 (IBM SPSS Statistics for Windows, Version 20.0, Armonk, NY, USA).

RESULTS

In all, 113 patients were consecutively assessed: 59 were excluded because they did not meet inclusion criteria ($n = 48$) or declined to participate ($n = 2$) or had difficulty arranging transportation to the study site ($n = 19$). A total of 44 patients were randomly assigned to either the EG ($n = 23$) or the CG ($n = 21$). Two patients in the EG and 3 in the CG subsequently withdrew; of the remaining 39 patients, 21 in the EG and 18 in the CG completed the study.

There were no significant between-group differences in demographics and clinical data (**Table 1**) or in primary and secondary outcome measures at baseline (T0). Cerebellar functions assessed with EDSS subitem were homogeneous between EG and CG and the median score was 1 corresponding to "Abnormal signs without disability."

Primary Outcome

There were no significant between-group differences in ARAT scores (**Table 2**). Both groups showed an overall significant improvement in performance at T1 and T2 ($p < 0.001$).

Secondary Outcomes

No adverse events or safety concerns arose during the conduction of study. Both groups showed an overall significant improvement on all secondary outcome measures without significant between-group differences (**Tables 2, 3**). Both groups presented at the enrollment a notable capacity at the UL FMA (29). Only the EG showed significant changes in the motor activity log-amount of use (MAL-AOU) at both T1 and T2 (**Table 3**). At T2 significant improvements in muscle strength during finger extension ($p = 0.02$) and flexion ($p < 0.001$) were noted in the EG. Preliminary observation of muscular function revealed abnormalities in lifting the wooden cube for both groups. After training, the EG showed increased extensor carpi activity similar to activation in healthy control subjects. These affects were maintained at the follow-up evaluation (**Figure 4**).

DISCUSSION

The main finding of this RCT is that upper limb activity and function improved after both robot-assisted hand training and robot-unassisted treatment in these patients with MS. Interestingly, only the group that received robot-assisted hand training reported significant improvements in the use of the treated upper limb and in the assessment of skills in the life habits domain (accomplishments). In addition, preliminary observation of muscular activity showed enhancement of extensor carpi activation only in the robot-assisted hand training group, suggesting a task-specific effect of this training mode on muscle activity.

TABLE 2 | Clinical outcome measures and inferential statistics.

		Intervention Phase						Repeated measures ANOVA		
		Before	After	FU	Mean between-group differences			Group between-participants	Time within-participants	Time x group interaction
					Before	After	FU			
Outcome Measure	Group	Mean (SD)	Mean (SD)	Mean (SD)	95% CI (LB, UB)	95% CI (LB, UB)	95% CI (LB, UB)	*p*	*p*	*p*
PRIMARY OUTCOME MEASURE										
ARAT	EG	41.57 (15.22)	46.52 (14.43)	45.76 (15.55)	0.02 (−9.69; 9.72)	1.41 (−7.63; 10.45)	0.32 (−9.31; 9.94)	n.s.	**<0.001***	n.s.
	CG	41.55 (14.62)	45.11 (13.39)	45.44 (14.01)						
SECONDARY OUTCOME MEASURES										
NHPT speed	EG	0.19 (0.10)	0.21 (0.11)	0.22 (0.12)	−0.004 (−0.07; 0.06)	−0.02 (−0.10; 0.06)	−0.02 (−0.10; 0.06)	n.s.	**<0.001***	n.s.
	CG	0.19 (0.10)	0.22 (0.13)	0.24 (0.13)						
FM	EG	51.71 (14.89)	54.56 (13.71)	55.61 (13.41)	−0.95 (−9.88; 7.97)	−2.55 (−10.65; 5.56)	−0.50 (−8.87; 7.87)	n.s.	**<0.001***	n.s.
	CG	52.67 (12.63)	57.11 (11.27)	56.11 (12.38)						
MI	EG	81.24 (17.11)	84.94 (14.20)	85.32 (14.69)	0.52 (−9.59; 10.63)	0.22 (−8.72; 9.15)	1.15 (−8.21; 10.51)	n.s.	**0.001***	n.s.
	CG	80.72 (14.04)	84.72 (13.31)	84.17 (14.10)						

EG, Experimental group; CG, Control group; FU, Follow Up; ARAT, Action Research Arm Test; NHPT, Nine Hole Peg Test; MI, Motricity Index.
**Statistically significant.*
°Trend toward statistical significance; for post-hoc analysis p significant if <0.025; 95% confidence interval (CI), lower bound (LB), upper bound (UB).

TABLE 3 | Clinical QOL, participation outcome measures and inferential statistics.

		Intervention Phase						Repeated measures ANOVA			*Post hoc* analysis	
		Before	After	FU	Mean between-group differences			Group between-participants	Time within-participants	Time x group interaction	within-group	
					Before	After	FU				T1-T0	T2-T0
Outcome Measure	Group	Mean (SD)	Mean (SD)	Mean (SD)	95% CI (LB, UB)	95% CI (LB, UB)	95% CI (LB, UB)	*p*	*p*	*p*	*p*	*p*
MAL-AoU	EG	96.31 (45.10)	100.71 (46.15)	100.92 (46.71)	−6.00 (−34.83; 22.84)	−4.07 (−32.87; 24.73)	−3.69 (−32.97; 25.60)	n.s.	**0.007***	n.s.	0.005*	0.016*
	CG	102.31 (43.58)	104.78 (42.55)	104.61 (43.45)							n.s.	n.s.
MAL-QoM	EG	96.95 (41.37)	102.15 (42.17)	101.68 (43.30)	1.01 (−25.44; 27.45)	1.43 (−25.76; 28.62)	1.79 (−25.99; 29.57)	n.s.	**<0.001***	n.s.	<0.001*	0.015*
	CG	95.94 (39.95)	100.72 (41.38)	99.89 (42.10)							0.013*	n.s.
MSQOL-54 (PH)	EG	42.46 (19.18)	44.77 (18.60)	45.59 (19.84)	−1.39 (−13.70; 10.92)	1.59 (−11.10; 14.27)	3.21 (−9.18; 15.60)	n.s.	n.s.	n.s.	–	–
	CG	43.85 (17.17)	43.18 (18.75)	42.48 (17.78)							–	–
MSQOL-54 (MH)	EG	54.61 (25.77)	58.78 (22.10)	58.85 (24.29)	−2.14 (−17.50; 13.23)	−1.99 (−17.40; 1.41)	2.29 (−13.52; 18.11)	n.s.	n.s.	n.s.	–	–
	CG	56.75 (19.38)	60.78 (23.19)	57.41 (23.30)							–	–
LIFE-H (acc.)	EG	7.22 (1.90)	7.42 (1.84)	7.36 (1.83)	−0.24 (−1.28; 0.81)	−0.13 (−1.13; 0.87)	−0.23 (1.23; 0.76)	n.s.	**0.01***	n.s.	0.002*	0.026°
	CG	7.45 (1.29)	7.55 (1.22)	7.6 (1.21)							n.s.	n.s.
LIFE-H (PS)	EG	3.96 (0.83)	4.29 (0.65)	4.29 (0.75)	−0.17 (−0.70; 0.36)	−0.09 (−0.54; 0.35)	−0.12 (−0.60; 0.37)	n.s.	**<0.001***	n.s.	0.001*	0.001*
	CG	4.13 (0.78)	4.38 (0.71)	4.41 (0.74)							0.001*	0.024*

EG, Experimental group; CG, Control group; FU, Follow Up; QOL, Quality Of Life; MAL-AoU, Motor Activity Log—Amount of Use; MAL-QoM, Motor Activity Log—Quality of Movement; MSQOL-54 (PH), Multiple Sclerosis Quality of Life (Physical Health); MSQOL-54 (MH), Multiple Sclerosis Quality of Life (Mental Health); LIFE-H (acc.), Life Habits (accomplishments); LIFE-H (PS), Life Habits (Patient Satisfaction).

*Statistically significant.

°*trend toward statistical significance; for post-hoc analysis p significant if <0.025; 95% confidence interval (CI), LB lower bound, UB upper bound.*

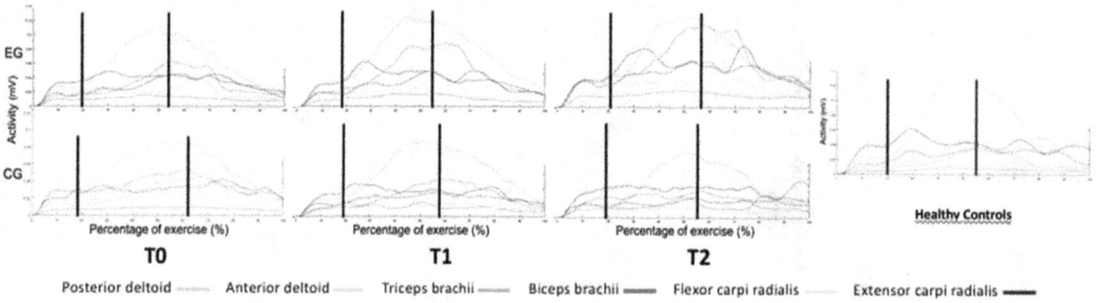

FIGURE 4 | EMG muscle activity during the reach-to-grasp task.

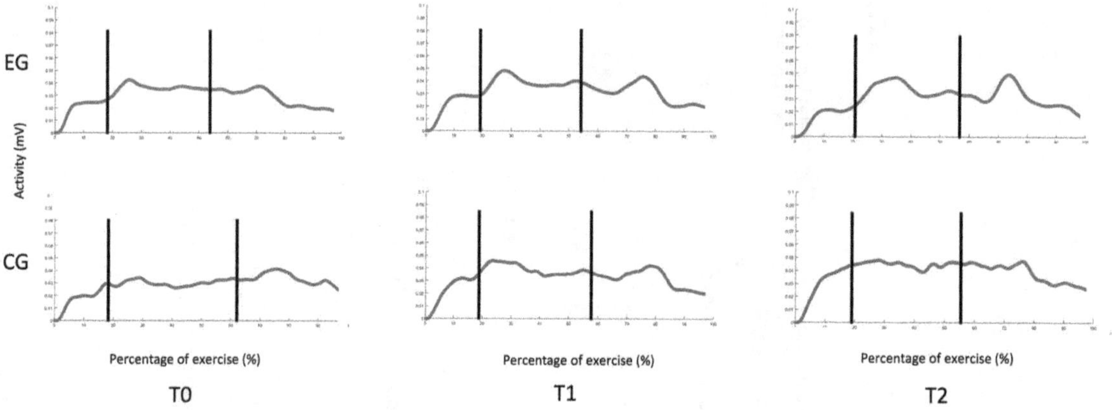

FIGURE 5 | EMG muscle activity of the Extensor Carpi Radialis.

Upper limb robot-assisted interventions have been increasingly applied in neurorehabilitation because they offer the advantage of high-intensity training, volume, and duration that can be delivered without the constant presence of a physiotherapist. However, several questions still need to be addressed: optimal therapy content and dosage according to degree of upper limb disability, effectiveness of rehabilitation strategies in improving upper limb function, and influence of type of training approach on increasing upper limb capacity and performance (8).

In a pilot RCT study conducted by Carpinella et al. 22 patients with MS were randomly assigned to receive either a robot-assisted reaching task (RT) training or robot-based training (RMT) in which objects had to be grasped and manipulated (Braccio di Ferro, Celin srl, La Spezia, Italy) (9). After 8 sessions, a significantly larger improvement in grasping was observed in the group assigned the RMT protocol. In a pilot study conducted by Feys et al. the effects of additional robot-supported virtual learning training added to conventional treatment were investigated (10). Seventeen patients received either 3 weekly sessions of conventional training alone or conventional training plus training with a 3-DoF haptic device (Haptic Master training, MOOG, the Netherlands). After 8 weeks, no significant changes in function and activity level were reported in either the intervention or the control group. However, a near-threshold significant between-group difference was measured for the MAL (amount of use and total). In their feasibility cross-over study, Vergaro et al. tested a robotic therapy protocol for rehabilitation of poor coordination in 8 patients with MS (30). No significant differences in the Nine Hole Peg test score were observed after administration of 8 training sessions of the two training protocols, though the movements became smoother after training.

While differences in sample and methods hamper comparisons between our and previous studies, our results provide evidence for a restorative potential of upper limb function after specific rehabilitation interventions in patients with MS. Both training protocols were administered to improve impairments in upper limb function (and hand dexterity), which would explain why no significant differences were detected between the two interventions. Training specificity differed slightly between the two approaches: the robot-assisted hand training was mainly focused on visual feedback and a task-specific approach, whereas the robot-unassisted training dealt with functional movement and context-specific training (3). Both training protocols shared common features such as unilateral training, mobility, stretching, and exercise progression (3). However, only with the more intensive, repetitive, and task-specific training did the amount of upper arm use and muscle activity improve, and continue through to follow-up assessment.

Chronic upper limb disuse might contribute to disability and explain the functional differences beyond the adaptive functional reorganization observed in clinical stages and forms of MS (2). Patients with MS may develop a negative learning phenomenon, which consists of relying on their less affected arm to perform activities of daily living with a progressive suppression of movements in the more affected arm (2, 25). Interference with this learned phenomenon may be the mechanism through which physical therapy can limit the extent of upper limb disability in stroke patients and in patients with MS (31–33).

Unfortunately, we were unable to identify the factors related to robot-assisted training that would have been crucial to this finding. Nevertheless, we argue that such training may boost more successful use of the hand that, in turn, could increase confidence in performing upper limb activity. The role of training intensity, along with the need to better balance uni- and bimanual upper limb exercise, may have contributed to successful outcomes. The visual feedback provided by the Amadeo system may have increased patient motivation during training and awareness of upper limb capacity Moreover, training intensity may have reduced the one's perception of difficulty and assistance required by the patient during upper limb activity assessed with LIFE-H-accomplishment section. Although both groups presented a notable capacity of the UL and minimal signs of cerebellar dysfunctions, the interactive feedback provided by the robotic training was a stimulating way to increase patient motivation, reduce effort and increase performance during ADLs (29). This finding suggests that the robotic training effects may be extended beyond the physical aspects. Literature supports a disagreement between MS patients and treating physician regarding factors affecting the quality of life (34). The changes observed in EMG activity may support this view and are in line with previous preliminary reports (35). A smaller difference between the maximum and the minimum of extensor carpi radialis (ECR) activation as compared with healthy subjects was observed after treatment and only the EG recovered ECR activity, improving its modularity. One possible explanation for this is the specific training of finger muscles, and wrist stabilizer muscles indirectly, with the Amadeo system (**Figure 5**).

The strengths of the present study are the relatively large patient sample and the low drop-out rate, which suggest the feasibility of robotic training in patients with MS. The comprehensive and multidisciplinary evaluation of upper limb disorders according to the ICF framework, and the EMG analysis using a standardized experimental protocol to investigate the training effects on muscle activity are further strengths of this study. The study limitations are the lack of patient stratification by degree of impairment, the lack of assessment of cognitive and mood decline and the lack of neuroimaging support.

To conclude, as a part of the multifaceted management of upper limb rehabilitation, robotics is a feasible and valid approach to improving upper limb function and enhance UL use in patients with MS. Robotics holds promise and potential to enrich rehabilitation care in MS, but issues such as optimal dosage according to degree of upper limb disability need still to be addressed.

AUTHOR CONTRIBUTIONS

MG and NS have made substantial contributions to conception and design. AG, MB, MatC, MarC, EC, and AP participated in the enrollment phase. JC and CD carried out the clinical assessment. NV, MF, and ED carried out the Instrumental assessments. SM and EB designed the algorithm for EMG data analysis. MG and NV participated in the statistical analysis and drafted the manuscripts. NV, FF, AW and LS participated in the manuscript revision process and gave the final approval of the version.

ACKNOWLEDGMENTS

We thank Giulia Dusi for her assistance in data collection. This work is part of the activity of the Gruppo Interdisciplinare Sclerosi Multipla (AOUI Verona, Italy).

REFERENCES

1. Atlas of Multiple Sclerosis 2013. *Mapping Multiple Sclerosis Around the World* (2014) (Accessed 01 June 2017). Available online at: http://www.msif.org/wp-content/uploads/2014/09/Atlas-of-MS.pdf.
2. Tomassini V, Matthews PM, Thompson AJ, Fuglø D, Geurts JJ, Johansen-Berg H, et al. Neuroplasticity and functional recovery in multiple sclerosis. *Nat Rev Neurol.* (2012) 8:635–46. doi: 10.1038/nrneurol.2012.179
3. Spooren AI, Timmermans AA, Seelen HA. Motor training programs of arm and hand in patients with MS according to different levels of the ICF: a systematic review. *BMC Neurol.* (2012) 12:49. doi: 10.1186/1471-2377-12-49
4. Kister I, Bacon TE, Chamot E, Salter AR, Cutter GR, Kalina JT, et al. Natural history of multiple sclerosis symptoms. *Int J MS Care* (2013) 15:146–58. doi: 10.7224/1537-2073.2012-053
5. Johansson S, Ytterberg C, Claesson IM, Lindberg J, Hillert J, Andersson M, et al. High concurrent presence of disability in multiple sclerosis. *J Neurol.* (2007) 254:767–73. doi: 10.1007/s00415-006-0431-5
6. Cattaneo D, Lamers I, Bertoni R, Feys P, Jonsdottir J. Participation restriction in people with multiple sclerosis: prevalence and correlations with cognitive, walking, balance, and upper limb impairments. *Arch Phys Med Rehabil.* (2017) 98:1308–15. doi: 10.1016/j.apmr.2017.02.015
7. Mehrholz J, Pohl M, Platz T, Kugler J, Elsner B. Electromechanical and robot-assisted arm training for improving activities of daily living, arm function, and arm muscle strength after stroke. *Cochrane Database Syst Rev.* (2015) 9:CD006876. doi: 10.1002/14651858.CD006876.pub4
8. Lamers I, Maris A, Severijns D, Dielkens W, Geurts S, Van Wijmeersch B, et al. Upper limb rehabilitation in people with multiple sclerosis: a systematic review. *Neurorehabil Neural Repair* (2016) 30:773–93. doi: 10.1177/1545968315624785
9. Carpinella I, Cattaneo D, Bertoni R, Ferrarin M. Robot training of upper limb in multiple sclerosis: comparing protocols with or without manipulative task components. *IEEE Trans Neural Syst Rehabil Eng.* (2012) 20:351–60. doi: 10.1109/TNSRE.2012.2187462
10. Feys P, Coninx K, Kerkhofs L, De Weyer T, Truyens V, Maris A, et al. Robot-supported upper limb training in a virtual learning environment: a pilot

randomized controlled trial in persons with MS. *J Neuroeng Rehabil.* (2015) 12:60. doi: 10.1186/s12984-015-0043-3

11. Balasubramanian S, Klein J, Burdet E. Robot-assisted rehabilitation of hand function. *Curr Opin Neurol.* (2010) 23:661–70. doi: 10.1097/WCO.0b013e32833e99a4
12. Stein J, Bishop L, Gillen G, Helbok R. Robot-assisted exercise for hand weakness after stroke: a pilot study. *Am J Phys Med Rehabil.* (2011) 90:887–94. doi: 10.1097/PHM.0b013e3182328623
13. Kurtzke JF. Rating neurologic impairment in multiple sclerosis: an Expanded Disability Status Scale (EDSS). *Neurology* (1983) 33:1444–52. doi: 10.1212/WNL.33.11.1444
14. Folstein MF, Folstein SE, McHugh PR. "Minimental state". A practical method for grading the cognitive state of patients for the clinician. *J Psychiatr Res.* (1975) 12:189–98.
15. Bohannon RW, Smith MB. Interrater reliability of a modified Ashworth scale of muscle spasticity. *Phys Ther.* (1987) 67:206–7. doi: 10.1093/ptj/67.2.206
16. Kamm CP, Mattle HP, Müri RM, Heldner MR, Blatter V, Bartlome S, et al. Home-based training to improve manual dexterity in patients with multiple sclerosis: a randomized controlled trial. *Mult Scler.* (2015) 21:1546–56. doi: 10.1177/1352458514565959
17. Kalron A, Greenberg-Abrahami M, Gelav S, Achiron A. Effects of a new sensory re-education training tool on hand sensibility and manual dexterity in people with multiple sclerosis. *NeuroRehabilitation* (2013) 32:943–8. doi: 10.3233/NRE-130917
18. Bain PG, Findley LJ, Atchison P, Behari M, Vidailhet M, Gresty M, et al. Assessing tremor severity. *J Neurol Neurosurg Psychiatry* (1993) 56:868–73. doi: 10.1136/jnnp.56.8.868
19. Lyle RC. A performance test for assessment of upper limb function in physical rehabilitation treatment and research. *Int J Rehabil Res.* (1981) 4:483–92. doi: 10.1097/00004356-198112000-00001
20. Mathiowetz V, Weber K, Kashman N, Volland G. Adult norms for the nine hole Peg test of finger dexterity. The occupational therapy. *J Res.* (1985) 5:24–33. doi: 10.1177/153944928500500102
21. Lamers I, Kelchtermans S, Baert I, Feys P. Upper limb assessment in multiple sclerosis: a systematic review of outcome measures and their psychometric properties. *Arch Phys Med Rehabil.* (2014) 95:1184–200. doi: 10.1016/j.apmr.2014.02.023
22. Feys P, Lamers I, Francis G, Benedict R, Phillips G, LaRocca N, et al. Multiple sclerosis outcome assessments consortium. the nine-hole Peg test as a manual dexterity performance measure for multiple sclerosis. *Mult Scler.* (2017) 23:711–20. doi: 10.1177/1352458517690824
23. Sanford J, Moreland J, Swanson LR, Stratford PW, Gowland C. Reliability of the Fugl-Meyer assessment for testing motor performance in patients following stroke. *Phys Ther.* (1993) 73:447–54. doi: 10.1093/ptj/73.7.447
24. Bohannon RW. Motricity Index scores are valid indicators of paretic upper extremity strength following stroke. *J Phys Ther Sci.* (1999) 11:59–61. doi: 10.1589/jpts.11.59
25. Taub E, Miller NE, Novack TA, Cook EW III, Fleming WC, Nepomuceno CS, et al. Technique to improve chronic motor deficit after stroke. *Arch Phys Med Rehabil.* (1993) 74:347–54.
26. Vickrey BG, Hays RD, Harooni R, Myers LW, Ellison GW. A health-related quality of life measure for multiple sclerosis. *Qual Life Res.* (1995) 4:187–206. doi: 10.1007/BF02260859
27. Fougeyrollas P, Noreau L, Bergeron H, Cloutier R, Dion SA, St-Michel G. Social consequences of long term impairments and disabilities: conceptual approach and assessment of handicap. *Int J Rehabil Res.* (1998) 21:127–41. doi: 10.1097/00004356-199806000-00002
28. Konrad P. *The ABC of EMG: A Practical Introduction to Kinesiological Electromyography.* Scottsdale, AZ (2006).
29. Hoonhorst MH, Nijland RH, van den Berg JS, Emmelot CH, Kollen BJ, Kwakkel G. How do Fugl-Meyer arm motor scores relate to dexterity according to the Action Research Arm Test at 6 months poststroke? *Arch Phys Med Rehabil.* (2015) 96:1845–9. doi: 10.1016/j.apmr.2015.06.009
30. Vergaro E, Squeri V, Brichetto G, Casadio M, Morasso P, Solaro C, et al. Adaptive robot training for the treatment of incoordination in Multiple Sclerosis. *J Neuroeng Rehabil.* (2010) 7:37. doi: 10.1186/1743-0003-7-37
31. Wolf SL, Winstein CJ, Miller JP, Taub E, Uswatte G, Morris D, et al. EXCITE investigators. Effect of constraint-induced movement therapy on upper extremity function 3 to 9 months after stroke: the EXCITE randomized clinical trial. *JAMA* (2006) 296:2095–104. doi: 10.1001/jama.296.17.2095
32. Smania N, Gandolfi M, Paolucci S, Iosa M, Ianes P, Recchia S, et al. Reduced-intensity modified constraint-induced movement therapy versus conventional therapy for upper extremity rehabilitation after stroke: a multicenter trial. *Neurorehabil Neural Repair* (2012) 26:1035–45. doi: 10.1177/1545968312446003
33. Mark VW, Taub E, Bashir K, Uswatte G, Delgado A, Bowman MH, et al. Constraint-Induced Movement therapy can improve hemiparetic progressive multiple sclerosis. Preliminary findings. *Mult Scler.* (2008) 14:992–4. doi: 10.1177/1352458508090223
34. Ysrraelit MC, Fiol MP, Gaitán MI, Correale J. Quality of life assessment in multiple sclerosis: different perception between patients and neurologists. *Front Neurol.* (2018) 8:729. doi: 10.3389/fneur.2017.00729
35. Pellegrino L, Stranieri G, Tiragallo E, Tacchino A, Brichetto G, Coscia M, et al. Analysis of upper limb movement in multiple sclerosis subjects during common daily actions. In: *Engineering in Medicine and Biology Society (EMBC), Procedings of the 37th Annual International Conference of the IEEE,* Milan: IEEE (2015) Aug 25–29, paper no. 15585597.

18

The Games for Older Adults Active Life (GOAL) Project for People with Mild Cognitive Impairment and Vascular Cognitive Impairment

Laura Fabbri, Irene Eleonora Mosca, Filippo Gerli, Leonardo Martini, Silvia Pancani, Giulia Lucidi, Federica Savazzi, Francesca Baglio, Federica Vannetti, Claudio Macchi and The GOAL Working Group*

IRCCS Fondazione Don Carlo Gnocchi, Milan, Italy

Correspondence:
Federica Vannetti
fvannetti@dongnocchi.it

Background: People living with Mild Cognitive Impairment (MCI) and Vascular Cognitive Impairment (VCI) are persons who do not fulfill a diagnosis of dementia, but who have a high risk of progressing to a dementia disorder. The most recent guidelines to counteract cognitive decline in MCI/VCI subjects suggest a multidimensional and multi-domain interventions combining cognitive, physical, and social activities. The purpose of this study is to test an innovative service that provides a multi-dimensional tele-rehabilitation program through a user-friendly web application. The latter has been developed through a participatory design involving MCI specialists, patients, and their caregivers. Particularly, the proposed tele-rehabilitation program includes cognitive, physical, and caregiver-supported social activities. The goal is to promote and preserve an active life style and counteract cognitive decline in people living with MCI/VCI.

Methods: The study is a randomized controlled trial. Sixty subjects will be randomly assigned to the experimental group, who will receive the tele-rehabilitation program, or the control group, who will not receive any treatment. The trial protocol comprises three steps of assessment for the experimental group: at the baseline (T_0), after tele-rehabilitation program (T_1) and at follow-up after 12-months (T_2). Differently, the control group will be assessed twice: at the baseline and at 12-months follow-up. Both the experimental and the control group will be assessed with a multidimensional evaluation battery, including cognitive functioning, behavioral, functional, and quality of life measures. The tele-rehabilitation program lasts 8 weeks and includes cognitive exercises 3 days a week, physical activities 2 days a week, and social activities once a week. In addition, group will be given an actigraph (GENEActiv, Activisinghts Ltd., Cambridgshire, UK) to track physical and sleep activity.

Discussion: Results of this study will inform on the efficacy of the proposed tele-rehabilitation to prevent or delay further cognitive decline in MCI/VCI subjects. The expected outcome is to counteract cognitive decline and improve both physical functioning and quality of life.

Ethics and Dissemination: The study is approved by the Local Ethics Committee and registered in https://clinicaltrials.gov (NCT03383549). Dissemination will include submission to a peer-reviewed journal, patients, and healthcare magazines and congress presentations.

Keywords: mild cognitive impairment, vascular cognitive impairment, cognitive training, tele-rehabilitation, web application

INTRODUCTION

Cognitive aging can be successful or lead to impairment depending on the interplay of a manifold of influencing factors. Among these factors, we can count genetic markers, cardiovascular status, neural functional plasticity mechanisms, as well as social, cognitive, and psychological status (1). Within unsuccessful aging paths, the balance between these factors orients toward Mild Cognitive Impairment (MCI) or Vascular Cognitive Impairment (VCI). Mild cognitive impairment (MCI) is a syndrome defined as a cognitive decline which is greater than expected for individual's age and education level but that does not interfere notably with activities of daily life (2). Since his definition in 1999 (3), MCI has been considered the transitional status between normal aging and the diagnosis of a mild dementia (4). MCI is consistently shown to have a high risk of progression to dementia (2, 5) and a pronounced risk of disability and loss of autonomy (6, 7). In addition, cerebrovascular disease that causes brain infarctions becomes more common with advancing age and represents a risk factor for the further development of vascular dementia (8, 9). The construct of VCI, a high-risk phenotype for the development of vascular dementia, has been introduced to capture the entire spectrum of cognitive disorders associated with all forms of cerebral vascular brain injury. There is evidence that about one third of dementia cases globally are attributable to potentially modifiable risk factors that include different daily habits (10, 11). Furthermore, in the study of successful aging compared to the pathological one, the fundamental role that the environment plays in counteracting cognitive decline through the activation of neuro-plasticity mechanisms for the recovery of alternative pathways has been demonstrated (12). Within a holistic framework, the adoption of an appropriate habits alongside cognitive training and enhancement activities can therefore activate brain compensation mechanisms to tackle the physiological and pathological neurodegeneration processes of the elderly, keeping the cognitive level high. On the one hand, there is rising evidence that cognitive training programs are effective in improving or at least maintaining cognitive performance and slowing the progression from MCI or VCI to mild dementia (13, 14). On the other hand, the importance of an intervention that takes into account, beside cognition, also of motor aspects in pre-clinical conditions and in the early stages of dementia has been highlighted (15). To maintain physical abilities and counteract the damage caused by the general physiological decline in the elderly, the adapted physical activity (APA) program has been recognized as an effective tool (16). Furthermore, from a holistic point of view, although social stimulation is often neglected in interventions, recent studies observed that being engaged in social activities represents a protective factor against cognitive decline (17). Therefore, promoting support from the caregivers in social activity participation has been recommended to retain the present abilities and sense of well-being in the persons with cognitive impairment (18). In line with this perspective, the most recent guidelines for the management of MCI/VCI suggest the importance of promoting multidimensional and multi-domain interventions. A multi-dimensional training program integrates different activities, such as the physical and the cognitive one. In addition, the latter could be multi-domains, including exercises that stimulate multiple cognitive domains (i.e., memory, attention, processing speed) (3, 7, 19). Finally, there is evidence that mental, physical, and social stimulation activities equally contribute to decrease dementia risk (20). How to include these activities in a feasible and sustainable rehabilitation service and how to deliver the latter to people living with MCI/VCI, still remains a debated issue. The advancement in technology has enhanced the possibility to provide remote tele-rehabilitation services through low-cost devices, that can ensure continuity of care and can easily reach people living in geographical remote areas. In fact, this kind of services supplies distant support, information exchange between patients and their clinical providers and promotes the administration of multi-dimensional activity programs (21, 22). The lack of familiarity with the technologic devices may constitute a limit to the implementation of technology enhanced services to supply a home-based tele-rehabilitation in people with advanced age or early cognitive impairment (23). For this reason, the development of an accessible service represents a design priority. The use of a participatory co-design process that follows an iterative development model might help in overcoming this limitation (24). The main aim of the proposed trial is to test the performance of a multi-dimensional tele-rehabilitation customized program, which contents are available by a user-friendly web application developed through a participatory design (involving patients, clinicians, technicians, and caregivers). The presented study would investigate whether subjects living with MCI/VCI condition participating in the tele-rehabilitation program will show improvements in cognition, quality of life, adherence, and engagement in the program with respect to subjects living with MCI/VCI condition of the control group.

METHODS AND ANALYSIS

Study Design

The proposed study is a randomized controlled clinical trial. A Consolidated Standards of Reporting Trials (CONSORT) flow diagram for enrollment and randomization in the GOAL study is showed in **Figure 1**. Subjects that, at the first screening will be deemed as eligible, according to the inclusion criteria, will undergo a baseline assessment (T_0). During the baseline a general cognitive and physical evaluation will be performed by using the scales, tests and questionnaires reported in the Participant's evaluation sub-paragraph. Participants will be then randomly assigned, through the use of a computer algorithm (http://www.graphpad.com/quikcalcs/randMenu/) to the control or treatment group. The tele-rehabilitation program will comprise the performing of cognitive exercises 3 days a week, APA activities 2 days a week, and social activities once a week. In addition, treatment group will be given an actigraph (GENEActiv, Activisinghts Ltd., Cambridgeshire, UK) to track physical and sleep activity. Those subjects will undergo a post-training assessment immediately at the end of the tele-rehabilitation program (T_1) and after 12 months (T_2). Participants belonging to the control group will be evaluated only at T_2.

Eligibility Criteria/Participants

Participants will be recruited from the Memory Clinic of University Hospital of Careggi (Florence, Italy), and the Don Carlo Gnocchi Foundation (Florence, Italy). Inclusion criteria

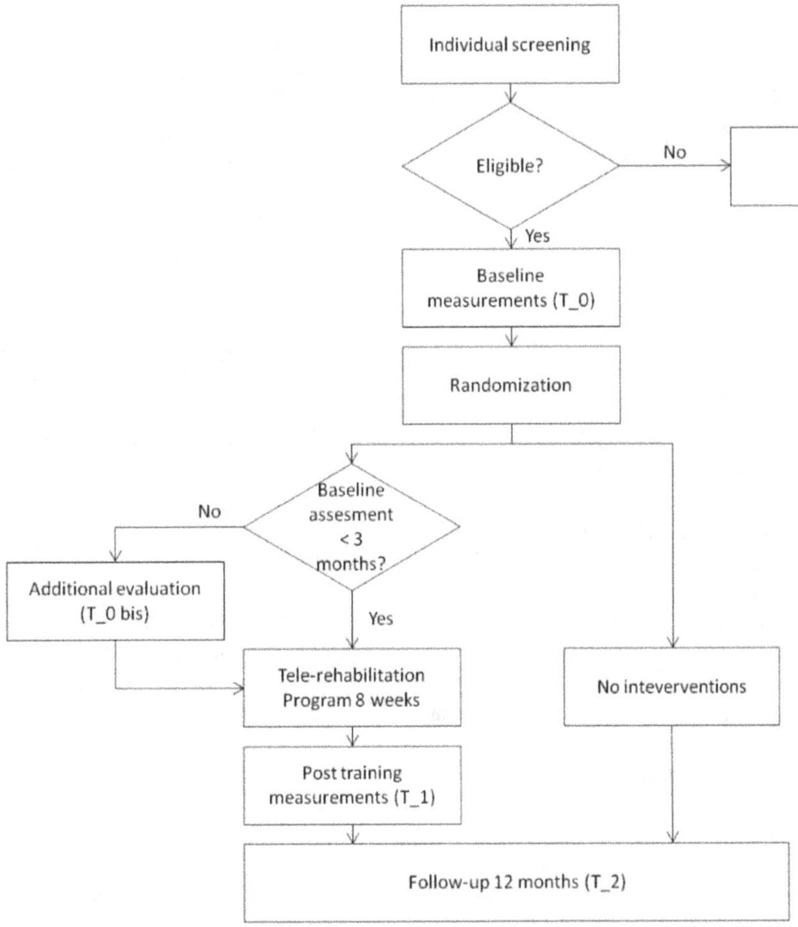

FIGURE 1 | CONSORT flow diagram. Consolidated Standards of Reporting Trials (CONSORT) flow diagram for enrollment and randomization GOAL study.

TABLE 1 | Criteria for MCI/VCI classification.

MCI due to AD	VCI
• Hachinski ischemic score ≤4 • Exclusion of other dementia-causes with cerebral TC or MRI • Fazekas score <2 • Biomarkers of neuronal injury (Rate of brain and hippocampal atrophy, FDG-PET imaging or CSF tau/phosphorylated-tau) OR • Biomarker of β amyloid deposition (CSF Ab42 ore PET amyloid imaging) compatible with MCI due to AD	• Hachinski ischemic score >4 • Fazekas score ≥2 • MRI or TC evidence of (one or more): - Multiple white matter lesions compatible with small vessel disease - Lacunar state - One or more ischemic lesions in strategic areas

will be the following: (a) diagnosis of MCI due to Alzheimer's Disease (AD), according to "Research Clinical Criteria" (25) or diagnosis of Vascular cognitive impairment (VCI) according to the harmonization standards from National Institute for Neurological Disorders and Stroke and the Canadian Stroke Network (8) (**Table 1**); (b) Mini Mental State Examination (MMSE) ≥24 (26); (c) aged 65–80 years old; (d) school attendance ≥3 years (to avoid both cultural bias and limits due to the neuropsychological instruments used); (e) right-handed according to the Edinburgh Scale (27). Exclusion criteria will be: (a) severe auditory and/or visual loss; (b) severe behavioral/psychiatric disturbances; (c) actual or anamnestic substance abuse disorder; (d) cognitive disturbances secondary to an acute or general medical disorders (e) stable medication of the following pharmacological treatments: cholinesterase inhibitor, memantine, antidepressant, or antipsychotic drugs.

Participants' Evaluation

Participants will be assessed through an extensive evaluation including cognitive functioning, behavioral, functional and perceived quality of life measures with the following tests (**Table 2**):

- The Montreal cognitive assessment [MoCA; (28)], which represents a sensitive tool in persons with MCI for a general cognitive assessment;
- The Digit span and the Corsi span tasks (backward and forward) (29), to assess both verbal and visuo-spatial short-term memory and working memory;
- The Free and Cued Selective Reminding Test [FCSRT; (30)] - Delayed Free Recall (DFR) and Immediate Free Recall (IFR) for verbal episodic memory evaluation;
- The Rey Complex Figure Test, copy and delayed recall [RCFT; (31)], to evaluate constructional skills, visuographic memory and some aspects of planning and executive function;
- The modified card sorting Test, short version [MCST; (32)] for the assessment of executive functions;
- The Trail Making Test [TMT; (33)] for the assessment of attention and -executive functions;
- The Stroop test, short version (34), to assess selective attention, cognitive flexibility and sensitivity to interference;
- The Semantic and Fonemic fluencies (35, 36) or the assessment of language skills;
- The Activities of Daily Living Inventory [ADCS/ADL; (37)] to assess patient's performance in the basic and instrumental activities of daily living.
- The center for Epidemiological Studies Depression scale [CES-D; (38)] to evaluate both the presence and the entity of depressive symptoms;
- The 36-Item Short Form Survey [SF-36; (39)] to assess the subjective perceived quality of live;
- The cognitive Reserve Index questionnaire [CRIq; (40)] for the evaluation of the cognitive reserve;
- The Short physical performance battery [SPPB; (41)], to measure functional status and physical performance;
- The Harvard Alumni Activity Survey [HAAS; (42)], to assess physical activity level;
- The International Physical Activity Questionnaire – Short Form [IPAQ; (43)], for health related physical activity evaluation.

Tele-Rehabilitation Program

On the basis of literature, the present protocol is designed aiming at affecting patients' on different domains in line with a holistic approach to promote well-being: cognition, motor skills, and social environment. The cognitive module integrates a collection of brain training exercises from BrainHQ, a third-party platform developed by Posit Science, that makes available Serious Games (SGs) for multidomain stimulation. The proposed SGs are adaptive type, i.e., the difficulty varies in relation to the user performance and becomes more demanding through both reductions in stimulus display duration and increases in task complexity. Difficulty is maintained immediately over the user comfort threshold, which according to several studies, efficaciously stimulates the neural plasticity (44–46). Cognitive activities are meant to reinforce attention, brain speed, memory, people skills, intelligence, and navigation. The physical module includes a training program of APA exercises (16), delivered through a guided video. Regular participation in an APA exercise program has been previously associated with improved self-rated health and improved mood (47). The proposed exercises aim to train trunk, upper, and lower limbs and are designed to require only: a chair, a gym-stick, two small bottles of water and a resistance band, to be performed. Each module comprises a warming-up, a strengthening and a stretching session, with a level of difficulty (basic and advanced) adjusted according to participants' training level and physical capabilities (e.g., participants with reduced ability in mobilizing the upper limbs may have a customized program comprising advanced/basic exercises only for the lower limbs and vice versa). Social level is addressed with the involvement of caregivers and patients in some leisure activities. The caregiver module includes suggestions of social activities to be carried out with the caregiver during the weekend, such as watching a movie, gardening, cooking etc. At the beginning and at the end of daily activity, participants are asked to fill a questionnaire on their self-perceived physical/emotional status.

TABLE 2 | Evaluation battery during the proposed trial.

Outcome measures	*T_0*	*T_1*	*T_2*
PRIMARY OUTCOME:			
General cognitive assessment	✓	✓	✓
• Montreal cognitive assessment (MoCA) (28)			
Memory	✓		✓
• The Digit span and the Corsi span tasks (backward and forward) (29)			
• Free and Cued Selective Reminding Test (FCSRT) (30)	✓		✓
• Recall of rey's figure (31)	✓	✓	✓
Attention and executive functions	✓		✓
• The modified card sorting Test, short version (MCST) (32)			
• The Trial Making Test (TMT) (33)	✓		✓
• Stroop test, short version (34)	✓	✓	✓
Visuospatial/constructional ability	✓	✓	✓
• Copy of rey's figure (31)			
Language	✓	✓	✓
• Semantic fluency (35)			
• Fonemic fluency (36)	✓	✓	✓
SECONDARY OUTCOMES:			
Activities of daily living inventory	✓	✓	✓
• The Activities of Daily Living Inventory (ADCS-ADL) (37)			
Depression symptoms	✓	✓	✓
• The center for Epidemiological Studies Depression scale (CES-D) (38)			
Health status	✓		✓
• The 36-Item Short Form Survey (SF-36) (39)			
Cognitive reserve	✓		
• The cognitive Reserve Index questionnaire (CRIq) (40)			
Physical activity level	✓	✓	✓
• The short Physcal performance battery (SPPB) (41)			
• The Harvard Alumni Activity Survey (HAAS) (42)	✓		✓
• The International Physical Activity Questionnaire (IPAQ) (43)	✓		✓

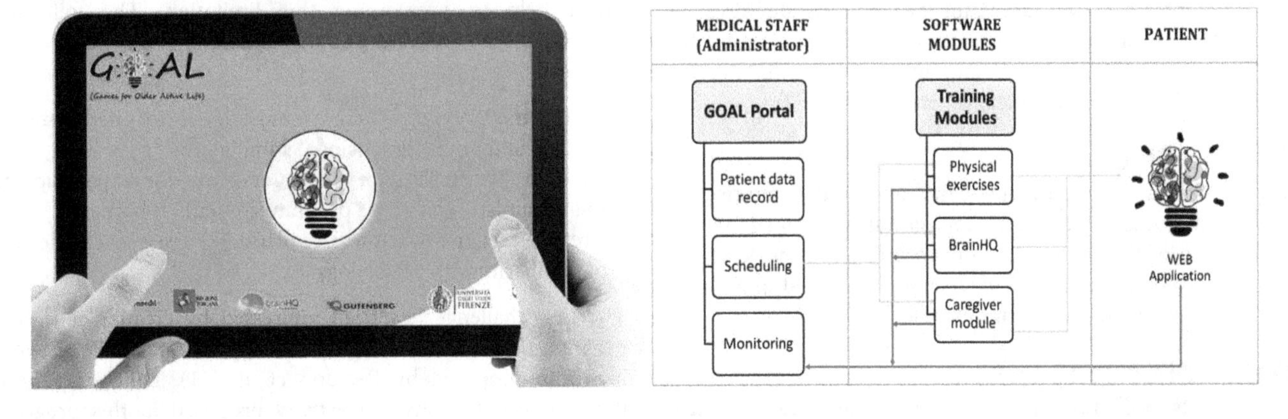

FIGURE 2 | WebApp interface and its functional architecture.

GOAL-App Architecture

A web-application, named GOAL-App, has been specifically designed to implement a weekly tele-rehabilitation program consisting of combined cognitive, physical and social activities (to be performed with the caregiver), according to the clinician indications. Scheduling and monitoring of activities are accessible by the GOAL-App administrator (**Figure 2**). Each activity is implemented in the three independent modules on cognition, motor skills and social level. The first realized web-app prototype was developed further through a series of design and feedback loops with MCI specialists, patients living with MCI and VCI and their caregivers. Thanks to this participatory design the following critical aspects emerged and were addressed:

- The need for a full screen interface with a few number of large buttons;
- The possibility to pause the physical module to take breaks during the exercises, if needed;
- The need for a user-manual and a Support Service Center for technical problems.

Patients, provided with a tablet, will access the final version of the tele-rehabilitation program through the GOAL-App. Before the beginning of the treatment, participants will be trained to use the tablet autonomously at their home. During the training sessions participants, with the support of their caregivers, will go through each module of the program, at least once, until they feel familiar with the use of the device. A mobile wifi router will be provided in case participants don't have access to internet connection. In addition, they will be given a kit, made up of a stick and a resistance band, to perform the physical exercises at home.

Outcomes Measures

As the aim of this program will be to involve the participants in multidimensional activities to counteract cognitive decline, the primary outcome of this study will be the changes of cognitive domains evaluated (such as general cognitive assessment, memory, attention, and executive functions, visuospatial/constructional ability, and language) of the whole sample through a comprehensive neuropsychological assessment at T_0 and at T_2 (see **Table 2** for a detailed list of the used neuropsychological tools). Together with the cognitive level, the following secondary outcomes will be evaluated in the whole sample at T_0 and T_2: independence, presence of depressive symptoms, quality of life and physical activity level through scales and actigraphic data (see **Table 2** for the used questionnaires). In addition, the primary and secondary outcomes will be evaluated in the treatment group before and after the tele-rehabilitation program using a reduced battery of tests (see **Table 2**).

Sample Size

Sample size has been estimated based on previous multicenter controlled studies (21, 48). Under the assumption of normal distribution of the primary outcome scores and considering an α level of 0.05, a sample size of 60 subjects resulted in a power >70% and was then chosen for this trial.

Data Collection

Assessments will take place at the Don Carlo Gnocchi Foundation (Florence, Italy). All assessors will receive proper instructions and guidance regarding all outcome parameters and assessments that will be taken. A reminder for each visit will be given to all patients to diminish retention and incomplete follow-up.

Data Management

Study data will be recorded in an access database. All participants will be registered with an identification code with a random order. Source data will include the original documents relating to the study, as well as the medical treatment and medical history of participant. The database will be kept current to reflect subject status at each phase during the course of the study.

Statistical Analyses

Statistical analysis on outcome measures will be conducted using SPSS version 24 (SPSS Inc, Chicago, IL). Baseline differences between groups will be tested by the independent-samples *t*-test for parametric data and the Mann-Whitney *U*-test for non-parametric data. According to data normality, a statistical test for independent samples will be performed to look at significant changes in primary and secondary outcome measures between control and treatment groups. Moreover, a statistical test for paired sample will be used to investigate the presence of significant changes in the treatment group cognitive and physical parameters before and after the tele-rehabilitation program. An alpha level of $\leq$0.05 will be considered as significant.

DISCUSSION AND CONCLUSIONS

In the context of cognitive decline, technologies have been increasingly conceived as a support for patients, their caregivers and the clinicians. The presented trial is claiming to provide MCI/VCI subjects together with their caregivers with an innovative customized tele-rehabilitation program, which contents are available by a user-friendly web application. However, the lack of familiarity with the technologic devices may constitute a limit to the implementation of technology enhanced services to supply a home-based tele-rehabilitation in people with advanced age or early cognitive impairment (23). For this reason, the use of a participatory co-design process that follows an iterative development model might help in overcoming this limitation. The following challenges to program implementation were successfully managed:

- Define the program contents most likely to offer a multi-domain and multi-dimensional stimulation;
- Develop a platform to enable the participants self-administration of the program contents at home;
- Create a user-friendly interface platform to ease a possible lack of familiarity with technology.

The first challenge has been addressed by creating a weekly program that combines cognitive and physical, similar to what has been proposed by Realdon et al. (21). Differently from their project, the physical activity proposed in this program is based on APA exercises and customized to the participant's training level and physical capability. In addition, this program promotes the participation of the subjects in social activities to be conducted with the support of the caregiver. The choice to include in the training program social activities originates from evidence in the literature showing the importance of social stimulation as protective factor against major cognitive decline (17, 49). The second challenge has been met by creating a web-app and providing participants with a tablet and an internet connection, if needed. The possibility to perform the exercises at home, will likely enhance participation in the program. Furthermore, the proposed tele-rehabilitation program leads to a significant reduction of costs compared to previously proposed trainings (50, 51), where participants attended a clinic and were supervised by medical staff. The third challenge has been dealt through a participatory co-design process, used to develop a platform shaped on the basis of user needs. The possible limitations of this study may stem from the restricted numbers of participants enrolled. A potential pitfall could be a drop-out of MCI, therefore the sample size will be increased. Data collection may be impacted by the adherence to the program, especially considering the age of participants, their compliance to the treatment and their medical condition. The monitoring of activity by the administrator is among the several strategies expected to help solve the possible problem of the adherence. However, a high adherence is expected due to the possibility to carry this out at home. To protect sensitive data that will be stored and processed through the web-application, all participants will be registered with an identification code with a random order. Another limitation could be a potential learning effect of neuropsychological instruments due to the timing of the project. This could be avoided by using parallel versions when possible and by a well-structured time scheduling. Some symptoms of apathy, a predictive factor of AD progression (52, 53), are indirectly tested by registering daytime motor activity with actigraphic measures (54, 55). Direct specific measures of apathy cannot be used because of administration issues. The next step is to test the proposed program on subjects living with MCI and VCI condition through the presented trial. The expectation is to counteract cognitive decline, improve physical functioning and quality of life.

ETHICS AND DISSEMINATION

The study will be carried out in compliance with the protocol approved by the previously mentioned ethical committee. A written informed consent will be given to each participant (**Appendix A** in Supplementary Material). The trial is registered at https://clinicaltrials.gov, unique identifier NCT03383549 (registration date: 26/dec/2017). Potentially eligible participants will be screened by the study site principal or sub-investigator for the confirmation of a diagnosis of MCI due to AD or VCI, with a MMSE score $\geq$24 (26), an age between 65 and 80 years old, a school attendance $\geq$3 years and with a right-dominant hand. Additionally, potential participants will be questioned and their medical record will be checked in regard to the other eligibility criteria. Given eligibility to take part in the study, they will be provided with further details and an informed consent form by one of the study members. The model consent form and other related documentation given to participants (all in Italian) can be obtained by the corresponding author upon request. The study clinicians will be responsible to explain and make sure the protocol is correctly understood by participants. A separate list with patients screened, but who are not enrolled will contain information regarding the number of patients and the reasons for not enrolling. In order to provide an equal and ethic treatment to all participants, the control group will receive the proposed program at a later date. All anonymized data will be stored in a secure database protected by a password. Only the research team will have access to the database. After the statistical analysis of this trial, the data will be published in a peer-reviewed medical journal, thereby adhering to the CONSORT reporting standards (56) and SPIRIT guidelines (57). The results will be disseminated through peer-reviewed publications, presentation at relevant scientific conferences and the general public.

AUTHOR CONTRIBUTIONS

LF, IEM, GL, FS, FB, FV, and CM developed the original concept of the trial. LF, FS, FB, FV, and CM drafted the original protocol. LF, IEM, FG, LM, SP, GL, FS, FB, FV, GWG, and CM developed the design. LF, GL, FS, FB, GWG, and CM developed the methodology. LF, IEM, FS, FB, FV, and CM developed the analysis plan. LF, IEM, FG, LM, FB, FV, and CM adapted the trial proposal as a protocol paper. LF, IEM, SP, FV, and CM did manuscript writing. All authors reviewed and commented on drafts of the protocol and paper. All authors read and approved the final manuscript.

GOAL WORKING GROUP

Sandro Sorbi, Camilla Ferrari, Gemma Lombardi: Università degli Studi di Firenze, NEUROFARBA, Firenze, Italy; **Andrea Stoppini, Stefania Pazzi, Tommaso Migliazza:** Consorzio di Bioingegneria e Informatica medica - CBIM, Pavia, Italy.

ACKNOWLEDGMENTS

We acknowledge the support of BANDO FAS SALUTE funding program.

REFERENCES

1. Reuter-Lorenz PA, Park DC. How does it STAC up? Revisiting the scaffolding theory of aging and cognition. *Neuropsychol Rev.* (2014) 24:355–70. doi: 10.1007/s11065-014-9270-9
2. Gauthier S, Reisberg B, Zaudig M, Petersen RC, Ritchie K, Broich K, et al. Mild cognitive impairment. *Lancet* (2006) 367:1262–70. doi: 10.1016/S0140-6736(06)68542-5
3. Petersen RC, Smith GE, Waring SC, Ivnik RJ, Tangalos EG, Kokmen E. Mild cognitive impairment: clinical characterization and outcome. *Arch Neurol.* (1999) 56:303–8. doi: 10.1001/archneur.56.3.303
4. Petersen RC. Mild cognitive impairment as a diagnostic entity. *J Intern Med.* (2004) 256:183–94. doi: 10.1111/j.1365-2796.2004.01388.x
5. Petersen RC, Lopez O, Armstrong MJ, Getchius TS, Ganguli M, Gloss D, et al. Practice guideline update summary: mild cognitive impairment: report of the guideline development, dissemination, and implementation Subcommittee of the American Academy of Neurology. *Neurology* (2018) 90:126–35. doi: 10.1212/WNL.0000000000004826
6. Petersen RC, Caracciolo B, Brayne C, Gauthier S, Jelic V, Fratiglioni L. Mild cognitive impairment: a concept in evolution. *J Intern Med.* (2014) 275:214–28. doi: 10.1111/joim.12190
7. Bruderer-Hofstetter M, Rausch-Osthoff AK, Meichtry A, Münzer T, Niedermann K. Effective multicomponent interventions in comparison to

active control and no interventions on physical capacity, cognitive function and instrumental activities of daily living in elderly people with and without mild impaired cognition–a systematic review and network meta-analysis. *Ageing Res Rev.* (2018) 45:1–14. doi: 10.1016/j.arr.2018.04.002
8. Hachinski V, Iadecola C, Petersen RC, Breteler MM, Nyenhuis DL, Black SE, et al. National institute of neurological disorders and stroke-canadian stroke network vascular cognitive impairment harmonization standards. *Stroke J Cereb Circ.* (2006) 37:2220–41. doi: 10.1161/01.STR.0000237236.88823.47
9. Gorelick PB, Scuteri A, Black SE, DeCarli C, Greenberg SM, Iadecola C, et al. Vascular contributions to cognitive impairment and dementia: a statement for healthcare professionals from the American Heart Association/American Stroke Association. Stroke *J Cereb Circ.* (2011) 42:2672–713. doi: 10.1161/STR.0b013e3182299496
10. Norton S, Matthews FE, Barnes DE, Yaffe K, Brayne C. Potential for primary prevention of Alzheimer's disease: an analysis of population-based data. *Lancet Neurol.* (2014) 13:788–94. doi: 10.1016/S1474-4422(14)70136-X
11. Livingston G, Sommerlad A, Orgeta V, Costafreda SG, Huntley J, Ames D, et al. Dementia prevention, intervention, and care. *Lancet* (2017) 390:2673–734. doi: 10.1016/S0140-6736(17)31363-6
12. Vance DE, Kaur J, Fazeli PL, Talley MH, Yuen HK, Kitchin B, et al. Neuroplasticity and successful cognitive aging: a brief overview for nursing. *J Neurosci Nurs.* (2012) 44:218–27. doi: 10.1097/JNN.0b013e3182527571
13. Gates N, Valenzuela M. Cognitive exercise and its role in cognitive function in older adults. *Curr Psychiatry Rep.* (2010) 12:20–7. doi: 10.1007/s11920-009-0085-y
14. Woods B, Aguirre E, Spector AE, Orrell M. Cognitive stimulation to improve cognitive functioning in people with dementia. *Cochrane Database Syst Rev.* (2012) 15:CD005562. doi: 10.1002/14651858.CD005562.pub2
15. Grande G, Vanacore N, Maggiore L, Cucumo V, Ghiretti R, Galimberti D, et al. Physical activity reduces the risk of dementia in mild cognitive impairment subjects: a cohort study. *J Alzheimers Dis.* (2014) 39:833–9. doi: 10.3233/JAD-131808
16. Macchi C. *Theory and Technique of Physical Activity Adult -Elder.* Firenze: Master Books (2012). p. 15–40.
17. Yaffe K, Fiocco AJ, Lindquist K, Vittinghoff E, Simonsick EM, Newman AB, et al. Predictors of maintaining cognitive function in older adults The Health ABC Study. *Neurology* (2009) 72:2029–35. doi: 10.1212/WNL.0b013e3181a92c36
18. Vikström S, Josephsson S, Stigsdotter-Neely A, Nygård L. Engagement in activities: experiences of persons with dementia and their caregiving spouses. *Dementia* (2008) 7:251–70. doi: 10.1177/1471301208091164
19. Karssemeijer EGA, Aaronson JA, Bossers WJ, Smits T, Olde Rikkert MGM, Kessels RPC. Positive effects of combined cognitive and physical exercise training on cognitive function in older adults with mild cognitive impairment or dementia: a meta-analysis. *Ageing Res Rev.* (2017) 40:75–83. doi: 10.1016/j.arr.2017.09.003
20. Gates N, Valenzuela M, Sachdev PS, Singh MAF. Psychological well-being in individuals with mild cognitive impairment. *Clin Interv Aging* (2014) 9:779–92. doi: 10.2147/CIA.S58866
21. Realdon O, Rossetto F, Nalin M, Baroni I, Cabinio M, Fioravanti R, et al. Technology-enhanced multi-domain at home continuum of care program with respect to usual care for people with cognitive impairment: the Ability-TelerehABILITation study protocol for a randomized controlled trial. *BMC Psychiatry* (2016) 16:425. doi: 10.1186/s12888-016-1132-y
22. Alloni A, Sinforiani E, Zucchella C, Sandrini G, Bernini S, Cattani B, et al. Computer-based cognitive rehabilitation: the CoRe system. *Disabil Rehabil.* (2017) 39:407–17. doi: 10.3109/09638288.2015.1096969
23. Richardson M, Zorn TE, Weaver CK. *Senior's Perspectives on the Barriers, Benefits and Negatives Consequences of Learning and Using Computers.* Department of Management Communication, University of Waikato (2002).
24. Mayer JM, Zach J. Lessons learned from participatory design with and for people with dementia. In: *Proceedings of the 15th International Conference on Human-Computer Interaction With Mobile Devices and Services.* New York, NY: ACM (2013). p. 540–5.
25. Albert MS, DeKosky ST, Dickson D, Dubois B, Feldman HH, Fox NC, et al. The diagnosis of mild cognitive impairment due to Alzheimer's disease: recommendations from the National Institute on Aging-Alzheimer's Association workgroups on diagnostic guidelines for Alzheimer's disease. *Alzheimer's Dement.* (2011) 7:270–9. doi: 10.1016/j.jalz.2011.03.008
26. Magni E, Binetti G, Bianchetti A, Rozzini R, Trabucchi M. Mini-mental state examination: a normative study in Italian elderly population. *Eur J Neurol.* (1996) 3:198–202. doi: 10.1111/j.1468-1331.1996.tb00423.x
27. Oldfield RC. The assessment and analysis of handedness: the Edinburgh inventory. *Neuropsychologia* (1971) 9:97–113. doi: 10.1016/0028-3932(71)90067-4
28. Conti S, Bonazzi S, Laiacona M, Masina M, Coralli MV. Montreal Cognitive Assessment (MoCA)-Italian version: regression based norms and equivalent scores. *Neurol Sci.* (2015) 36:209–14. doi: 10.1007/s10072-014-1921-3
29. Monaco M, Costa A, Caltagirone C, Carlesimo GA. Forward and backward span for verbal and visuo-spatial data: standardization and normative data from an Italian adult population. *Neurol Sci.* (2013) 34:749–54. doi: 10.1007/s10072-012-1130-x
30. Frasson P, Ghiretti R, Catricalà E, Pomati S, Marcone A, Parisi L. et al. Free and cued selective reminding test: an Italian normative study. *Neurol Sci.* (2011) 32:1057–62. doi: 10.1007/s10072-011-0607-3
31. Caffarra P, Vezzadini G, Dieci F, Zonato F, Venneri A. Rey-Osterrieth complex figure: normative values in an Italian population sample. *Neurol Sci.* (2002) 22:443–7. doi: 10.1007/s100720200003
32. Caffarra P, Vezzadini G, Dieci F, Zonato F, Venneri A. Modified card sorting test: normative data. *J Clin Exp Neuropsychol.* (2004) 26:246–50. doi: 10.1076/jcen.26.2.246.28087
33. Giovagnoli AR, Del Pesce M, Mascheroni S, Simoncelli M, Laiacona M, Capitani E. Trail making test: normative values from 287 normal adult controls. *Ital J Neurol Sci.* (1996) 17:305–9. doi: 10.1007/BF01997792
34. Caffarra P, Vezzadini G, Dieci F, Zonato F, Venneri A. Una versione abbreviata del test di Stroop: dati normativi nella popolazione italiana. *Nuova Riv Neurol.* (2002) 12:111–5.
35. Novelli G, Papagno C, Capitani E, Laiacona M. Tre test clinici di ricerca e produzione lessicale. Taratura su sogetti normali. *Archivio di psicologia, Neurologia e Psichiatria* (1986).
36. Carlesimo GA, Caltagirone C, Gainotti G, Fadda L, Gallassi R, Lorusso S, et al. The mental deterioration battery: normative data, diagnostic reliability and qualitative analyses of cognitive impairment. *Eur Neurol.* (1996) 36:378–84. doi: 10.1159/000117297
37. Galasko D, Bennett D, Sano M, Ernesto C, Thomas R, Grundman M, Ferris S. An inventory to assess activities of daily living for clinical trials in Alzheimer's disease. *Alzheimer Dis Assoc Disord.* (1997). doi: 10.1007/978-1-4612-4116-4_62
38. Radloff LS. The CES-D scale: a self-report depression scale for research in the general population. *Appl Psychol Meas.* (1977) 1:385–401. doi: 10.1177/014662167700100306
39. Apolone G, Mosconi P. The Italian SF-36 Health Survey: translation, validation and norming. *J Clin Epidemiol.* (1998) 51:1025–36. doi: 10.1016/S0895-4356(98)00094-8
40. Nucci M, Mapelli D, Mondini S. Cognitive Reserve Index questionnaire (CRIq): a new instrument for measuring cognitive reserve. *Aging Clin Exp Res.* (2012) 24:218–26.
41. Guralnik JM, Simonsick EM, Ferrucci L, Glynn RJ, Berkman LF, Blazer DG, et al. A short physical performance battery assessing lower extremity function: association with self-reported disability and prediction of mortality and nursing home admission. *J Gerontol.* (1994) 49:M85–94. doi: 10.1093/geronj/49.2.M85
42. Paffenbarger RS Jr, Wing AL, Hyde RT. Physical activity as an index of heart attack risk in college alumni. *Am J Epidemiol.* (1978) 108:161–75. doi: 10.1093/oxfordjournals.aje.a112608
43. Mannocci A, Di Thiene D, Del Cimmuto A, Masala D, Boccia A, De Vito E, et al. International Physical Activity Questionnaire: validation and assessment in an Italian sample. *Ital J Public Health* (2012) 7.
44. Lumsden J, Edwards EA, Lawrence NS, Coyle D, Munafò MR. Gamification of cognitive assessment and cognitive training: a systematic review of applications and efficacy. *JMIR Serious Games* (2016) 4:e11. doi: 10.2196/games.5888
45. Smith-Ray RL, Irmiter C, Boulter K. Cognitive training among cognitively impaired older adults: a feasibility study assessing the potential improvement in balance. *Front Public Health* (2016) 4:219. doi: 10.3389/fpubh.2016.00219

46. Li H, Li J, Li N, Li B, Wang P, Zhou T. Cognitive intervention for persons with mild cognitive impairment: a meta-analysis. *Ageing Res Rev.* (2011) 10:285–96. doi: 10.1016/j.arr.2010.11.003
47. Hicks GE, Benvenuti F, Fiaschi V, Lombardi B, Segenni L, Stuart M, et al. Adherence to a community-based exercise program is a strong predictor of improved back pain status in older adults: an observational study. *Clin J Pain* (2012) 28:195–203. doi: 10.1097/AJP.0b013e318226c411
48. Farina E, Mantovani F, Fioravanti R, Rotella G, Villanelli F, Imbornone E, et al. Efficacy of recreational and occupational activities associated to psychologic support in mild to moderate Alzheimer disease: a multicenter controlled study. *Alzheimer Dis Assoc Disord.* (2006) 20:275–82. doi: 10.1097/01.wad.0000213846.66742.90
49. Karp A, Paillard-Borg S, Wang HX, Silverstein M, Winblad B, Fratiglioni L. Mental, physical and social components in leisure activities equally contribute to decrease dementia risk. *Dement Geriatr Cogn Disord.* (2006) 21:65–73. doi: 10.1159/000089919
50. Singh MAF, Gates N, Saigal N, Wilson GC, Meiklejohn J, Brodaty H, Baker MK. The Study of Mental and Resistance Training (SMART) study—resistance training and/or cognitive training in mild cognitive impairment: a randomized, double-blind, double-sham controlled trial. *J Am Med Direct Assoc.* (2014) 15:873–80. doi: 10.1016/j.jamda.2014.09.010
51. Maffei L, Picano E, Andreassi MG, Angelucci A, Baldacci F, Baroncelli L, et al. Randomized trial on the effects of a combined physical/cognitive training in aged MCI subjects: the Train the Brain study. *Sci Rep.* (2017) 7:39471. doi: 10.1038/srep39471
52. Palmer K, Di Iulio F, Varsi AE, Gianni W, Sancesario G, Caltagirone C, et al. Neuropsychiatric predictors of progression from amnestic-mild cognitive impairment to Alzheimer's disease: the role of depression and apathy. *J Alzheimers Dis.* (2010) 20:175–83. doi: 10.3233/JAD-2010-1352
53. Di Iulio F, Palmer K, Blundo C, Casini AR, Gianni W, Caltagirone C, et al. Occurrence of neuropsychiatric symptoms and psychiatric disorders in mild Alzheimer's disease and mild cognitive impairment subtypes. *Int Psychogeriatr.* (2010) 22:629–40. doi: 10.1017/S1041610210000281
54. Müller U, Czymmek J, Thöne-Otto A, Yves von Cramon D. Reduced daytime activity in patients with acquired brain damage and apathy: a study with ambulatory actigraphy. *Brain Injury* (2006) 20:157–60. doi: 10.1080/02699050500443467
55. David R, Mulin E, Friedman L, Le Duff F, Cygankiewicz E, Deschaux O, et al. Decreased daytime motor activity associated with apathy in Alzheimer disease: an actigraphic study. *Am J Geriatr Psychiatry* (2012) 20:806–14. doi: 10.1097/JGP.0b013e31823038af
56. Schulz KF, Altman DG, Moher D. CONSORT 2010 statement: updated guidelines for reporting parallel group randomised trials. *BMC Med.* (2010) 8:18. doi: 10.1186/1741-7015-8-18
57. Chan AW, Tetzlaff JM, Gøtzsche PC, Altman DG, Mann H, Berlin JA, et al. SPIRIT 2013 explanation and elaboration: guidance for protocols of clinical trials. *BMJ* (2013) 346:e7586. doi: 10.1136/bmj.e7586

19

Snx27 Deletion Promotes Recovery from Spinal Cord Injury by Neuroprotection and Reduces Macrophage/Microglia Proliferation

Yuzhe Zeng [1], Nawen Wang [2], Tiantian Guo [2], Qiuyang Zheng [2], Shuang Wang [1], Songsong Wu [1], Xi Li [1], Jin Wu [1], Zhida Chen [1], Huaxi Xu [3], Xin Wang [2,4] and Bin Lin [1]**

[1] Department of Orthopaedics, The Affiliated Southeast Hospital of Xiamen University, Orthopaedic Center of People's Liberation Army, Zhangzhou, China, [2] Fujian Provincial Key Laboratory of Neurodegenerative Disease and Aging Research, Institute of Neuroscience, College of Medicine, Collaborative Innovation Center for Brain Science, Xiamen University, Xiamen, China, [3] Neuroscience Initiative, Sanford Burnham Prebys Medical Discovery Institute, La Jolla, CA, United States, [4] State Key Laboratory of Cellular Stress Biology, Xiamen University, Xiamen, China

***Correspondence:**
Xin Wang
wangx@xmu.edu.cn
Bin Lin
linbin813@163.com

Sorting nexin 27 (SNX27) is an endosome-associated cargo adaptor that is involved in various pathologies and development of neurological diseases. However, the role of SNX27 in spinal cord injury (SCI) remains unclear. In this study, we found that SNX27 was up-regulated in injured mice spinal cords by western blot and immunofluorescence. A comparative analysis of Basso mouse scale (BMS), footprint test and corticospinal tract (CST) tracing in *Snx27*$^{+/+}$ and *Snx27*$^{+/-}$ mice revealed that haploinsufficiency of SNX27 ameliorated the clinical symptoms of SCI. Based on the results of western blot and immunofluorescence, mechanistically, we found that SNX27 deficiency suppresses apoptotic caspase-3 induced neuronal death. In addition, SNX27 haploinsufficiency lowers the infiltration and activation of macrophage/microglia by suppressing their proliferation at the SCI lesion site. Together, these results suggest that down-regulation of SNX27 is a potential therapy targeting both acute neuronal death and chronic neuroinflammation, and promoting nerve repair after SCI.

Keywords: sorting nexin 27, neuroprotection, macrophage/microglia, functional recovery, spinal cord injury

INTRODUCTION

Spinal cord injury (SCI) is a traumatic event resulting in sensory, motor, and autonomic dysfunction and has direct impacts on the quality of life of affected individuals (1), pharmacological treatments for SCI are still very limited (2). In addition, secondary injuries (such as edema, ischemia, glial activation, neuroinflammation, and excitotoxicity) can further exacerbate the damage to the cord itself (3–5). However, the underlying mechanisms are still largely unknown, many factors could be involved in this process (6). Among these factors, excitotoxicity and neuroinflammation are two main mechanisms that cause the overall effects to the spinal cord (3).

Excitotoxicity is a kind of neuronal cell death caused by excessive activation of glutamate receptors due to increasing levels of extracellular glutamate at the lesion site. Additionally, the increased activation of NMDA receptors contributes to extensive spinal dysfunction. Previous studies show that neuronal death due to CNS injury can be decreased by down-regulation of NMDA receptors such as GluN1 and GluN2B (7, 8). Neuroinflammation responses involve inflammatory cell infiltration (such as neutrophils and macrophages), in addition to microglia activation.

Together these cells release a large number of pro-inflammatory cytokines and neurotoxins leading to neuronal death, axonal interruption adjacent to the primary lesion, and hindered axonal regeneration (9–12). It has been shown that regulation of posttraumatic inflammation is required to improve functional recovery (13, 14), such as through depletion of macrophages (15) and delivery of anti-inflammatory chemicals to the spinal cord lesion site (16, 17). Therefore, SCI treatment strategies should not only focus on removal of injury factors but also need to suppress the excitotoxicity and the activation of macrophage/microglias (18–21).

Sorting nexin 27 (SNX27) is an endosome-associated cargo adaptor (22) that is involved in the development and pathologies of neurological diseases (23). SNX27-deficiency causes cognitive impairment and contributes to the pathologies of Down syndrome by regulating glutamate receptor recycling (24) and contributes to Alzheimer disease pathologies by controlling APP processing (25, 26). Furthermore, the contributions of SNX27 in a wide range of neurological diseases have been characterized ranging from infantile myoclonic epilepsy (27) and hydrocephalus (28), to drug addiction (29), and neuropathic pain (30). Together, these findings demonstrate the vital role of SNX27 in neurological disorders and neuropathic injuries such as SCI.

Despite its well-characterized roles in various neurological disorders, the role of SNX27 in SCI remains unclear. Previous studies show that nerve ligation induces allodynia related to elevated expression of SNX27 and knock down of spinal SNX27 ameliorates allodynia induced by spinal nerve ligation (30), suggesting a potential role of SNX27 in SCI. In this study, we took advantage of a compression model which clinically resembles SCI by fracture dislocations and burst fractures (31). We found that SNX27 was up-regulated in injured mouse spinal cords. SNX27 haploinsufficiency reduced neuronal loss and cleaved caspase 3, as well as the infiltration and proliferation of macrophage/microglia. Moreover, haploinsufficiency of SNX27 improved motor function recovery and corticospinal axon regeneration in $Snx27^{+/-}$ mice after SCI. These findings suggest that down regulation of SNX27 is a potential therapeutic target to overcome the two main obstacles to nerve repair after SCI.

MATERIALS AND METHODS

Animals

$Snx27^{+/+}$ and $Snx27^{+/-}$ mice were generated by crossing heterozygotes in the C57BL/6 background and were bred in the Animal Center of Xiamen University. All mice used for experiments were females between the ages of 10 and 14 weeks (weight 20–25 g). Pairs of female $Snx27^{+/+}$ and $Snx27^{+/-}$ mice were matched by age with maximum differences of 2 weeks (24). All mice were housed in a specific pathogen-free laboratory animal room and given access to a 12 h light-dark cycle in a 18∼22°C facility, with free access to food and water. $Snx27^{+/+}$ and $Snx27^{+/-}$ mice were randomly assigned into two groups: the sham group and SCI group, through a completely randomized digital table. Observers were blinded to the grouping and experimental design during data collection and analysis. The total number of animals has been summarized in **Table 1**.

Antibody

The antibodies used were as follows: rabbit anti-mouse SNX27 (1:50, Thermo Fisher Scientific, #23025), rabbit anti-mouse Glial Fibrillary Acidic Protein, GFAP (1:500, WAKO, #Z0334), rabbit anti-mouse Ionized calcium-binding adapter molecule 1, Iba1 (1:250, DAKO, #019-19741), rabbit anti-mouse cleaved-caspase3 (1:800, Cell Signaling Technology, #9664S), mouse anti-mouse NeuN (1:400, EMD Millipore, #MAB377), rabbit anti-mouse β-actin (1:5,000, proteintech, #20536-1-AP), Alexa-fluor-488-conjugated goat anti-rabbit IgG (1:500, Thermo Fisher Scientific, #11034), Alexa-fluor-546-conjugated goat anti-mouse IgG (1:500, Thermo Fisher Scientific, #11081), HRP-conjugated goat anti-rabbit IgG (H + L) (1:10,000, Thermo Fisher Scientific, #31460), and HRP-conjugated goat anti-mouse IgG (H +L) (1:10 000, Thermo Fisher Scientific, #31430).

Compressive Injury and Surgical Procedures

The surgical procedures for SCI were described previously (32). After mice were anesthetized with ketamine (100 mg/kg, *i.p.*) and xylazine (15 mg/kg, *i.p.*), the T9 lamina was removed and a compressive injury to the spinal cord was inflicted with No. 5 Dumont forceps (Fine Science Tools) modified with a spacer making the maximal closure 0.4 mm, which was applied for 60 s. Surgeries were performed by a surgeon who was blinded to the group allocation. The incision was closed in layers. Postoperatively, 1 mL of saline solution was administered to prevent dehydration. The bladder was pressed 2 times per day until the bladder reflex was re-established. All animals were housed 3 per cage in a controlled environment on a 12/12-h dark and light cycle.

Behavioral Assessment

Basso Mouse Scale (BMS)

BMS, a standardized locomotor rating scale, was used to examine the motor recovery of injured animals (33). Before surgical procedures, mice were acclimated to the open field environment for 1 week. This rating scale assesses not only limb movement, stepping, and coordination, but also trunk stability in an open field. Animals with better locomotor recovery are given a higher score. The test was performed before the surgical procedures (day−1) and on days 1, 7, 14, 21, and 28 after the injury.

Footprint Test (33)

For footprint analysis, the hind paws were painted with black ink to record the walking pattern across a paper runway (3 × 30 cm) during continuous locomotion 4 weeks after the injury. The stride lengths and widths were measured and analyzed only when the mice ran at a constant velocity.

The data were collected by two researchers blinded to the experiment design.

BDA Tracing

Mice were anesthetized and placed on a rodent stereotaxic frame, and a midline incision was made to reveal the bregma. Four small holes in the skull were bored with a microdrill and biotinylated dextran amine (BDA, 10% solution in 0.1 M PBS, Invitrogen,

TABLE 1 | Summary of the total number of animals.

	Groups	C57BL/6	SCI		Sham		Total
			Snx27$^{+/+}$	*Snx27*$^{+/-}$	*Snx27*$^{+/+}$	*Snx27*$^{+/-}$	
Experiment	Behavioral assessment	0	12	12	12	12	48
	BDA tracing (followed by behavioral assessment)	0	0	0	0	0	0
	Immunohistochemistry	6	19	19	0	0	44
	Immunoblotting	20	11	11	0	0	42
Total		26	42	42	12	12	134

D1956) was injected into the right motor cortex using a Hamilton syringe. Four injections of 0.5 μL were injected at a rate of 0.05 μL/min. The coordinates were as follows: 1.5 mm lateral, 0.6 mm deep, and 0.5 mm anterior; 0.0, 0.5, and 1.0 mm caudal to the bregma. The mice were sacrificed 14 days after BDA injection to visualize the corticospinal tract (CST) axons (34, 35).

BDA-Labeled Axon Counts

BDA-labeled axons were detected by application of Streptavidin-Alexa 488 (Thermo Fisher Scientific) in the sagittal section. The number of fibers was analyzed with a confocal microscope. BDA-labeled axons were quantified between the track end and the lesion site. The number of BDA labeled axons at different distances from the lesion center were quantified. BDA labeled axons were counted from five to seven adjacent sections per animal by a person blinded to the experiment design.

Histology

Anesthetized mice were transcardially perfused with ice-cold PBS (0.1 M; pH 7.4) followed by 4% paraformaldehyde (PFA) in PBS. The thoracic area of the spinal cord was removed and cleaved into a 1 cm segment. The tissues were post-fixed in 4% PFA overnight followed by cryoprotection in 30% sucrose for another 48 h. Then, the tissues were embedded in OCT and serially sectioned into 15 μm slices with a Leica CM1860 Cryostat.

Immunohistochemistry

Before staining, spinal cord sections were dried at 60°C for 1 h, and then rinsed with 0.1 M PBS 3 times. After blocking in 5% goat serum, the sections were incubated with indicated primary antibodies at 4°C overnight. The next day, the slides were rinsed with 0.1 M PBS and incubated for 1 h in secondary antibodies. After rinsing with 0.1 M PBS, the sections were counterstained with DAPI and mounted with fluoromount G. Images were acquired by confocal fluorescence microscopy (Nikon Microsystems). All the measurements were made by a person blinded to this experiment design.

Immunoblotting

Animals were sacrificed and the spinal cord tissue was quickly dissected. A segment 0.5 cm long centered at the lesion site was removed. Tissues were lysed in RIPA lysis buffer (25 mM Tris-HCl, pH 7.6, 150 mM NaCl, 1% sodium deoxycholate, 1% Nonidet P-40, 0.1% sodium dodecyl sulfate), supplemented with protease inhibitors (Roche). Equal amounts of protein lysates were subjected to SDS-polyacrylamide gel electrophoresis, transferred to a PVDF membrane (EMD Millipore), and blotted with indicated antibodies. The protein levels were quantified by Image J software by a person blinded to the experiment design and the acquired data were normalized to β-actin.

Statistical Analysis

Statistical differences between groups were calculated with an unpaired two-tailed Student's *t*-test. Other analyses were performed using two-way analysis of variance (ANOVA) with Tukey's *post-hoc* multiple-comparison test as appropriate to the design. The variance similarity between samples was confirmed using *t*-tests. All analyses were conducted using GraphPad Prism software version 7.0. All data are presented as mean ± S.E.M.

RESULTS

Expression of SNX27 Is Up-Regulated in the Injured Spinal Cord

To assess the pathological function of SNX27 following SCI, we analyzed the expression of SNX27 in the spinal cord of sham and injured mice. Expression levels of SNX27 were significantly increased in the lesion sites of the SCI-group, but not the sham-groups at days 3, 7, and 14 after injury (**Figure 1A**). This up-regulation of SNX27 protein levels was detected on day 3 after SCI and reached its peak on day 7 post-injury (**Figure 1B**). Furthermore, immunofluorescence analysis indicated that SNX27 expression was strongly upregulated in SCI-groups compared to the sham-groups on day 7 post-injury (**Figure 1C**). Interestingly, the expression of SNX27 was particularly concentrated in the lesion site and was upregulated in the early stage of SCI, which suggests that SNX27 might have an impact on neuronal death and inflammation.

SNX27 Haploinsufficiency Promotes Functional Recovery After SCI

We investigate the roles of SNX27 in the pathogenesis of SCI using *Snx27*$^{+/-}$ mice, as homozygous knockout of SNX27 results in severe developmental retardation and early lethality in *Snx27*$^{-/-}$ mice, making it impossible to determine whether SNX27 influences functional recovery after SCI (24). The Tail DNA products from *Snx27*$^{+/+}$ and *Snx27*$^{+/-}$ mice were

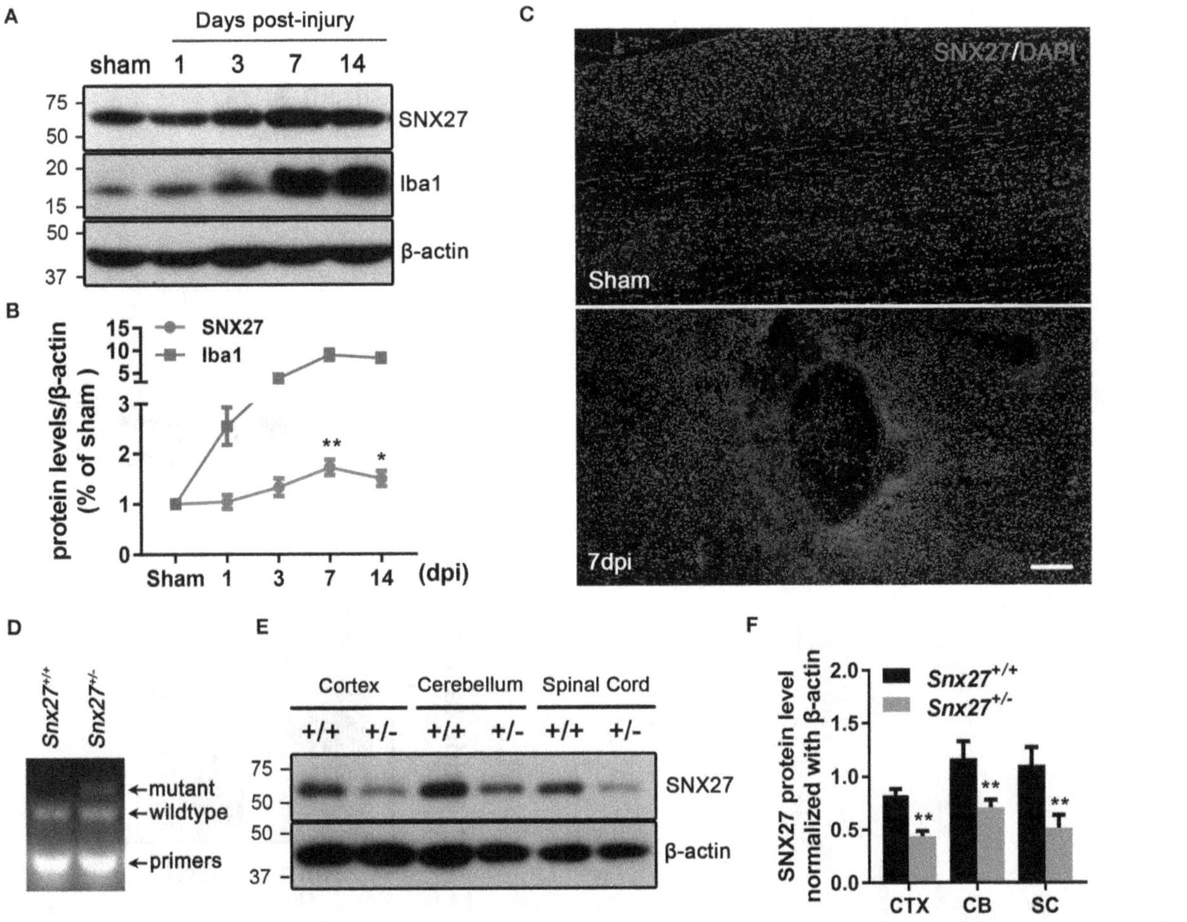

FIGURE 1 | Expression of SNX27 in the injured spinal cord and the identification of *Snx27*$^{+/-}$ mice. **(A)** Western Blot analysis of SNX27 and Iba1 levels in spinal cords from sham SCI treated mice. **(B)** Time course analysis of SNX27 expression at the SCI lesion site, $n = 4$ mice per time point. **(C)** Histological analysis of SNX27 expression in the spinal cords from sham and SCI mice 7 days post injury. Scale bar = 200 μm. **(D)** PCR genotyping of *Snx27*$^{+/+}$ and *Snx27*$^{+/-}$ mice. **(E,F)** Western Blot analysis of SNX27 in *Snx27*$^{+/+}$ and *Snx27*$^{+/-}$ mice. The results were represented as the mean ± SEM and data were evaluated by One-way ANOVA with Tukey *post-hoc* test, $^*p < 0.05$, $^{**}p < 0.01$. dpi, days post injury. CTX, Cortex; CB, Cerebellum; SC, Spinal Cord.

genotyped by PCR (**Figure 1D**). Meanwhile, SNX27 protein expression in spinal cord, cortex and cerebellum of *Snx27*$^{+/+}$ and *Snx27*$^{+/-}$ mice was evaluated by western blot analysis and we found a reduction of SNX27 expression (about 50%) in *Snx27*$^{+/-}$ mice compared to that in *Snx27*$^{+/+}$ mice (**Figures 1E,F**).

To investigate the effects of SNX27 on motor recovery after SCI, footprint analysis, and open field locomotion tests were performed to objectively assess the functional improvements in *Snx27*$^{+/+}$ and *Snx27*$^{+/-}$ mice at week 4 after SCI. The sham groups of both *Snx27*$^{+/+}$ and *Snx27*$^{+/-}$ mice displayed normal functional outcomes. On day 1 post-injury, both genotypes displayed significant hind limb paralysis. However, most *Snx27*$^{+/-}$ mice showed consistent plantar stepping and consistent coordination (BMS score: 6 or 7) on day 28 post-injury. In contrast, *Snx27*$^{+/+}$ mice had little to no coordination and rotated paw position (BMS score: 4 or 5) although they displayed frequent or consistent plantar stepping (**Figure 2A**). In contrast to *Snx27*$^{+/+}$ mice, *Snx27*$^{+/-}$ mice exhibited longer stride length and width of the hind limb in footprint analyses at week 4 post-injury. Together, these data indicate that SNX27 is involved in functional disabilities of the spine and recovery of hind limb motor function, which was significantly improved in *Snx27*$^{+/-}$ mice after SCI (**Figures 2B–D**).

SNX27 Haploinsufficiency Increases Axon Regeneration After SCI

Corticospinal tract (CST) growth is correlated with functional recovery after SCI (36). Therefore, we wondered whether SNX27 is involved in the recovery of CST after SCI. We injected biotinylated dextran amine (BDA) into the right sensorimotor cortex of mice to label the CST on day 28 post-injury and all mice were sacrificed after 2 weeks. The number of BDA$^+$ nerve fibers crossing the compressive injury lesion site were quantified to evaluate functional improvement. In *Snx27*$^{+/+}$ mice, most of the BDA$^+$ nerve fibers retracted from the lesion site (**Figure 3A**). In contrast, *Snx27*$^{+/-}$ mice displayed vigorous regrowth of

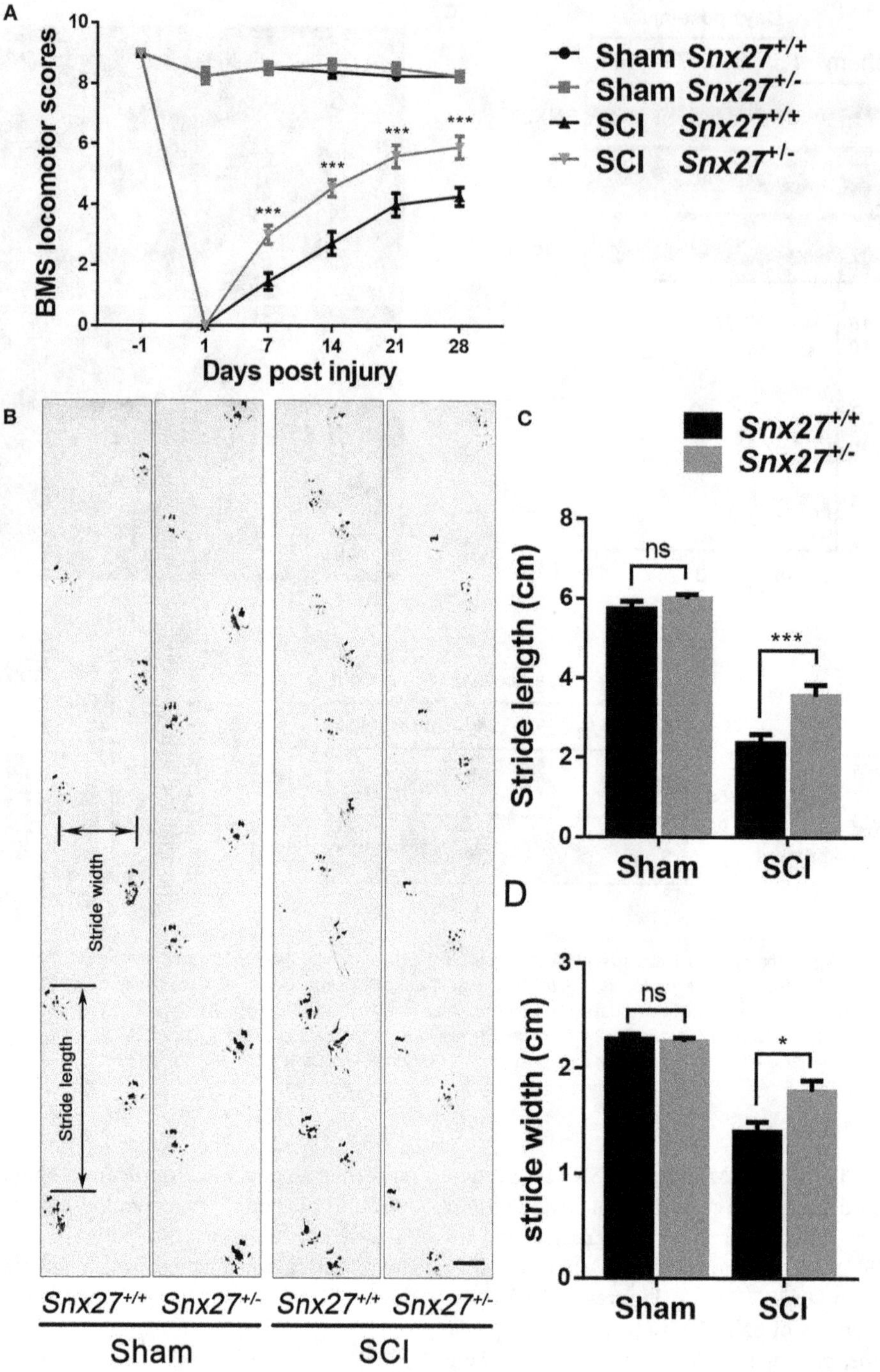

FIGURE 2 | SNX27 haploinsufficiency promotes functional recovery after SCI. **(A)** Evaluating functional recovery of $Snx27^{+/+}$ and $Snx27^{+/-}$ mice after SCI using BMS scoring, $n = 12$. Scale bar = 1cm. **(B)** Representative images of footprint analysis 28 days post injury. **(C,D)** Quantification of stride width and stride length in the footprint analysis 28 days post injury, $n = 12$. Values are expressed as mean ± SEM, Data were analyzed using repeated measures ANOVA followed by Bonferroni's *post-hoc* test, $^{*}p < 0.05$, $^{***}p < 0.001$.

nerve fibers (**Figure 3A′**), with more continuous BDA^+ axons traversing the lesion site and growing into the distal spinal cord about 0.8 mm to the caudal lesion site (**Figure 3B′,C′**). Quantification of the BDA^+ axons of CST caudal to the lesion site showed that $Snx27^{+/-}$ mice had significantly more axons in the spinal cords 2 mm away from the lesion site than $Snx27^{+/+}$ mice (**Figure 3D**). All these data imply that SNX27-deficiency might enhance corticospinal axon regeneration after SCI.

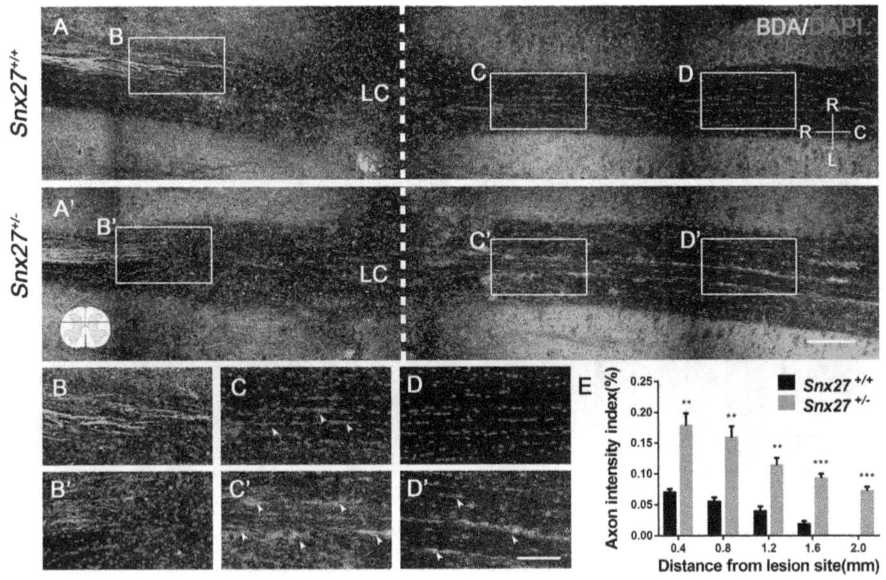

FIGURE 3 | SNX27 haploinsufficiency increases axon regeneration after SCI. **(A)** Overview of BDA-labeled nerve fibers (green) in horizontal sections of *Snx27*$^{+/+}$ mice and *Snx27*$^{+/-}$ mice dorsal columns, ranging from rostral 1,500 μm (−1,500 μm) to caudal 2,000 μm (+2,000 μm) around the LC, Scale bar = 200 μm. R-C, Rostral–caudal; R-L, right–left. Dashed lines indicate the lesion center (LC). **(B,B′,C,C′,D,D′)** Higher magnification of the boxed areas in A. Arrowheads indicate BDA-labeled nerve fibers. Scale bar = 100 μm. **(E)** Quantification of BDA-labeled nerve fibers crossing the lesion site. $n = 8$ mice per genotype. Values are expressed as mean ± SEM and data were evaluated by One-way ANOVA with Tukey *post-hoc* test. $^{**}p < 0.01$, $^{***}p < 0.001$. LC, Lesion Center.

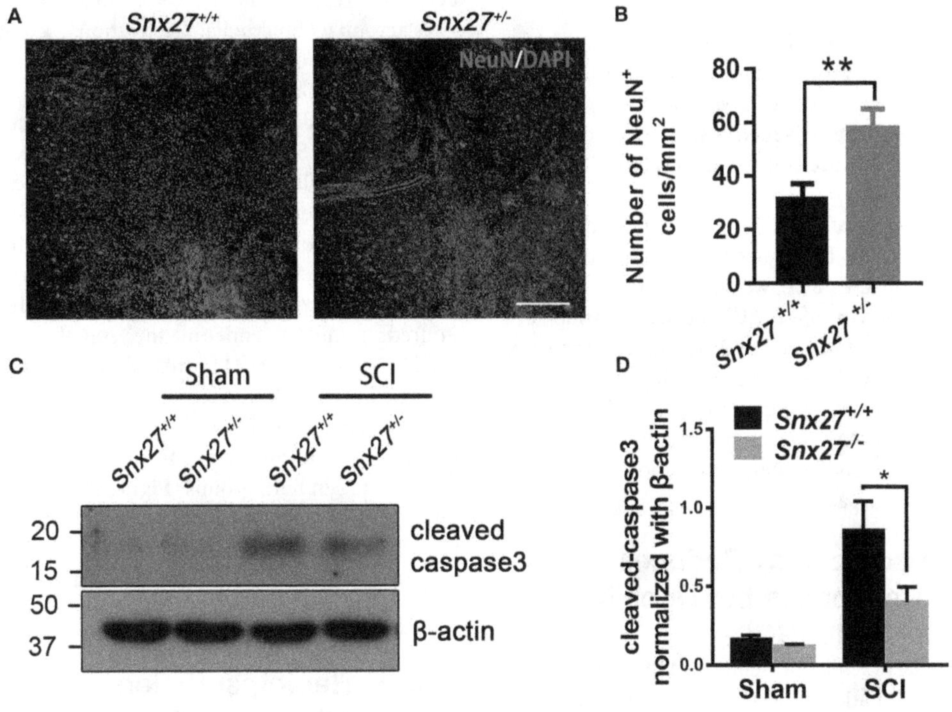

FIGURE 4 | SNX27 haploinsufficiency prevents neuronal death and caspase-3 activation after SCI. **(A)** Representative images of the lesion center in the spinal cords from *Snx27*$^{+/+}$ mice and *Snx27*$^{+/-}$ mice 7 days post injury, Scale bar = 200 μm. **(B)** NeuN^{+} cell quantification of the lesion center in the spinal cords from *Snx27*$^{+/+}$ mice and *Snx27*$^{+/-}$ mice 7 days post injury, $n = 4$. **(C)** Western blot analysis of cleaved caspase-3 levels in the spinal cord of *Snx27*$^{+/+}$ mice and *Snx27*$^{+/-}$ mice 3 days post injury. **(D)** Quantitative analysis of cleaved caspase-3 expression in the spinal cord of *Snx27*$^{+/+}$ mice and *Snx27*$^{+/-}$ mice 3 days post injury, $n = 4$. Values are expressed as mean ± SEM and were evaluated by Student's independent sample *t*-test. $^{*}p < 0.05$, $^{**}p < 0.01$.

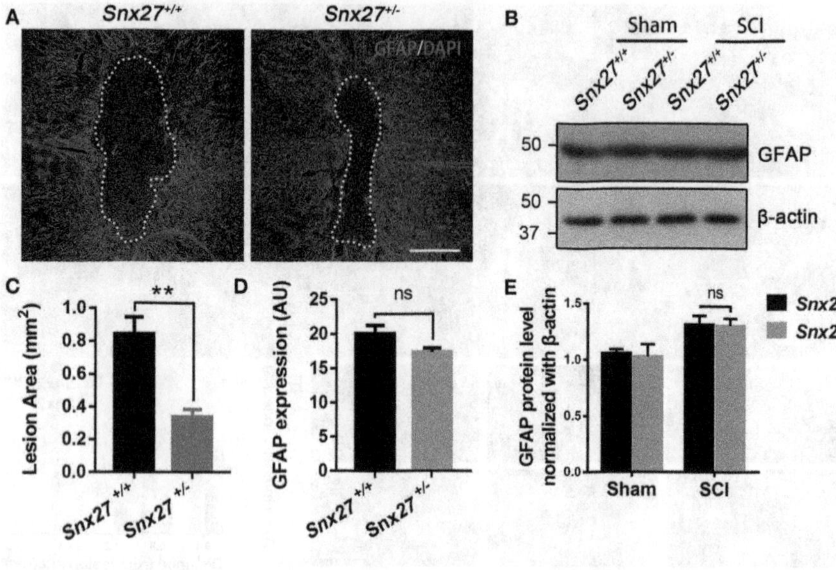

FIGURE 5 | SNX27 haploinsufficiency reduces the size of lesion region without influencing gliosis after SCI. **(A)** Representative images of GFAP staining indicating the lesion region 7 days post injury, $n = 6$, Scale bar = 200 μm. Dashed lines indicate the lesion area. **(B)** Western blot analysis of GFAP in the spinal cord of *Snx27*$^{+/+}$ mice and *Snx27*$^{+/-}$ mice 7 days post injury. **(C,D)** Quantification of GFAP-negative area (lesion region) and GFAP protein expression, $n = 6$. **(E)** Quantitative analysis of GFAP expression, $n = 3$. Values are expressed as mean ± SEM and were evaluated by Student's independent sample *t*-test. $^{**}p < 0.01$.

SNX27 Haploinsufficiency Prevents Neuronal Death and Caspase-3 Activation After SCI

To determine the effects of SNX27 on neuronal survival after SCI, the number of NeuN-positive cells adjacent to the lesion site was counted on day 3 post-injury. Consistent with the behavioral data, there were more NeuN-positive cells adjacent to the lesion site in *Snx27*$^{+/-}$ mice compared with *Snx27*$^{+/+}$ mice (**Figures 4A,B**).

Caspase-3 is activated after SCI as a key execution in neuronal apoptosis (37, 38). To investigate the effect of SNX27 on apoptotic cell death after SCI, we tested for the presence of active cleaved caspase-3 after SCI in each group and found that the level of cleaved caspase-3 was indeed increased after SCI. However, cleaved caspase-3 was highly decreased in the SCI-*Snx27*$^{+/-}$ group compared with SCI-*Snx27*$^{+/+}$ group (**Figures 4C,D**). Taken together, our results indicate that SNX27 haploinsufficiency confers neuroprotection possibly via decreasing activation of caspase 3.

SNX27 Haploinsufficiency Reduces Inflammatory Responses but Does Not Influence Gliosis After SCI

Increased glial fibrillary acidic protein (GFAP) expression is associated with scar formation, a secondary damage after SCI, and is an indicator of reactive gliosis. Sagittal sections were stained for GFAP to examine the pathological effects of SNX27 on lesion size and astrocyte reactivity after SCI. The lesion volume, of the GFAP-negative area, was comparable between *Snx27*$^{+/+}$ and *Snx27*$^{+/-}$ mice on day 7 after SCI, but the GFAP-negative area was significantly smaller in *Snx27*$^{+/-}$ mice (**Figures 5A,C**). However, there was no difference in reactive astrocytes indicated by GFAP expression in the regions adjacent to the lesion sites between *Snx27*$^{+/+}$ and *Snx27*$^{+/-}$ mice (**Figures 5B,D,E**).

Macrophage/microglia activation contributes to the development of secondary injury after SCI. Therefore, we analyzed the expression pattern of Iba1, a marker for macrophage/microglia activation and accumulation, in the spinal cord of SCI mouse models. Increased number of round and amoeboid-like Iba1$^+$ cells (activated macrophage/microglia) have been observed in the injured boundary zone and lesion center, but the Iba1$^+$ cells in the non-injury site remained ramified (quiescent macrophage/microglia). In addition, we found that *Snx27*$^{+/-}$ mice had reduced Iba1 density in the injured boundary zone of the spinal cord compared with *Snx27*$^{+/+}$ littermates (**Figures 6A,A′,D**), but had no difference in the zones of the lesion center (**Figures 6B,B′**) or the non-injury sites on day 7 post-injury (**Figures 6C,C′**). Expression of Iba1 was 5- to 6-fold higher in injured spinal cords compared with sham tissues in both groups (**Figures 6E,F**). However, *Snx27*$^{+/-}$ mice had significantly reduced Iba1 upregulation than *Snx27*$^{+/+}$ mice. These results indicate that SNX27 haploinsufficiency suppresses inflammatory responses but not scar formation after SCI.

SNX27 Haploinsufficiency Suppresses the Proliferation of Macrophage/Microglia After SCI

SNX27 haploinsufficiency suppresses inflammatory responses but not scar formation after SCI, implying that SNX27 might be involved in the proliferation of microglial/macrophage cells that migrate toward and infiltrate the lesion site. Therefore,

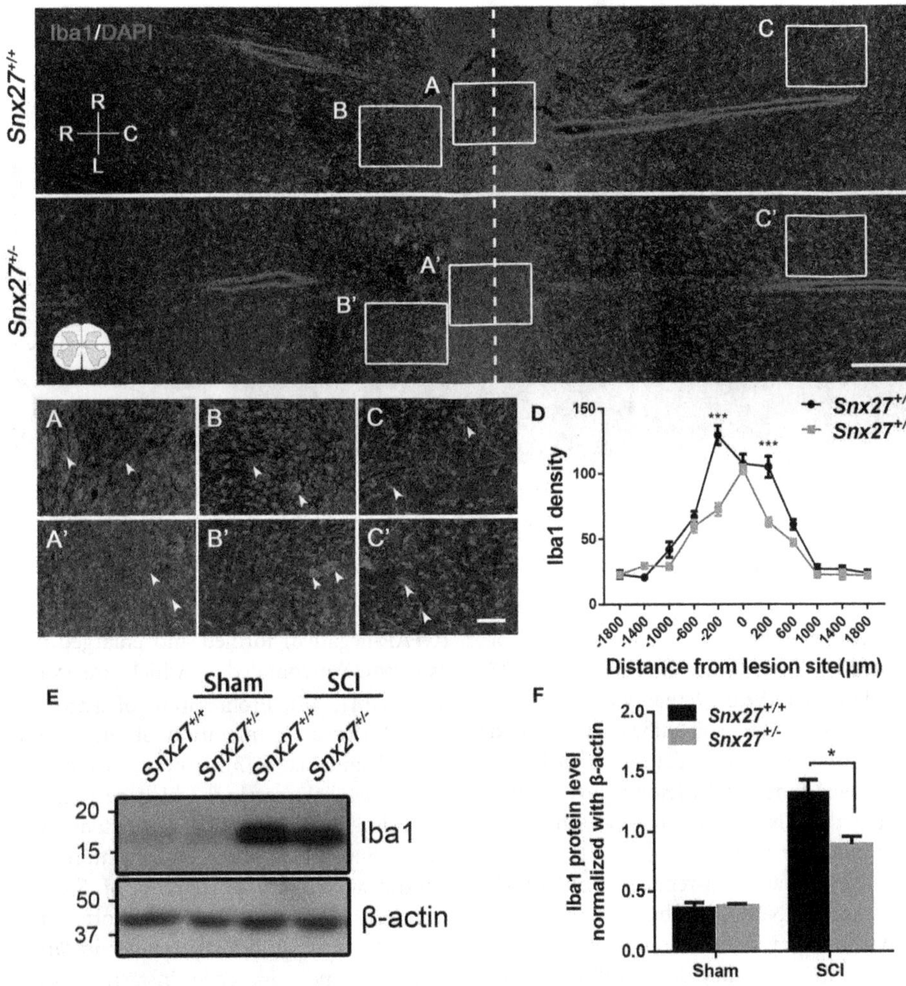

FIGURE 6 | SNX27 haploinsufficiency reduces the activation of macrophage/microglia in the injured spinal cord. Top, Overview of Iba1-positive cell in horizontal sections of *Snx27*$^{+/+}$ mice and *Snx27*$^{+/-}$ mice dorsal spinal columns, ranging from rostral 1,500 μm (–1,500 μm) to caudal 1,500 μm (+1,500 μm) around the LC. $n = 6$. Scale bar = 200 μm. R-C, Rostral–caudal; R-L, right–left. Dashed lines indicate the lesion center. Below, Higher magnification of the different zones: the lesion centers **(A,A′)**; the injury boundary zones **(B,B′)**; the non-injury zones **(C,C′)**, Scale bar = 50 μm. Arrowheads indicate the quiescent and activated microglia. **(D)** Quantification of Iba1 density. **(E)** Western blot analysis of Iba1 expression in the spinal cords from *Snx27*$^{+/+}$ mice and *Snx27*$^{+/-}$ mice 7 days post injury. **(F)** Quantitative analysis of Iba1 expression, $n = 4$. Values are expressed as mean ± SEM and data were evaluated by One-way ANOVA with Tukey *post-hoc* test. $^{*}p < 0.05$, $^{***}p < 0.001$.

double immunostaining for Ibal and Ki67, a cellular marker for proliferation (39), was performed in sagittal sections of the spinal cords on day 7 post-injury. In contrast to *Snx27*$^{+/+}$ littermates, *Snx27*$^{+/-}$ mice exhibited fewer Ki67^{+} cells in the lesion site (**Figure 7A**), indicating that SNX27 haploinsufficiency suppresses the proliferation of cells in injured spinal cords. Furthermore, fewer cells positive for both Ibal and Ki67 was observed in the lesion site of *Snx27*$^{+/-}$ mice following SCI, compared with those in *Snx27*$^{+/+}$ littermates (**Figure 7B**). Therefore, SNX27 haploinsufficiency suppresses proliferation of macrophage/microglia following SCI.

DISCUSSION

SNX27, an endosome-associated cargo adaptor, is involved in developmental and neurological diseases, such as Down syndrome, Alzheimer's disease, infantile myoclonic epilepsy, hydrocephalus, and neuropathic pain (24–26, 30). Previous reports found that SNX27 is involved in neuropathic pain in a mouse spinal nerve ligation model (30). However, before our study, the physiological function of SNX27 in SCI has not been investigated. For the first time, we determined the roles of SNX27 in SCI, which will extend our understanding the functional regulation of SNX27 in spinal cord injury.

In this study, we found that SNX27 expression starts to increase on day 3 and reached the plateau on day 7 after SCI (**Figure 1B**). Moreover, we found that the expression of SNX27 was markedly upregulated around the lesion site where the necrotic neurons and activated microglia/macrophage emerged after spinal cord injury (**Figure 1C**). These results suggest that SNX27 is associated with neuronal death and neuroinflammation, and may function in the early stage of

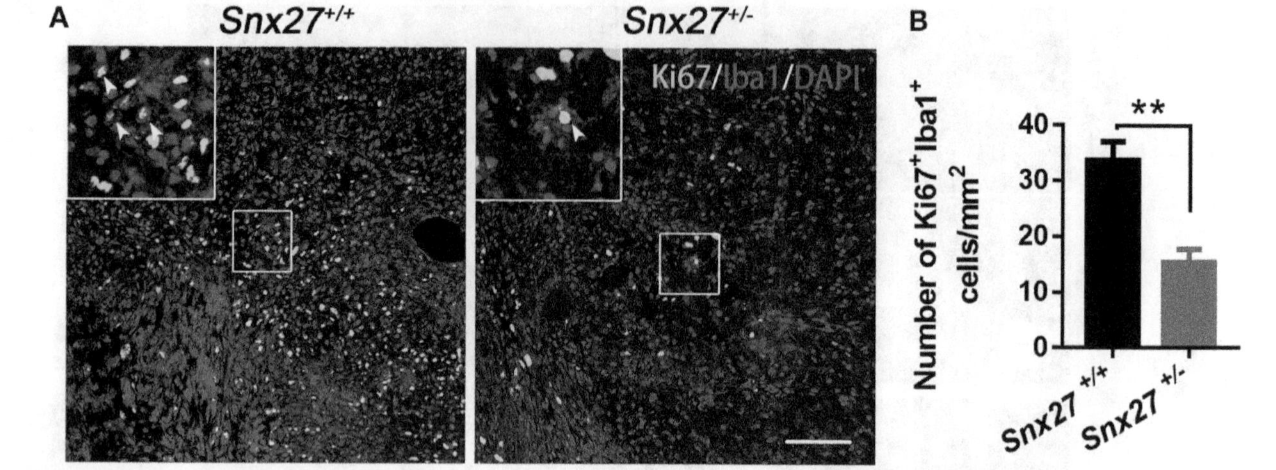

FIGURE 7 | SNX27 haploinsufficiency suppresses the proliferation of macrophage/microglia after SCI. **(A)** Immunohistological analysis of horizontal spinal cord sections from $Snx27^{+/+}$ mice and $Snx27^{+/-}$ mice 7 days post injury using antibodies against Iba1 and Ki67 in horizontal sections. Arrowheads indicate $Ki67^+Iba1^+$ cells. **(B)** Quantification of $Ki67^+Iba1^+$ cells at the area which is ranging from rostral 400 μm (−400 μm) to caudal 400 μm (+400 μm) around the LC, $n = 3$. Values are expressed as mean ± SEM and were evaluated by Student's independent sample *t*-test. $^{**}p < 0.01$.

SCI. Furthermore, we investigate the physiological function of SNX27 in SCI using $Snx27^{+/-}$ mice since that loss of Snx27 results in severe neuronal death and early lethality in $Snx27^{-/-}$ mice. We have found that SNX27 haploinsufficiency elevated corticospinal axon regeneration from the caudal area to the lesion area (**Figure 3**) and improved functional motor recovery after SCI (**Figure 2**), suggesting that SNX27 may have an effect on functional recovery after spinal cord injury.

Previous studies have shown that down-regulation of NMDA receptors, such as GluN1 and GluN2B, contributes to reduction of neuronal death due to CNS injury, but is accompanied by side-effects (7, 8). Moreover, SNX27-deficiency decreased glutamate receptor recycling to the post-synaptic surface (24). Therefore, we put forward the hypothesis that deficiency of SNX27 might protect neurons from Glutamate-induced excitotoxicity in SCI damage by reducing the surface expression of NMDA receptors. We found that SNX27 haploinsufficiency significantly promoted neuronal survival adjacent to the lesion site and reduced expression of apoptotic cleaved caspase-3 after SCI (**Figure 4**). This indicates SNX27 haploinsufficiency protects neurons from SCI-induced apoptotic cell death and possibly by blocking NMDA receptor activation.

A sequential inflammatory cascade is initiated after spinal cord injury (40), microglia and astrocyte, two types of glial cells reside in the spinal cord are likely contributors. They can be activated to various degrees after spinal cord injury (41, 42). Although there are different functional states of macrophage/microglia activated after SCI, treatments aimed at anti-inflammatory pathways have been a mainstay of pre-clinical SCI research for many years (43). Macrophage/microglia that infiltrate in the injured area can secrete inflammatory factors such as TNFα, IL-1, IL-6, aggravating neuronal damage and cavity formation, while suppressing neurogenesis and axonal regeneration (36, 44). In the days following the initial damage to the spinal cord, secondary damage continues in the tissue surrounding the original site of injury, spinal cavity (GFAP-negative) formed and enlarged gradually with reactive astrocytes surrounded it, which are exacerbating neurological defects (41, 45). Proliferation of astrocytes at the early stage of SCI can limit migration of the immune cells toward the injured spinal cord (3). However, over time, astrocytes produce extensive glial scarring, which restricts the regeneration and extension of axons (3). Consistent with previous reports, we found that there were more macrophage/microglia infiltrating in the spinal cord of $Snx27^{+/+}$ mice compared with $Snx27^{+/-}$ mice (**Figure 6**). Moreover, the lesion site (GFAP-negative) was significantly smaller in $Snx27^{+/-}$ mice, although there was no difference in astrogliosis between $Snx27^{+/+}$ and $Snx27^{+/-}$ mice (**Figure 5**). SNX27 haploinsufficiency reduced the number of infiltrating $Iba1^+/Ki67^+$ cells (newborn microglia/macrophage) in the lesion sites after SCI (**Figure 7**). Thus, SNX27 haploinsufficiency suppresses the inflammatory response by inhibiting the macrophage/microglia proliferation after SCI, but SNX27 has no effect on astrogliosis in this SCI model.

CONCLUSION

In summary, our findings demonstrate a pathological function of SNX27 in spinal cord injury by increasing neuroinflammation and neuronal apoptotic death. The details of the underlying mechanism deserve further scrutiny.

AUTHOR CONTRIBUTIONS

YZ, XW, and BL conceived the study. YZ designed and performed the experiments. TG, ShW, SoW, XL, JW, and ZC provided additional advice in experimental design and execution. HX provided discussion. YZ, XW, and BL wrote the manuscript. NW and QZ edited the manuscript. XW and BL supervised the project.

ACKNOWLEDGMENTS

We thank W. Hong for providing *Snx27* KO mice, P. Slesinger for providing the rabbit anti-SNX27 antibody. This work was supported in part by National Natural Science Foundation of China (81571176, 31871077, and 81822014 to XW), National Key R&D Program of China (2016YFC1305900 to XW), Natural Science Foundation of Fujian Province of China (2017J06021 to XW and 2017J01163 to BL), the Fundamental Research Funds for the Chinese Central Universities (20720150061 to XW), 2016 military logistics research program (CNJ16J012 to BL) and Multi-disciplinary joint research of the Affiliated Southeast Hospital of Xiamen University (14YLG001 to BL).

REFERENCES

1. Fehlings M, Singh A, Tetreault L, Kalsi-Ryan S, Nouri A. Global prevalence and incidence of traumatic spinal cord injury. *Clin Epidemiol.* (2014) 6:309–31. doi: 10.2147/CLEP.S68889
2. Manzhulo O, Tyrtyshnaia A, Kipryushina Y, Dyuizen I, Manzhulo I. Docosahexaenoic acid induces changes in microglia/macrophage polarization after spinal cord injury in rats. *Acta Histochem.* (2018) 120:741–7. doi: 10.1016/j.acthis.2018.08.005
3. Gomes-Leal W, Corkill DJ, Freire MA, Picanco-Diniz CW, Perry VH. Astrocytosis, microglia activation, oligodendrocyte degeneration, and pyknosis following acute spinal cord injury. *Exp Neurol.* (2004) 190:456–67. doi: 10.1016/j.expneurol.2004.06.028
4. Jia YF, Gao HL, Ma LJ, Li J. Effect of nimodipine on rat spinal cord injury. *Genet Mol Res.* (2015) 14:1269–76. doi: 10.4238/2015.February.13.5
5. Li Y, Gu R, Zhu Q, Liu J. Changes of spinal edema and expression of aquaporin 4 in methylprednisolone-treated rats with spinal cord injury. *Ann Clin Lab Sci.* (2018) 48:453–9.
6. Becker D, Sadowsky CL, McDonald JW. Restoring function after spinal cord injury. *Neurologist* (2003) 9:1–15. doi: 10.1097/01.nrl.0000038587.58012.05
7. Huang M, Cheng G, Tan H, Qin R, Zou Y, Wang Y, et al. Capsaicin protects cortical neurons against ischemia/reperfusion injury via down-regulating NMDA receptors. *Exp Neurol.* (2017) 295:66–76. doi: 10.1016/j.expneurol.2017.05.001
8. Zhang Z, Liu J, Fan C, Mao L, Xie R, Wang S, et al. The GluN1/GluN2B NMDA receptor and metabotropic glutamate receptor 1 negative allosteric modulator has enhanced neuroprotection in a rat subarachnoid hemorrhage model. *Exp Neurol.* (2017) 301(Pt A):13–25. doi: 10.1016/j.expneurol.2017.12.005
9. Horn KP, Busch SA, Hawthorne AL, van Rooijen N, Silver J. Another barrier to regeneration in the CNS: activated macrophages induce extensive retraction of dystrophic axons through direct physical interactions. *J Neurosci.* (2008) 28:9330–41. doi: 10.1523/JNEUROSCI.2488-08.2008
10. Beattie MS. Inflammation and apoptosis: linked therapeutic targets in spinal cord injury. *Trends Mol Med.* (2004) 10:580–3. doi: 10.1016/j.molmed.2004.10.006
11. Slaets H, Nelissen S, Janssens K, Vidal PM, Lemmens E, Stinissen P, et al. Oncostatin M reduces lesion size and promotes functional recovery and neurite outgrowth after spinal cord injury. *Mol Neurobiol.* (2014) 50:1142–51. doi: 10.1007/s12035-014-8795-5
12. Bethea JR. Spinal cord injury-induced inflammation: a dual-edged sword. *Progr Brain Res.* (2000) 128:33–42. doi: 10.1016/S0079-6123(00)28005-9
13. Donnelly DJ, Longbrake EE, Shawler TM, Kigerl KA, Lai W, Tovar CA, et al. Deficient CX3CR1 signaling promotes recovery after mouse spinal cord injury by limiting the recruitment and activation of Ly6Clo/iNOS+ macrophages. *J Neurosci.* (2011) 31:9910–22. doi: 10.1523/JNEUROSCI.2114-11.2011
14. Courtine G, van den Brand R, Musienko P. Spinal cord injury: time to move. *Lancet* (2011) 377:1896–8. doi: 10.1016/S0140-6736(11)60711-3
15. Gris D, Marsh DR, Oatway MA, Chen Y, Hamilton EF, Dekaban GA, et al. Transient blockade of the CD11d/CD18 integrin reduces secondary damage after spinal cord injury, improving sensory, autonomic, and motor function. *J Neurosci.* (2004) 24:4043–51. doi: 10.1523/JNEUROSCI.5343-03.2004
16. Popovich PG, Guan Z, Wei P, Huitinga I, van Rooijen N, Stokes BT. Depletion of hematogenous macrophages promotes partial hindlimb recovery and neuroanatomical repair after experimental spinal cord injury. *Exp Neurol.* (1999) 158:351–65. doi: 10.1006/exnr.1999.7118
17. Stirling DP, Khodarahmi K, Liu J, McPhail LT, McBride CB, Steeves JD, et al. Minocycline treatment reduces delayed oligodendrocyte death, attenuates axonal dieback, and improves functional outcome after spinal cord injury. *J Neurosci.* (2004) 24:2182–90. doi: 10.1523/JNEUROSCI.5275-03.2004
18. Mallory GW, Grahn PJ, Hachmann JT, Lujan JL, Lee KH. Optical Stimulation for Restoration of Motor Function After Spinal Cord Injury. *Mayo Clin Proc.* (2015) 90:300–7. doi: 10.1016/j.mayocp.2014.12.004
19. Estrada V, Muller HW. Spinal cord injury - there is not just one way of treating it. *F1000Prime Rep.* (2014) 6:84. doi: 10.12703/P6-84
20. Wang J, Pearse DD. Therapeutic hypothermia in spinal cord injury: the status of its use and open questions. *Int J Mol Sci.* (2015) 16:16848–79. doi: 10.3390/ijms160816848
21. de Rivero Vaccari JP, Dietrich WD, Keane RW. Therapeutics targeting the inflammasome after central nervous system injury. *Transl Res.* (2016) 167:35–45. doi: 10.1016/j.trsl.2015.05.003
22. Gallon M, Clairfeuille T, Collins BM, Cullen PJ. A unique PDZ domain and arrestin-like fold interaction reveals mechanistic details of endocytic recycling by SNX27-retromer. *Mol Biol Cell* (2014) 111:E3604–13. doi: 10.1073/pnas.1410552111
23. Cai L, Loo LS, Atlashkin V, Hanson BJ, Hong W. Deficiency of sorting nexin 27 (SNX27) leads to growth retardation and elevated levels of N-methyl-D-aspartate receptor 2C (NR2C). *Mol Cell Biol.* (2011) 31:1734–47. doi: 10.1128/MCB.01044-10
24. Wang X, Zhao Y, Zhang X, Badie H, Zhou Y, Mu Y, et al. Loss of sorting nexin 27 contributes to excitatory synaptic dysfunction by modulating glutamate receptor recycling in Down's syndrome. *Nat Med.* (2013) 19:473–80. doi: 10.1038/nm.3117
25. Wang X, Huang T, Zhao Y, Zheng Q, Thompson RC, Bu G, et al. Sorting nexin 27 regulates Abeta production through modulating gamma-secretase activity. *Cell Rep.* (2014) 9:1023–33. doi: 10.1016/j.celrep.2014.09.037
26. Huang TY, Zhao Y, Li X, Wang X, Tseng IC, Thompson R, et al. SNX27 and SORLA interact to reduce amyloidogenic subcellular distribution and processing of amyloid precursor protein. *J Neurosci.* (2016) 36:7996–8011. doi: 10.1523/JNEUROSCI.0206-16.2016
27. Damseh N, Danson CM, Al-Ashhab M, Abu-Libdeh B, Gallon M, Sharma K, et al. A defect in the retromer accessory protein, SNX27, manifests by infantile myoclonic epilepsy and neurodegeneration. *Neurogenetics* (2015) 16:215–21. doi: 10.1007/s10048-015-0446-0
28. Wang X, Zhou Y, Wang J, Tseng IC, Huang T, Zhao Y, et al. SNX27 Deletion causes hydrocephalus by impairing ependymal cell differentiation and ciliogenesis. *J Neurosci.* (2016) 36:12586–97. doi: 10.1523/JNEUROSCI.1620-16.2016
29. Munoz MB, Slesinger PA. Sorting nexin 27 regulation of G protein-gated inwardly rectifying K(+) channels attenuates *in vivo* cocaine response. *Neuron* (2014) 82:659–69. doi: 10.1016/j.neuron.2014.03.011
30. Lin TB, Lai CY, Hsieh MC, Wang HH, Cheng JK, Chau YP, et al. VPS26A-SNX27 Interaction-dependent mGluR5 recycling in dorsal horn neurons mediates neuropathic pain in rats. *J Neurosci.* (2015) 35:14943–55. doi: 10.1523/JNEUROSCI.2587-15.2015
31. Cheriyan T, Ryan DJ, Weinreb JH, Cheriyan J, Paul JC, Lafage V, et al. Spinal cord injury models: a review. *Spinal Cord* (2014) 52:588–95. doi: 10.1038/sc.2014.91
32. Mostacada K, Oliveira FL, Villa-Verde DM, Martinez AM. Lack of galectin-3 improves the functional outcome and tissue sparing by modulating inflammatory response after a compressive spinal cord injury. *Exp Neurol.* (2015) 271:390–400. doi: 10.1016/j.expneurol.2015.07.006
33. Wang SM, Hsu JC, Ko CY, Chiu NE, Kan WM, Lai MD, et al. Astrocytic CCAAT/enhancer-binding protein delta contributes to glial scar formation and impairs functional recovery after spinal cord injury. *Mol Neurobiol.* (2016) 53:5912–27. doi: 10.1007/s12035-015-9486-6
34. Danilov CA, Steward O. Conditional genetic deletion of PTEN after a spinal cord injury enhances regenerative growth of CST axons and motor function recovery in mice. *Exp Neurol.* (2015) 266:147–60. doi: 10.1016/j.expneurol.2015.02.012

35. Liu K, Lu Y, Lee JK, Samara R, Willenberg R, Sears-Kraxberger I, et al. PTEN deletion enhances the regenerative ability of adult corticospinal neurons. *Nature Neurosci.* (2010) 13:1075–81. doi: 10.1038/nn.2603
36. Du K, Zheng S, Zhang Q, Li S, Gao X, Wang J, et al. Pten deletion promotes regrowth of corticospinal tract axons 1 year after spinal cord injury. *J Neurosci.* (2015) 35:9754–63. doi: 10.1523/JNEUROSCI.3637-14.2015
37. Lee JY, Chung H, Yoo YS, Oh YJ, Oh TH, Park S, et al. Inhibition of apoptotic cell death by ghrelin improves functional recovery after spinal cord injury. *Endocrinology* (2010) 151:3815–26. doi: 10.1210/en.2009-1416
38. Lee JY, Kang SR, Yune TY. Fluoxetine prevents oligodendrocyte cell death by inhibiting microglia activation after spinal cord injury. *J Neurotrauma* (2015) 32:633–44. doi: 10.1089/neu.2014.3527
39. Scholzen T, Gerdes J. The Ki-67 protein: from the known and the unknown. *J Cell Physiol.* (2000) 182:311–22. doi: 10.1002/(SICI)1097-4652(200003)182:3<311::AID-JCP1>3.0.CO;2-9
40. Gensel JC, Zhang B. Macrophage activation and its role in repair and pathology after spinal cord injury. *Brain Res.* (2015) 1619:1–11. doi: 10.1016/j.brainres.2014.12.045
41. Fan H, Zhang K, Shan L, Kuang F, Chen K, Zhu K, et al. Reactive astrocytes undergo M1 microglia/macrohpages-induced necroptosis in spinal cord injury. *Mol Neurodegener.* (2016) 11:14. doi: 10.1186/s13024-016-0081-8
42. Gaudet AD, Mandrekar-Colucci S, Hall JCE, Sweet DR, Schmitt PJ, Xu X, et al. miR-155 deletion in mice overcomes neuron-intrinsic and neuron-extrinsic barriers to spinal cord repair. *J Neurosci.* (2016) 36:8516–32. doi: 10.1523/JNEUROSCI.0735-16.2016
43. Squair JW, Ruiz I, Phillips AA, Zheng MMZ, Sarafis ZK, Sachdeva R, et al. Minocycline reduces the severity of autonomic dysreflexia after experimental spinal cord injury. *J Neurotrauma* (2018). doi: 10.1089/neu.2018.5703.[Epub ahead of print].
44. Lopes RS, Cardoso MM, Sampaio AO, Barbosa MS Jr, Souza CC, MC DAS, et al. Indomethacin treatment reduces microglia activation and increases numbers of neuroblasts in the subventricular zone and ischaemic striatum after focal ischaemia. *J Biosci.* (2016) 41:381–94. doi: 10.1007/s12038-016-9621-1
45. Boato F, Hendrix S, Huelsenbeck SC, Hofmann F, Grosse G, Djalali S, et al. C3 peptide enhances recovery from spinal cord injury by improved regenerative growth of descending fiber tracts. *J Cell Sci.* (2010) 123(Pt 10):1652–62. doi: 10.1242/jcs.066050

20

Using the Technology Acceptance Model to Identify Factors that Predict Likelihood to Adopt Tele-Neurorehabilitation

***Marlena Klaic*[1]* *and Mary P. Galea*[2]**

[1] Allied Health Department, Royal Melbourne Hospital, Parkville, VIC, Australia, [2] Department of Medicine (Royal Melbourne Hospital), University of Melbourne, Parkville, VIC, Australia

***Correspondence:**
Marlena Klaic
marlena.klaic@mh.org.au

Tele-neurorehabilitation has the potential to reduce accessibility barriers and enhance patient outcomes through a more seamless continuum of care. A growing number of studies have found that tele-neurorehabilitation produces equivalent results to usual care for a variety of outcomes including activities of daily living and health related quality of life. Despite the potential of tele-neurorehabilitation, this model of care has failed to achieve mainstream adoption. Little is known about feasibility and acceptability of tele-neurorehabilitation and most published studies do not use a validated model to guide and evaluate implementation. The technology acceptance model (TAM) was developed 20 years ago and is one of the most widely used theoretical frameworks for predicting an individual's likelihood to adopt and use new technology. The TAM3 further built on the original model by incorporating additional elements from human decision making such as computer anxiety. In this perspective, we utilize the TAM3 to systematically map the findings from existing published studies, in order to explore the determinants of adoption of tele-neurorehabilitation by both stroke survivors and prescribing clinicians. We present evidence suggesting that computer self-efficacy and computer anxiety are significant predictors of an individual's likelihood to use tele-neurorehabilitation. Understanding what factors support or hinder uptake of tele-neurorehabilitation can assist in translatability and sustainable adoption of this technology. If we are to shift tele-neurorehabilitation from the research domain to become a mainstream health sector activity, key stakeholders must address the barriers that have consistently hindered adoption.

Keywords: stroke, neurorehabilitation after stroke, tele-neurorehabilitation, technology—ICT, telehealth acceptance

STROKE

Great advances have been made in acute stroke management, which has led to a marked decrease in mortality rates (1). However, incidence remains high with almost 14 million new strokes occurring annually and more than 80 million prevalent cases globally in 2016. The annual cost to society for first-ever stroke in Australia is AUD $5 billion and in the United States USD $50 billion and includes hospitalization, informal care and loss of productivity (2, 3).

Stroke is the main cause of acquired disability in the adult population with high numbers of survivors experiencing sensorimotor impairment, reduced cognition, and reduced function (4–7). There is strong evidence showing that neurorehabilitation in the acute, subacute, and chronic phases of recovery improves patient outcomes across numerous domains including activities of daily living and health-related quality of life (8–13). Improvement in function and subsequent reduction of disability, by as little as 1-point on the Modified Rankin Scale (mRS), can reduce the costs of care by 85% (2). Despite the evidence of the effectiveness of neurorehabilitation and the potential to reduce burden of care and associated costs, access to rehabilitation is inequitable. A recent audit of acute stroke care in Australia found that only 39% of patients admitted with a primary diagnosis of stroke were assessed for rehabilitation yet 75% were found to have rehabilitation needs (14). This suggests that a large number of Australian stroke survivors may be missing out on the opportunity to maximize their recovery. An Australian study exploring rehabilitation referral patterns for stroke survivors found there were significant variations in selection resulting in inequitable access to rehabilitation (15–17). The reasons for the variation in referrals for neurorehabilitation are multiple and include clinical and non-clinical factors such as reduced workforce capacity and limited access to rehabilitation beds requiring a prioritization approach (17).

Factors that impact on the provision of specialize neurorehabilitation are common across both developing and developed countries (14–18). In Australia, funding models typically emphasize reducing length of stay in an effort to reduce the cost of an episode of rehabilitation. In developing countries, access to organized stroke care, particularly neurorehabilitation, is limited (1, 19, 20). The need for alternative models of neurorehabilitation that are effective and efficient and can overcome current barriers has become an urgent priority, particularly in the more recent context of the COVID-19 pandemic where the demand for remote healthcare has increased rapidly. Telehealth strategies have shown great potential globally as an effective strategy to improve accessibility to healthcare (21, 22). Neurorehabilitation delivered using a telehealth platform, known as tele-neurorehabilitation, may overcome some of the barriers evident in more traditional, center-based models of care. This is particularly true for low and middle-income countries where access to specialized health and rehabilitation services is limited but information and communication technologies (ICT) are readily available and commonly used (23).

TELE-NEUROREHABILITATION

Tele-neurorehabilitation refers to a model of care that uses ICT to deliver clinical rehabilitation and education to patients with a neurological condition at a remote location, such as the patient's home (24, 25). There is a broad range of ICT that may be used in tele-neurorehabilitation from simple devices such as telephones and videoconferencing, up to more complex sensor-based systems with inertial measurement units (25–28).

The number of studies exploring effectiveness of tele-neurorehabilitation has grown over the last 10 years. This increased focus reflects advances in ICT and the growing need to find efficient, effective and economical models of care in the context of fiscally constrained healthcare settings. Laver et al. recently completed a systematic review of tele-neurorehabilitation for stroke services which included evidence from 22 randomized controlled trials with a total of 1,937 participants (29). The studies encompassed a large range of interventions such as mobility retraining, communication therapy and upper limb programs. The technologies used were equally varied and included telephone follow ups, electrical stimulation, IMU sensors and a virtual online library. The authors of the review found there was moderate-quality evidence that tele-neurorehabilitation for stroke survivors achieves results equivalent to usual care for activities of daily living, depressive symptoms, and health related quality of life. However, Laver et al. noted that the studies included in the systematic review did not address feasibility of ICT from the perspective of either the participants or the prescribing clinicians. This raises questions regarding what type of patient is most appropriate for a tele-neurorehabilitation program, how much training is needed for both user and prescriber and what infrastructure is necessary to support sustainable implementation of this model. The large body of research on implementation science suggests that a theoretical model can provide a framework to guide both implementation and evaluation of tele-neurorehabilitation and potentially enhance sustainable adoption of this model (30).

TELE-NEUROREHABILITATION AND TECHNOLOGY ACCEPTANCE

The technology acceptance model (TAM) is one of the most widely utilized theoretical models explaining an individual's intention to use new technology (31, 32). The first iteration of the TAM was developed in the 1980's and proposed that a person's intention to use and subsequent use of technology can be predicted two beliefs: (1) their perception of how useful the technology is, and (2) their perception as to whether it is easy to use. A large body of research on the TAM found that it consistently predicted 40% of the variance in the intention to use and subsequent use of technology (31). Twenty years later, the TAM was extended to become the TAM2 and included output quality, results demonstrability, job relevance, subjective norm and perceived ease of use as determinants of perceived usefulness. Another model, the determinants of perceived ease of use, was developed at the same time and included factors that anchor beliefs about technology, including computer self-efficacy, computer anxiety, computer playfulness and perceptions of external control (31). Furthermore, experience and voluntary use of the technology were considered to be factors that moderated perceived usefulness.

Most recently, the TAM2 and the determinants of perceived ease of use have been combined to become the TAM3. This integrated model proposes that perceived usefulness is influenced by a number of factors including the quality of output from the technology and how relevant it is to the needs of the user. Perceived ease of use is determined by the person's beliefs about their own skills and includes computer self-efficacy and anxiety. Importantly, both perceived usefulness and perceived ease of use can be mediated through external factors such as increased practice / experience using the technology and adequate resources to support the person's use of technology (31).

There is a significant body of research on application of all iterations of the TAM in health settings, particularly in relation to the adoption of electronic health records and telehealth (33, 34). A recent study used the TAM to predict if a group (n = 325) of Canadians would use electronic medical health records to manage health information such as making future appointments (35). The authors found that perceived ease of use was the strongest predictor of perceived usefulness. The users' prior experiences with technology, needs and values all correlated with intention to use the electronic medical health record. Another study exploring patient uptake of electronic health records found that difficulties logging in and a complex user interface impacted on adoption (36). Despite the growing evidence-base using the TAM to predict user adoption of technology, none of the published studies focus on tele-neurorehabilitation. The aim of this perspective is to explore if published studies on tele-neurorehabilitation can be mapped onto the variables in the TAM3.

METHODS

A systematic mapping review approach was selected as the intention was to describe and categorize the body of tele-neurorehabilitation evidence using the TAM3 framework. A traditional systematic review aims to identify and assess the quality of published literature in order to answer a very specific question. By contrast, a systematic mapping review characterizes the literature and catalogs it according to a criteria or framework or model. In this study, the published literature on tele-neurorehabilitation will be described and categorized using the TAM3 framework. A systematic mapping review process is particularly useful when the topic area is broad and the quality and range of studies is diverse (37–39). This approach can provide information about knowledge gaps and therefore direct future research, including systematic reviews.

The methods applied to a systematic mapping review process are as follows: (1) literature search, (2) literature selection, and (3) literature mapping to the TAM3.

Literature Search

Databases relevant to the health sciences were searched including CINAHL (EBSCO), PsycINFO (EBSCO), PubMed (National Center for Biotechnology Information), and SCOPUS. Search terms were telerehabilitation or tele-rehabilitation or telehealth or remote rehabilitation AND stroke or cerebrovascular accident or CVA AND home or remote. Limitations included English-language, adult population and peer-reviewed papers. The search date was for studies published from 2000 to July 2020.

Literature Selection

The aim of this study was to determine if the existing literature on tele-neurorehabilitation could be mapped using the TAM3, with a specific focus on the user experience. Therefore, studies which included any information on patient or therapist experience of tele-neurorehabilitation, were a particular target. Following removal of protocols, center-based interventions and systematic reviews, a total of 22 studies were identified. **Table 1** presents data extracted from the studies including aims, population and outcomes. The studies included pre/post-studies, evaluation of devices, and qualitative exploration of user experience with tele-neurorehabilitation. Participants were stroke survivors in acute, sub-acute or chronic phases of recovery and varied in their impairments. Consequently, the tele-neurorehabilitation interventions included sit-to-stand practice, communication therapies, psychosocial interventions and activities of daily living practice. The type of ICT used also varied widely from telephones to apps with associated sensor data.

Literature Mapping to TAM3

All 22 studies were readily able to be mapped on to the TAM3 and revealed patterns in relation to the barriers and facilitators for tele-neurorehabilitation. **Figure 1** displays the findings using the TAM3 model which is expanded on in the following sections.

RESULTS

Tele-Neurorehabilitation and Perceived Usefulness

Do Stroke Survivors and Clinicians Perceive That Tele-Neurorehabilitation Will Be Beneficial?

The majority of studies found that tele-neurorehabilitation interventions were not inferior to conventional center-based models of care (41, 42, 46, 47, 50, 54–56, 60). Patients and carers/family reported subjective improvements in communication, gait, activities of daily living, and motivation. Only one study found that patients preferred a conventional home exercise program over tele-neurorehabilitation due to the perception that the tele-neurorehabilitation was too complex (59). None of the studies explored therapist perceptions of the usefulness of tele-neurorehabilitation, particularly in comparison to conventional models of center-based neurorehabilitation.

Tele-Neurorehabilitation and Perceived Ease of Use

Do Stroke Survivors and Clinicians Perceive That Tele-Neurorehabilitation Is Easy to Use?

A number of studies found that participants enjoyed gaming technology associated with some of the tele-neurorehabilitation interventions and found them easy to use, engaging and motivating (41, 43, 47, 48, 52, 54). Experiences with both hardware and software had a marked effect on the user perception of tele-neurorehabilitation. For example, hands-free systems were perceived as easier to use (60) than those that required the participant to don/doff splints, sensors, and other similar hardware (40–42, 45, 56, 57).

TABLE 1 | Data extraction for studies included in the mapping review.

Author (date, country)	Study design sample	Study aim	Intervention	Outcomes measured	Results
Burdea et al. (40)	Pre/post Stroke survivors and their caregivers ($n = 8 + 8$)	To evaluate the feasibility of a tele-neurorehabilitation system developed for the study	4-weeks (20 sessions) participating in serious gaming with Grasp game controller	Motor function and impairment Emotion and cognition Survey of user experience	High rate of compliance Improvement in mood and cognition Participants had an overall positive attitude to the system Both carers and participants scored technical problems as the lowest
Chen et al. (41)	Qualitative Stroke survivors $N = 13$ participants	To investigate patient perceived benefits of and barriers to using a telerehabilitation system at home	6-weeks using a home-based telerehabilitation system with serious gaming 18 sessions supervised 18 sessions unsupervised	Semi-structured interviews exploring attitudes, motivation and usage	Perceived improvement in physical abilities, psycho-social health and well-being Participants intended to continue to use the system provided improvements in games and progress feedback were made
Cherry et al. (42)	Qualitative Stroke survivors $N = 10$	To determine participants' general impressions about the benefits and barriers of using robotic therapy devices for in-home rehabilitation	2-h daily robotic assisted therapy for a maximum period of 3-months	Direct observation In-depth semi structured interviews exploring the user experience	Benefits included increased mobility, sense of control over therapy and outlet for stress and tension Barriers were donning the hardware (arm device) and technical difficulties
Cronce et al. (43)	Case Report Stroke survivor $N = 1$	To evaluate the feasibility of a virtual rehabilitation system developed for the study	7 × 30-min training sessions using the VR system and serious gaming	Questionnaire exploring system use	Easy to use system that was highly engaging and motivating
Deng et al. (44)	Pilot RCT Stroke survivors Experimental $N = 8$ Control $N = 8$	To explore feasibility of using telerehabilitation to improve ankle dorsiflexion and to compare complex vs. simple movements of the ankle	4-weeks of telerehabilitation using a computerized system	Gait 10-meter walk test fMRI Participant feedback	Improved ankle dorsiflexion Difficulties donning hardware but overall
Deutsch et al. (45)	Case Report Stroke Survivor Clinician ($N = 1 + 1$)	To describe the outcomes of using motor imagery via a telerehabilitation platform	3 × 45–60-min sessions over 4-weeks using motor imagery delivered in the home with telerehabilitation	Imagery ability Motor behavior Fugl-Meyer Timed up and Go Questionnaire on system usability	Improvement in gait and balance Both patient and clinician found the system useful Lowest score for functions and capabilities of the system
Dodakian et al. (46)	Pre/Post Stroke survivors $N = 12$	To assess feasibility and motor gains of a telerehabilitation system developed for the study	28-days of home-based telerehabilitation delivered in 2 × 14-day blocks System consisted of specialized computer, table and set up for serious gaming	Vital signs Arm motor function Mood QoL Survey of patient experience with the technology	Improvement in arm motor function compliance and satisfaction with the system Improved stroke prevention knowledge No correlation between computer literacy and outcomes
Ellington et al. (47)	Pre/Post Stroke survivors $N = 14$	To investigate the behavioral intention to use a virtual system for practicing instrumental activities of daily living	4 × 1 h sessions using affected upper limb to practice two virtual activities e.g., meal preparation	Questionnaire based on the TAM Semi-structured interview	Positive attitude and intention to use technology Relationship between perceived usefulness and intention to use

(Continued)

TABLE 1 | Continued

Author (date, country)	Study design sample	Study aim	Intervention	Outcomes measured	Results
Flynn et al. (48)	Case report Stroke survivor $N = 1$	To explore the use of a low-cost virtual reality device	20 × 1-h sessions using a low-cost virtual reality device with associated serious gaming	Fugl-Meyer Timed up and go Daily logs of system use In-depth interview	Improvement in motor function, mood, mobility and gait Reported the system was motivating
Kurland et al. (49)	Pre/Post Stroke survivors $N = 21$	To determine if a table-based home practice program could enable maintenance of treatment gains in post-stroke aphasia	6-month home practice program with weekly teletherapy sessions	% accuracy on naming Boston naming test	Greater number of training sessions with the technology resulted in fewer gains in naming accuracy
Lai et al. (50)	Pre/Post Stroke survivors $N = 21$	To evaluate the feasibility of using videoconferencing for community-based stroke rehabilitation	8-week intervention delivered at a community center for seniors via videoconferencing. Included education modules, exercise and psychosocial support	Balance Self esteem Stroke Knowledge Mood ADL Focus group discussions exploring satisfaction	Improvements in balance, self-esteem, stroke knowledge and quality of life. 67% rated clinical effectiveness of the system as good
Langan et al. (51)	Cross-sectional study Therapists $N = 107$	To examine the extent to which physical and occupational therapists use technology in clinical stroke rehabilitation programs	N/A	Survey measuring use of technology	Poor use of technology even when available
Piron et al. (52)	Pilot study Stroke survivors $N = 10$	To compare degree of satisfaction of patients using virtual reality therapy programmed at home with those using the same system in a hospital setting	1-h of rehabilitation daily for 1 month involving virtual tasks practiced in a VR system	Fugl-Meyer scale Questionnaire measuring degree of satisfaction	High compliance Tele-neurorehabilitation group had a lower score for therapist explanation of the treatment, higher outcome for UL motor
Rogerson et al. (53)	Mixed-methods evaluation Chronic stroke survivors $N = 19$	To assess the feasibility and acceptability of a smart home system that monitors users' activity	Installation of a system and participant education on how to use it	Interview on user experience of the system	The technology gave peace of mind Engagement with the system was variable
Seo et al. (54)	Pre/Post Chronic stroke survivors $N = 10$	To assess usability of a virtual reality rehabilitation system	Not described	Survey of user experience	Preference for easy to use games
Simpson et al. (55)	Pre/Post Stroke survivors $N = 8$	To investigate the feasibility of a phone-monitored home exercise program for the upper limb following stroke	8-week home exercise program with weekly telephone contact with therapist	Chedoke arm and hand inventory Motor activity log Grip strength Occupational performance Feasibility outcomes	Did not achieve exercise adherence or goal rates Motor improvement maintained at 3 and 6 month follow up
Simpson et al. (56)	Pre/Post Stroke survivors $N = 10$	To determine whether telerehabilitation is feasible in monitoring adherence and progressing functional exercises at home	4-weeks of telerehabilitation using an app with serious gaming and sensor system to monitor movements	Short physical performance battery (SPPB) Timed sit-to-stand test Satisfaction questionnaire	High compliance with the program High ratings for system usability, enjoyment and perceived benefits Improvement in SPPB
Standen et al. (57)	Prospective cohort study Stroke survivors $N = 17$	To investigate patient use of a low-cost virtual reality system	Equipment left in patient homes for 8-weeks with advice to use 3 times per day for maximum 20 min	Duration, frequency and intensity of use	Lack of familiarity with technology impacted use

(Continued)

TABLE 1 | Continued

Author (date, country)	Study design sample	Study aim	Intervention	Outcomes measured	Results
Threapleton et al. (58)	Cross-sectional study Acute stroke survivors ($N = 4$) Chronic stroke survivors ($N = 8$) Occupational therapists ($N = 13$)	To explore the value of virtual reality in preparing patients for discharge following stroke	Demonstration of a virtual home application prior to the interview	Semi structured interviews	Occupational therapists felt the system had the potential to educate and engage the patients in preparing for discharge home but may not be suitable for all patients Stroke survivors felt the system was not representative of their own homes
Triandafilou et al. (59)	Pre/Post Stroke survivors $N = 15$	To evaluate a virtual environment system developed for the trial and compare to an existing virtual reality system and a home exercise program (HEP)	1-week participation in each of the three interventions (total of 3-weeks)	Arm displacement Survey to measure participation and satisfaction	Low satisfaction with time spent in training for the VR system Preference for HEP over the other two systems
Warland et al. (60)	Pre/Post Chronic stroke $N = 12$	To establish feasibility, acceptability and preliminary efficacy of an adapted version of a commercially available, virtual-reality gaming system for upper-limb rehabilitation	9 × 40-min exercise sessions utilizing the system for 30 days per week over 3-weeks	Semi structured interview to explore feasibility and acceptability Fugl-Meyer Assessment Action research arm test Motor activity log Participation	High level of enjoyment Improvement in all motor and function outcomes
Woolf et al. (61)	Quasi-randomized controlled feasibility study Chronic stroke survivors with aphasia $N = 21$	To test the feasibility of a randomized controlled trial comparing face to face and remotely delivered word finding therapy for people with aphasia	8 × 1 h therapy delivered using videoconferencing technology compared to face to face therapy and an attention control condition	Word retrieval Recruitment and attrition rates Participant observation and interviews Treatment fidelity	Treatment fidelity was high Compliance and satisfaction with the intervention were good Picture naming improved but not naming in conversation

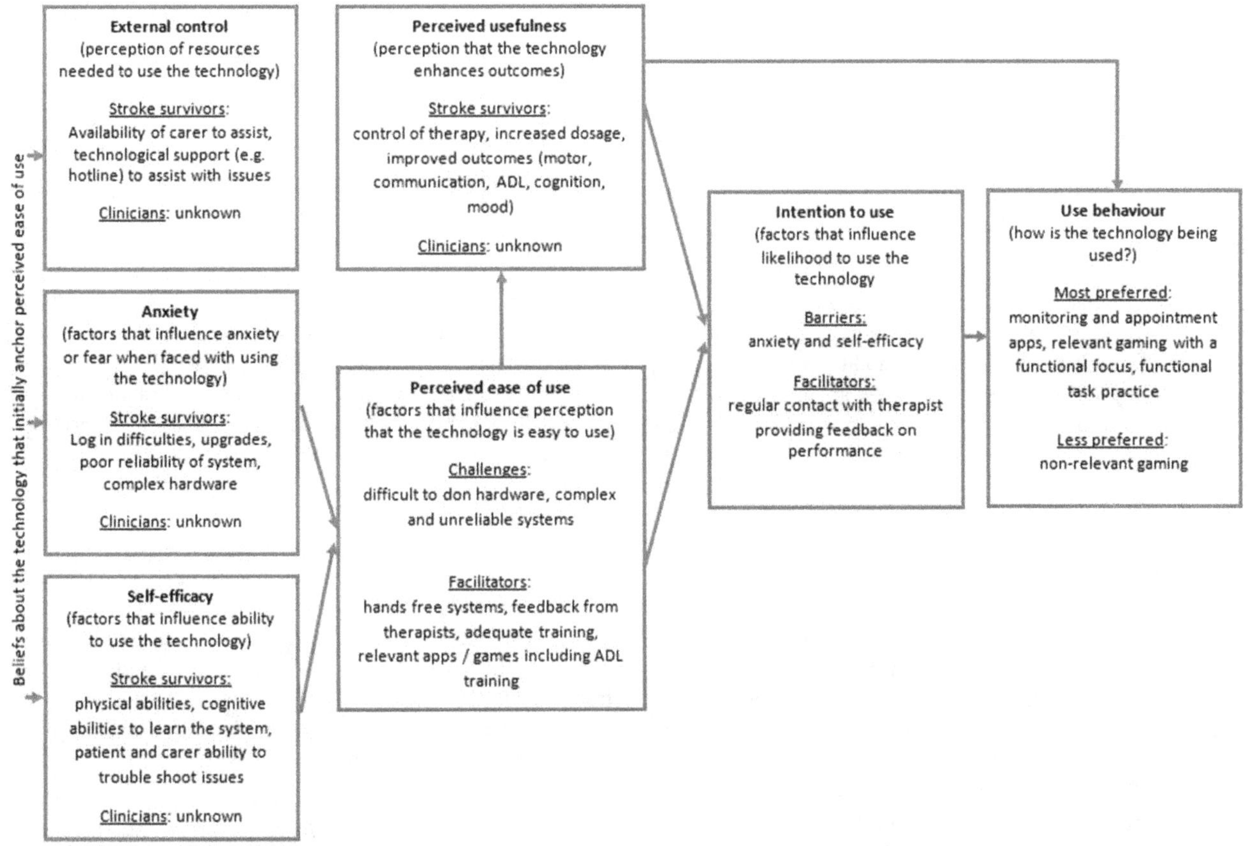

FIGURE 1 | Result of mapping the 22 studies to the variables of the TAM3 (31).

Low self-efficacy related to the tele-neurorehabilitation system used was a frequently reported problem that affected perception of ease of use, compliance, and subsequent intention to continue using the system in the future (57, 60). Conversely, prior experience with relevant technology, such as computers, correlated to improved compliance and perceptions of ease of use (46, 53).

Anxiety and frustration with tele-neurorehabilitation was apparent when more complex ICT and hardware was used (42, 44, 46). Unreliable internet bandwidth, and technical issues which were not easily resolved further contributed to anxiety and perceptions of ease of use (46). Studies where the ICT was familiar (e.g., telephones) and consisted of easy to understand tasks (e.g., sit-to-stand practice) appeared to reduce anxiety secondary to the perception that they were easier to use (47, 56).

Increased exposure and practice with tele-neurorehabilitation systems improved compliance and reduced anxiety related to low confidence and proficiency with technology (46, 48, 49, 59). However, the amount of experience necessary to reduce technology-related anxiety remains unclear with studies reporting variable amounts of time spent on training participants and therapists. Conversely, one study found there was a correlation between number of training sessions to achieve proficiency in using the technology and poorer outcomes, indicating that the technology may not be suitable for all disorders or patients (49).

The most commonly reported external variable necessary to support engagement in tele-neurorehabilitation was the presence of a carer/family member (44, 46, 61, 62). This was the case irrespective of the nature of intervention being delivered or the type of ICT being used.

Tele-Neurorehabilitation and Behavioral Intentions

Are Stroke Survivors and Clinicians Motivated or Willing to Exert the Effort to Engage in Tele-Neurorehabilitation?

A number of studies found that participants reported an intention to continuing engaging in tele-neurorehabilitation, with some provisos, including a request for easier and more reliable technology and access to their performance results (40, 41, 47, 52, 53).

Tele-Neurorehabilitation and Use Behavior

How Are Stroke Survivors and Clinicians Using Tele-Neurorehabilitation?

Tele-neurorehabilitation with a focus on relevant, easy to use components was rated more highly by participants than complex systems with multiple componentry (46, 53). For example, appointment reminder systems, monitoring apps and ADL focused gaming was selected more often than motor-based gaming. Participants also preferred tele-neurorehabilitation systems where the therapist could observe and provide feedback and encouragement via a videoconferencing or other interactive system (41, 45, 54, 56).

DISCUSSION

It is anticipated that the demand for neurorehabilitation will continue to grow due to an aging population and high incidence rates of diseases such as stroke. Rehabilitation resources in both developing and developed countries are limited and the need to find alternative yet effective and efficient models is imperative. Tele-neurorehabilitation has great potential to increase accessibility to rehabilitation for individuals with neurological impairments. However, consideration must be given for both human and ICT factors that can hinder or facilitate adoption of tele-neurorehabilitation.

A review of the published evidence on tele-neurorehabilitation through the lens of TAM3 reveals that perception of ease of use is influenced by the user's belief that they have the requisite skills and ability to use the technology (computer self-efficacy) and the degree of apprehension or fear they experience when faced with learning to use the technology (computer anxiety). Easy to use ICT and adequate experience using the technology assists the user to adjust their beliefs about computer self-efficacy and reduces computer anxiety (46, 63). Some studies found that patients were open to and excited about tele-neurorehabilitation but experienced numerous technological malfunctions which increased computer anxiety and reduced perceived enjoyment (64). Nearly all studies found that carers were critical to ensure that patients were able to overcome barriers related to system set-up, thus reducing computer anxiety (63).

There is little to no evidence on the feasibility of tele-neurorehabilitation for the "typical" stroke survivor who is likely to have cognitive impairment. Published studies have found that patients with cognitive impairment can benefit from computer training programs, suggesting that at least some of these patients may have computer self-efficacy and be appropriate for a tele-neurorehabilitation intervention. There is little to no evidence on how much experience or practice and training with a system is needed for the stroke survivor to become a confident user. Understanding the type and frequency of training necessary to establish and maintain computer self-efficacy would contribute to a more informed implementation and sustainable adoption of tele-neurorehabilitation.

Although gains have been made in design of ICT to potentially enhance tele-neurorehabilitation, barriers to adoption that were identified more than 20 years ago remain apparent today (65). These barriers are relevant for both patients and prescribing clinicians and include poor computer self-efficacy, high computer anxiety, low perception of usefulness and a belief that the technology is not user-friendly (65, 66). If we are to realize the full potential of tele-neurorehabilitation, it is of critical importance that we approach the topic using a validated and well-tested theoretical framework to guide and evaluate implementation. This would make a significant contribution to the evidence-base on tele-neurorehabilitation.

AUTHOR CONTRIBUTIONS

MK and MG conceived the ideas presented. MK completed the initial draft of the manuscript which was reviewed and edited by MG resulting in the final manuscript. All authors contributed to the article and approved the submitted version.

REFERENCES

1. Johnson CO, Nguyen M, Roth GA, Nichols E, Alam T, Abate D, et al. Global, regional, and national burden of stroke, 1990–2016: a systematic analysis for the global burden of disease study 2016. *Lancet Neurol.* (2019) 18:439–58. doi: 10.1016/S1474-4422(19)30034-1
2. Majersik JJ, Woo D. The enormous financial impact of stroke disability. *Neurology.* (2020) 94:377–8. doi: 10.1212/WNL.0000000000009030
3. Cadilhac DA, Carter R, Thrift AG, Dewey HM. Estimating the long-term costs of ischemic and hemorrhagic stroke for Australia: new evidence derived from the North East Melbourne stroke incidence study (NEMESIS). *Stroke.* (2009) 40:915–21. doi: 10.1161/STROKEAHA.108.526905
4. Sun JH, Tan L, Yu JT. Post-stroke cognitive impairment: epidemiology, mechanisms and management. *Ann Transl Med.* (2014) 2:80. doi: 10.3978/j.issn.2305-5839.2014.08.05
5. Douiri A, Rudd AG, Wolfe CD. Prevalence of poststroke cognitive impairment: South London stroke register 1995–2010. *Stroke.* (2013) 44:138–45. doi: 10.1161/STROKEAHA.112.670844
6. Langhorne P, Coupar F, Pollock A. Motor recovery after stroke: a systematic review. *Lancet Neurol.* (2009) 8:741–54. doi: 10.1016/S1474-4422(09)70150-4
7. Crichton SL, Bray BD, McKevitt C, Rudd AG, Wolfe CD. Patient outcomes up to 15 years after stroke: survival, disability, quality of life, cognition and mental health. *J Neurol Neurosurg Psychiatry.* (2016) 87:1091–8. doi: 10.1136/jnnp-2016-313361
8. Hubbard IJ, Harris D, Kilkenny MF, Faux SG, Pollack MR, Cadilhac DA. Adherence to clinical guidelines improves patient outcomes in Australian audit of stroke rehabilitation practice. *Arch Phys Med Rehabil.* (2012) 93:965–71. doi: 10.1016/j.apmr.2012.01.011
9. Hubbard IJ, Parsons MW, Neilson C, Carey LM. Task-specific training: evidence for and translation to clinical practice. *Occup Ther Int.* (2009) 16:175–89. doi: 10.1002/oti.275
10. Wright L, Hill KM, Bernhardt J, Lindley R, Ada L, Bajorek BV, et al. Stroke management: updated recommendations for treatment along the care continuum. *Intern Med J.* (2012) 42:562–9. doi: 10.1111/j.1445-5994.2012.02774.x
11. Korner-Bitensky N. When does stroke rehabilitation end? *Int J Stroke.* (2013) 8:8–10. doi: 10.1111/j.1747-4949.2012.00963.x
12. Granger CV, Markello SJ, Graham JE, Deutsch A, Ottenbacher KJ. The uniform data system for medical rehabilitation: report of patients with stroke discharged from comprehensive medical programs in 2000-2007. *Am J Phys Med Rehabil.* (2009) 88:961–72. doi: 10.1097/PHM.0b013e3181c1ec38
13. Andrusin J, Breen JC, Keenan J, Monico S, Garth H. Abstract TP181: community based outpatient stroke rehabilitation program achieve excellent outcomes including return to work, driving, stroke education knowledge, and other rehabilitation outcomes. *Stroke.* (2019) 50(Suppl. 1):ATP181. doi: 10.1161/str.50.suppl_1.TP181

14. National Stroke Audit. *Acute Services Report.* (2019). Melbourne, VIC (2019).
15. Hakkennes SJ, Brock K, Hill KD. Selection for inpatient rehabilitation after acute stroke: a systematic review of the literature. *Arch Phys Med Rehabil.* (2011) 92:2057–70. doi: 10.1016/j.apmr.2011.07.189
16. Ilett PA, Brock KA, Graven CJ, Cotton SM. Selecting patients for rehabilitation after acute stroke: are there variations in practice? *Arch Phys Med Rehabil.* (2010) 91:788–93. doi: 10.1016/j.apmr.2009.11.028
17. Kennedy GM, Brock KA, Lunt AW, Black SF. Factors influencing selection for rehabilitation after stroke: a questionnaire using case scenarios to investigate physician perspectives and level of agreement. *Arch Phys Med Rehabil.* (2012) 93:1457–9. doi: 10.1016/j.apmr.2011.11.036
18. Jørgensen HS, Kammersgaard LP, Houth J, Nakayama H, Raaschou HO, Larsen K, et al. Who benefits from treatment and rehabilitation in a stroke unit? A community-based study. *Stroke.* (2000) 31:434–9. doi: 10.1161/01.STR.31.2.434
19. Pandian JD, Sudhan P. Stroke epidemiology and stroke care services in India. *J Stroke.* (2013) 15:128–34. doi: 10.5853/jos.2013.15.3.128
20. Wissel J, Olver J, Sunnerhagen KS. Navigating the poststroke continuum of care. *J Stroke Cerebrovasc Dis.* (2013) 22:1–8. doi: 10.1016/j.jstrokecerebrovasdis.2011.05.021
21. Moffatt JJ, Eley DS. The reported benefits of telehealth for rural Australians. *Aust Health Rev.* (2010) 34:276–81. doi: 10.1071/AH09794
22. Bagayoko CO, Traore D, Thevoz L, Diabate S, Pecoul D, Niang M, et al. Medical and economic benefits of telehealth in low- and middle-income countries: results of a study in four district hospitals in Mali. *BMC Health Serv Res.* (2014) 14(Suppl. 1):S9. doi: 10.1186/1472-6963-14-S1-S9
23. Combi C, Pozzani G, Pozzi G. Telemedicine for developing countries. A survey and some design issues. *Appl Clin Inform.* (2016) 7:1025–50. doi: 10.4338/ACI-2016-06-R-0089
24. Brennan DM, Barker LM. Human factors in the development and implementation of telerehabilitation systems. *J Telemed Telecare.* (2008) 14:55–8. doi: 10.1258/jtt.2007.007040
25. Russell TG. Physical rehabilitation using telemedicine. *J Telemed Telecare.* (2007) 13:217–20. doi: 10.1258/135763307781458886
26. Hoffmann T, Russell T, Cooke H. Remote measurement via the internet of upper limb range of motion in people who have had a stroke. *J Telemed Telecare.* (2007) 13:401–5. doi: 10.1258/135763307783064377
27. Crocher V, Fong J, Klaic M, Oetomo D, Tan Y. A tool to address movement quality outcomes of post-stroke patients. *Replace, Repair, Restore, Relieve – Bridging Clinical and Engineering Solutions in Neurorehabilitation 2014.* Cham: Springer International Publishing (2014). doi: 10.1007/978-3-319-08072-7_53
28. Holden M, Dyar T, Dayan-Cimadoro L, Schwamm L, Bizzi E. Virtual environment training in the home via telerehabilitation. *Arch Phys Med Rehabil.* (2004) 85:E12. doi: 10.1016/j.apmr.2004.06.046
29. Laver KE, Adey-Wakeling Z, Crotty M, Lannin NA, George S, Sherrington C. Telerehabilitation services for stroke. *Cochrane Database Syst Rev.* (2020) 1:CD010255. doi: 10.1002/14651858.CD010255.pub3
30. Grimshaw JM, Eccles MP, Lavis JN, Hill SJ, Squires JE. Knowledge translation of research findings. *Implement Sci.* (2012) 7:50. doi: 10.1186/1748-5908-7-50
31. Venkatesh V, Bala H. Technology acceptance model 3 and a research agenda on interventions. *J Decis Sci Inst.* (2008) 39:273–315. doi: 10.1111/j.1540-5915.2008.00192.x
32. Davis FD, Bagozzi RP, Warshaw PR. User acceptance of computer technology: a comparison of two theoretical models. *Manag Sci.* (1989) 35:982–1003. doi: 10.1287/mnsc.35.8.982
33. Rahimi B, Nadri H, Lotfnezhad Afshar H, Timpka T. A systematic review of the technology acceptance model in health informatics. *Appl Clin Inform.* (2018) 9:604–34. doi: 10.1055/s-0038-1668091
34. Holden RJ, Karsh BT. The technology acceptance model: its past and its future in health care. *J Biomed Inform.* (2010) 43:159–72. doi: 10.1016/j.jbi.2009.07.002
35. Razmak J, Bélanger C. Using the technology acceptance model to predict patient attitude toward personal health records in regional communities. *Inform Technol People.* (2018) 31:306–326. doi: 10.1108/ITP-07-2016-0160
36. Portz JD, Bayliss EA, Bull S, Boxer RS, Bekelman DB, Gleason K, et al. Using the technology acceptance model to explore user experience, intent to use, and use behavior of a patient portal among older adults with multiple chronic conditions: descriptive qualitative study. *J Med Internet Res.* (2019) 21:e11604. doi: 10.2196/11604
37. Grant MJ, Booth A. A typology of reviews: an analysis of 14 review types and associated methodologies. *Health Inform Librar J.* (2009) 26:91–108. doi: 10.1111/j.1471-1842.2009.00848.x
38. Hammick M. A BEME review: a little illumination. *Med Teach.* (2005) 27:1–3. doi: 10.1080/01421590500046858
39. Clapton J, Rutter D, Sharif N. *SCIE Systematic Mapping Guidance.* London: SCIE (2009).
40. Burdea GC, Grampurohit N, Kim N, Polistico K, Kadaru A, Pollack S, et al. Feasibility of integrative games and novel therapeutic game controller for telerehabilitation of individuals chronic post-stroke living in the community. *Top Stroke Rehabil.* (2020) 27:321–36. doi: 10.1080/10749357.2019.1701178
41. Chen Y, Chen Y, Zheng K, Dodakian L, See J, Zhou R, et al. A qualitative study on user acceptance of a home-based stroke telerehabilitation system. *Top Stroke Rehabil.* (2020) 27:81–92. doi: 10.1080/10749357.2019.1683792
42. Cherry CO, Chumbler NR, Richards K, Huff A, Wu D, Tilghman LM, et al. Expanding stroke telerehabilitation services to rural veterans: a qualitative study on patient experiences using the robotic stroke therapy delivery and monitoring system program. *Disabil Rehabil Assist Technol.* (2017) 12:21–7. doi: 10.3109/17483107.2015.1061613
43. Cronce A, Gerald Fluet P, Patel J, Alma Merians PJJOAMR. Home-based virtual rehabilitation for upper extremity functional recovery post-stroke. *J Alt Med Res.* (2018) 10:27–35.
44. Deng H, Durfee WK, Nuckley DJ, Rheude BS, Severson AE, Skluzacek KM, et al. Complex versus simple ankle movement training in stroke using telerehabilitation: a randomized controlled trial. *Physical Ther.* (2012) 92:197–209. doi: 10.2522/ptj.20110018
45. Deutsch JE, Maidan I, Dickstein R. Patient-centered integrated motor imagery delivered in the home with telerehabilitation to improve walking after stroke. *Physical Ther.* (2012) 92:1065–77. doi: 10.2522/ptj.20110277
46. Dodakian L, McKenzie AL, Le V, See J, Pearson-Fuhrhop K, Burke Quinlan E, et al. A home-based telerehabilitation program for patients with stroke. *Neurorehabil Neural Repair.* (2017) 31:923–33. doi: 10.1177/1545968317733818
47. Ellington A, Adams R, White M, Diamond P. Behavioral intention to use a virtual instrumental activities of daily living system among people with stroke. *Am J Occupat Ther.* (2015) 69:6903290030p1–8. doi: 10.5014/ajot.2015.014373
48. Flynn S, Palma P, Bender A. Feasibility of using the sony playstation 2 gaming platform for an individual poststroke: a case report. *J Neurol Phys Ther.* (2007) 31:180–9. doi: 10.1097/NPT.0b013e31815d00d5
49. Kurland J, Liu A, Stokes P. Effects of a tablet-based home practice program with telepractice on treatment outcomes in chronic aphasia. *J Speech Lang Hear Res.* (2018) 61:1140–56. doi: 10.1044/2018_JSLHR-L-17-0277
50. Lai JC, Woo J, Hui E, Chan W. Telerehabilitation—a new model for community-based stroke rehabilitation. *J Telemed Telecare.* (2004) 10:199–205. doi: 10.1258/1357633041424340
51. Langan J, Subryan H, Nwogu I, Cavuoto L. Reported use of technology in stroke rehabilitation by physical and occupational therapists. *Disabil Rehabil Assist Technol.* (2018) 13:641–7. doi: 10.1080/17483107.2017.1362043
52. Piron L, Turolla A, Tonin P, Piccione F, Lain L, Dam M. Satisfaction with care in post-stroke patients undergoing a telerehabilitation programme at home. *J Telemed Telecare.* (2008) 14:257–60. doi: 10.1258/jtt.2008.080304
53. Rogerson L, Burr J, Tyson S. The feasibility and acceptability of smart home technology using the Howz system for people with stroke. *Disabil Rehabil Assist Technol.* (2020) 15:148–52. doi: 10.1080/17483107.2018.1541103
54. Seo NJ, Arun Kumar J, Hur P, Crocher V, Motawar B, Lakshminarayanan K. Usability evaluation of low-cost virtual reality hand and arm rehabilitation games. *J Rehabil Res Dev.* (2016) 53:321–34. doi: 10.1682/JRRD.2015.03.0045
55. Simpson LA, Eng JJ, Chan M. H-GRASP: the feasibility of an upper limb home exercise program monitored by phone for individuals post stroke. *Disabil Rehabil.* (2017) 39:874–82. doi: 10.3109/09638288.2016.1162853
56. Simpson DB, Bird ML, English C, Gall SL, Breslin M, Smith S, et al. Connecting patients and therapists remotely using technology is feasible and facilitates exercise adherence after stroke. *Top Stroke Rehabil.* (2020) 27:93–102. doi: 10.1080/10749357.2019.1690779

57. Standen PJ, Threapleton K, Connell L, Richardson A, Brown DJ, Battersby S, et al. Patients' use of a home-based virtual reality system to provide rehabilitation of the upper limb following stroke. *Physical Ther.* (2015) 95:350–9. doi: 10.2522/ptj.20130564
58. Threapleton K, Newberry K, Sutton G, Worthington E, Drummond A. Virtually home: Exploring the potential of virtual reality to support patient discharge after stroke. *Br. J. Occup. Ther.* (2017) 80:99–107.
59. Triandafilou KM, Tsoupikova D, Barry AJ, Thielbar KN, Stoykov N, Kamper DG. Development of a 3D, networked multi-user virtual reality environment for home therapy after stroke. *J Neuroeng Rehabil.* (2018) 15:88. doi: 10.1186/s12984-018-0429-0
60. Warland A, Paraskevopoulos I, Tsekleves E, Ryan J, Nowicky A, Griscti J, et al. The feasibility, acceptability and preliminary efficacy of a low-cost, virtual-reality based, upper-limb stroke rehabilitation device: a mixed methods study. *Disabil Rehabil.* (2019) 41:2119–34. doi: 10.1080/09638288.2018.1459881
61. Woolf C, Caute A, Haigh Z, Galliers J, Wilson S, Kessie A, et al. A comparison of remote therapy, face to face therapy and an attention control intervention for people with aphasia: a quasi-randomised controlled feasibility study. *Clin Rehabil.* (2016) 30:359–73. doi: 10.1177/0269215515582074
62. Standen PJ, Threapleton K, Richardson A, Connell L, Brown DJ, Battersby S, et al. A low cost virtual reality system for home based rehabilitation of the arm following stroke: a randomised controlled feasibility trial. *Clin Rehabil.* (2017) 31:340–50. doi: 10.1177/0269215516640320
63. Cikajlo I, Hukić A, Dolinšek I, Zajc D, Vesel M, Krizmanič T, et al. Can telerehabilitation games lead to functional improvement of upper extremities in individuals with Parkinson's disease? *Int J Rehabil Res.* (2018) 41:230–8. doi: 10.1097/MRR.0000000000000291
64. Brown EVD, Dudgeon BJ, Gutman K, Moritz CT, McCoy SW. Understanding upper extremity home programs and the use of gaming technology for persons after stroke. *Disabil Health J.* (2015) 8:507–13. doi: 10.1016/j.dhjo.2015.03.007
65. Standing C, Standing S, McDermott ML, Gururajan R, Kiani Mavi R. The paradoxes of telehealth: a review of the literature 2000–2015. *Syst Res Behav Sci.* (2018) 35:90–101. doi: 10.1002/sres.2442
66. Seelman KD, Hartman LM. Telerehabilitation: policy issues and research tools. *Int J Telerehabil.* (2009) 1:47–58. doi: 10.5195/IJT.2009.6013

21

An Italian Neurorehabilitation Hospital Facing the SARS-CoV-2 Pandemic: Data from 1207 Patients and Workers

Antonino Salvia, Giovanni Morone, Marco Iosa, Maria Pia Balice, Stefano Paolucci, Maria Grazia Grasso, Marco Traballesi, Ugo Nocentini, Rita Formisano, Marco Molinari, Angelo Rossini and Carlo Caltagirone*

Fondazione Santa Lucia, IRCCS, Rome, Italy

***Correspondence:**
Giovanni Morone
g.morone@hsantalucia.it

Objective: The aim of the present observational study is to report on the data from a large sample of inpatients, clinical staff and other workers at an Italian neurorehabilitation hospital dealing with SARS-CoV-2 infections, in order to analyze how it might have affected the management and the effectiveness of neurorehabilitation.

Methods: The data on infection monitoring, obtained by 2,192 swabs, were reported and compared among 253 patients, 722 clinical professionals and 232 other hospital workers. The number of admissions and neurorehabilitation sessions performed in the period from March-May 2020 was compared with those of the same period in 2019.

Results: Four patients and three clinical professionals were positive for COVID-19 infection. Six out of these seven people were from the same ward. Several measures were taken to handle the infection, putting in place many restrictions, with a significant reduction in new admissions to the hospital ($p < 0.001$). However, neither the amount of neurorehabilitation for inpatients ($p = 0.681$) nor the effectiveness of treatments ($p = 0.464$) were reduced when compared to the data from 2019.

Conclusions: Our data show that the number of infections was contained in our hospital, probably thanks to the protocols adopted for reducing contagion and the environmental features of our wards. This allowed inpatients to continue to safely spend more than 3 hours per day in neurorehabilitation, effectively improving their independence in the activities of daily living.

Keywords: coronavirus, COVID-19, rehabilitation, molecular test, swab, SARS-CoV-2, hospital design and construction

INTRODUCTION

The World Health Organization (WHO) characterized the novel severe acute respiratory syndrome coronavirus-2 (SARS-CoV-2) outbreak as a pandemic on March 11th 2020 (1). In response to this, many governments implemented a series of emergency containment measures, including social restrictions and the quarantine of positive and suspect cases. Italy was the first Western country with a wide diffusion of coronavirus disease (COVID-19), so it could be important for other countries to analyze in depth the Italian case-study (2). In April, Iosa and coworkers suggested a dynamic analysis of the Italian case-fatality ratio to gain deeper insight into the course of the COVID-19 pandemic, and we anticipated the need to prepare rehabilitation units. Both people with COVID-19 sequelae related to motor and respiratory functions and patients with neurological disorders (3), not infected but needing neurorehabilitation in the time of this pandemic, could not wait to be treated (4–6). Several measures, including those imposed by the Decrees of the Italian President of the Council of Ministers, were taken to tackle the infection in rehabilitation hospitals with the aim of monitoring the insurgence of epidemic outbreaks (4). As nosocomial transmission is a severe problem in relation to the condition of inpatients, any action should be taken to minimize the risk of transmission among patients and clinical staff (7). However, an analysis of the impact of these measures is lacking in the literature. A recent study analyzed the outcomes of outpatients with pre-existing neurological disorders reporting the prevalence of symptoms of COVID-19 infection (8). The authors found that the presence of neurological chronic diseases did not increase the prevalence of COVID-19 infection, but the burden of neurological disorders was worsened by the lockdown. These problems could be even more dramatic for inpatients. Indeed, hospital access to people with neurological impairments due to brain or spinal cord injury in the subacute phase was often postponed as a consequence of infection. However, the neurorehabilitation of these patients is time-dependent and cannot be delayed, nor can it be reduced in intensity (9, 10). Furthermore, in Italy, there was an increased pressure on high specialty neurorehabilitation wards to admit patients with severe neurological disabilities (sometimes even with unstable vital functions and a high risk of medical complications) due to the sudden need for intensive care units to free up beds for COVID-19 positive patients with respiratory insufficiency. Other countries are now facing the same problem. In this scenario, there is a need for a quantitative analysis of the impact of the adopted restriction measures on inpatients needing neurorehabilitation, especially in hospitals exposed to the risk of COVID-19 infection.

The aim of the present observational study is to report on the data regarding COVID-19 infection monitoring in a large sample of inpatients needing neurorehabilitation, clinical staff and other hospital workers, analyzing how it might have affected the management and the efficacy of neurorehabilitation.

MATERIALS AND METHODS

This was an observational study performed on data collected during the monitoring of hospitalized inpatients and people working in our hospital from April 30th to May 26th 2020. People were classified into three categories: inpatients, clinical staff (medical doctors, psychologists, nurses, therapists, health care assistants, etc.) and other hospital workers (administrative staff, cleaners, etc.). They underwent repetitive series of swabs related to the program monitoring at out hospital during the COVID-19 pandemic.

Protocols

During the SARS-CoV-2 pandemic, the Italian Society of Neurological Rehabilitation indications were followed for the reorganization of neuro-rehabilitation activities (4). Moreover, we also changed our protocols in the following aspects:

- Our neurorehabilitation units admitted patients with subacute neurological impairments due to severe acquired brain lesions or stroke coming from an acute unit only if they were not affected or suspected to be infected with COVID-19 (with two negative nasal swabs performed within the last 48 h before discharge from acute wards).
- Our hospital is formed by six identical wards for inpatients, with 26 bedrooms having only two beds each (each room was 46 square meters with a bathroom inside), according to the requirements defined by Italian law, plus one room with negative pressure, and the availability of a gym in each ward (as shown in **Figure 1**). We planned three different pathways for human traffic within each ward: one for entering, one for exit, and one specific for isolated patient with different elevators just used for them, as shown in **Figure 1**. This figure also shows that each ward has a gym in which there were two rooms for speech therapy. The detail of one bed-room and of the isolation room with negative pressure were also shown in that figure.
- Healthy people, such as workers and allowed visitors, could enter into the hospital only if their body temperature was lower than 37.5°C (if higher, home isolation was suggested). Employees commute from home, no specific restrictions to social activities were required by the hospital direction, but they were required to strictly follow the restrictions of the lockdown programmed by Italian government for all the citizens (for example, in the study period, in Italy most of the shops were closed, restaurants were closed, religious meetings were forbidden).
- Posters with behavioral/health general rules (such as about social distancing in rooms, maximum number of people allowed into elevators at the same time, hand hygiene recommendations, use of protective devices, and so on) were positioned at each entrance and within all the complex operative units and the number of hand-sanitizing gel dispensers in the whole hospital was increased.
- A specific guideline has been drawn up describing prevention and control measures during the management of suspected and confirmed cases of COVID-19 in our facility, and several training sessions have been held with the health care professionals for the correct use of SARS-CoV-2 personal protective equipment (PPE) such as surgical masks, whereas suspected cases were cared by clinical staff using medical cap, eye-visor, face shield, N95 respiratory mask, double disposable gloves, medical protecting coverall, leg cover waterproof boots.
- Reorganization of work shifts (medical and non-medical staff) with a reduction in some activities in order to reduce contact and movements (for example, encouraging staff to work from home for administrative activities).
- After the first case of a positive swab in our hospital (April 30th), neither new admissions (up to May 21st) nor visitors

(for the entire month of May and the first weeks of June, with only a few exceptions for caregivers staying in the same room of patients needing continuous assistance after two consecutive negative swabs) were allowed. An extraordinary plan for daily cleaning and sanitization of the wards was putted in action.

- Outpatient activities and/or day hospital rehabilitation were reduced (only activities that cannot be postponed according to regional guidelines were maintained in different areas and different clinical staff from those of inpatients to avoid contacts between these two populations).
- Strengthening of patient and caregiver support networks, also through information technologies and an emphasis on the role of tele-rehabilitation.
- Seven sessions of swab analyses for monitoring patients and workers were carried out from the end of April to the end of May.

Epidemiological Analysis

From 30th April, we started an epidemiological analysis on the inpatients and employers of our hospital with the main aim to identify asymptomatic subjects. The whole sample was formed of 1,207 people: 253 inpatients, 722 clinical professionals and 232 other hospital workers. Among the patients, 153 were affected by stroke, 54 by traumatic brain injury, 31 by spinal cord injury, 9 by multiple sclerosis, 2 by Parkinson's disease, and 4 by orthopedic problems. Our hospital provides six wards for inpatients. Workers and patients were assigned to the same ward for the entire investigation period, in order to limit transfers.

Data Analysis

Data are reported in terms of mean and standard deviation for continuous measures, absolute frequency for counted discrete measures, median and interquartile range (IQR = third–first quartiles) for ordinal measures of clinical scales and not normally distributed variables. Odds ratios were computed together with relevant 95% confidence intervals (95% CI) and inferred by the chi-squared test. Paired t-tests were performed to compare the data related to March, April and May 2020 and 2019 in terms of time spent in neurorehabilitation activities. Mann–Whitney U-tests were performed for comparing the Barthel Index (BI) score at admission and discharge, effectiveness and length of stay in the period from March to May 2020 vs. the same period in 2019. The effectiveness was computed as the percentage improvement obtained in terms of the BI-score with respect to the maximum achievable one. The level of statistical significance was set at 5%.

RESULTS

Epidemiological Data of Swab Analysis

During the study period, the statistics of the outbreak in Italy reported 104,664 new contagions in March, 99,671 in April, and 27,534 in May. In Lazio (the Italian region of our hospital and in which resided our employees) the number of contagions were 3,092 in March, 3,521 in April and 1,112 in May, on a population of about 5.9 million of people (11).

In our hospital, a total of 2,192 nasal swabs were performed in <1 month: 13 swabs on April 30th finding one nurse positive; 62 swabs on May 2nd finding another nurse and two stroke patients positive (these patients came from the same ward as the first positive case); 1,093 swabs on May 4th and 5th with positive findings in other two stroke patients (from the same ward) and one therapist (from another ward); no more positive cases were found in the subsequent analysis of 31 swabs on May 7th, 151 swabs between 11th and 12th, 738 between 18th and 19th, 104 swabs on 26th May. All seven positive cases (corresponding to a prevalence of 0.6%) were asymptomatic. Familiars were advised. According to the regional guidelines, positive patients were immediately isolated in the special room with negative pressure and transferred within 6 h to a regional dedicated Covid-hospital (during this short time, the patients did not receive any rehabilitation session). After the recovery in that hospital and the following negativization of two consecutive swabs, two out of the four patients were discharged at home and the other two were re-admitted to our hospital to continue the neurorehabilitation. The cases of positive employers were notified to the competent authorities, and these subjects were quarantined at home for 14 days in charge to family physician, and they were allowed to return to work after 2 negative nasal swabs performed within the last 48 h.

The cumulative data are reported in **Table 1**. The odds ratio of being infected by SARS-CoV2 was not statistically different between patients and clinical staff, although it was close to the significance threshold (OR = 3.85; 95% CI: 0.86–17.3; $p = 0.0588$). Conversely, an odds ratio of 64.8 (95% CI: 7.7–545; $p < 0.001$) was found in favor of being hospitalized or working in the same ward. For a comparison with the data of the outbreak during the study period, in Italy there were 104,664 new contagions in March, 99,671 in April and 27,534 in May. In Lazio (the Italian region of our hospital and in which resided our employees) the number of contagions were 3,092 in March, 3,521 in April and 1,112 in May.

Number of Treated Patients

The admission of patients to the hospital was stopped immediately after the first positive swab. This measure implies a reduction in inpatients, as shown in **Figure 2**. During the period from March to May 2020, 89 patients were admitted (median BI-score = 12, IQR = 26). In the same period of 2019 the number of admissions were 180; however, the median BI-score was not significantly different (BI-score = 13, IQR = 30, $p = 0.468$).

The hospital bed occupancy was significantly different in the entire period from March to May 2020 with respect to the same period in 2019 ($p < 0.001$), especially after the first positive case, when the temporary halt to new admissions occurred, as shown in **Figure 2**. The rehabilitation of outpatients (day hospital) was even more significantly decreased: it was 36% of planned occupancy in March, 3.8% in April and 8.6% in May, whereas the matching percentages in 2019 were 106, 102.1, and 103.6%, respectively ($p = 0.010$).

From an economic point of view, the amount of loss of income related to the reduction of Day Hospital was 64% in March, 96% in April, and 92% in May; whereas that of inpatients was 5, 6,

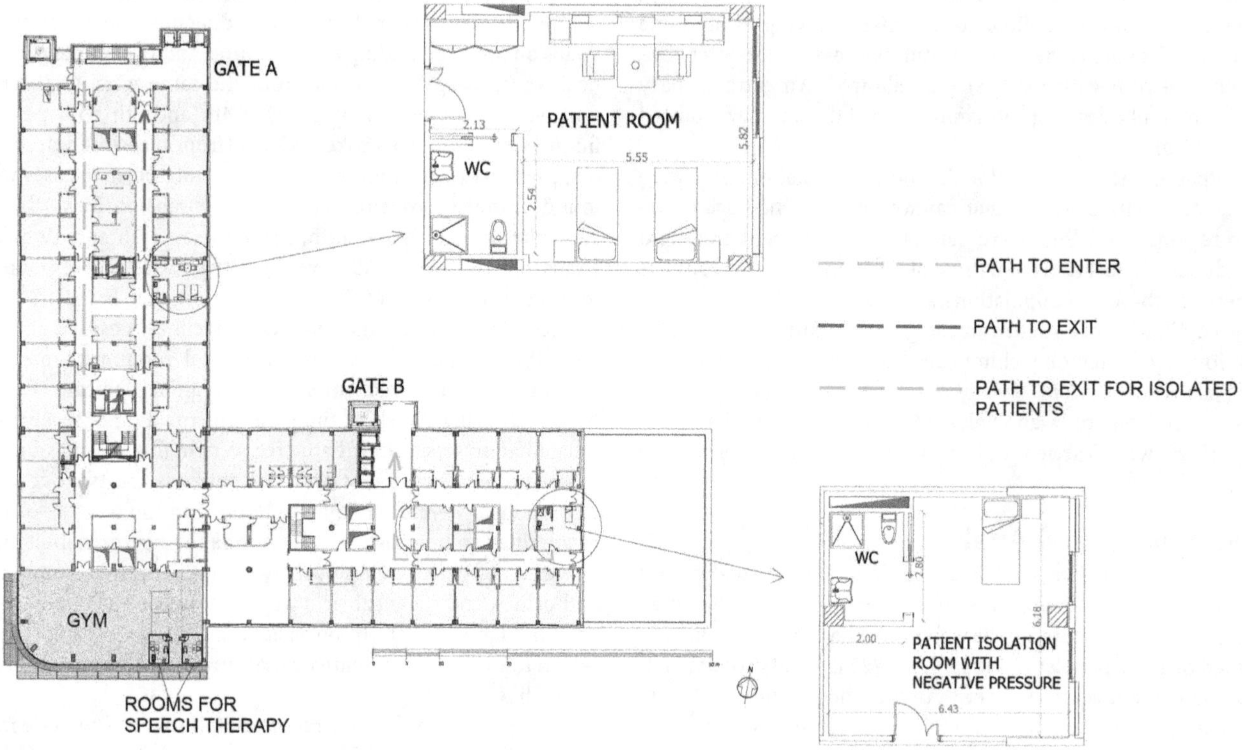

FIGURE 1 | The planimetry of one of the six identical wards of our hospital. In details are also shown the planimetry of one of the twenty-seven standard patient's rooms of the ward (in yellow) and the special isolation room with negative pressure. In blue the rooms of doctors and in pink the gym. Stairs and elevators are located in proximity to each gate. The dotted rows show the pathway defined for human traffic during the analyzed period: the blue pathway is that for entering into the ward, the red one for exit from the ward, and the green one that related to a patient isolated in the special room. All the measures are expressed in meters.

TABLE 1 | Data on subjects classified as patients, clinical staff or other hospital workers.

Categories of people	Age (years old)	Sample *N*	Gender (female %)	Number of tests	Positive swab
Patients	66.3 ± 16.2	253	35%	560	4
Clinical staff	44.0 ± 11.8	722	64%	1,361	3
Other workers	47.6 ± 12.4	232	59%	271	0
Total	50.7 ± 16.4	1207	57%	2,192	7

15%, respectively. The loss related to other outpatient hospital services were 73, 81, and 61%, respectively.

Number of Treatments and Their Effectiveness in Inpatients

The mean time spent by each patient in neurorehabilitation activities was not reduced in the period from March to May 2020 (global mean: 213 ± 15 min) with respect to the same period in 2019 (211 ± 10 min, $p = 0.558$), nor in the period after the first positive cases with the temporary halt to new admissions (211 ± 11 vs. 215 ± 10 min, $p = 0.681$). The number of patients discharged in the period from March to May 2020 was 71; their median BI-score was 69 (IQR = 50) with a treatment effectiveness of 48 ± 40% and a median length of stay of 49 days (IQR = 42). In the same period in 2019, the number of discharged patients was much higher at 233, with a median BI-score of 54 (IQR = 67, $p = 0.049$), an effectiveness of 47 ± 36% ($p = 0.464$) and a median length of stay of 63 days (IQR = 52, $p = 0.001$), as shown in **Figure 3**.

DISCUSSION

The aim of the present observational study was to report on how COVID-19 infections were monitored and contained in a large sample of inpatients and workers, and how infection management might have affected neurorehabilitation activities. Our results highlight three important findings about the management of the COVID-19 outbreak in neurorehabilitation.

First of all, the safety protocol and continuous monitoring performed with nasal swabs allowed us to identify 7 cases in 1,207 screened people. All the positive cases were asymptomatic, and only the planned monitoring allowed us to discover the presence

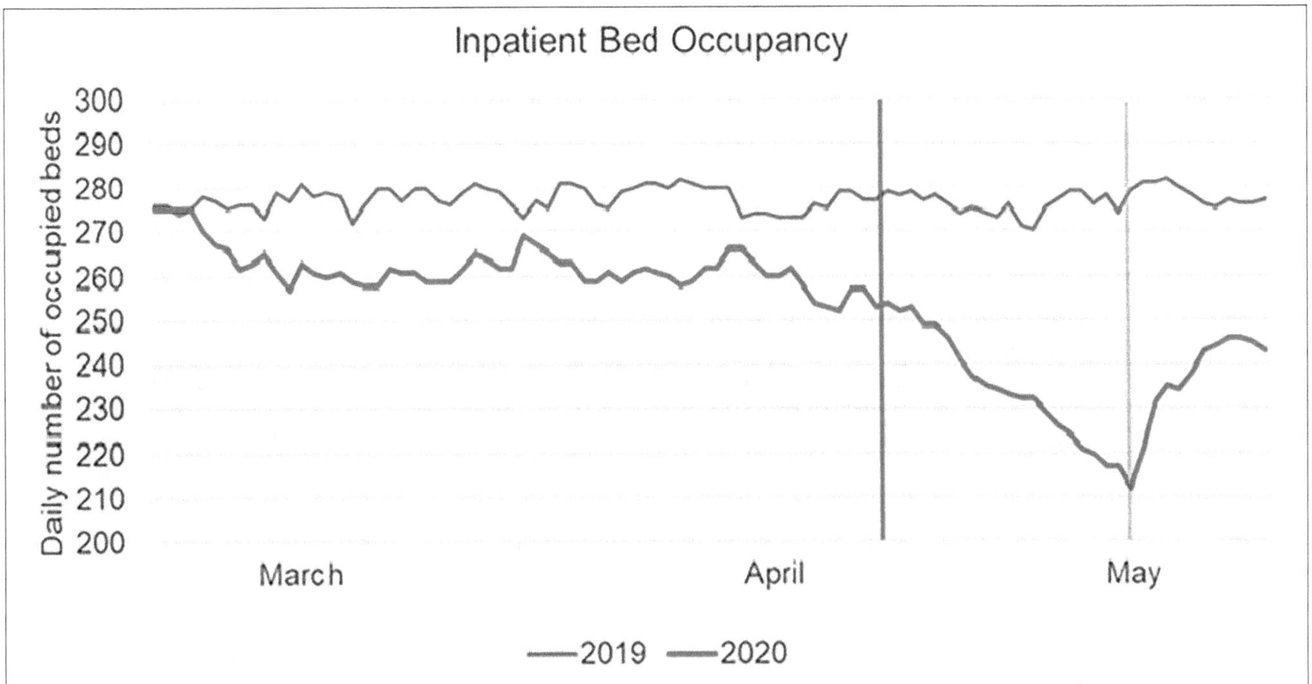

FIGURE 2 | Hospital bed occupancy in 2019 (blue line) and in 2020 (red line) for the period from March to May. The vertical red line represents the day of the first positive case in our hospital, corresponding to the beginning of the temporary halt to new admissions. The green line represents the last day of this period of halted admissions.

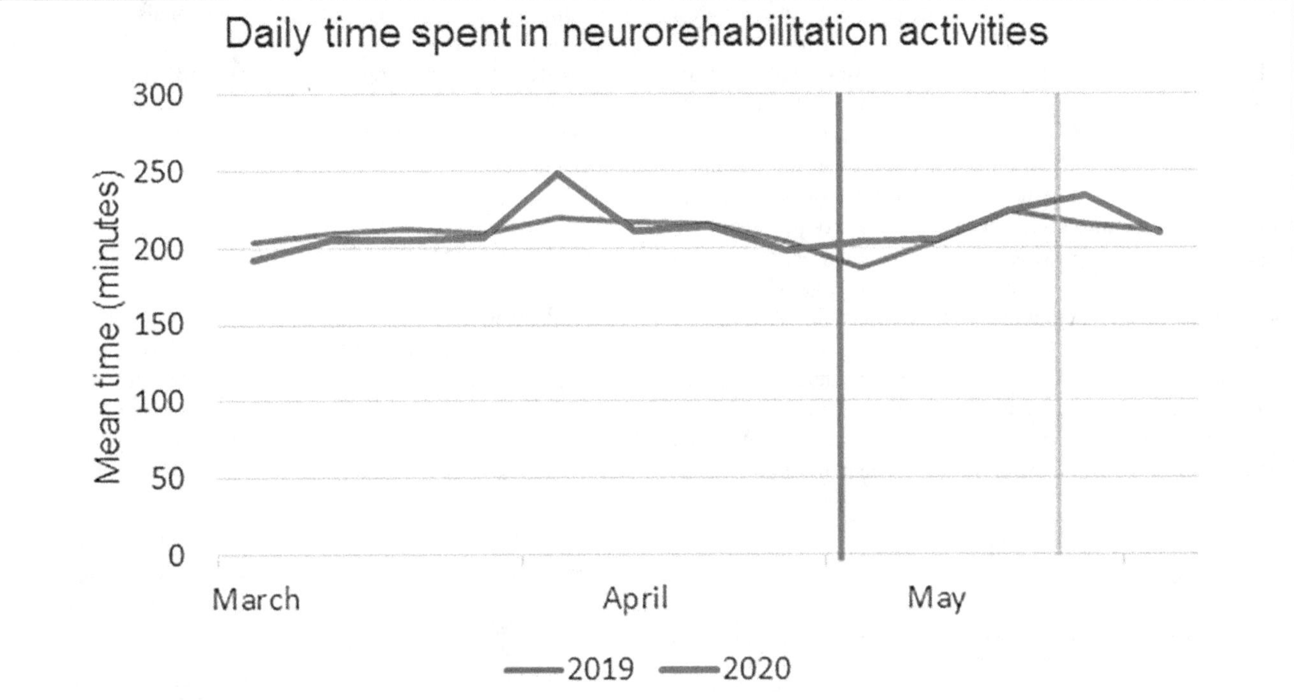

FIGURE 3 | Mean time spent by patients in neurorehabilitation activities (in minutes), averaged by week in 2019 (blue line) and 2020 (red line). The vertical red line represents the day of the first positive case in our hospital, corresponding to the beginning of the temporary halt to new admissions. The green line represents the last day of this period of halted admissions.

of positive cases in the hospital. The prevalence of COVID-19 on the screened population in our hospital (0.6%) was slightly higher than that of the Italian population at 0.2% (11), but this was due to the fact that our sample was related to a hospital population.

The second finding is related to the clusterization of positive cases, with 6 out of 7 coming from the same ward. The odds ratio related to the environmental factor was 64.8 vs. an odds ratio of 3.85 for the category of persons (patients vs. clinical staff). This effect was already well-known and at the basis of social distancing and isolation of infected patients (12). Furthermore, this odds ratio may suggest the need to isolate the different wards of a hospital, reducing possible contacts among patients and/or workers in different wards. The protocols related to internal transfers, inspired by the Decrees of the Italian President of the Council of Ministers together with the scientific literature (4, 10), adopted severe measures and allowed us to counteract the pandemic. Among the adjunctive measures, it is important to mention the requirement of two negative nasal swabs within the last 48 h before discharge from acute wards for being admitted in our hospital, even if this was not required by the World Health Organization guidelines.

Moreover, the prompt interdiction of visitor entry, although this rule enormously overwhelmed nursing staff and neurorehabilitation professionals regarding the management of daily activities and the psychological isolation of inpatients with severe neurological disabilities and common neuropsychological disorders. Another factor that may have contributed to containing the outbreak could be the architectural structure of our wards, with wide bedrooms having only two beds each and the availability of a wide gym in each ward. Before COVID-19, some authors (13) reported that the architecture of hospital facilities does not influence nosocomial infection rates, concluding that there is a lack of stringent evidence to link hospital design and construction with the prevention of nosocomial infection. However, further studies (14–16) support the opposite idea, i.e., that the design of the physical environment influences nosocomial infection rates. The safety protocols, the large rooms and the presence of a gym in each ward, together with the presence of six isolation rooms with negative pressure, could be the key factors that limited the outbreak of SARS-CoV-2 in our hospital.

Finally, the third main finding of our study was that, during the containment of the pandemic in our hospital, the admissions were significantly reduced due to the temporary halt on admissions, but the mean time spent by inpatients in rehabilitation was not reduced by the emergency. It allowed us to provide the same level of treatment effectiveness. Despite many difficulties in discharging patients from our neurorehabilitation hospital due to the problems with managing the chronic phase of neurological diseases, the length of stay was shorter than that in 2019, according to a general process of reduction of length of stay already occurring before pandemic. The main problem was the dramatic reduction in amount of care reserved to outpatients, as also observed elsewhere (8).

Our study has some limits, the main of which is that the present study is an observational study based only on one hospital, without a population-based analysis and with some populations (i.e., stroke patients) that could be overrepresented. However, our study is similar to a previous one analyzing rehabilitation of outpatients, although ours is more focused on inpatients. The presence of COVID-19, its management and the contemporary management of neurorehabilitation makes this study important for other similar hospitals.

In conclusion, the prevalence of COVID-19 infection in our inpatient neurorehabilitation hospital was effectively managed, affecting the number of admissions and the rehabilitation of outpatients, but not that of inpatients, who achieved a good level of independence in the activities of daily living, similar to that of hospitalized patients in the same period in 2019. Six out of seven positive cases of SARS-CoV-2 were recorded in the same ward, and wide screening allowed us to contain the infection by isolating and transferring positive professionals and patients, respectively. These results suggest the need for repetitive and systematic screening of patients and clinical staff in neurorehabilitation hospitals to prevent outbreaks and to maintain a high amount of effective neurorehabilitation for inpatients.

AUTHOR CONTRIBUTIONS

GM and MI wrote the first draft of this manuscript. MI and SP performed all the data analysis. CC, AS, and AR conceptualized and supervised the study. SP, MG, MT, UN, RF, and MM revised the manuscript and provided important contributions. MB was responsible of all the swab analysis. All authors contributed to the article and approved the submitted version.

REFERENCES

1. The World Health Organization (2020). Available online at: https://www.who.int/emergencies/diseases/novel-coronavirus-2019 (accessed June 10, 2020).
2. Lazzerini M, Putoto G. COVID-19 in Italy: momentous decisions and many uncertainties. *Lancet Glob Health.* (2020) 8:e641–2. doi: 10.1016/S2214-109X(20)30110-8
3. Iosa M, Paolucci S, Morone G. Covid-19: a dynamic analysis of fatality risk in Italy. *Front Med.* (2020) 7:185. doi: 10.3389/fmed.2020.00185
4. Bartolo M, Intiso D, Lentino C, Sandrini G, Paolucci S, Zampolini M, et al. Urgent measures for the containment of the coronavirus (Covid-19) epidemic in the neurorehabilitation/rehabilitation departments in the phase of maximum expansion of the epidemic. *Front Neurol.* (2020) 11:423. doi: 10.3389/fneur.2020.00423
5. Stillman MD, Capron M, Alexander M, Di Giusto ML, Scivoletto G. COVID-19 and spinal cord injury and disease: results of an international survey. *Spinal Cord Ser Cases.* (2020) 6:21. doi: 10.1038/s41394-020-0275-8
6. Baricich A, Santamato A, Picelli A, Morone G, Smania N, Paolucci S, et al. Spasticity treatment during COVID-19 pandemic: clinical recommendations. *Front. Neurol.* (2020) 11:719. doi: 10.3389/fneur.2020.00719
7. Wang Y, Wang Y, Chen Y, Qin Q. Unique epidemiological and clinical features of the emerging 2019 novel coronavirus pneumonia (COVID-19)

implicate special control measures. *J Med Virol.* (2020) 92:568–76. doi: 10.1002/jmv.25748

8. Piano C, Stasio ED, Primiano G, Janiri D, Luigetti M, Frisullo G, et al. An Italian neurology outpatient clinic facing SARS-CoV-2 pandemic: data from 2,167 patients. *Front Neurol.* (2020) 11:564. doi: 10.3389/fneur.2020.00564
9. Paolucci S, Antonucci G, Grasso MG, Morelli D, Troisi E, Coiro P, et al. Early vs. delayed inpatient stroke rehabilitation: a matched comparison conducted in Italy. *Arch Phys Med Rehabil.* (2000) 81:695–700. doi: 10.1016/S0003-9993(00)90095-9
10. Leocani L, Diserens K, Moccia M, Caltagirone C. Disability through COVID-19 pandemic: neurorehabilitation cannot wait. *Eur J Neurol.* (2020) 27:e50–1. doi: 10.1111/ene.14320
11. Available online at: https://www.epicentro.iss.it/coronavirus/sars-cov-2-sorveglianza-dati (accessed June 10, 2020).
12. Jarvis CI, Van Zandvoort K, Gimma A, Prem K, CMMID COVID-19 working group, Klepac P, et al. Quantifying the impact of physical distance measures on the transmission of COVID-19 in the UK. *BMC Med.* (2020) 18:124. doi: 10.1186/s12916-020-01597-8
13. Dettenkofer M, Seegers S, Antes G, Motschall E, Schumacher M, Daschner FD. Does the architecture of hospital facilities influence nosocomial infection rates? A systematic review. *Infect Control Hosp Epidemiol.* (2004) 25:21–5. doi: 10.1086/502286
14. Iyendo TO, Uwajeh PC, Ikenna ES. The therapeutic impacts of environmental design interventions on wellness in clinical settings: a narrative review. *Complementary Ther Clin Pract.* (2016) 24:174–88. doi: 10.1016/j.ctcp.2016.06.008
15. Anåker A, Heylighen A, Nordin S, Elf M. Design quality in the context of healthcare environments: a scoping review. *HERD.* (2017) 10:136–50. doi: 10.1177/1937586716679404
16. Ulrich RS, Zimring C, Zhu X, DuBose J, Seo HB, Choi YS, et al. A review of the research literature on evidence-based healthcare design. *HERD.* (2008) 1:61–125. doi: 10.1177/193758670800100306

Permissions

All chapters in this book were first published by Frontiers; hereby published with permission under the Creative Commons Attribution License or equivalent. Every chapter published in this book has been scrutinized by our experts. Their significance has been extensively debated. The topics covered herein carry significant findings which will fuel the growth of the discipline. They may even be implemented as practical applications or may be referred to as a beginning point for another development.

The contributors of this book come from diverse backgrounds, making this book a truly international effort. This book will bring forth new frontiers with its revolutionizing research information and detailed analysis of the nascent developments around the world.

We would like to thank all the contributing authors for lending their expertise to make the book truly unique. They have played a crucial role in the development of this book. Without their invaluable contributions this book wouldn't have been possible. They have made vital efforts to compile up to date information on the varied aspects of this subject to make this book a valuable addition to the collection of many professionals and students.

This book was conceptualized with the vision of imparting up-to-date information and advanced data in this field. To ensure the same, a matchless editorial board was set up. Every individual on the board went through rigorous rounds of assessment to prove their worth. After which they invested a large part of their time researching and compiling the most relevant data for our readers.

The editorial board has been involved in producing this book since its inception. They have spent rigorous hours researching and exploring the diverse topics which have resulted in the successful publishing of this book. They have passed on their knowledge of decades through this book. To expedite this challenging task, the publisher supported the team at every step. A small team of assistant editors was also appointed to further simplify the editing procedure and attain best results for the readers.

Apart from the editorial board, the designing team has also invested a significant amount of their time in understanding the subject and creating the most relevant covers. They scrutinized every image to scout for the most suitable representation of the subject and create an appropriate cover for the book.

The publishing team has been an ardent support to the editorial, designing and production team. Their endless efforts to recruit the best for this project, has resulted in the accomplishment of this book. They are a veteran in the field of academics and their pool of knowledge is as vast as their experience in printing. Their expertise and guidance has proved useful at every step. Their uncompromising quality standards have made this book an exceptional effort. Their encouragement from time to time has been an inspiration for everyone.

The publisher and the editorial board hope that this book will prove to be a valuable piece of knowledge for researchers, students, practitioners and scholars across the globe.

List of Contributors

Adam Buchwald and Carolyn Falconer
Department of Communicative Sciences and Disorders, New York University, New York, NY, United States

Avrielle Rykman-Peltz and Gary W. Thickbroom
Restorative Neurology Clinic, Burke Neurological Institute, White Plains, NY, United States
Weill Cornell Medicine, New York City, NY, United States

Linda M. Gerber and Clara Oromendia
Weill Cornell Medicine, New York City, NY, United States

Mar Cortes
Restorative Neurology Clinic, Burke Neurological Institute, White Plains, NY, United States
Weill Cornell Medicine, New York City, NY, United States
Icahn School of Medicine at Mount Sinai, New York City, NY, United States

Alvaro Pascual-Leone
Berenson-Allen Center for Noninvasive Brain Stimulation, Beth Israel Deaconess Medical Center, Harvard Medical School, Boston, MA, United States
Fundación Institut Guttmann, Institut Universitari de Neurorehabilitació Adscrit a la UAB, Barcelona, Spain

Hermano Igo Krebs
Department of Mechanical Engineering, Massachusetts Institute of Technology, Cambridge, MA, United States

Felipe Fregni
Spaulding Rehabilitation Hospital, Harvard Medical School, Cambridge, MA, United States

Johanna Chang and Bruce T. Volpe
Center for Biomedical Science, Feinstein Institute for Medical Research, Manhasset, NY, United States

Dylan J. Edwards
Restorative Neurology Clinic, Burke Neurological Institute, White Plains, NY, United States
Weill Cornell Medicine, New York City, NY, United States
Moss Rehabilitation Research Institute, Elkins Park, PA, United States
School of Medical and Health Sciences, Edith Cowan University, Joondalup, WA, Australia

Rosanne B. van Dijsseldonk, Brenda E. Groen and Noel L. W. Keijsers
Department of Research, Sint Maartenskliniek, Nijmegen, Netherlands
Department of Rehabilitation, Cognition and Behavior, Radboud University Medical Center, Donders Institute for Brain, Nijmegen, Netherlands

Lysanne A. F. de Jong
Department of Research, Sint Maartenskliniek, Nijmegen, Netherlands

Alexander C. H. Geurts
Department of Rehabilitation, Cognition and Behavior, Radboud University Medical Center, Donders Institute for Brain, Nijmegen, Netherlands
Department of Rehabilitation, Sint Maartenskliniek, Nijmegen, Netherlands

Marije Vos-van der Hulst
Department of Rehabilitation, Sint Maartenskliniek, Nijmegen, Netherlands

Sophie Schneider, Michael Brogioli, Urs Albisser, László Demkó and Armin Curt
Spinal Cord Injury Center, Balgrist University Hospital, Zurich, Switzerland

Roger Gassert
Rehabilitation Engineering Laboratory, Department of Health Sciences and Technology, ETH Zurich, Zurich, Switzerland

Werner L. Popp
Spinal Cord Injury Center, Balgrist University Hospital, Zurich, Switzerland
Rehabilitation Engineering Laboratory, Department of Health Sciences and Technology, ETH Zurich, Zurich, Switzerland

Isabelle Debecker
REHAB Basel, Clinic for Neurorehabilitation and Paraplegiology, Basel, Switzerland

Inge-Marie Velstra
Clinical Trial Unit, Swiss Paraplegic Center, Nottwil, Switzerland

Eliana Berra, Silvano Cristina, Claudio Pacchetti and Mauro Fresia
Neurorehabilitation Unit and Parkinson Unit, IRCCS Mondino Foundation, Pavia, Italy

Roberto De Icco, Micol Avenali, Carlotta Dagna and Cristina Tassorelli
Neurorehabilitation Unit and Parkinson Unit, IRCCS Mondino Foundation, Pavia, Italy
Department of Brain and Behavioral Sciences, University of Pavia, Pavia, Italy

Mariella Pazzagli
Department of Psychology, University of Rome "La Sapienza," Rome, Italy
IRCCS Fondazione Santa Lucia, Rome, Italy

Giulia Galli
IRCCS Fondazione Santa Lucia, Rome, Italy

Luca Falsiroli Maistrello, Tommaso Geri and Marco Test
Department of Neuroscience, Rehabilitation, Ophthalmology, Genetics, Maternal and Child Health, University of Genova, Genoa, Italy

Silvia Gianola
Unit of Clinical Epidemiology, IRCCS Galeazzi Orthopaedic Institute, Milan, Italy
Center of Biostatistics for Clinical Epidemiology, School of Medicine and Surgery, University of Milano-Bicocca, Monza, Italy

Martina Zaninetti
Department of Neuroscience, Rehabilitation, Ophthalmology, Genetics, Maternal and Child Health, University of Genova, Genoa, Italy
UOC di Recupero e Rieducazione Funzionale, Ospedale Policlinico Borgo Roma, Azienda Ospedaliera Universitaria Integrata di Verona, Verona, Italy

Qingcong Wu, Bai Chen and Hongtao Wu
College of Mechanical and Electrical Engineering, Nanjing University of Aeronautics and Astronautics, Nanjing, China

Xingsong Wang
College of Mechanical Engineering, Southeast University, Nanjing, China

Hanneke J. R. van Duijnhoven, Jolanda M. B. Roelofs, Jasper J. den Boer and Geert E. A. van Bon
Department of Rehabilitation, Donders Institute for Brain, Cognition and Behaviour, Radboud University Medical Center, Nijmegen, Netherlands

Frits C. Lem
Department of Rehabilitation, Sint Maartenskliniek, Nijmegen, Netherlands

Rifka Hofman
Rehabilitation Medical Centre Klimmendaal, Arnhem, Netherlands

Vivian Weerdesteyn
Department of Rehabilitation, Donders Institute for Brain, Cognition and Behaviour, Radboud University Medical Center, Nijmegen, Netherlands
Research, Sint Maartenskliniek, Nijmegen, Netherlands

Chiara Zucchella
Neurology Unit, University Hospital of Verona, Verona, Italy

Elena Sinforiani and Sara Bernini
Alzheimer's Disease Assessment Unit, Laboratory of Neuropsychology, IRCCS Mondino Foundation, Pavia, Italy

Stefano Tamburin
Neurology Unit, University Hospital of Verona, Verona, Italy
Department of Neurosciences, Biomedicine and Movement Sciences, University of Verona, Verona, Italy

Angela Federico and Elisa Mantovani
Department of Neurosciences, Biomedicine and Movement Sciences, University of Verona, Verona, Italy

Roberto Casale and Michelangelo Bartolo
Neurorehabilitation Unit, Department of Rehabilitation, HABILITA, Bergamo, Italy

Robert Schulz, Bastian Cheng, Christian Gerloff and Götz Thomalla
Department of Neurology, University Medical Center Hamburg-Eppendorf, Hamburg, Germany

Clemens G. Rung
Department of Neurology, University Medical Center Hamburg-Eppendorf, Hamburg, Germany
Department of Neurology, University Medical Center Schleswig-Holstein, Lübeck, Germany

Marlene Bönstrup
Department of Neurology, University Medical Center Hamburg-Eppendorf, Hamburg, Germany
Human Cortical Physiology and Neurorehabilitation Section, National Institute of Neurological Disorders and Stroke, National Institutes of Health, Bethesda, MD, United States

Friedhelm C. Hummel
Defitech Chair of Clinical Neuroengineering, Center for Neuroprosthetics and Brain Mind Institute, Swiss Federal Institute of Technology (EPFL), Geneva, Switzerland
Defitech Chair of Clinical Neuroengineering, Clinique Romande de Réadaptation, Center for Neuroprosthetics and Brain Mind Institute, Swiss Federal Institute of Technology Valais (EPFL Valais), Sion, Switzerland
Clinical Neuroscience, University of Geneva Medical School, Geneva, Switzerland

Takashi Takebayashi
Department of Occupational Therapy, School of Health Science and Social Welfare, Kibi International University, Takahashi, Japan

Kayoko Takahashi
Department of Rehabilitation, School of Allied Health Science, Kitasato University, Sagamihara-shi, Japan

Satoru Amano
Department of Rehabilitation, The Hospital of Hyogo College of Medicine, Nishinomiya-shi, Japan

Yuki Uchiyama
Department of Rehabilitation, Hyogo College of Medicine, Nishinomiya-shi, Japan

Masahiko Gosho
Department of Biostatistics, Faculty of Medicine University of Tsukuba, Tsukuba, Japan

Kazuhisa Domen
Department of Rehabilitation Medicine, Hyogo College of Medicine, Nishinomiya, Japan

Kenji Hachisuka
Kyushu Rosai Hospital, Moji Medical Center, Kitakyushu-shi, Japan

Dongmei Ye, Hongwei Liu, Surui Zhang, Hong Zhang, Jingya Li and Wenfei Yu
Department of Rehabilitation, Affiliated Zhongshan Hospital of Dalian University, Dalian, China

Chen Chen
Department of Anatomy, Medical College of Dalian University, Dalian, China

Dongdong Song
Department of Imaging, Affiliated Zhongshan Hospital of Dalian University, Dalian, China

Mei Shen
Department of Rehabilitation, People's Hospital of Longhua District of Shenzhen, Shenzhen, China

Qiwen Wang
Department of Rehabilitation, Affiliated Zhongshan Hospital of Dalian University, Dalian, China
Department of Rehabilitation, People's Hospital of Longhua District of Shenzhen, Shenzhen, China

Bia Lima Ramalho, Maria Luíza Rangel, Ana Carolina Schmaedeke and Claudia D. Vargas
Laboratory of Neurobiology of Movement, Institute of Biophysics Carlos Chagas Filho, Federal University of Rio de Janeiro, Rio de Janeiro, Brazil
Laboratory of Neuroscience and Rehabilitation, Institute of Neurology Deolindo Couto, Federal University of Rio de Janeiro, Rio de Janeiro, Brazil

Fátima Smith Erthal
Laboratory of Neurobiology II, Institute of Biophysics Carlos Chagas Filho, Federal University of Rio de Janeiro, Rio de Janeiro, Brazil

Alessandro Rossi, Giorgia Varallo, Margherita Novelli, Valentina Villa and Federica Scarpina
Istituto Auxologico Italiano IRCCS, Psychology Research Laboratory, San Giuseppe Hospital, Verbania, Italy

Gianluca Castelnuovo, Emanuele Maria Giusti, Giada Pietrabissa, Roberto Cattivelli, Chiara Anna Maria Spatola, Guido Edoardo D'Aniello, Giuseppe Riva and Enrico Molinari
Istituto Auxologico Italiano IRCCS, Psychology Research Laboratory, San Giuseppe Hospital, Verbania, Italy
Department of Psychology, Catholic University of Milan, Milan, Italy

Cesare Cavalera, Daniele Di Lernia, Claudia Repetto and Camillo Regalia
Department of Psychology, Catholic University of Milan, Milan, Italy

Gian Mauro Manzoni
Istituto Auxologico Italiano IRCCS, Psychology Research Laboratory, San Giuseppe Hospital, Verbania, Italy
Faculty of Psychology, eCampus University, Novedrate, Italy

Donatella Saviola
Cardinal Ferrari Rehabilitation Center, Santo Stefano Rehabilitation Istitute, Fontanellato, Italy

Samantha Gabrielli and Marco Lacerenza
Pain Medicine Center, San Pio X Clinic, Humanitas, Milan, Italy

Francesca Luzzati and Andrea Cottini
IRCCS Galeazzi Orthopedic Institute, Milan, Italy

Carlo Lai
Department of Dynamic and Clinical Psychology, Sapienza University of Rome, Rome, Italy

Eleonora Volpato
Department of Psychology, Catholic University of Milan, Milan, Italy
HD Respiratory Rehabilitation Unit, IRCCS Fondazione Don Carlo Gnocchi, Milan, Italy

Francesco Pagnini
Department of Psychology, Catholic University of Milan, Milan, Italy
Department of Psychology, Harvard University, Cambridge, MA, United States

Valentina Tesio and Lorys Castelli
Department of Psychology, University of Turin, Turin, Italy

Mario Tavola
Anesthesia and Intensive Care, ASST Lecco, Lecco, Italy

Riccardo Torta and Fabrizio Benedetti
Department of Neuroscience "Rita Levi Montalcini", University of Turin, Turin, Italy

Marco Arreghini, Loredana Zanini, Amelia Brunani, Ionathan Seitanidis, Giuseppe Ventura and Paolo Capodaglio
Istituto Auxologico Italiano IRCCS, Rehabilitation Unit, San Giuseppe Hospital, Verbania, Italy

Andrea Brioschi and Matteo Bigoni
Istituto Auxologico Italiano IRCCS, Department of Neurology and Neurorehabilitation, San Giuseppe Hospital, Verbania, Italy

Lorenzo Priano and Alessandro Mauro
Department of Neuroscience "Rita Levi Montalcini", University of Turin, Turin, Italy
Istituto Auxologico Italiano IRCCS, Department of Neurology and Neurorehabilitation, San Giuseppe Hospital, Verbania, Italy

Paolo Notaro
Pain Medicine, Anesthesiology Department, A.O. Ospedale Niguarda ca Granda, Milan, Italy

Giorgio Sandrini
Neurorehabilitation Unit and Parkinson Unit, IRCCS Mondino Foundation, Pavia, Italy
C. Mondino National Neurological Institute, Pavia, Italy
Department of Brain and Behavioral Sciences, University of Pavia, Pavia, Italy

Susan Simpson
University of South Australia, Adelaide, SA, Australia
Regional Eating Disorders Unit, NHS Lothian, Livingston, United Kingdom

Brenda Kay Wiederhold
Virtual Reality Medical Institute, Brussels, Belgium

Santino Gaudio
Department of Neuroscience, Functional Pharmacology, Uppsala University, Uppsala, Sweden

Jeffrey B. Jackson
Virginia Tech, Falls Church, VA, United States

Cleo D. Bol
Neurocenter, Lucerne Cantonal Hospital, Lucerne, Switzerland

Judith J. W. van Beek and Tim Vanbellingen
Neurocenter, Lucerne Cantonal Hospital, Lucerne, Switzerland
Gerontechnology and Rehabilitation Group, University of Bern, Bern, Switzerland

Erwin E. H. van Wegen and Marc B. Rietberg
Department of Rehabilitation Medicine, Amsterdam Movement Sciences, MS Center Amsterdam, Amsterdam University Medical Center VUmc, Amsterdam, Netherlands

Christian P. Kamm
Neurocenter, Lucerne Cantonal Hospital, Lucerne, Switzerland
Department of Neurology, Inselspital University Hospital Bern, University of Bern, Bern, Switzerland

Sung Ho Jang and Jeong Pyo Seo
Department of Physical Medicine and Rehabilitation, College of Medicine, Yeungnam University, Daegu, South Korea

Marialuisa Gandolfi, Nicola Valè, Eleonora Kirilova Dimitrova, Maria Donata Benedetti, Alberto Gajofatto, Mirko Filippetti, Carola De Paoli, Elena Chemello and Jessica Corradi
Department of Neurosciences, Biomedicine and Movement Sciences, University of Verona, Verona, Italy

Stefano Mazzoleni and Elena Battini
The Bio Robotics Institute, Scuola Superiore Sant' Anna, Polo Sant' Anna Valdera, Pontedera, Italy

Francesco Ferraro
Section of Neuromotor Rehabilitation, Department of Neuroscience, ASST Carlo Poma, Mantova, Italy

Matteo Castelli and Maruo Camin
Centro di riabilitazione Franca Martini—ATSM ONLUS, Trento, Italy

Alessandro Picelli and Nicola Smania
Department of Neurosciences, Biomedicine and Movement Sciences, University of Verona, Verona, Italy
UOC Neurorehabilitation, AOUI Verona, Verona, Italy

Andreas Waldner
Department of Neurological Rehabilitation, Private Hospital Villa Melitta, Bolzano, Italy

Leopold Saltuari
Research Department for Neurorehabilitation South Tyrol, Bolzano, Italy
Department of Neurology, Hochzirl Hospital, Zirl, Austria

Fabbri, Irene Eleonora Mosca, Filippo Gerli, Leonardo Martini, Silvia Pancani, Giulia Lucidi, Federica Savazzi, Francesca Baglio, Federica Vannetti and Claudio Macchi
IRCCS Fondazione Don Carlo Gnocchi, Milan, Italy

Yuzhe Zeng, Shuang Wang, Songsong Wu, Xi Li, Jin Wu, Zhida Chen and Bin Lin
Department of Orthopaedics, The Affiliated Southeast Hospital of Xiamen University, Orthopaedic Center of People's Liberation Army, Zhangzhou, China

Nawen Wang, Tiantian Guo and Qiuyang Zheng
Fujian Provincial Key Laboratory of Neurodegenerative Disease and Aging Research, Institute of Neuroscience, College of Medicine, Collaborative Innovation Center for Brain Science, Xiamen University, Xiamen, China

Huaxi Xu
Neuroscience Initiative, Sanford Burnham Prebys Medical Discovery Institute, La Jolla, CA, United States

Xin Wang
Fujian Provincial Key Laboratory of Neurodegenerative Disease and Aging Research, Institute of Neuroscience, College of Medicine, Collaborative Innovation Center for Brain Science, Xiamen University, Xiamen, China
State Key Laboratory of Cellular Stress Biology, Xiamen University, Xiamen, China

Marlena Klaic
Allied Health Department, Royal Melbourne Hospital, Parkville, VIC, Australia

Mary P. Galea
Department of Medicine (Royal Melbourne Hospital), University of Melbourne, Parkville, VIC, Australia

Antonino Salvia, Giovanni Morone, Marco Iosa, Maria Pia Balice, Stefano Paolucci, Maria Grazia Grasso, Marco Traballesi, Ugo Nocentini, Rita Formisano, Marco Molinari, Angelo Rossini and Carlo Caltagirone
Fondazione Santa Lucia, IRCCS, Rome, Italy

Index